Artificial Intelligence in Adaptive Radiation Therapy

Online at: https://doi.org/10.1088/978-0-7503-6119-4

About the Series

The series in Physics and Engineering in Medicine and Biology will allow the Institute of Physics and Engineering in Medicine (IPEM) to enhance its mission to 'advance physics and engineering applied to medicine and biology for the public good'.

It is focused on key areas including, but not limited to:
- clinical engineering
- diagnostic radiology
- informatics and computing
- magnetic resonance imaging
- nuclear medicine
- physiological measurement
- radiation protection
- radiotherapy
- rehabilitation engineering
- ultrasound and non-ionising radiation.

A number of IPEM–IOP titles are being published as part of the EUTEMPE Network Series for Medical Physics Experts.

A full list of titles published in this series can be found here: https://iopscience.iop.org/bookListInfo/physics-engineering-medicine-biology-series.

Artificial Intelligence in Adaptive Radiation Therapy

Edited by
Yi Wang
Department of Radiation Oncology, Massachusetts General Hospital,
Harvard Medical School, 100 Blossom Street, Boston, MA 02114, USA

X. Sharon Qi
Department of Radiation Oncology, University of California, Los Angeles,
200 Medical Plaza Driveway, Los Angeles, CA 90095, USA

IOP Publishing, Bristol, UK

ISBN   978-0-7503-6119-4 (ebook)
ISBN   978-0-7503-6117-0 (print)
ISBN   978-0-7503-6120-0 (myPrint)
ISBN   978-0-7503-6118-7 (mobi)

DOI   10.1088/978-0-7503-6119-4

Version: 20251101

IOP ebooks

British Library Cataloguing-in-Publication Data: A catalogue record for this book is available from the British Library.

Published by IOP Publishing, wholly owned by The Institute of Physics, London

IOP Publishing, No.2 The Distillery, Glassfields, Avon Street, Bristol, BS2 0GR, UK

US Office: IOP Publishing, Inc., 190 North Independence Mall West, Suite 601, Philadelphia, PA 19106, USA

To my beloved wife, Ying, whose love and support give meaning to every endeavor, and to my inspiring son, Lucas, whose dream of one day landing on Mars reminds me always to reach higher.

—Yi Wang

*To my husband, Yan,
to my daughter, Isabella,
and to my parents, for their love, patience and inspiration.*

—X. Sharon Qi

.

Contents

6   Introduction to adaptive radiotherapy   6-1
Jack Neylon, Michael Vincent Lauria and Yi Lao

11 Artificial intelligence-based intrafraction motion monitoring for precise adaptive radiation therapy delivery 11-1

Lianli Liu and James M Balter

12 Artificial intelligence for quality assurance in adaptive radiation therapy 12-1

Sang Kyu Lee and Maria Chan

15 Offline computed tomography-based and online cone beam computed tomography-based adaptive radiation therapy 15-1

Joel A Pogue, Natalie Viscariello, Dennis N Stanley, Joseph Harms, Richard A Popple and Carlos E Cardenas

20 Safety and training considerations in the clinical implementation of artificial intelligence adaptive radiation therapy   20-1

Kelly Nealon and Jennifer Pursley

21 Ethical and regulatory considerations in artificial intelligence for adaptive radiation therapy   21-1

Dandan Zheng, Megan Hyun and Andrew Fanning

Preface

Artificial Intelligence (AI) is playing a transformative role in healthcare, particularly in the field of radiation therapy (RT). Adaptive radiation therapy (ART), a complex and dynamic treatment approach that incorporates feedback mechanisms to account for patient-specific anatomic, biological, and functional changes during the course of treatment, holds significant promise. The integration of AI into ART heralds a new era of enhanced precision, efficiency, and personalization in cancer care.

This book, *Artificial Intelligence in Adaptive Therapy*, is a comprehensive and timely exploration of how AI technologies are reshaping the landscape of ART from data acquisition and image processing to decision-making and treatment delivery. This book is designed to serve as a foundational and forward-looking resource for medical physicists, radiation oncologists, researchers, and clinicians interested in understanding and leveraging the power of AI in RT and ART.

The book begins with the fundamental concepts of AI (chapter 1) and gradually builds toward advanced clinical applications (section II) in ART, and clinical applications in ART (section III), providing a structured and in-depth view of the entire AI–ART ecosystem.

Early chapters lay the groundwork by introducing AI in the context of radiation therapy, including imaging technologies, big data utilization, image registration and segmentation, dose prediction, and motion monitoring, etc. Subsequent chapters dive into the technical pillars of each step of the ART workflow. This book also addresses the growing role of AI in quality assurance, treatment adaptation, response prediction, and clinical trials.

Recognizing the real-world challenges of implementation, later chapters (section III) provide critical discussions on ethical, regulatory, safety, and training considerations. The book concludes with a vision of recent advances and the future of AI-augmented ART, highlighting promising research directions and emerging innovations.

Our goal is to equip clinicians, researchers, and trainees with the knowledge to critically engage with AI technologies and thoughtfully incorporate them into clinical practice. As adaptive therapy continues to evolve, AI will be a key enabler of innovation, efficiency, and improved patient outcomes. Whether you are new to the field or an experienced practitioner seeking to stay current, this book aims to inform, inspire, and guide your journey through the rapidly evolving world of AI-powered adaptive therapy. We hope this book will serve as both a guide and a catalyst for further advancement in this exciting and fast-moving field.

Foreword

In the ever-advancing field of radiation oncology, the integration of artificial intelligence (AI) promises transformative change, particularly in the realm of adaptive radiation therapy (ART). The recent advances in AI have come just in time to bring ART to clinical reality and represents a significant leap forward in personalizing treatment plans, optimizing radiation therapy delivery, and improving patient outcomes. *Artificial Intelligence in Adaptive Radiation Therapy* serves as the first comprehensive guide to understand and apply AI-driven techniques in radiation oncology as they relate to ART, providing a deep dive into both the theoretical underpinnings and practical implementations of the topic.

The chapters within this book cover a wide array of topics, from the basics of AI and its introduction into radiation therapy to more advanced applications of AI-driven imaging, treatment planning, and real-time adaptation. Each chapter is meticulously crafted by leading experts in the field, offering insights into how AI can enhance every step of the ART workflow, from simulation to quality assurance. The discussions are grounded in the latest research and clinical practice, making this book an invaluable resource for clinicians, researchers, and trainees alike.

As you dive into the pages of *Artificial Intelligence in Adaptive Radiation Therapy*, you will not only discover the profound impact that AI is having on the highly technical field of radiation oncology, but also in the way we approach cancer treatment in general. The innovations discussed here not only push the boundaries of what is possible in radiation oncology, but also pave the way for future technological advancements that will continue to enhance the precision and effectiveness of radiation oncology and cancer care.

This book is much more than just a compilation of knowledge; it is a testament to the collaborative efforts of scientists, clinicians, and engineers who are dedicated to advancing the field of radiation therapy. It is hoped that the insights shared in these pages will inspire further exploration and innovation, ultimately leading to better outcomes for cancer patients worldwide.

Welcome to the future of radiation therapy—where AI plays a central role in shaping the next generation of cancer treatment.

Michael Steinberg, MD
Professor and Chair
Department of Radiation Oncology
David Geffen School of Medicine at UCLA

Acknowledgments

The editors gratefully acknowledge the contributions of all chapter authors, whose expertise and dedication have been essential to the creation of this book. Their collective scholarship has brought together a comprehensive and timely perspective on this rapidly evolving field.

We extend our sincere appreciation to the reviewers, whose thoughtful and constructive feedback greatly enhanced the scientific rigor and clarity of the work. We are also thankful to the IOP Publishing team for their consistent guidance and support throughout the publication process.

Our deepest appreciation to our families for their patience, understanding and unwavering support throughout the preparation of this book.

Editor biographies

Yi Wang

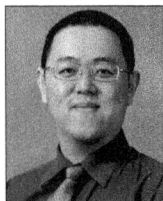

Dr Yi Wang is a medical physicist from the Department of Radiation Oncology at Massachusetts General Hospital (MGH) and an Assistant Professor of Radiation Oncology at Harvard Medical School (HMS) in Boston, MA, USA. He earned his BEng in Automation from the Beijing University of Aeronautics and Astronautics (China) in 2002, and his MS and PhD in Biomedical Engineering from the University of Michigan (Ann Arbor, MI, USA) in 2004 and 2009, respectively. He completed the three-year residency in therapeutic medical physics at the Harvard Medical Physics Residency Program in 2012, including a year of postdoctoral fellowship at the Francis H Burr Proton Therapy Center at MGH. Since then, he has been working as a faculty physicist in the Department of Radiation Oncology at MGH. Locally, he leads an AI Lab and serves as the Director of the Mass General Brigham (MGB) Undergraduate Fellowship Program in Medical Physics. As an internationally recognized expert on AI for radiation therapy, he serves in multiple AI-related committees, task groups, and working groups in the American Association of Physicists in Medicine (AAPM), including the Machine Intelligence Subcommittee, Ad Hoc Advisory Committee on Artificial Intelligence Boot Camps, the Vice Chair of Task Group 384 (Clinical Implementation of Automated Segmentation for Adaptive Radiation Therapy), and the Chair of the Working Group on Generative Artificial Intelligence. He has authored and co-authored over 40 journal articles, conference papers, and book chapters.

X. Sharon Qi

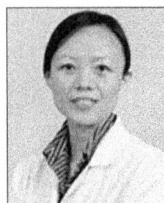

X. Sharon Qi, PhD, is a Professor of Medical Physics in the Department of Radiation Oncology at the University of California Los Angeles (UCLA). She is an affiliated faculty member of UCLA's CAMPEP-accredited Physics and Biology in Medicine Interdisciplinary Graduate Program. Dr. Qi is board-certified in Therapeutic Radiologic Physics by the American Board of Radiology and is a Fellow of the American Association of Physicists in Medicine (AAPM).

Dr. Qi earned her bachelor's degree in physics and her PhD degree in Experimental Particle Physics from the Institute of High Energy Physics, Chinese Academy of Sciences in Beijing, China. She pursued her doctoral research as a scientist at Fermi National Accelerator Laboratory (Fermilab) in Batavia, Illinois, before completing a postdoctoral fellowship in Medical Physics at the Medical College of Wisconsin. She served as a faculty member in the Department of Radiation Oncology at the University of Colorado Denver prior to joining UCLA.

Dr. Qi has served as both principal investigator and co-investigator on various research projects and clinical trials. She has published more than 130 peer-reviewed journal articles, over 220 peer reviewed abstracts, and 7 book chapters. Her research focuses on image-guided radiation therapy and adaptive radiation therapy, outcome modeling and response prediction, big data analytics, and the application of AI in radiotherapy oncology.

As an internationally recognized expert in AI for radiation therapy, Dr. Qi contributes actively to multiple AI-focused committees, working groups, and task groups with the AAPM. Her roles include serving on the Machine Intelligence Subcommittee (MIS) and the Therapy Physics Committee (TPC), Chairing Task Group 384 on the clinical implementation of automated segmentation for adaptive radiation therapy, and acting as Vice Chair of the Working Group on Generative Artificial Intelligence. Beyond AAPM, she also contributes to broader national initiatives through the American Society for Radiation Oncology (ASTRO) and NRG Oncology.

Beyond her research and committee service, Dr. Qi actively contributes to scientific publishing, serving as Deputy Editor and Associate Editor for the Journal of Medical Physics, and holding editorial and peer review roles for other journals in radiation therapy.

List of contributors

Brian Anderson
University of North Carolina, 101 Manning Drive, Chapel Hill, NC 27514, USA

Parsa Bagherzadeh
McGill University, 3755 Ch de la Côte Ste-Catherine Montréal, Québec, H3T 1E2, Canada

James M Balter
University of Michigan, 1500 E Medical Center Drive, Ann Arbor, MI, USA

Kristy Brock
The University of Texas MD Anderson Cancer Center, 1400 Pressler Street, FCT 14.6048, Unit 1902, Houston, TX 77030, USA

Jing Cai
The Hong Kong Polytechnic University, Y921, Block Y, The Hong Kong Polytechnic University, No 11 Yuk Choi Road, Hung Hom, Kowloon, Hong Kong

Carlos Eduardo Cardenas
University of Alabama at Birmingham, 1700 6th Avenue Street, Birmingham, AL 35233, USA

Maria Chan
Memorial Sloan Kettering Cancer Center, 136 Mountainview Blvd, Basking Ridge, NJ 07920, USA

Xinru Chen
The University of Texas MD Anderson Cancer Center, 1400 Pressler Street, Houston, TX 77030, USA

Laurence Court
The University of Texas MD Anderson Cancer Center, 1515 Holcombe Boulevard, Houston, Texas 77030, USA

Sunan Cui
University of Washington, 1959 NE Pacific Street Box Number 356043, Seattle, WA 98195, USA

Xianjin Dai
Stanford University, 875 Blake Wilbur Drive, Stanford, CA 94305, USA

Denis Dudas
Czech Technical University in Prague, Břehová 78/7, 115 19 Prague, Czech Republic

Issam El Naqa
H Lee Moffitt Cancer Center and Research Institute, 12902 Magnolia Drive, Tampa, FL 33612, USA

Shirin Abbasinejad Enger
McGill University, 3755 Ch de la Côte Ste-Catherine Montréal, Québec, H3T 1E2, Canada

Andrew Fanning
University of Nebraska Medical Center, 986861 Nebraska Medical Center, Omaha, NE 68198-6861, USA

Jie Fu
University of Washington, 1959 NE Pacific Street Box Number 356043, Seattle, WA 98195, USA

Yu Gao
Stanford University, 875 Blake Wilbur Drive, Palo Alto, CA, USA

Huaizhi Geng
University of Pennsylvania, 3400 Civic Center Boulevard, TRC-2 West, Philadelphia, PA 19104, USA

Andrew Godley
University of Texas Southwestern Medical Center, 2280 Inwood Rd, Dallas, TX 75235, USA

Bin Han
Stanford University, 875 Blake Wilbur Drive, Palo Alto, CA, USA

Joseph Harms
University of Alabama at Birmingham, 1700 6th Avenue Street, Birmingham, AL 35233, USA

Elizabeth Huynh
London Health Sciences Centre, 800 Commissioners Road East, London, ON, N6A 5W9, Canada

Megan Hyun
Memorial Sloan Kettering Cancer Center, 1275 York Avenue, New York, NY 10065, USA

Yi Lao
City of Hope National Medical Center, 1500 East Duarte Road, Duarte, CA 91010, USA

Michael Vincent Lauria
University of California, Los Angeles, 200 Medical Plaza Driveway Suite B265, Los Angeles, CA 90095, USA

Sang Ho Lee
University of Pennsylvania, 3400 Civic Center Boulevard, TRC-2 West, Philadelphia, PA 19104, USA

Sang Kyu Lee
Memorial Sloan Kettering Cancer Center, 480 Red Hill Road, Middletown, NJ 07748, USA

Mu-Han Li
University of Texas Southwestern Medical Center, 2280 Inwood Rd, Dallas, TX 75235, USA

Lianli Liu
Stanford University, 875 Blake Wilbur Drive, Palo Alto, CA, USA

Kelly Nealon
Massachusetts General Hospital, Harvard Medical School, 55 Fruit Street, Boston, MA 02114, USA

Jack Neylon
University of California, Los Angeles, 200 Medical Plaza Driveway, Suite B265, Los Angeles, CA 90095, USA

Oscar Pastor-Serrano
Stanford University, 3145 Porter Drive, Wing A, Palo Alto CA 94304, USA

Joel Anthony Pogue
University of Alabama at Birmingham, 1700 6th Avenue Street, Birmingham, AL 35233, USA

Richard Allen Popple
University of Alabama at Birmingham, 1700 6th Avenue Street, Birmingham, AL 35233, USA

Jennifer Pursley
Mayo Clinic, Rochester, 200 1st Street SW, Rochester, MN 55905, USA

X. Sharon Qi
University of California, Los Angeles, 200 Medical Plaza Driveway, Suite B265, Los Angeles, CA 90095, USA

Laya Rafiee Sevyeri
Medical Physics Unit, Department of Oncology, McGill University, Montreal, Canada

Gregory Sharp
Massachusetts General Hospital, Harvard Medical School, 55 Fruit Street, Boston, MA 02114, USA

Chenyang Shen
University of Texas Southwestern Medical Center, 2280 Inwood Rd, Dallas, TX 75235, USA

Lauren Smith
Memorial Sloan Kettering Cancer Center, 1275 York Avenue, New York, NY 10065, USA

Dennis Nichols Stanley
University of Alabama at Birmingham, 1700 6th Avenue Street, Birmingham, AL 35233, USA

Xinzhi Teng
The Hong Kong Polytechnic University, Y921, Block Y, The Hong Kong Polytechnic University, No.11 Yuk Choi Road, Hung Hom, Kowloon, Hong Kong

Ivan Vazquez
The University of Texas MD Anderson Cancer Center, 1840 Old Spanish Trl, Houston, TX 77054, USA

Justin Visak
University of Texas Southwestern Medical Center, 2280 Inwood Rd, Dallas, TX 75235, USA

Natalie Nicole Viscariello
University of Alabama at Birmingham, 1700 6th Avenue Street, Birmingham, AL 35233, USA

Tonghe Wang
Memorial Sloan Kettering Cancer Center, 1275 York Avenue, New York, NY 10065, USA

Yi Wang
Massachusetts General Hospital, Harvard Medical School, 100 Blossom Street, Boston, MA 02114, USA

Brian Winey
Massachusetts General Hospital, Harvard Medical School, 100 Blossom Street, Cox 3, Boston, MA 02114, USA

Jinzhong Yang
The University of Texas MD Anderson Cancer Center, 1400 Pressler Street, Houston, TX 77030, USA

Ming Yang
The University of Texas MD Anderson Cancer Center, 1840 Old Spanish Trl, Houston, TX 77054, USA

Xiaofeng Yang
Emory University, 1365 Clifton Road NE, Building C, Atlanta, GA 30322, USA

Cenji Yu
Mayo Clinic, Rochester, 200 First Street SW, Rochester, MN 55905, USA

Ying Xiao
University of Pennsylvania, 3400 Civic Center Boulevard, TRC-2 West, Philadelphia, PA 19104, USA

Lei Xing
Stanford University, 875 Blake Wilbur Drive, Stanford, CA 94305, USA

Jiang Zhang
The Hong Kong Polytechnic University, Y921, Block Y, The Hong Kong Polytechnic University, No 11 Yuk Choi Road, Hung Hom, Kowloon, Hong Kong

Xinyu Zhang
The Hong Kong Polytechnic University, Y921, Block Y, The Hong Kong Polytechnic University, No 11 Yuk Choi Road, Hung Hom, Kowloon, Hong Kong

Yuanpeng Zhang
The Hong Kong Polytechnic University, Y921, Block Y, The Hong Kong Polytechnic University, No 11 Yuk Choi Road, Hung Hom, Kowloon, Hong Kong

Yao Zhao
The University of Texas MD Anderson Cancer Center, 1400 Pressler Street, Houston, TX 77030, USA

Dandan Zheng
University of Rochester, 601 Elmwood Avenue, Rochester, NY 14642, USA

Yujing Zou
McGill University, 3755 Ch de la Côte Ste-Catherine Montréal, Québec, H3T 1E2, Canada

Chapter 1

Fundamentals of artificial intelligence

Parsa Bagherzadeh, Laya Rafiee Sevyeri, Yujing Zou and Shirin Abbasinejad Enger

Artificial Intelligence (AI) is transforming healthcare, with adaptive radiotherapy standing out as a key area where AI is reshaping cancer treatment. By leveraging real-time data, AI enables more personalized and precise treatment plans, improving patient outcomes. This chapter introduces the fundamentals of AI, focusing on machine learning (ML) and deep learning (DL), which drive innovations in radiotherapy. It covers the evolution of AI from rule-based systems to advanced learning algorithms, exploring their applications in clinical settings. It will discuss the ethical considerations surrounding AI in healthcare, including transparency, bias, and data privacy, setting the stage for a deeper dive into AI's role in adaptive radiotherapy.

1.1 A brief introduction to AI

Artificial intelligence (AI), a subfield of computer science, focuses on developing systems capable of performing tasks that typically require human intelligence. Such tasks include problem-solving, learning, perception, and language understanding. AI systems leverage algorithms, statistical models, and machine learning techniques to analyse and interpret data, enabling them to make decisions, recognize patterns, and improve performance over time. AI applications range from virtual assistants and recommendation systems to complex tasks in various fields. In particular, AI plays a significant role in healthcare, transforming medical decision-making and treatment strategies by changing the existing landscape. In the context of adaptive radiotherapy, an intricate interplay of AI methodologies is reshaping how we approach cancer treatments. The term 'artificial intelligence' was coined at the Dartmouth Conference in 1956, where researchers aimed to explore how machines could simulate human intelligence. In the 1960s and 1970s, AI research mainly focused on logic-based symbolic reasoning, which involves representing knowledge using symbols and rules, allowing machines to manipulate these symbols to derive logical conclusions and make decisions [1]. During this period, AI found its

doi:10.1088/978-0-7503-6119-4ch1

applications in medicine through systems such as MYCIN [2], a system for diagnosing bacterial infections and recommending antibiotic treatments.

In parallel with symbolic reasoning, AI research also focused on optimization and handling uncertainty, both important for developing intelligent systems. Fuzzy logic, for instance, is a mathematical framework that deals with uncertainty as well as imprecision, allowing for the representation of partial truths [3]. This flexibility makes it particularly suitable for systems where variables may have ambiguous or overlapping boundaries. Genetic algorithms are examples of evolutionary optimization techniques inspired by principles of natural selection and genetics [4]. They employ a population of potential solutions, subjecting them to genetic operations such as crossover, mutation, and selection to evolve toward an optimal solution over successive generations.

The development of reasoning systems continued in the 1980s as expert systems. Expert systems serve as digital counterparts to human domain experts, leveraging a comprehensive knowledge base to guide decision-making processes. These systems bring a wealth of rules and domain-specific knowledge into play, enhancing the precision of decision-making [5].

ONCOCIN [6] is an example of a system designed to assist oncologists in the treatment of cancer patients. Note that the rules in expert systems are predefined and programmed into the system, outlining how the system needs to behave in different situations. Expert systems, thus, lack the ability to adapt or learn from new data, and they operate within the boundaries of the predetermined rules set by human experts and the initial knowledge programmed into the system.

The limitations of expert systems later motivated the development of machine learning (ML) models in the 1990s and 2000s. In contrast to expert systems, ML models extrapolate from data. ML involves the development of algorithms that enable machines to learn and improve from experience. In adaptive radiotherapy, ML algorithms can leverage extensive patient data to discern patterns and forecast customized treatment plans [7]. For example, these algorithms can be used in segmentation tasks to help delineate volumes concerning the tumor and organs at risk. This progresses to treatment management, addressing motion during the treatment and treatment plan optimization. Ultimately, decisions are interconnected through reviewing treatment specifics, enabling adaptive changes.

While classical ML models do not have predefined rules such as expert systems, they still require human expert efforts to design a feature set. These features, specific attributes or characteristics selected from input data, provide structured information to help algorithms discern and differentiate between data inputs, enhancing pattern recognition and prediction capabilities. Deep learning (DL), a subfield of ML, employs neural networks with multiple layers to extract representations from raw data [8] without explicit feature engineering. DL has dominated AI research since 2010. DL, with its capacity to autonomously acquire hierarchical features from intricate data, has the potential to enhance precision and efficiency across all stages of radiotherapy treatment and its automation.

The landscape of AI in healthcare has undergone a transformative shift with the rise of ML and DL techniques. This chapter focuses on ML and DL, describing their capacity to discern intricate patterns, adapt to dynamic patient conditions, and optimize and automate radiotherapy treatments. The nuances of these data-driven approaches within the context of adaptive radiotherapy are explored. A practical understanding of these AI approaches is provided from classical ML to DL and generative models. An overview of ethical considerations regarding transparency and bias is also provided.

1.2 Machine learning basics

This section briefly introduces basic definitions of ML, including different learning strategies, feature representation, feature selection, and classical ML models.

1.2.1 Learning paradigms

An ML algorithm refers to a type of algorithm that can learn from experience. The learning process can occur in various ways. Considering the data and the type of information it provides, three main learning paradigms can be defined: (i) supervised, (ii) unsupervised, and (iii) self-supervised learning.

Supervised learning is the most commonly used ML paradigm. It earns its name as it resembles a teacher guiding a student's progress. Here, the algorithm learns from a training dataset, with known correct answers, by making predictions iteratively, which are then corrected. This process continues until the algorithm achieves a satisfactory performance level. Formally, supervised learning involves training a model on a dataset $D_{\text{train}} = \{(x_1, y_1), (x_2, y_2),...,(x_n, y_n)\}$, where each sample $(x_i \in X)$ is paired with its corresponding ground-truth label $(y_i \in Y)$. In summary, the goal of supervised learning is to learn a function f that accurately maps input x to an output y, where $\hat{y} = f(x)$ provides a reliable prediction of y [9].

Unsupervised learning assumes that access is limited to the input variables, and their corresponding ground truth remains unavailable ($D_{\text{train}} = \{x_1, x_2,...,x_n\}$). The objective of unsupervised learning is to model the underlying structure or distribution of the data to gain insights. Unlike supervised learning, no supervision is provided for the given training data. Unsupervised learning problems extend beyond traditional clustering, which involves grouping similar samples into distinct clusters, and association problems, which discover interesting relationships or patterns among variables in large datasets. Unsupervised models include dimensionality reduction models, such as principal component analysis (PCA) [10], as well as generative models such as autoencoders [11] and generative adversarial networks (GANs) [12], which are widely used to generate examples resembling the training data.

Self-supervised learning is a fairly new ML paradigm where a model learns from the data without relying on externally provided labeled annotations. Instead of using labeled data created by human annotators, self-supervised learning leverages the inherent structure or information within the data to generate supervisory signals. The model is tasked with predicting certain parts or properties of the input data based on other parts, creating a pretext task such as jigsaw puzzle [13] or rotations detection [14]. This process enables the model to learn useful representations or features from the input data, which can later be utilized for downstream tasks such as classification or regression. Self-supervised learning is particularly valuable in scenarios where obtaining labeled data is challenging or expensive.

In addition to these three paradigms, one may also consider semi-supervised learning and reinforcement learning paradigms. In semi-supervised learning, we typically have access to a small set of labeled data along with a large set of unlabeled data, while in reinforcement learning an agent learns a task by interacting with an environment and updates its approach based on the positive or negative rewards it receives.

1.2.2 Regression versus classification

Classification and regression are two fundamental types of supervised ML tasks. Classification aims to assign input data points to predefined categories or classes, as illustrated in figure 1.1(a). Classifying tissue samples as normal, benign, or malignant based on histopathological images, identifying the presence or absence of specific genetic mutations, distinguishing between different stages of cancer progression based on imaging data, and detecting cancer recurrence or metastasis from medical imaging scans, are examples of classification tasks in precision oncology. In contrast, in regression the goal is to predict a continuous numeric output based on input features, as shown in figure 1.1(b). A regression model may use features such as patient age, sex, tumor size, Gleason score, stage, and grade to predict radiation dose, which is a continuous numeric value.

1.2.3 Feature engineering and representation

Representing real-world samples using structures understandable by computers (often vectors or matrices) is the first step in developing an ML model. Considering the task at hand, domain experts define a set of features that capture the most important characteristics of a sample. Such features serve as the descriptors that constitute the input for ML algorithms. This step in developing ML models is often referred to as feature engineering and representation. A sample dataset for the

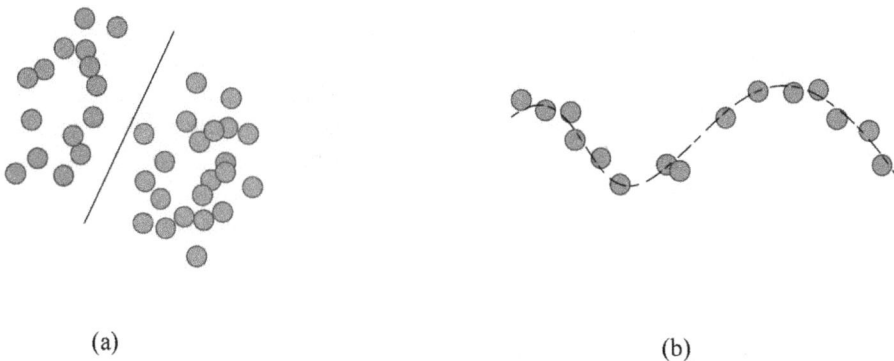

(a)   (b)

Figure 1.1. Classification versus regression. (a) A sample classification example of two classes with a clear decision boundary. (b) A regression model fitted on a sample dataset.

Table 1.1. A sample dataset for predicting the therapeutic role of radiotherapy.

ID	Age	Sex	Time since 1st RT	Dose/fraction (Gy)	Region	Site	T stage	Output
1	45	Male	120	2.5	Chest	Lung	T2	Curative
2	62	Female	90	1.8	Abdomen	Kidney	T1	Palliative
3	55	Male	150	1.9	Neck	Thyroid	T3	Curative
4	70	Female	180	2.2	Pelvis	Prostate	T2	Palliative
5	38	Male	75	1.6	Extremities	Arm	T1	Curative
6	48	Female	110	2.3	Chest	Breast	T2	Curative
7	64	Male	200	2.8	Neck	Tongue	T3	Palliative
8	58	Male	130	2.1	Abdomen	Pancreas	T2	Palliative
9	50	Female	160	2.4	Pelvis	Ovary	T3	Curative
10	42	Male	85	1.9	Extremities	Leg	T1	Curative

task of predicting the therapeutic role of radiotherapy is provided in table 1.1. The expert has designed/engineered a set of $d_{in} = 8$ features (the first eight columns) as predictive features for the output (the last column). Each entity in the world, in this case a patient, is then characterized using the feature set.

1.2.3.1 Feature encoding

As table 1.1 shows, the features are inherently different in terms of the values they can take. Features such as sex, region, site, etc, are nominal categorical and comprise a finite set of discrete values with no inherent ranking or order. An ordinal variable also comprises a finite set of discrete values, but it has a clear ranked ordering between the values, such as ratings (e.g. low, medium, high) or stages (e.g. T1, T2, T3). Another feature type is numerical features such as age, dose, time, etc, that take continuous values from a domain. As the name suggests, such features are characterized by numeric values and can represent a wide range of data types, such as integers, real numbers, or ratios.

Identifying and understating different feature types is important since it determines which type of ML models might be applicable. Different ML models require different encoding schema for their inputs. As introduced in section 1.2.5, decision trees, for instance, assume that all features are categorical, while models such as k-nearest neighbors and support vector machines that operate on vector spaces require the features to be numerical.

Ordinal encoding, for instance, is used when the categorical values have a clear order or rank. It assigns a unique numerical value to each category based on its position in the order as shown in the feature stage in table 1.2. On the other hand, one-hot encoding is used for categorical variables that do not have a natural rank ordering. Assuming m different categories, each category can be encoded by a one-hot vector $\{0, 1\}^m$, where each dimension corresponds to a category. For instance, in table 1.2, the category 'Male' for sex is encoded as $\langle 1, 0 \rangle$.

Table 1.2. Different encoding schema.

Feature	Categorical	Numerical
Stage	T1, T2, T3	1, 2, 3
Sex	Male, female	$<1, 0>$, $<0, 1>$
Age	R	$[1, 20)$, $[20, 40)$, $[40, 60)$

Converting numerical features to categorical features, on the other hand, often involves discretization of the domain into intervals, each of which is considered a category (see 'Age' in table 1.2). When discretizing numerical features, an important design decision is the number of intervals, which can affect the model's performance. For instance, if the number of intervals is too low, the categorical feature may oversimplify the underlying numerical distribution, losing important information and patterns. Discretizing numerical features can also be used for data de-identification [15]. This reduction in granularity serves as a privacy-enhancing mechanism, especially in medical applications where the disclosure of fine-grained details could lead to the re-identification of individuals.

1.2.3.2 Feature selection

Medical data are inherently complex, often characterized by many features, and patient information extends far beyond basic demographics, comprising variables such as genetic markers, vital signs, medical history, diagnostic results, etc. The number of features in adaptive radiotherapy is even larger since it requires monitoring changes over time. Patients' anatomy, for instance, may evolve during the course of treatment due to weight loss, tumor regression/progression, and each time point adds new features. Moreover, radiotherapy involves a large set of dosimetric features, including dose distributions and dose–volume histograms, which leads to an increase in the number of features.

Many features, however, can lead to computational inefficiencies, resulting in long training and prediction times. Moreover, it might increase the risk of over-fitting (discussed in section 1.4), as the model may capture noise and intricacies specific to the training data, hindering its ability to generalize to new instances. The complexity imposed by numerous features impedes computational efficiency and hampers model interpretability. Thus, pre-processing is required to select a subset of features to mitigate these challenges and enhance the overall performance of the ML model. Feature selection involves choosing a subset of the original features from the dataset based on their relevance to the task at hand [16]. The goal is to retain the most informative features while discarding irrelevant or redundant ones, reducing the complexity of the model, and potentially improving its interpretability. As an example, in some datasets, features such as patient ID often carry random values without meaningful patterns for predictive purposes. Including such features may introduce noise and deteriorate the predictive ability. Therefore, careful feature selection is crucial to exclude random-valued features. Note that patient IDs may contain some information. For instance, some databases might incrementally assign IDs, meaning that the ID is correlated with the date of diagnosis. In other cases where certain features are constant or nearly constant across a patient cohort, including all instances of these features, they may not add value and could be considered redundant. For instance, body site might be highly correlated with sex. An example is the ovary, specific to the female reproductive system, rendering the sex feature redundant. Finally, some features may bear some information for output prediction. Their contribution as strong predictors needs to be evaluated to avoid overemphasizing less impactful variables. Feature selection involves using various measures to assess the relevance and importance of features in a dataset. Common techniques include evaluating features based on feature correlation coefficients or statistical measures such as mutual information.

Pearson correlation, for instance, is a statistical measure that quantifies the strength and direction of a linear relationship between two variables x and y:

$$r_{xy} = \frac{\sum_{i=1}^{n}(x_i - \bar{x})(y_i - \bar{y})}{\sum_{i=1}^{n}(x_i - \bar{x})^2 \sum_{i=1}^{n}(x_i - \bar{y})^2}, \tag{1.1}$$

where $\bar{x}$ and $\bar{y}$ are the mean values for x and y. The correlation coefficient is a dimensionless value that ranges from -1 to 1. A coefficient of 1 indicates a perfect positive linear relationship, meaning that as one variable increases, the other also increases proportionally. Conversely, a coefficient of -1 signifies a perfect negative linear relationship, where one variable decreases as the other increases. A coefficient of 0 implies no linear correlation between the variables.

Mutual information, on the other hand, can capture non-linear relationships between features. Assuming $u_1, \ldots, u_{|x|}$ as possible values for feature x and $v_1, \ldots, v_{|y|}$ as possible values for y, mutual information $I(x, y)$ is an information-theoretic measure which is defined based on individual and joint entropies of two random variables:

$$I(x, y) = H(x) + H(y) - H(x, y) \tag{1.2}$$

$$H(x) = \sum_{j=1}^{|x|} P(x = u_j) \log \log P(x = u_j),$$

$$H(y) = \sum_{k=1}^{|y|} P(y = v_k) \log \log P(y = v_k).$$

This formulation of the mutual information is only applicable to categorical features. For numerical continuous features, an estimate is used, which is implemented in most of the existing ML libraries such as scikit-learn [17].

Feature selection is a subset of the broader dimensionality reduction paradigm [18]. In fact, any feature subset selection is a dimensionality reduction but not vice versa. Some dimensionality reduction methods, such as PCA and autoencoders,

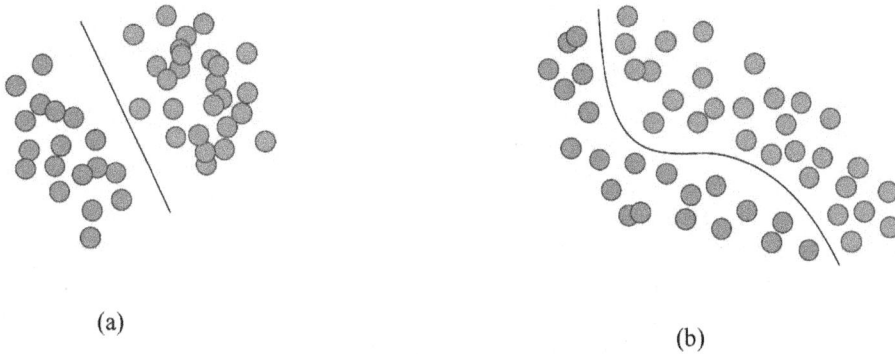

(a)

(b)

Figure 1.2. Two different geometric distributions of data: (a) linear separable and (b) linear non-separable.

transform the original feature space into a lower-dimensional representation by creating new composite features. In medical applications, feature selection might be preferable to such approaches to enhance interpretability. Feature selection retains a subset of the original features, providing transparency in the model's decision-making process. This transparency is important in medical contexts where understanding the relationship between input features and predictions is essential for gaining trust from clinicians and ensuring the responsible adoption of the model in clinical practice.

1.2.4 Linear separability

When designing an ML model, an important consideration is the geometric distribution of data in terms of linear (non-)separability. Linear separability and linear non-separability refer to the inherent structure of a dataset in relation to a classification task. In a scenario of linear separability, classes within the data can be effectively separated by a hyperplane—a geometric construct in the feature space as presented in figure 1.2(a). This means that a straight line or plane can distinguish between different classes, allowing the application of linear classification algorithms such as linear support vector machines or logistic regression. On the other hand, in cases of linear non-separability, a single hyperplane cannot accurately separate the classes, requiring more complex decision boundaries, such as curves or non-linear surfaces as illustrated in figure 1.2(b). In such cases, non-linear classification techniques such as kernel methods or DL models may be more appropriate to capture the intricate relationships within the data. Understanding whether a dataset exhibits linear separability or not is important in selecting the most suitable ML approach for a given classification problem.

1.2.5 Classical models

Classical ML models have been foundational in the evolution of AI, serving as powerful tools for data analysis and decision-making across various domains, including healthcare. These models rely on predefined features as described in section 1.2.3 and statistical techniques to identify patterns and make predictions. Understanding these models is important since it provides a knowledge of the principles and methods widely used in the field, enabling practitioners to appreciate the evolution of ML.

1.2.5.1 Decision trees

Decision trees are a fundamental concept in ML, widely employed for their intuitive and transparent representation of decision-making processes. Serving as predictive models, decision trees navigate through a series of (often binary) choices based on input features to reach a final decision or prediction. Figure 1.3 shows a decision tree learned based on the dataset provided in table 1.1. Decision trees are composed of three types of nodes: root, internal nodes, and leaves. All root and internal nodes correspond to features, and depending on the feature value, one of the sub-trees is traversed. The sub-trees are iteratively traversed until a leaf node is reached, corresponding to a classification decision.

The training process of a decision tree is often referred to as tree induction [20]. During the induction, at each root/internal node, the decision tree tries to partition the training samples (based on feature value) such that the subsets have the least impurity regarding class labels. The class impurity can be quantified using measures such as entropy or Gini index. Assuming a binary classification problem, the maximum entropy and Gini values are 1.0 and 0.5, respectively. The minimum value for these measures often occurs for the leaf nodes—the least impurity and the most certainty for the classification. In some cases, however, the designer might prefer to

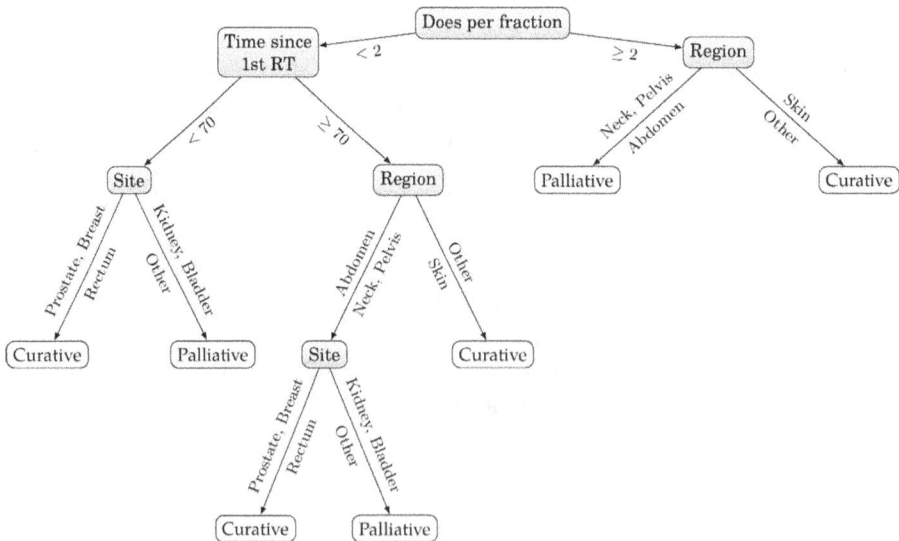

Figure 1.3. A decision tree for predicting the therapeutic role of radiotherapy (inspired by [19]). Based on the value of features, the branches are iteratively traversed until a leaf node is reached.

terminate the induction process to keep the tree below a certain height[1] (for instance, to avoid over-fitting). In such cases, some leaf nodes might have a non-zero impurity value. Note that the induction process may ignore some of the features. For instance, in figure 1.3, features such as sex or age do not appear in the tree. This means that the decision tree has implicitly performed a feature subset selection.

1.2.5.2 Random forests

Decision trees, while powerful, suffer from limitations. Their tendency to overfit (discussed in section 1.4.4) and sensitivity to data variations can lead to unreliable predictions. Moreover, decision trees have a greedy optimization scheme and they have limited ability to capture complex relationships.

Random forests represent an ensemble machine learning method that leverages the collective power of multiple decision trees. Each tree is constructed from a random subset of features, introducing an element of stochasticity that enhances generalization. By aggregating the predictions from this ensemble, random forests achieve robustness to over-fitting and improve overall prediction accuracy compared to individual decision trees. This technique has gained widespread adoption due to its effectiveness in various classification and regression tasks.

1.2.5.3 Support vector machines

Assuming a linear separable distribution for data, the classes can be separated using a line or hyperplane characterized as $x. \ w + b = 0$, where $w \in R^{d_{in}}$ and $b \in R$ are the slope and intercept parameters of the hyperplane. There are, however, infinite possible values for the parameters, resulting in many potential discriminators as shown in figure 1.4(a). While all the hyperplanes effectively separate the training samples, some of them may misclassify test samples, leading to poor generalization.

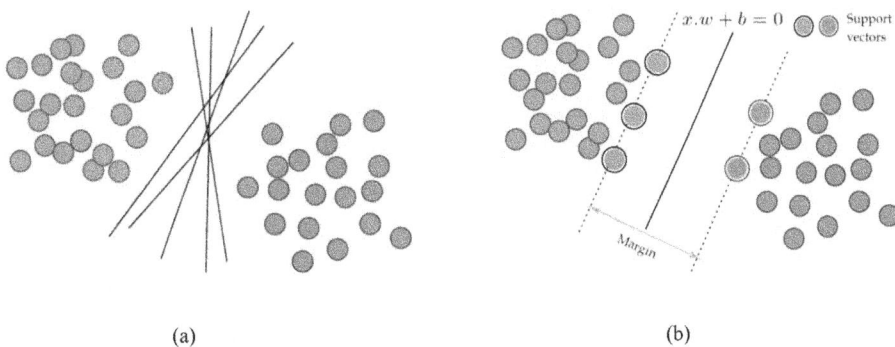

(a)   (b)

Figure 1.4. Support vector machine. (a) Several possible separating lines and (b) the separating line with the largest margin.

---

[1] The height of a tree is defined as the maximum number of internal nodes on the longest path from the root to any leaf node.

Support vector machines (SVMs), on the other hand, try to identify a hyperplane that not only accurately classifies training data points but also maintains a significant distance, or margin, to the nearest data points of each class, which are called support vectors as presented in figure 1.4(b). Acting as a buffer zone, this margin provides robustness to variations in the data and improves the model's generalization ability. By maximizing this margin, an SVM aims to achieve a clear separation between classes, reducing the risk of misclassification and enhancing the model's ability to generalize well to unseen data.

Support vectors are embedded within the model after the training in an SVM. In the context of sensitive medical data, this can potentially violate patient privacy due to the inclusion of support vectors in the model. In particular, if the support vectors correspond to specific individuals in the dataset, it may inadvertently disclose sensitive information about those patients, compromising their privacy. This means that these models should not be trained on identifiable data.

1.2.5.4 k-nearest neighbors

k-nearest neighbors (kNN) is a simple ML algorithm that operates on the principle of proximity. The intuition behind kNN is that similar data points in a feature space tend to belong to the same class or category. Distance metrics often measure this similarity in vector space. A common distance metric is Euclidean distance, which measures the straight-line distance between points in a vector space. Other popular distances include Manhattan distance, which calculates the sum of absolute differences along each dimension. Other metrics, such as Minkowski distance, allow a tunable parameter to adjust the emphasis on different dimensions [20].

An illustration of the kNN classification of a test sample (the point with no color) with different k values is provided in figure 1.5. The prediction is often made by a majority voting of the labels that fall within the neighborhood. Note how the decision changes with increasing k value. For a binary classification task, choosing an even or odd value for k is important since it impacts the resolution of ties as shown in figure 1.5(b). An odd k value is preferred to avoid ties (figure 1.6(c)), ensuring a clear majority decision when voting among the nearest neighbors. Note that in multi-label classification a tie situation may occur when multiple neighbors have the same number of occurrences for different labels, and the resolution of the tie does not depend on the specific value of k. In general, a smaller k value tends to

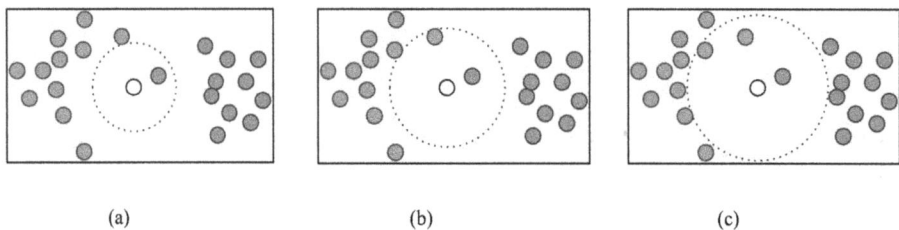

| (a) | (b) | (c) |

Figure 1.5. Different neighborhoods of an arbitrary test sample: (a) 1NN classifying as blue, (b) 2NN, no classification due to tie, and (c) 3NN classifying as red.

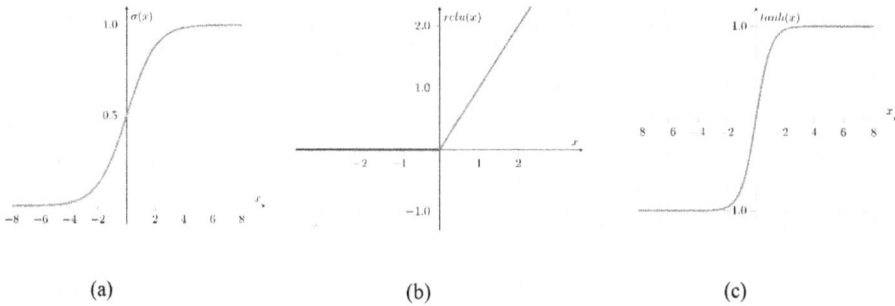

Figure 1.6. Different activation functions: (a) sigmoid, (b) ReLu, and (c) hyperbolic tangent [22].

result in a more flexible and low-bias model, allowing it to adapt well to intricate patterns in the data, but it might be sensitive to noise [21]. On the other hand, a larger k value leads to a smoother decision boundary, reducing sensitivity to noise but potentially introducing bias.

While simple, kNN can be a powerful and effective algorithm for certain types of datasets, in particular when the underlying relationships are based on local patterns and proximity. kNN can be categorized as a *lazy learner* [20], where it learns by memorizing the training data and classifying new instances based on their proximity to known examples. This means that the training data must always be available to the model even when the model is deployed. An important consideration when using such models is the privacy of patients.

1.3 Artificial neural networks

Artificial neural networks (ANNs), inspired by the human brain, consist of interconnected layers of artificial neurons. While traditional models such as decision trees and SVMs require handcrafted features, neural networks can automatically learn complex and hierarchical representations through multiple layers of inter-connected neurons.

1.3.1 Feed-forward neural networks

Feed-forward neural networks are the most basic form of neural nets which express a mapping:

$$y = f(xW + b), \tag{1.3}$$

where $f(\cdot)$ is an activation function, $x \in R^{d_{in}}$ is the input vector, $y \in R^{d_{out}}$ is the output. The mapping is characterized by two learnable parameters $W \in R^{d_{in} \times d_{out}}$ (weight matrix) and $b \in R^{d_{out}}$ (bias vector). If $f(\cdot) = I(\cdot)$ (identity function), equation (1.3) expresses a linear mapping. In this case, the neural net can only approximate linear functions. On the other hand, if a non-linear activation is used, the network can approximate more sophisticated functions. Examples of non-linear activations such as sigmoid, rectified linear units (ReLU), and hyperbolic tangent (tanh) are provided in figure 1.6.

A problem with sigmoid and hyperbolic tangent functions is that they can easily saturate, i.e. large input values converge to 1.0, and small values converge to -1 or 0 for hyperbolic tangent and sigmoid, respectively. Once saturated, it becomes challenging for the learning algorithm to continue to adapt the weights to improve the model's performance. The ReLU, on the other hand, is a piecewise linear function and has greatly improved the performance of neural networks. Since rectified linear units are nearly linear, they preserve many properties that make linear models easy to optimize [8].

Another common activation function is softmax, which is often used to obtain probability values from a vector $\boldsymbol{h} = [h_1, h_2, ..., h_d]$:

$$
\mathrm{softmax}(h) = \left[\frac{\exp(h_1)}{\sum_j \exp(h_j)}, \cdots, \frac{\exp(h_d)}{\sum_j \exp(h_j)} \right]. \tag{1.4}
$$

The softmax function is often applied to the output layer of a network and yields class probabilities for a multi-class classification problem.

1.3.2 Recurrent neural networks

The primary assumption of feed-forward networks is that the features of a sample do not change over time; thus, their input is often represented by a single feature vector. Many phenomena, however, have temporal dynamics where the behavior changes through time. A patient, for instance, might have new tests, radiation dose, changes in organs, etc, which means that a sequence of feature vectors $x_1, x_2, ..., x_T$ now describes the patient where x_t denotes a time-dependent feature. A predictive system should consider such changes to provide a personalized treatment recommendation.

Recurrent neural networks (RNNs) are a class of networks introduced for processing sequences [23] where the current state $\boldsymbol{h}_t \in R^{d_h}$ is a function of the current input $x_t \in R^{d_{in}}$, and previous hidden state $\boldsymbol{h}_{t-1}$. Note that the term *state* is borrowed from the terminology used in control theory, where a system is often described by its state, which represents a set of variables that describe the system at a particular point in time [22]. Figure 1.7 shows a recurrent network. Note the feedback loop, which allows a memory of different time steps/positions.

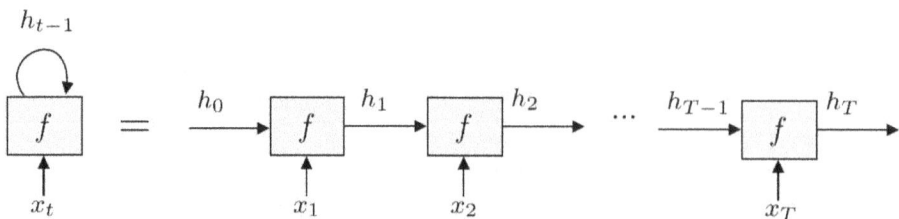

Figure 1.7. A recurrent network unfolded through time. The hidden representation at time step t (h_t) is a function of x_t and h_{t-1}. Reproduced with permission from [22].

The network can be unfolded through time/positions, showing that a recurrent net is, in fact, a feed-forward network that is applied over all positions.

Formally, an RNN can be characterized as

$$h_t = f(x_t, h_{t-1}) = f(x_t W + h_{t-1}\widetilde{W} + b). \tag{1.5}$$

The function is characterized by two weight matrices $W \in R^{d_{in} \times d_h}, \widetilde{W} \in R^{d_h \times d_h}$ that are learning parameters, as well as a bias vector $b \in R^{d_h}$. In a recurrent net, the hidden state h_t represents a history of observed inputs from the beginning of a sequence up to the current input. The h_t corresponding to the final position (h_T) is assumed to represent the whole sequence and can be followed by a simple classifier to determine the label for the desired task. The weight matrix then needs to be updated based on the error of the classifier's prediction. In recurrent nets, particularly with long sequences, the vanishing gradient problem can occur, leading to difficulties in preserving relevant information across distant time steps/positions, hindering the network's ability to effectively capture long-term dependencies. This issue can result in diminished learning capabilities for tasks requiring the retention of context over extended temporal spans.

1.3.3 Convolutional neural networks

Convolutional neural networks (CNNs) were introduced for pattern recognition tasks to process spatial data, such as images [24] and have been exponentially applied in the medical computer vision domain. A major difference between a neuron in a CNN from a regular ANN is that its neurons are designed to be three-dimensional with width, height, and depth. A CNN comprises layers where each layer transforms a 3D (i.e. RGB channels) input to a 3D output. The basic components of a CNN are the convolutional, pooling, and fully connected layers.

Convolution layers use filters or kernels, which are spatially small 3D matrices, to convolve or slide across through the width and height of the input volume. The resulting output is then passed to an activation function (see section 1.3.1), producing a 2D feature map or activation map for each filter that learns visual patterns.

Pooling layers downsample an input volume to decrease the size of feature representation progressively, hence reducing the number of parameters and the computational time. It is commonly followed by a convolution layer, achieving spatial invariance. Average pooling computes the average value in a sliding window while preserving general information. Max pooling selects the maximum value in a sliding window, effectively capturing the most prominent features and patterns during down-sampling.

The **fully connected** (FC) **layer** flattens the output of the final convolutional or pooling layers into a vector h. An output layer is responsible for producing the final predictions or classifications (elaborated in section 1.3.5). In a CNN, the initial layers often detect general patterns (image edges and colors) and deeper layers learn task-specific representations. Figure 1.8 illustrates a simple example of a

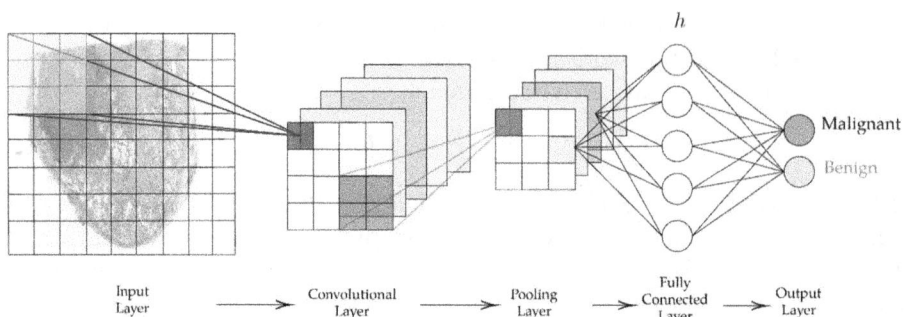

Figure 1.8. A CNN architecture comprising five stacked layers: input layer of a histopathology whole slide image, convolutional layer, pooling layer, fully connected layer, and output layer to predict a class.

classification task predicting cancer malignancy from an H&E histopathology whole slide image (WSI) using a CNN-based architecture.

While CNN is often applied to classify entire images, a specific architecture of CNNs designed for pixel-wise biomedical image segmentation is U-Net [25]. It has become the basis of many auto-segmentation algorithms applied to medical images [26]. In this design, the encoder network or the contracting path is a feature extractor. It acquires an abstract representation of the input image through a series of encoder blocks comprising convolutions while the spatial dimensions of the input volume are gradually reduced. The decoder network or the expanding path increases the spatial dimensions of the extracted features, localizing these features in the image and producing a segmentation map.

1.3.4 Attention

CNNs effectively capture local spatial information through convolutional filters but face challenges in capturing global context and long-range dependencies within data [27]. Their limited receptive fields (due to filters with small window size) can hinder understanding complex scenes where relationships between distant elements are crucial. Adaptive attention to local and global context is required to address these challenges. This has motivated the development of architecture such as transformers [28] that use the attention mechanism.

1.3.4.1 Self-attention

The attention mechanism resembles a spotlight that an ML model can use to focus on specific parts of input data when making predictions. Instead of treating all parts of the input equally (equal weights), the model can assign different levels of importance or 'attention' to different elements [29]. While different forms of attention mechanism exist, one of its most well-known and widely used forms is self-attention, defined as

$$\underbrace{[\tilde{x}_1; \ldots; \tilde{x}_T]}_{\tilde{x}} \tilde{x} = \text{softmax}(XW^q(XW^k)^T) \underbrace{}_{A} XW^v, \tag{1.6}$$

where W^q, W^k, and W^v are training parameters and $X = [x_1; ...; x_T]$ is a matrix of input representations (positions/time steps 1 to T). In this formalism, the product $XW^q(XW^k)^T$ represents the similarity between inputs at different positions, resulting in a square matrix $A \in R^{T \times T}$, where $A_{t, k}$ represents the amount of attention that the tth input element pays to the kth element. A softmax activation is then applied to A (row-level) to obtain a probability distribution. The self-attention mechanism results in a matrix of contextualized representations $\widetilde{X} = [\tilde{x}_1; ...; \tilde{x}_T]$, where each row is obtained using an adaptive weighted average of x_1, ... , x_T, enabling the model to focus on different input elements.

1.3.4.2 Positional encoding

Although a self-attention mechanism captures relationships between different elements in a sequence, it does not account for positional information. Thus, additional positional encoding is often introduced before applying self-attention to ensure the model can discern the sequence's order and the relative positions of elements. This positional encoding matrix P (often a constant matrix) is added to matrix X. A common form of positional encoding is sinusoidal, which is represented as

$$P_{t, 2j} = \sin(t/10000^{2j/d}) \qquad (1.7)$$

$$P_{t, 2j+1} = \cos(t/10000^{2j/d}),$$

where t is the position index and d is the number of input dimensions. An illustration of a positional encoding matrix P for 15 positions ($t = 0, ..., 14$) and $d = 100^2$ is provided in figure 1.9(a). Note that the representations corresponding to adjacent positions (rows) are similar while distance positions have dissimilar representations, allowing the position of each element in a sequence to be captured explicitly.

1.3.4.3 Transformer encoder

Transformers are attention-based networks introduced to address the problem of vanishing long-distance information that exists in RNNs and CNNs [28]. Figure 1.9(b) illustrates the transformer architecture, where its input is the matrix $X = [x_1; ...; x_T]$. In contrast to a recurrent net, where the input is processed one position at a time, in transformers, the inputs at all positions are fed into the network simultaneously. A self-attention layer obtains the new contextual representations. A residual connection is used for each layer to avoid issues such as exploding gradient. The final output of the transformer is a matrix of hidden representations h_t ($t = 1, ..., T$).

Modern neural network architectures are versatile, and advancements in different domains within the broader field of DL are interconnected. CNNs, for instance, were originally introduced for image data, and their success sparked interest in exploring their adaptability to other domains such as natural language processing

---

[2] The number of positions and the value of d are chosen arbitrarily.

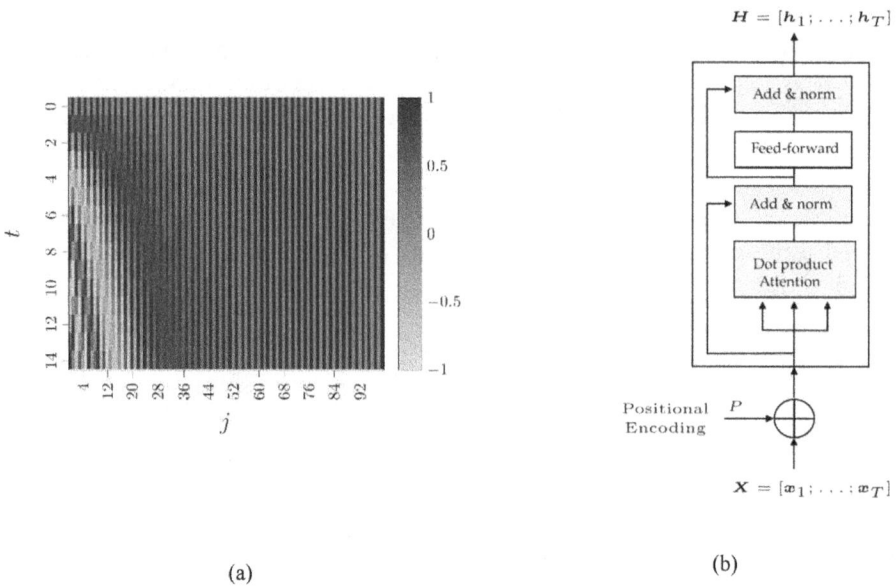

(a)

(b)

Figure 1.9. Transformer architecture: (a) positional encoding and (b) transformer encoder.

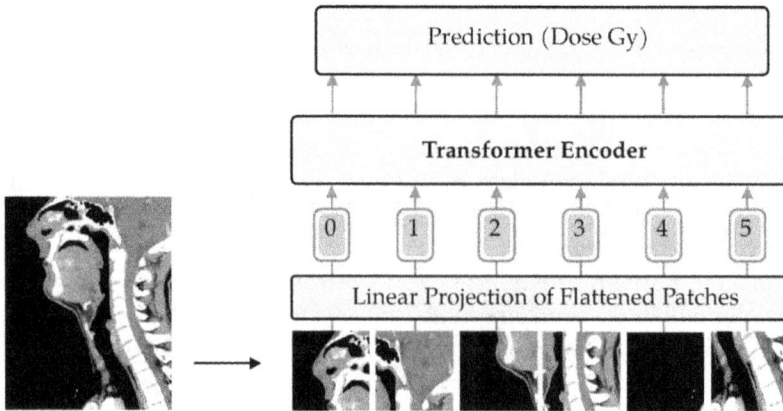

Figure 1.10. A vision transformer.

(NLP) [30]. On the other hand, transformers, initially developed by the NLP community, marked a significant paradigm shift in sequence modeling. Surprisingly, their capabilities transcended their original NLP domain and were later successfully applied to computer vision tasks. This adaptation is called the vision transformer, where an image is seen as a sequence of patches, as shown in figure 1.10 [31]. Benefiting from the attention mechanism, a vision transformer allows adaptive attention to local and global contexts, often leading to superior performances compared to CNNs.

1.3.5 Training neural networks

Making predictions in neural nets involves using learned representations to generate outputs. The neural layers discussed in the previous sections are mostly encoders that try to learn a representation from an input. The learned representation h (usually a vector) is then used as input to a classifier/regressor to make predictions. For classification, a simple projection $z = hW^{cls}$ can be used, where $W^{cls} \in R^{d_h \times N_c}$ and N_c is the number of classes.

The projection results in a vector $z \in R^{N_c}$ of logits where each dimension corresponds to a class. A softmax activation is then used to convert the logit values to class probabilities $p = \text{softmax}(z)$ and the dimension with highest p_c probability corresponds to the predicted class. For regression, a projection $z = hW^{reg}$ is often used to map h to a single scalar value where $W^{reg} \in R^{d_h \times 1}$.

Loss functions are mathematical measures that quantify the difference between predicted values and actual values in an ML model, serving as a guide for adjusting model parameters. The goal is to minimize the loss function during the training process to improve the accuracy of the model. For classification tasks, a commonly used loss function is cross-entropy loss. The cross-entropy loss $L(y, p) = -\sum_{c=1}^{N_c} y_c \log \log (p_c)$, has two input arguments $y \in \{0,1\}^{N_c}$, a one-hot vector representing the true class, and p as the probability vector (softmax output). For regression tasks, squared error $L(y, z) = (y - z)^2$ is a commonly used form.

Gradient descent is an iterative approach for training neural nets and the minimization of their prediction error (over training data). The loss L is a function of the network's trainable parameters W (see figure 1.11). Therefore, the minimization involves finding an optimal W^* that minimizes the error. Most neural networks describe non-convex functions, meaning that several local minima exist. In this case, a minimum is found using a gradient descent approach that relies on

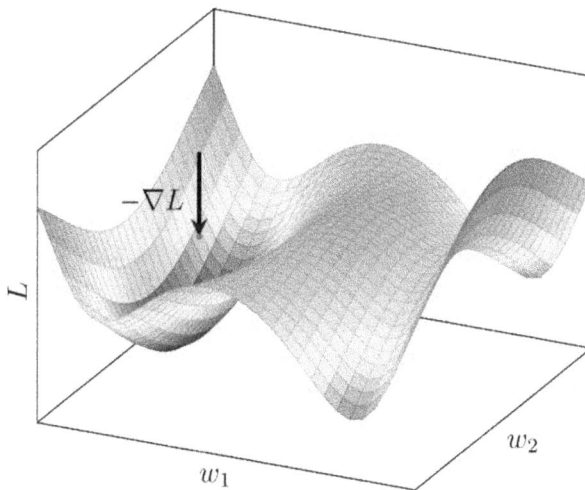

Figure 1.11. An error/loss surface as a function of training parameters (here w_1 and w_2).

∇L, the gradient of loss L with respect to the set of trainable parameters W. The gradient represents the direction and the magnitude of the ascent of the loss function. In each iteration, trainable parameters are updated with a step-size $\eta > 0$ (also known as the learning rate):

$$W_{\text{new}} = W_{\text{old}} - \eta \nabla L. \tag{1.8}$$

As illustrated in figure 1.11, $-\nabla L$ directs the training process towards a descending direction of the loss [22].

1.3.6 Applications and use cases of deep learning

Dosimetry utilizing the Monte Carlo (MC) method is widely regarded as the gold standard and the most precise approach for calculating absorbed radiation dose in heterogeneous materials such as human tissue. This method accurately models fundamental physical processes within the context of patient-specific anatomy, source and applicator geometry, and the presence of tissue and material variations [32]. Monte Carlo simulations, however, involve the stochastic sampling of numerous particle tracks, making them time-consuming. DL, with its capacity to learn from large amounts of data, has the potential to approximate the complex physics involved in radiation interactions. By training neural networks on large datasets of simulated radiation scenarios, these models can potentially learn to predict dose distributions with faster speed while significantly reducing the computational burden associated with Monte Carlo simulations. An example of such DL systems is RapidBrachyDL [33], which is a 3D deep CNN. RapidBrachyDL calculates dose distributions for high dose rate (HDR) brachytherapy, with patient CT images and treatment plans used as inputs, while accelerating the simulation process by 300 times.

In addition to dose prediction, deep models can also be used for predicting possible side effects of a prescribed dose. For instance, early detection of toxicities in radiotherapy is crucial for ensuring the safety and well-being of patients undergoing cancer treatment. An example is the architecture proposed by Elhaminia *et al* which is a CNN- and attention-based model for prediction of toxicity in pelvic radiotherapy [34], demonstrating an 80% accuracy. Investigation of attention weights in this model provides insight on which anatomical regions are associated with high risk of toxicity, and how dose maps impact the network's prediction.

DL has shown significant promise in adaptive radiotherapy when applied to various image modalities such as CT, MRI, and PET. One key application is in image segmentation, where deep learning models can accurately delineate organs at risk and target volumes. For example, in head and neck cancer treatment, precise segmentation of critical structures such as the spinal cord or salivary glands is crucial to avoid unnecessary radiation exposure and minimize side effects. Another application is in image registration, where deep learning can align images from different time points to track changes in tumor size and position. This is particularly important for tumors that exhibit significant intrafractional motion, such as lung tumors. By accurately registering images, clinicians can adapt the treatment plan to ensure that the tumor receives the intended dose while sparing healthy tissue.

Despite the novel applications of deep learning models, the moderate-sized datasets in the medical domain pose challenges for training robust ML models. Transfer learning is a technique widely used in medical computer vision tasks with limited datasets and computational resources. It involves utilizing a pre-trained model, trained on a large dataset, as a starting point for a new task with a smaller dataset. In this approach, a large number of parameters in the pre-trained model are frozen (not updated by gradient descent) to retain learned representations, and fine-tuning allows updating a small subset of parameters during training to learn task-specific features. This approach promotes faster model convergence and improved performance by leveraging general knowledge gained from the original large dataset [35]. VGGNet [36] is a well-known CNN, pre-trained on an extensive image classification task, ImageNet [37], which comprises 1000 classes. This pre-training facilitates the deployment of VGGNet in segmentation tasks, a common requirement in many medical imaging applications [38].

1.4 Model training and evaluation

1.4.1 Hyperparameters

Hyperparameters are external configuration settings that are not learned from the data but are set prior to the training process (by an ML expert). These parameters play a crucial role in determining the model's performance. In kNNs, for instance, the primary hyperparameter is the k itself, as well as the choice for the distance metric. Other examples of a hyperparameter are the maximum depth of a decision tree, the minimum number of samples required to split an internal node in a decision tree, and for random forests, the number of estimators (decision trees).

For deep learning models, there are several key hyperparameters that play a crucial role in determining their performance and behavior. The architecture-related hyperparameters include the number of layers, the size of each layer (number of neurons or units), the activation function used in each layer (e.g. ReLU, sigmoid, tanh), and the type of layers used (e.g. dense, convolutional, recurrent). These hyperparameters collectively define the model's capacity to learn complex patterns and representations from the data. Additionally, hyperparameters such as the learning rate (η), batch size, the type of optimizer (e.g. Adam, SGD) are related to the training process.

Hyperparameters are tuned during the training process, allowing the adjustment of these external configuration settings to achieve optimal results. This iterative tuning helps to find a middle ground between model complexity and generalization, enhancing the overall performance of the ML model.

1.4.2 Data split

When humans learn, the process of acquiring knowledge and skills involves both training and testing. Just as students need to undergo exams to demonstrate their understanding and proficiency, ML models require testing to evaluate their performance on new, unseen data. Thus, in addition to a training set, two other hold-out sets, namely validation and test sets, are used. While a training set directly influences the learning process of a model, a validation set is used to evaluate the performance of the model during the learning, to tune hyperparameters, and select the best performing model. The test set on the other hand is never disclosed to the model during the learning process and is only used to evaluate the performance once the training is finished. In ML it is common to have a small sized dataset. This might pose a challenge when splitting the data, since the performance estimates might be misleading due the small size of partitions. Techniques such as k-fold cross-validation and stratified k-fold cross-validation mitigate issues related to small or moderate-sized datasets, offering more accurate estimates of generalization error [39].

1.4.3 Evaluation metrics

Once an ML model is developed, its performance needs to be evaluated, using quantitative measures. The performance of a predictive model is often measured on a hold-out test set, i.e. a set that has not been exposed to the model during its training process. This allows informed decisions to be made in comparing different models and choosing the one that has the best performance for unseen data (generalization capability).

The **confusion matrix** provides detailed insights into predictive model performance, which shows correct and incorrect predictions for each class. Figure 1.12(a) shows a sample confusion matrix for a binary classification problem. Each entry in the matrix counts the number of correct/incorrect classifications for each class. True positive (TP) is the number of positive test samples correctly classified as positive.

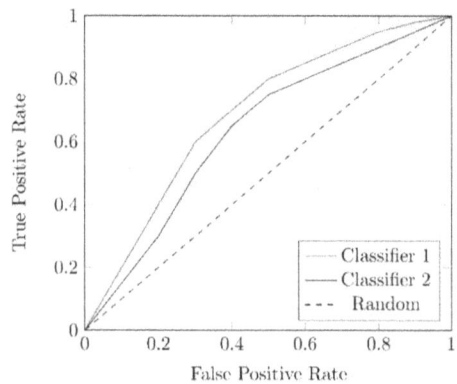

Figure 1.12. Performance evaluation: (a) a confusion matrix and (b) an ROC curve.

Likewise, true negative (TN) is the number of negative samples correctly classified as negative. False positive (FP) corresponds to the number of negative test samples misclassified as positive, and false negative (FN) is the number of positive samples misclassified as negative.

A set of performance measures can be defined to aggregate the matrix entries and provide more focused insight into a model's performance, especially in cases of imbalanced distributions. Three of the most common metrics are recall, precision, and F1 score.

Recall is the ratio of true positive predictions to the total number of actual positives:

$$R = \frac{TP}{TP + FN}.$$ (1.9)

Recall measures the ability of a model to capture all positive instances. High recall means that the model has fewer false negatives. In the example provided in figure 1.13(a) the model has few false negatives (FN = 3) leading to a relatively high recall ($R = 0.84$). Note that a model can have a perfect recall ($R = 1$) by predicting all samples as positive (i.e. FN = 0).

Precision, on the other, is the ratio of true positive predictions to the total number of positive predictions:

$$P = \frac{TP}{TP + FP}.$$ (1.10)

Precision measures the accuracy of positive predictions, and a high precision means that the model has fewer false positives. In figure 1.13(a), while the model demonstrated high recall, it shows a poor precision (only slightly better than random) due to the relatively large number of false positives. The emphasis on precision or recall depends on the domain and the task at hand. For instance, when identifying treatment options, it is crucial to have a high precision while for identifying high-risk patients for screening, a high recall is important.

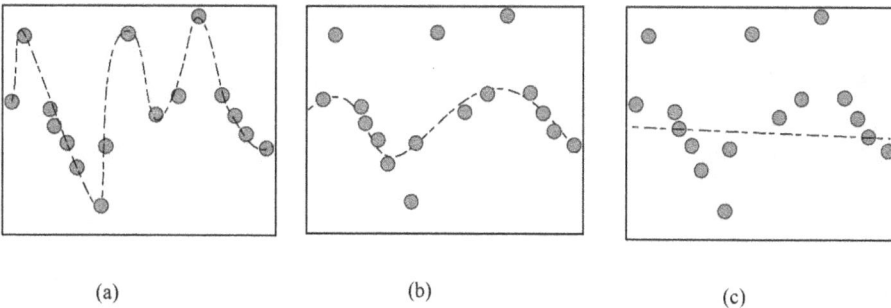

(a)	(b)	(c)

Figure 1.13. Different fitting scenarios: (a) over-fitting, (b) proper fitting, and (c) under-fitting.

The **F1** score combines precision and recall using their harmonic mean:

$$\text{F1} = 2\frac{P \times R}{P + R}. \tag{1.11}$$

The F1 score provides a balanced measure of a model's performance by considering both false positives and false negatives. It is particularly useful in cases with an imbalanced class distribution or when both types of classification errors have significant implications. Figure 1.13(a) shows that the model has a moderate F1 due to low precision.

The **receiver operating characteristics** (ROC) curve is a valuable tool for assessing a model's ability to discriminate between classes, visualizing the tradeoff between the false positive rate (FPR) and true negative rate (TPR) (see figure 1.13(b)). The area under the curve (AUC) quantifies model performance, with perfect prediction yielding an AUC of 1 and random prediction an AUC of 0.5. As figure 1.13(b) shows, the AUC for classifier 1 is bigger than the AUC for classifier 2, suggesting a better performance for classifier 1.

1.4.4 Overfitting versus under-fitting

The development of an ML model involves striking a balance between complexity and simplicity. Neglecting this balance may lead to under-fitting or over-fitting. Under-fitting means the model is too simplistic to capture the underlying patterns in the training data, e.g. using a linear classifier for linear non-separable data (see figure 1.13(a)). An indicator of under-fitting is a low performance or high error rate on the training data, let alone test data. This is because the model fails to grasp even the most basic patterns present in the training data.

Conversely, over-fitting occurs when the model has a high learning capacity, and the training data has a relatively simple distribution (see figure 1.13(b)). High performance (low error) on training data, but a low performance on test data are indicators of over-fitting. Hyperparameter tuning is a common approach to prevent over-fitting. In decision trees, for instance, techniques such as pruning, which involves limiting the growth of the tree by setting a maximum depth or restricting the minimum number of samples required to split a node can be used [20].

1.5 Generative models

Generative models are a class of ML models designed to learn and mimic the underlying distribution of a given dataset. Unlike discriminative models, which focus on predicting labels or classifying data ($p(y|x)$), generative models aim to capture the joint probability distribution of the input data and the corresponding labels ($p(x, y)$).

The primary purpose of generative models is to generate new data samples that are similar to the training data. These models can generate new examples from scratch by sampling from the learned distribution, allowing them to create realistic data that preserves the statistical properties of the original dataset. Generative models have various applications, including data augmentation, image and text synthesis, anomaly detection, and semi-supervised learning. They are particularly useful in scenarios where obtaining labeled data is expensive or impractical, as they can generate synthetic data for training discriminative models. While various deep generative models have been proposed in the literature, we focus solely on introducing the two most prominent and recent techniques in this discussion.

1.5.1 Generative adversarial networks

A generative adversarial network (GAN) [12] is a deep generative model where its primary goal is to mimic the distribution of training data and, consequently, generate samples drawn from the learned distribution. GAN is a two-player minimax game involving two opposing models: a generator G and a discriminator D, as shown in figure 1.14. In this framework, both models are trained simultaneously. The discriminator aims to distinguish between samples from the true data distribution and the generator distribution. In contrast, the generator seeks to minimize the likelihood of being identified as fake by approximating the data distribution from a simpler distribution, such as Gaussian or uniform.

During training, the generator tries to mislead the discriminator, while the discriminator endeavors to maximize the probability of accurately predicting true labels for both real and generated samples. The competitive dynamic between these two components encourages continual improvement. The ideal stopping point is reached when G captures the distribution of the training data ($p_g = p_{\text{data}}$), and D can no longer differentiate between generated and training data, resulting in a probability close to 0.5 for each sample.

Given G and D as neural networks, the training of GANs is formulated as follows. The generator G aims to learn the distribution over data x and a prior on the input noise variable, defined as $p_z(z)$. $G(z; \theta_g)$ is the mapping function, where G is a neural network parameterized by θ_g. Conversely, $D(x; \theta_d)$ defines the mapping function for the discriminator D. Here, p_g and p_{data} represent the generated and training data distributions, respectively. The discriminator's output is a scalar representing the label of the input data; that is, $D(x)$ indicates the probability of x belonging to the training data distribution rather than p_g. While D maximizes the probability of assigning true labels to both training and generated samples, G minimizes $\log(1 - D(G(z)))$. Thus, D and G engage in a minimax game to optimize the following objective function:

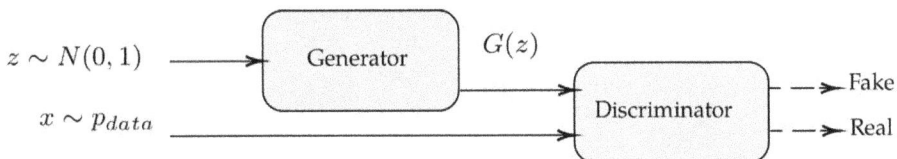

Figure 1.14. GAN architecture; z represents noise sampled from a Gaussian distribution, $G(z)$ denotes the generated image from the noise z, and x represents a training sample drawn from the p_{data} distribution. (Reproduced with permission from [42].)

$$\sim V(D, G) = E_{x \sim P_{\text{data}}(x)}[\log \log D(x)] + E_{z \sim P_{z}(z)}[\log \log (1 - D(G(z)))]. \quad (1.12)$$

Given that discrimination is inherently easier than generation, this objective function might result in a suboptimal generator. Goodfellow *et al* [12] proposed reformulating equation (1.12) by replacing the minimization of log(1 − $D(G(z))$) with the maximization of log($D(G(z))$).

This zero-sum game between these two components can lead to rich representations of the training data, which can be further utilized for downstream tasks [40, 41]. While GANs have demonstrated great success in generating high-quality samples, they have limitations. Due to their adversarial training nature, they are known for potentially unstable training and limited diversity in generation.

1.5.2 Diffusion models

While existing deep generative models excel at image generation, they encounter certain challenges. A diffusion model [43], belonging to the class of generative models, was introduced to address these challenges by generating high-fidelity images. Diffusion models contain two main processes: forward diffusion process and reverse diffusion process. They define a chain of diffusion steps to slowly add random noise to data and then learn to reverse the diffusion process to construct desired data samples from the noise.

In the forward diffusion process shown in figure 1.15, we slowly and gradually add Gaussian noise to the input image x_0 through a series of T steps. We start with sampling a data point x_0 from the real data distribution $q(x)$ ($x_0 \sim q(x)$) and then add some Gaussian noise with variance β_t to x_{t-1}, producing a new latent variable x_t with distribution $q(x_{t-1})$

$$q(x_t \mid x_{t-1}) = N(x_t; \sqrt{1 - \beta_t} x_{t-1}, \beta_t I)$$

$$q(x_{1:T} \mid x_0) = \prod_{t=1}^{T} q(x_{t-1}), \quad (1.13)$$

where I and N denote the identity matrix and Gaussian distribution, respectively. The data sample x_0 gradually loses its distinguishable features as the step increases.

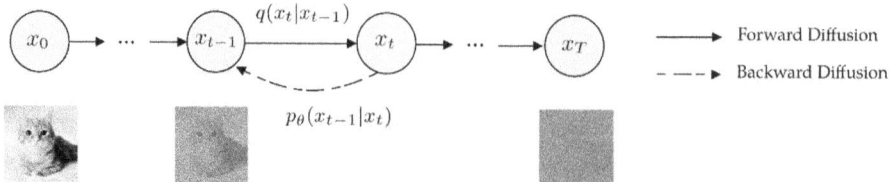

Figure 1.15. Diffusion process: through the forward process, noise is added to a given image x, drawn from q (x), through T steps. x_0 and x_T represent the original image and the image after T steps of adding noise, respectively. Through the reverse process, the given image x is reconstructed through a denoising process from step T to 0.

Eventually, when $T \to \infty$, it becomes equivalent to an isotropic Gaussian distribution.

The reverse diffusion process involves training a neural network to restore the original data by reversing the noise applied during the forward pass (see figure 1.15). Estimating $q(x_{t-1}|x_t)$ can be challenging as it can require the entire dataset. To address this, the reparameterization technique is employed, utilizing a parameterized model p_θ in the form of a neural network to learn the parameters. For sufficiently small β_t, the distribution becomes Gaussian, allowing the mean and variance to be parameterized easily:

$$p_\theta(x_{0:T}) = p(x_T) \prod_{t=1}^{T} p_\theta(x_{t-1} \mid x_t)$$

$$p_\theta(x_t) = N(x_{t-1}; \mu_\theta(x_t, t), \Sigma_\theta(x_t, t)). \tag{1.14}$$

The network is trained to predict the mean and variance for each time step. Here $\mu_\theta(x_t, t)$ and $\Sigma_\theta(x_t, t)$ define the mean and the covariance matrix, respectively.

There are different varieties of diffusion models such as diffusion probabilistic models (DPM) [45], noise-conditioned score network [44], and denoising diffusion probabilistic models (DDPM) [45].

1.5.3 Applications and use cases

Generative models such as GANs, autoencoders, variational autoencoders, and diffusion models have been used extensively in the literature for the medical domain, mainly for image generation to mitigate the limited and imbalanced data problems in developing AI tools for medical problems [42]. Han *et al* [46] utilized the DCGAN and Wasserstein GAN (WGAN) [47] for medical image generation. Nie *et al* [48] suggested an adversarial model to generate magnetic resonance imaging (MRI) images from computed tomography (CT) images, whereas recently the authors of [49] suggested using denoising diffusion models to generate high-quality MRI and CT. GANs have also been used for synthetic generation in structured data [50].

Aside from image generation, transfer learning and domain adaptation models using generative models such as GANs have found widespread application in the medical field. Domain adaptation is a subcategory of transfer learning when we aim to learn a model from a source data distribution and apply that model to a different target data distribution. Yaqoub *et al* [51] proposed using transfer learning in MR image reconstruction trained with GANs to mitigate the limited data problem in medical imaging tasks. Recent studies have applied domain adaptation approaches to address distribution shifts while leveraging existing medical data. Several studies considered working on MR images as the source domain and CT images as the target domain using adversarial training to generate synthetic CT images [52], cardiac structure segmentation [53], and image registration [54].

Generative models have also been used for anomaly detection. Anomaly detection, also known as out-of-distribution detection, focuses on recognizing samples that diverge from the rest of the data, signaling variations in measurement, experimental errors, or novel occurrences. This proves valuable in uncovering unknown anomalies in the medical field, where acquiring a suitable annotated dataset is consistently a challenge. This approach is also relevant in situations where information about the specific types of anomalies is scarce. The first anomaly detection model in medical imaging using GAN was proposed to find anomalies in optical coherence tomography [55]. While GANs were used mostly for detecting anomalies a few years ago, more recently, diffusion models have become the dominant approach. Wolleb *et al* [56] proposed a novel weakly supervised anomaly detection method based on denoising diffusion models to address the difficulties of anomaly detection models based on GANs in preserving fine details in the image. Pinaya *et al* [57] proposed a method based on diffusion models to detect and segment anomalies in brain imaging. Aside from images, anomaly detection using generative models in time-series data also gained attention [58].

In addition to potential applications of generative models, they gained attention in other medical imaging tasks. Wolterink *et al* [59] proposed an adversarial model by training two separate generators with two different losses and combining them to reduce the noise in low-dose CT images. Image super-resolution using GANs has also been investigated in medical images [60]. Different generative models have also been used extensively for image and video segmentation. Wu *et al* [61] combined diffusion and transformer models for medical image segmentation. In another study, a denoising diffusion probabilistic model was integrated into standard U-Net [62] models for medical image segmentation [63]. Generative models, specifically GANs, have been used for other modalities such as text. Even though generating discrete data such as text with GANs is challenging, several studies investigated using them for text generation purposes [64].

1.6 Ethical consideration and bias

AI has significantly transformed various aspects of our lives, holding great potential for societal benefits, ranging from healthcare applications to biomedical data analysis. In healthcare, AI has the capacity to enhance diagnostic accuracy, personalize treatment plans, improve patient outcomes, and streamline administrative tasks. Despite these positive impacts, there is also the potential for unintended harm and misuse. In the following, some of the most important of these potential harms and misuses will be explained.

1.6.1 Transparency and explainability

A computational system is considered transparent when every detail of its operation is known, whereas we refer to a system as explainable when humans can understand how it makes decisions. Transparency in a system does not necessarily ensure explainability. Understanding how a model operates can be particularly challenging, especially in the case of DL models with many parameters.

While explainability in DL models is often achieved through techniques such as layer-wise relevance propagation or attention mechanisms [30] to enhance their interpretability or model-agnostic approaches such as LIME [65], many classical

ML models, such as decision trees, SVMs, rule-based systems, and symbolic AI, inherently offer a certain level of explainability

1.6.2 Bias and fairness

Bias typically denotes a statistical deviation from a defined norm. In AI applications, this divergence often arises from illegitimate or unrelated factors influencing the output. For instance, gender is irrelevant to job performance; therefore, using gender as a basis for hiring a candidate is considered irrelevant (example: Amazon recruiting ML tool)[3]. Similarly, race is unrelated to criminality, making it irrelevant to incorporate race as a feature for predicting recidivism [66]. While bias can take various forms in AI models, it is mainly influenced by our data selection strategy.

Data selection bias occurs when the training data are incomplete and comprise only specific distributions, such as race, gender, ethnicity, etc, making algorithmic bias likely. In a study by Obermeyer *et al* [67], an algorithm used in healthcare to identify and assist patients with complex medical needs was investigated. The study revealed racial bias in the algorithm, as it systematically underestimated the healthcare needs of black patients compared to white patients. In another study, commercial gender classification systems were evaluated [68]. The findings showed that these systems exhibited higher accuracy for lighter-skinned and male faces compared to darker-skinned and female faces. The reason behind both models' biases were traced back to the imbalanced dataset used for training, which primarily featured specific race or gender categories. As a result, the AI model struggled to accurately classify in the case of underrepresented groups. In addition to data selection bias, a model's goals and validation metrics might impose biases on the model. Each of these biases can negatively impact marginalized and underrepresented groups, resulting in an unfair AI model.

To mitigate data selection bias and ensure that AI models in healthcare are fair and effective, it is crucial to train them on large and diverse datasets that accurately represent the patient population. This diversity needs to encompass various social statuses, minority groups, age groups, genders, races, and other relevant factors. By training on such datasets, AI models can learn to make decisions that are more inclusive and representative of the population they are intended to serve. This approach not only allows to reduce bias but also ensures that the resulting models are more robust and applicable across different patient demographics.

1.6.3 Data privacy violation

Modern DL methods heavily depend on large crowd-sourced datasets, which may contain sensitive or private information. Despite efforts to eliminate sensitive details, the presence of auxiliary knowledge and redundant encodings poses a risk of de-anonymizing datasets. Therefore, prioritizing a privacy-centric design is essential to safeguard individuals' information, especially in applying DL techniques to critical

---

[3] https://www.ml.cmu.edu/news/news-archive/2016–2020/2018/october/amazon-scraps-secret-artificial-intelligence-recruiting-engine-that-showed-biases-against-women.html

domains such as healthcare. Employing methods such as differential privacy and semantic security ensures data security throughout the model training process [69].

1.6.4 Risk and misuse

The aforementioned issues are primarily linked to poorly defined objectives and informational imbalances. However, even in cases where a system operates correctly, it can cause unethical conduct or deliberate misuse [70]. AI models trained on medical records might memorize patients' personal information. This means that the AI could potentially recreate a patient's data, raising privacy issues and making it difficult to ensure anonymity when using this data for research or development. In the worst-case scenario, AI memorizing patient data could be exploited by malicious actors, leading to situations where sensitive details are used for blackmail or other criminal purposes. Such models may also be misused by insurance companies to deny coverage or raise premiums based on pre-existing conditions gleaned from the memorized data. This could disproportionately harm patients with sensitive health histories.

In healthcare, the misuse of AI models can also have fatal consequences, such as intentionally manipulated AI algorithms used for medical diagnosis or treatment planning, leading to incorrect or harmful recommendations and patient outcomes [71]. Given the potential risks and misuse of AI applications, regulating these models seems necessary [72]. AI regulation refers to the establishment and enforcement of rules, standards, and guidelines governing the development, deployment, and use of AI systems. These regulations help to (i) ensure that AI systems are developed and used ethically and responsibly, (ii) safeguard individuals' privacy such as patients' data, and (iii) establish accountability and liability in cases of AI-related incidents or harm.

1.7 Summary

This chapter provided a comprehensive overview of the foundational concepts of AI, focusing particularly on machine learning and neural networks. It covered the basics of machine learning, discussing various learning paradigms, such as supervised and unsupervised learning. The importance of feature engineering, linear separability, and classical models was emphasized, providing readers with a good understanding of the essential components of machine learning.

The chapter also explored artificial neural networks, detailing the structure and function of different types of neural nets, including feed-forward, recurrent, convolutional networks, and transformers. Attention mechanisms and the training process for these networks were also covered. Applications and use cases of deep learning were highlighted, illustrating the practical impact of these technologies. Additionally, the chapter addressed model training and evaluation, discussing hyperparameters, data splits, evaluation metrics, and the common challenges of over-fitting and under-fitting. Finally, we touched on advanced topics such as generative models and their applications, and concluded with a critical examination of ethical considerations in AI, such as transparency, bias, data privacy, and the risks of misuse.

References

[1] Russell S and Norvig P 2011 *Artificial Intelligence: A Modern Approach* (Englewood Cliffs, NJ: Prentice-Hall)

[2] Shortliffe E H 1974 MYCIN: a rule-based computer program for advising physicians regarding antimicrobial therapy selection *PhD Thesis* Stanford University, Stanford, CA

[3] Zadeh L A 1965 Fuzzy sets *Inf. Control* **8** 338–53

[4] Holland J H 1975 *Adaptation in Natural and Artificial Systems* (Ann Arbor, MI: University of Michigan Press)

[5] Wells D M, Walrath D and Craighead P S 20000 Improvement in tangential breast planning efficiency using a knowledge-based expert system *Med. Dosim.* **25** 133–8

[6] Shortliffe E H, Scott A C, Bischoff M B, Campbell A B, van Melle W and Jacobs C D 1981 ONCOCIN: an expert system for oncology protocol management *Proc. IJCAI* **81** 876–81

[7] Roberfroid B, Lee J A, Geets X, Sterpin E and Barragán-Montero A M 2024 DIVE-ART: a tool to guide clinicians towards dosimetrically informed volume editions of automatically segmented volumes in adaptive radiation therapy *Radiother. Oncol.* **192** 110108

[8] Goodfellow I, Bengio Y, Courville A and Bengio Y 2016 *Deep Learning* **vol 1** (Cambridge, MA: MIT Press)

[9] Bishop C M 2006 *Pattern Recognition and Machine Learning (Information Science and Statistics)* (Berlin: Springer)

[10] Wold S, Esbensen K and Geladi P 1987 Principal component analysis *Chemometr. Intell. Lab. Syst.* **2** 37–52

[11] Ballard D H 1987 Modular learning in neural networks *AAAI* **647** 279–84

[12] Goodfellow I, Pouget-Abadie J, Mirza M, Xu B, Warde-Farley D, Ozair S, Courville A and Bengio Y 2014 Generative adversarial nets *Advances in Neural Information Processing Systems* vol 27 (Red Hook, NY: Curran Associates) pp 2672–80

[13] Noroozi M and Favaro P 2016 Unsupervised learning of visual representations by solving jigsaw puzzles *European Conf. on Computer Vision* (Berlin: Springer) pp 69–84

[14] Gidaris S, Singh P and Komodakis N 2018 Unsupervised representation learning by predicting image rotations arXiv: 1803.07728v1

[15] Gal T S, Tucker T C, Gangopadhyay A and Chen Z 2014 A data recipient centered de-identification method to retain statistical attributes *J. Biomed. Inform.* **50** 32–45

[16] Theodoridis S and Koutroumbas K 2009 *Pattern Recognition* (Amsterdam: Elsevier)

[17] Pedregosa F *et al* 2011 Scikit-learn: machine learning in Python *J. Mach. Learn. Res.* **12** 2825–30

[18] Duda R O *et al* 2006 *Pattern Classification* (New York: Wiley)

[19] Zhang-Salomons J and Salomons G 2015 Determine the therapeutic role of radiotherapy in administrative data: a data mining approach *BMC Med. Res. Method.* **15** 1–9

[20] Tan P-N, Steinbach M, Karpatne A and Kumar V 2016 *Introduction to Data Mining* (New York: Pearson Education)

[21] Bagherzadeh P and Sadoghi Yazdi H 2017 Label denoising based on Bayesian aggregation *Int. J. Mach. Learn. Cybern.* **8** 903–14

[22] Parsa B 2022 Studies on decoupled modules for integration of extant knowledge sources *PhD Thesis* Concordia University, Montreal

[23] Zadeh L and Desoer C 2008 *Linear System Theory: The State Space Approach* (Garden City, NY: Courier Dover)

[24] LeCun Y *et al* 1995 Convolutional networks for images, speech, and time series *The Handbook of Brain Theory and Neural Networks* **vol 3361** (Cambridge, MA: MIT Press)

[25] Ronneberger O, Fischer P and Brox T 2015 U-Net: convolutional networks for biomedical image segmentation arXiv:1505.04597

[26] Isensee F, Jaeger P F, Kohl S A A, Petersen J and Maier-Hein K H 2021 nnU-Net: a self-configuring method for deep learning-based biomedical image segmentation *Nat. Methods* **18** 203–11

[27] Zeiler M D and Fergus R 2014 Visualizing and understanding convolutional networks *Proc. Computer Vision–ECCV 2014: 13th European Conf. (Zurich, Switzerland, 6–12 September 2014)* (Berlin: Springer) pp 818–33

[28] Vaswani A, Shazeer N, Parmar N, Uszkoreit J, Jones L, Gomez A N, Kaiser Ł and Polosukhin I 2017 Attention is all you need *Advances in Neural Information Processing Systems* (Red Hook, NY: Curran Associates) pp 5998–6008

[29] Bahdanau D, Cho K and Bengio Y 2015 Neural machine translation by jointly learning to align and translate *Proc. of the 3rd Int. Conf. on Learning Representations, ICLR'15 (Vancouver, BC, Canada)*

[30] Kim Y 2014 Convolutional neural networks for sentence classification *Proc. of the 2014 Conf. on Empirical Methods in Natural Language Processing (EMNLP)* pp 1746–51

[31] Dosovitskiy A *et al* 2021 An image is worth 16x16 words: transformers for image recognition at scale *Proc. of the 9th Int. Conf. on Learning Representations, ICLR'21*

[32] Enger S A, Vijande J and Rivard M J 2020 Model-based dose calculation algorithms for brachytherapy dosimetry *Semin. Radiat. Oncol.* **30** 77–86

[33] Mao X, Pineau J, Keyes R and Enger S A 2020 RapidBrachyDL: rapid radiation dose calculations in brachytherapy via deep learning *Int. J. Radiat. Oncol. Biol. Phys.* **108** 802–12

[34] Elhaminia B, Gilbert A, Lilley J, Abdar M, Frangi A F, Scarsbrook A, Appelt A and Gooya A 2023 Toxicity prediction in pelvic radiotherapy using multiple instance learning and cascaded attention layers *IEEE J. Biomed. Health Inform.* **27** 1958–66

[35] Chen Y *et al* 2023 Patient-specific auto-segmentation on daily kVCT images for adaptive radiation therapy *Int. J. Radiat. Oncol. Biol. Phys.* **117** 505–14

[36] Simonyan K, Vedaldi A and Zisserman A 2014 Deep inside convolutional networks: visualising image classification models and saliency maps arXiv:1312.6034

[37] Krizhevsky A, Sutskever I and Hinton G E 2012 ImageNet classification with deep convolutional neural networks *Advances in Neural Information Processing Systems* **vol 25** (Red Hook, NY: Curran Associates)

[38] Chen Q, Bernard M E, Duan J and Feng X 2021 A transfer learning approach for improving OAR segmentation in the adaptive therapy or retreatment of head and neck cancer *Int. J. Radiat. Oncol. Biol. Phys.* **111** e125–6

[39] Maleki F, Ovens K, Najafian K, Forghani B, Reinhold C and Forghani R 2020 Overview of machine learning. Part 1 *Neuroimaging Clin. N. Am.* **30** e17–32

[40] Zhou C and Paffenroth R C 2017 Anomaly detection with robust deep autoencoders *Proc. of the 23rd ACM SIGKDD Int. Conf. on Knowledge Discovery and Data Mining* (New York: ACM) pp 665–74

[41] Han X, Chen X and Liu L P 2021 GAN ensemble for anomaly detection *Proc. of the AAAI Conf. on Artificial Intelligence* **35** 4090–7

[42] Laya R S 2023 Tackling distribution shift-detection and mitigation *PhD Thesis* Concordia University, Montreal

[43] Sohl-Dickstein J, Weiss E, Maheswaranathan N and Ganguli S 2015 Deep NN supervised learning using nonequilibrium thermodynamics *Int. Conf. on Machine Learning* **37** 2256–65

[44] Song Y and Ermon S 2019 Generative modeling by estimating gradients of the data distribution *Adv. Neural Inf. Process. Syst.* **32** 11918–30

[45] Ho J, Jain A and Abbeel P 2020 Denoising diffusion probabilistic models *Adv. Neural Infor. Process. Syst.* **33** 6840–51

[46] Han C, Hayashi H, Rundo L, Araki R, Shimoda W, Muramatsu S, Furukawa Y, Mauri G and Nakayama H 2018 GAN-based synthetic brain MR image generation *Proceedings of ISBI* (Piscataway, NJ: IEEE) pp 734–8

[47] Arjovsky M, Chintala S and Bottou L 2017 Wasserstein generative adversarial networks *Proc. of the 34th Int. Conf. on Machine Learning, Proc. of Machine Learning Research* vol 70D Precup and Y W Teh pp 214–23

[48] Nie D, Trullo R, Lian J, Petitjean C, Ruan S, Wang Q and Shen D 2017 Medical image synthesis with context-aware generative adversarial networks *Int. Conf. on Medical Image Computing and Computer-Assisted Intervention* (Berlin: Springer) pp 417–25

[49] Khader F *et al* 2023 Denoising diffusion probabilistic models for 3D medical image generation *Sci. Rep.* **13** 7303

[50] Jordon J, Yoon J and Van Der Schaar M 2018 PATE-GAN: generating synthetic data with differential privacy guarantees *Int. Conf. on Learning Representations*

[51] Yaqub M, Jinchao F, Ahmed S, Arshid K, Bilal M A, Akhter M P and Zia M S 2022 GAN-TL: generative adversarial networks with transfer learning for MRI reconstruction *Appl. Sci.* **12** 8841

[52] Abbas A, Abdelsamea M M and Gaber M M 2020 DETRAC: transfer learning of class decomposed medical images in convolutional neural networks *IEEE Access* **8** 74901–13

[53] Dou Q, Ouyang C, Chen C, Chen H and Heng P A 2018 Unsupervised cross-modality domain adaptation of convnets for biomedical image segmentations with adversarial loss arXiv:1804.10916

[54] Mahapatra D and Ge Z 2020 Training data independent image registration using generative adversarial networks and domain adaptation *Pattern Recognit.* **100** 107109

[55] Schlegl T, Seebӧck P, Waldstein S M, Schmidt-Erfurth U and Langs G 2017 Unsupervised anomaly detection with generative adversarial networks to guide marker discovery *Proceedings of IPMI* (Berlin: Springer) pp 146–57

[56] Wolleb J, Bieder F, Sandkühler R and Cattin P C 2022 Diffusion models for medical anomaly detection *Int. Conf. on Medical Image Computing and Computer-Assisted Intervention* (Berlin: Springer) pp 35–45

[57] Pinaya W H L *et al* 2022 Fast unsupervised brain anomaly detection and segmentation with diffusion models *Int. Conf. on Medical Image Computing and Computer-Assisted Intervention* (Berlin: Springer) pp 705–14

[58] Esteban C, Hyland S L and Rätsch G 2017 Real-valued (medical) time series generation with recurrent conditional GANs arXiv:1706.02633

[59] Wolterink J M, Leiner T, Viergever M A and Isgum I 2017 Generative adversarial networks for noise reduction in low-dose CT *IEEE Trans. Med. Imaging* **36** 2536–45

[60] Mahapatra D, Bozorgtabar B and Garnavi R 2019 Image super-resolution using progressive generative adversarial networks for medical image analysis *Comput. Med. Imaging Graph.* **71** 30–9

[61] Wu J, Fu R, Fang H, Zhang Y and Xu Y 2023 MedSegDiff-V2: diffusion based medical image segmentation with transformer arXiv:2301.11798

[62] Ronneberger O, Fischer P and Brox T 2015 U-Net: convolutional networks for biomedical image segmentation *Proc. Medical Image Computing and Computer-Assisted Intervention– MICCAI 2015: 18th Int. Conf.* vol 18 *(Munich, Germany, 5–9 October)* (Berlin: Springer) pp 234–41

[63] Zhang Z, Fan G, Liu T, Li N, Liu Y, Liu Z, Dong C and Zhou S 2023 Introducing shape prior module in diffusion model for medical image segmentation arXiv:2309.05929

[64] Kasthurirathne S N, Dexter G and Grannis S J 2021 Generative adversarial networks for creating synthetic free-text medical data: a proposal for collaborative research and re-use of machine learning models *AMIA Summits Transl. Sci. Proc.* **2021** 335

[65] Ribeiro M T, Singh S and Guestrin C 2016 'Why should I trust you?' Explaining the predictions of any classifier *Proc. of the 22nd ACM SIGKDD Int. Conf. on Knowledge Discovery and Data Mining* pp 1135–44

[66] Alikhademi K, Drobina E, Prioleau D, Richardson B, Purves D and Gilbert J E 2022 A review of predictive policing from the perspective of fairness *Artif. Intell. Law* **30** 1–17

[67] Obermeyer Z, Powers B, Vogeli C and Mullainathan S 2019 Dissecting racial bias in an algorithm used to manage the health of populations *Science* **366** 447–53

[68] Buolamwini J and Gebru T 2018 Gender shades: intersectional accuracy disparities in commercial gender classification *Conf. on Fairness, Accountability, and Transparency* (PMLR) pp 77–91

[69] Mireshghallah F, Taram M, Vepakomma P, Singh A, Raskar R and Esmaeilzadeh H 2020 Privacy in deep learning: a survey arXiv:2004.12254

[70] Ferrara E 2023 GenAI against humanity: nefarious applications of generative artificial intelligence and large language models arXiv:2310.00737

[71] Finlayson S G, Bowers J D, Ito J, Zittrain J L, Beam A L and Kohane I S 2019 Adversarial attacks on medical machine learning *Science* **363** 1287–9

[72] Hacker P, Engel A and Mauer M 2023 Regulating ChatGPT and other large generative AI models *Proc. of the 2023 ACM Conf. on Fairness, Accountability, and Transparency* pp 1112–23

Chapter 2

Introduction to artificial intelligence in radiation therapy

Elizabeth Huynh

The radiation therapy workflow is complex, involving many steps to see a patient through from pre-treatment initial consultation to post-treatment follow-up appointments. Each of these steps is labor intensive and involves decision-making guided by a vast amount of information. This information has the potential to be used by artificial intelligence (AI) to inform decision making, automate and improve processes, decrease appointment times, and ultimately improve the workflow to provide better care for cancer patients. This chapter provides an overview of the radiation therapy workflow and highlights points throughout the workflow where AI is currently being used clinically, and has the potential to be used in the future.

2.1 Introduction

Radiation therapy (RT) is a critical treatment for patients with cancer. While RT is most commonly recognized for treating cancerous lesions and improving symptoms from growing tumors, RT is also a treatment option for non-cancerous medical conditions such as cardiac radioablation for ventricular tachycardia [1], trigeminal neuralgia [2], and arteriovenous malformations [3]. The clinical RT workflow is complex, involving the expertise of multiple role groups including radiation oncologists, medical physicists, dosimetrists, therapists, and administrative staff. Each step of the workflow involves manual input into various hardware and software technologies to prepare, plan, and deliver radiation to the intended target within the patient and minimize the dose to healthy tissue. In this chapter we provide an overview of the RT workflow, staff roles within RT, and examples of how AI can transform, and in some cases already has, the field of RT.

2.1.1 Radiation therapy workflow

The RT workflow for each patient can be broken down into seven steps: the decision to treat with RT, simulation imaging, treatment planning, plan approval, plan

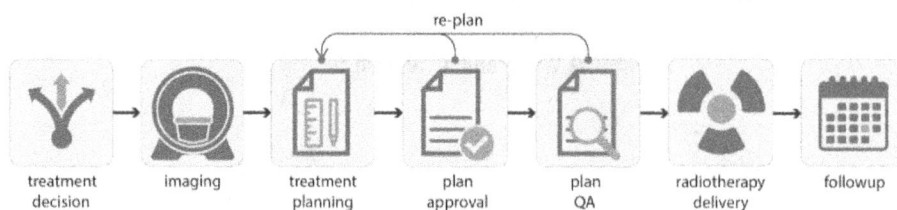

Figure 2.1. Overview of the RT workflow. (Reproduced and adapted with permission from [4]. Copyright 2020 Springer Nature.)

quality assurance (QA), delivery of radiation, and follow-up care (figure 2.1). The clinical workflow begins when the patient is referred to a radiation oncologist for consideration of RT, where the radiation oncologist reviews a wealth of the patient's data. For example, the radiation oncologist will perform a review of the patient's symptoms, comorbidities, medical history, and a physical examination. The patient's prior diagnostic imaging studies, pathological and genomic data are also evaluated. Using all this information, the radiation oncologist will assess the risk and severity of potential side effects from RT and the potential benefit from RT for their disease. The radiation oncologist will then formulate a plan for RT by determining the dose to prescribe to the target, the number of treatment fractions and frequency (e.g. daily, every other day, twice daily, etc), and the dose limits for surrounding normal tissues, or organs-at-risk (OARs). The radiation oncologists use information from nationally accepted standards, evidence from clinical trials, and evaluation of the individual patient's anatomy to determine the optimal dose to give to the target over a certain number of fractions and how much dose to limit to the OARs. This treatment intent is then presented to the patient for consent.

After the patient has consented to RT, the patient will attend simulation appointments to gather the data necessary to create the treatment plan tailored to the individual patient, primarily images to create the treatment plan. At the simulation appointment, the patient will be put in the position they will be treated in, and in most cases, the patient will be immobilized to reduce the likelihood of the patient moving during radiation delivery at treatment. The position the patient will be treated in is dependent on many factors such as the area in the body that will be treated, the radiation technique that will be used to treat the patient, and patient tolerability, that is, will the patient be able to remain in that position for the duration of the treatment. Patients to be treated with RT often have comorbidities, prior surgery or previous injuries that make certain positions intolerable for long durations of time; in these cases, exceptions from the standard treatment position will be made to accommodate patient comfort. Immobilization devices are hardware that facilitate positioning the patient in a reproducible manner for treatment. For example, for head and neck cancer patients, patients may be immobilized in a thermoplastic mask that covers the patient's head and neck and attaches to the treatment couch, which ensures that the patient's head and neck are in a consistent position throughout simulation and treatment.

Modern RT treatment planning requires a three-dimensional image of the patient, to identify and delineate the target and OARs, and a method for performing dose calculation. Currently, the majority of patients will receive a computed tomography (CT) scan where the target and OARs are contoured, and the Hounsfield units are used for determining the electron density for dose calculation. After the patient is immobilized in the treatment position, they will have a CT scan in the treatment position which is used for treatment planning. Due to the improved soft-tissue contrast of magnetic resonance imaging (MRI) over CT, patients may also receive an MRI either in the treatment position or a diagnostic MRI may be registered with the CT to provide more information for contouring. Additional diagnostic scans such as positron emission tomography (PET) that provide functional imaging may also be used. The use of additional imaging scans requires the image to be fused to the CT to align the anatomy of concern between the two images. The collective information from these images is used to define the target to be treated or gather information regarding the intrafraction motion of internal organs.

The target and OARs are contoured on the CT scan, and a treatment plan is created using computer software. The computer software, known as the treatment planning system (TPS), has the radiation treatment machine (linac) and radiation interactions modeled to determine the machine parameters required for treatment delivery and provide a visual depiction of the radiation dose distribution within the patient. The TPS receives input for each patient, including the CT scan, contours and dose prescribed. Various manual inputs are entered to assign beam parameters such as the gantry angle range, collimator angle, couch angle, jaw positions, beam energy, etc, that are optimal for the individual patient's plan. The treatment plan is designed with an optimization engine that determines the optimal positions of the multileaf collimators with the appropriate radiation fluence emanating from each gantry angle. This complex process requires the expertise of a dosimetrist that can change the optimization parameters to achieve the desired result as prescribed by the radiation oncologist for the target to receive a pre-specified dose and minimize dose to the OARs. The optimal plan is then approved by the radiation oncologist. While reviewing the treatment plan, the radiation oncologist may request changes resulting in a re-plan, in which the optimization parameters may be further changed by the dosimetrist. The final approved treatment plan is a representation of the radiation dose that will be delivered to the patient. This treatment plan is then sent to the record and verify system whose main purpose is to reduce the risk of treatment errors in RT. However, the record and verify system may also integrate the TPS, and interface with the treatment imaging and delivery systems.

Before the patient is treated with the treatment plan, the plan undergoes various QA procedures. A physicist reviews the plan ensuring that it meets all the technical requirements for treatment and the plan is delivering the intended dose to the target and adequately sparing OARs as prescribed by the radiation oncologist. If the physicist identifies errors in the plan, the plan may be requested to be re-planned. Further QA procedures may take place on the plan to verify that the plan as modeled in the TPS is what will be delivered by the linac, a procedure known as patient-specific IMRT or VMAT QA where the treatment plan is delivered to a phantom and a comparison of the delivered dose is made with the TPS planned dose.

Each piece of hardware and software that is part of the RT workflow, such as the linac, CT scanners, and TPS, also undergo periodic routine QA measurements to ensure that they are performing as expected, and if they are not, that appropriate measures are taken to adjust the hardware or software to realign them with their expected performance.

When the patient arrives at the linear accelerator for treatment delivery, the therapists set up the patient in the treatment position with the immobilization devices that were determined at simulation. The therapists take a series of images using the imaging capabilities available on the linac to ensure that the patient is in the same position that they were simulated in. For example, conventionally, linacs are equipped with x-ray based imaging methods such as 2D kilovoltage or megavoltage radiographs or cone beam CTs (CBCTs) that can acquire images before, after or during treatment. More recently, linacs equipped with an MRI imaging system (MRI-linacs) have become available and are seeing increased clinical use for MRI-guided set-up, monitoring motion during treatment, and adaptive RT. Other systems are available that can also assist in setting up the patient and monitoring motion during treatment, for example surface monitoring systems such as VisionRT [3, 5] or respiratory management systems such as the Varian real-time position management (RPM) systems [6]. The radiation treatment plan that was created specifically for the patient is then delivered.

The time from simulation to treatment delivery can range from hours to weeks. During this time, the tumor can grow and OARs change position, resulting in different anatomical positions from the treatment plan. Furthermore, the majority of treatments occur over multiple fractions, where changes in anatomical position and geometry can occur between fractions. Adaptive RT involves changing the patient's treatment plan based on updated information of their current anatomy on that particular treatment day. More details on adaptive RT are provided in chapter 6.

While the patient is on treatment, their chart and images are reviewed by RT staff periodically throughout their treatment (e.g. weekly), to ensure that they are receiving the treatment as intended. The radiation oncologist and other RT staff, such as nurses, also meet with the patient throughout the course of their treatment to discuss the treatment and any concerning side effects. After treatment, the patient attends a series of follow-up appointments with the radiation oncologist to review their response to RT including both toxicities and tumor response.

While the RT clinical workflow varies slightly at every institution, the general steps of consultation, simulation, treatment planning, plan approval, plan QA, treatment delivery and follow-up are foundational to the RT workflow.

2.1.2 Staff roles in radiation therapy

RT is a highly technical field involving the expertise and interactions of multiple role groups and technologies. Each role group is highly trained in their particular role through the clinical workflow. Staff that interact with the patient are considered

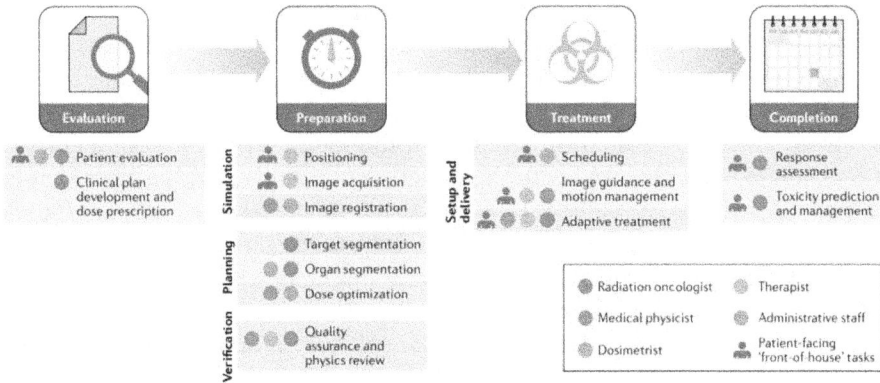

Figure 2.2. Representative example of staff role assignments throughout the RT workflow. (Reproduced with permission from [4]. Copyright 2020 Springer Nature.)

patient-facing 'front-of-house' roles, while staff roles that primarily do not interact with the patient are considered back-of-house roles (figure 2.2).

Administrative staff are involved in booking the multiple patient appointments for simulation, treatment, and on-treatment and follow-up visits with nursing and radiation oncologists. They follow guidelines to determine the appropriate timing and sequencing for multiple appointments for each patient. In a cancer center with hundreds or thousands of patients each year and a series of different appointments depending on disease site, cancer staging, and treatment plan, the manual booking of these appointments can be challenging. The booking of these appointments may occur in multiple softwares, such as the hospital electronic health record and the record and verify system used by the cancer center. These staff must interact with multiple softwares and with patients to discuss their appointments with them.

Radiation oncologists perform the initial consultation with the patient and using the patient data available to them, evaluate the patient's suitability for RT and determine the radiation dose, fractionation, frequency of treatment, and limiting doses to relevant OARs. After simulation, the radiation oncologist will determine and contour the treatment target and relevant OARs. While other role groups may contour OARs for the purposes of efficiency and workload, the radiation oncologist is ultimately responsible for reviewing and finalizing these contours. The radiation oncologist discusses and reviews the treatment plan with the dosimetrist, and takes into consideration the medical condition and history of the patient. The radiation oncologist approves the dose distribution to be delivered to the patient. They meet with the patient throughout their treatment for management of side effects and patient concerns, and follow-up with the patient after their treatment is complete for continued management of side effects and assess treatment response.

Dosimetrists generate treatment plans based on the radiation oncologist's contours, and the prescribed dose to the treatment target and OARs, maximizing the dose to the target and minimizing the dose to the OARs. This is a predominantly manual trial-and-error process in which the dosimetrist chooses the appropriate beam parameters for the treatment plan based on the patient's geometry and anatomy. The dosimetrist will then manually optimize the treatment plan by inputting objective functions, manipulating optimization tools available in the TPS, and utilizing optimization contours created by the dosimetrist. Through dosimetrist experience and consultation with the radiation oncologist, a treatment plan is generated and reviewed with the radiation oncologist. For patients that have been previously treated with RT, dosimetrists may need to utilize the dose distribution from the previous treatment to adjust the current treatment plan to achieve acceptable cumulative doses to the relevant OARs. This information is also reviewed and approved by the radiation oncologist.

Physicists are responsible for ensuring the software and hardware technologies being used in RT are safe and accurate. When a new technology is introduced in the clinic, a physicist must perform rigorous testing on the technology to ensure that the technology is performing as expected, a process known as commissioning. For example, when a new linac is commissioned, physicists perform numerous measurements on the linac and compare these results to how the radiation beam is modeled in the TPS and expected performance. Once the technology is being used clinically, routine QA measurements are either performed by the physicist or overseen by the physicist on these software and hardware technologies at various frequencies. For example, therapists may perform the daily QA on the linac, but the results are reviewed by a physicist, whereas a physicist will perform annual QA measurements on the linac. Patient-specific QA measurements may also be performed for a treatment plan, and while these measurements may be performed by a physics associate, assistant or trainee, a physicist provides the final approval before patient treatment. Physicists review treatment plans prior to treatment to evaluate the technical aspects of the treatment plan for suitability for treatment, and ensure that the treatment plan is fulfilling the desired intentions of the radiation oncologist through reviewing the contours, dose distribution, beam, and optimization parameters. The role of physicists is largely back-of-house working closely with the technology involved in RT.

Therapists have a predominantly patient-facing role. At the treatment simulation appointment, therapists are responsible for setting up the patient in the appropriate treatment position, and acquiring identifying information about the patient such as a photo for the patient records. Therapists also administer the radiation treatment at each fraction and are responsible for patient safety and avoiding misadministration of radiation. They set up the patient in the treatment position on the linac, acquire images to ensure the patient is in the correct position, prompt the linac to deliver the radiation treatment plan, and monitor the patient while treatment is being delivered. Therapists have the most interaction with the patient out of all the role groups, and are responsible for overseeing the patient's health during treatment. If patient concerns are noted during treatment, the therapists are responsible for advising the patient if the concern is within their area of expertise, or to refer them to nurses or the radiation oncologists. Therapists interact with the hardware and software technologists involved in RT, they are the primary users of the linac on a daily basis, and interact with the TPS and record and verify systems to perform QA tasks such as checking-in new patient charts to ensure all the required information is present and accurate or complete tasks related to a patient completing treatment. In some institutions, therapists may also be responsible for contouring OARs where the radiation oncologist performs a final review of these contours, and generate simple treatment plans for palliative patients.

While there are several other important role groups involved in RT such as nurses, dietitians, information technology personnel, and engineers, the focus of AI applications in RT have predominantly been to address challenges encountered by the aforementioned role groups.

2.2 Overview of AI in radiation therapy

Numerous steps are required for treating a single patient in the RT workflow, multiplied by the hundreds or thousands of patients that are treated at a single cancer center, which can lead to variability in the quality of care among all staff involved in the RT workflow. Throughout this overview of AI in RT, a glimpse of where AI can be used to improve efficiency, accuracy, and standardization of patient care are provided through examples at each step in the workflow. Greater detail on the applications of AI in RT are provided in the following chapters.

2.2.1 Patient evaluation and dose prescription

The challenge for radiation oncologists as they evaluate the patient at consultation is the myriad of available data related directly to the patient (e.g. medical history, pathological and genomic data, etc) and clinical evidence from previous patients through clinical trials detailing the risk of toxicities and benefits of treatment. As the magnitude of these data continue to increase, AI tools have the potential to automatically determine the most important clinical data to support radiation oncologists in their clinical decision making. While at present, there are no commercially available AI tools to do so, AI tools have been developed to assess medical images [7] and electronic medical records [8–10], and have shown the potential for predicting treatment outcomes [11–13]. Further development of these AI tools for RT specific patients are required for the application of guiding decisions on the treatment regime for RT patients.

While radiation oncologists use nationally accepted standards and evidence from clinical trials to prescribe radiation dose to the tumor and dose constraints to the OARs, often these goals for the treatment plan are not achievable due to the arrangement of the tumor and surrounding anatomy, which is highly patient dependent. Often, what is achievable for a particular treatment plan is only determined after the treatment plan has been created and multiple iterations are often required. AI tools can be applied to identify the achievable dose prescription for a patient based on the particular patient's anatomy [14], prior to treatment planning, which would inform radiation oncologists and dosimetrists to develop a clinically acceptable and achievable treatment plan with greater efficiency.

2.2.2 Treatment simulation

Currently, CT is the gold standard imaging acquired for radiation therapy. However, CT images are prone to metal artifacts from metal implants such as metal screws in the spine and metal dental fillings, which obscure the imaging field of view and clinically relevant structures, which can make contouring in these areas challenging. While many commercial CT scanners have metal artifact reduction softwares, these softwares improve the image quality but some artifacts are still present and these softwares can also create their own types of artifacts [15]. AI algorithms have been developed to generate metal artifact free CT images without introducing other artifacts [16–18].

These CT images are often registered to other imaging modalities, such as MRI and PET, to assist contouring treatment targets, or previous RT CTs to assess dose contributions from previous treatments in re-irradiation scenarios. The process of aligning the two images during image registration can be challenging as the patient may be in a different position in each scan; for example, the patient may have their arms up in one scan versus arms down in another, or on a rounded couch top as in diagnostic images versus a flat couch top in CT simulations. These differences can introduce uncertainties in the treatment planning process [19]. Commercially available automatic registration tools have challenges when attempting to register images of different modalities or in the presence of imaging artifacts. AI tools have been developed to achieve better accuracy and robustness for image registration [20, 21].

MRI has increasingly been utilized in RT, with MRI simulators accompanying CT simulators becoming more common in RT departments. The improved soft-tissue visualization of MRI over CT enables radiation oncologists to better distinguish tumors from surrounding OARs. However, these approaches require an additional imaging scan and also introduce uncertainties due to image registration. MR-only clinical workflows have gained increasing interest as the patient undergoes only a single MRI simulation and eliminates the MRI–CT registration uncertainty. However, CT is still required for electron density information for the dose calculation. There has been considerable work on creating synthetic CTs from MRIs (CTs generated from only MRI information) [22], and even commercial softwares are now available that have leveraged AI to create synthetic CTs for disease sites such as the brain and pelvis [23, 24]. These AI tools use specialized MRI sequences such as Dixon to generate synthetic CTs that have been reported to accurately duplicate CT images, even in challenging areas such as the brain where there may have been bone resection from surgery [25] (figure 2.3).

2.2.3 Contouring

Contouring the treatment target and relevant OARs has historically been a very manual process, requiring hours of work. Contouring the treatment target involves utilizing the collection of medical information for the patient as well as an understanding of the predicted progression of the cancer and any potential motion that the target may undergo during treatment. The accuracy of the contours is

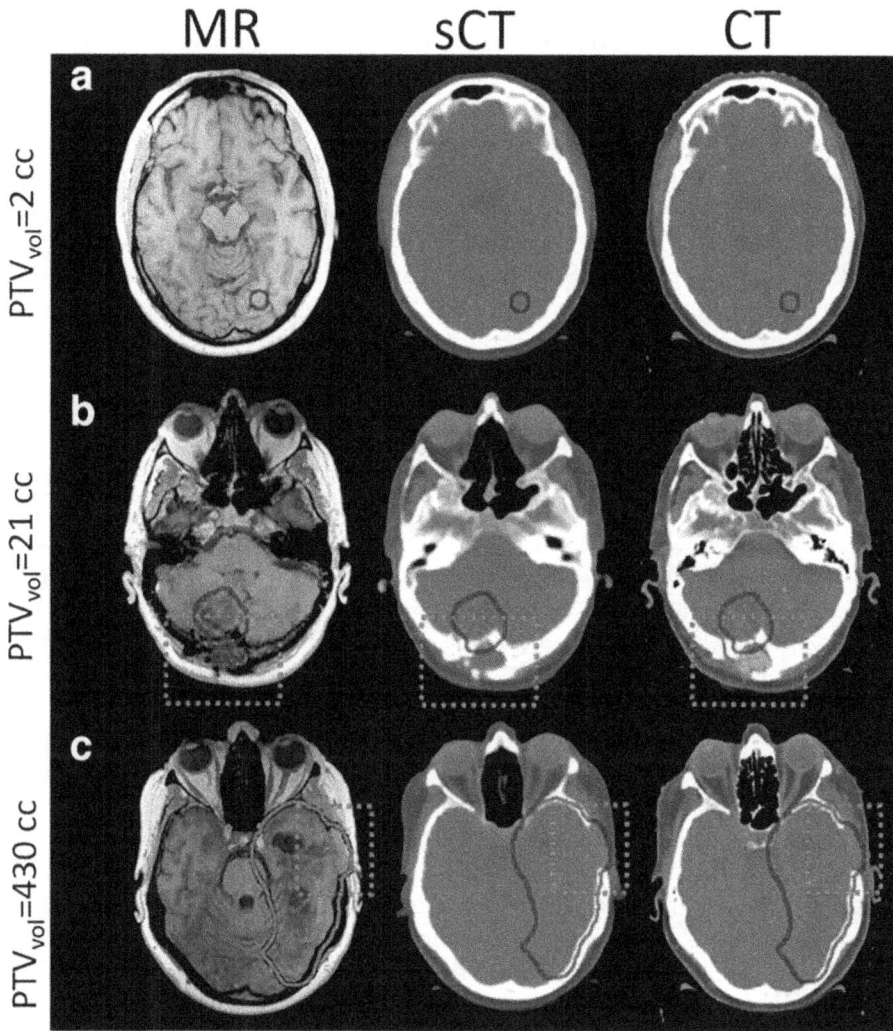

Figure 2.3. Example of synthetic CT (sCT) generation for three patients (a-c), with the MRI using the Dixon sequence, sCT and CT. Blue region is the planning target volume (PTV) with the corresponding volumes on the leftmost column, and the red box indicates the region of bone resection due to surgery. (Reproduced with permission from [25]. Copyright 2021 Springer Nature.)

important as the treatment plan dose distribution and analysis of this distribution is dependent on the contours, and ultimately drives the dose delivered to the patient.

OAR contouring is often delegated to other role groups such as radiation therapists or dosimetrists in the interest of efficiency and reducing workload for the radiation oncologist. The radiation oncologist is ultimately responsible for reviewing and approving these contours, if they were not completed by themselves. A significant variation in OAR contouring exists among clinicians, and the degree of variation is organ-dependent [26, 27]. The under- or over contouring of an OAR can result in unnecessary increased dose to the critical organ or under treatment of the target. Analysis of the treatment plan, assessing the dose to organs and treatment target, and their acceptability is heavily reliant on the dose volume histogram (DVH), which is dependent on the OAR contouring. Many research groups have developed AI tools to contour various organs throughout the body such as in the head and neck region [28–30], thoracic [31] and abdominal organs [32], and cardiac substructures [33, 34]. Several radiation oncology focused commercially available AI-based auto contouring solutions are available such as Contour ProtegeAI+ by MiM (OH, USA), Limbus AI (Canada), Deep Learning Segmentation within the RayStation Treatment Planning System (RaySearch Laboratories, Stockholm, Sweden), and AutoContour from Radformation (New York, USA). These AI auto contouring softwares have been developed for nearly all relevant OARs in RT, primarily on CT scans but also for MRI for some disease sites, and have offered substantial time savings ranging from 15 to 90 min depending on the disease site [35]. Despite automation, staff are still required to review these contours after applying the AI tools, as the contours may not be of sufficient accuracy for clinical use. AI tools have also been developed to automate QA of OAR contouring to ensure consistency and standardization [36].

Variation in tumor segmentation can result in a decrease in the likelihood of tumor control in the case of under contouring the target, and overdosing critical OARs in the case of over contouring the target. Interclinician variation in tumor segmentation exists among radiation oncologists, leading to a difference in treatment plan quality and resulting in clinical outcomes such as survival [37–39]. AI auto contouring tools for treatment targets have been developed by the scientific community for various cancers such as nasopharyngeal carcinomas [40] (figure 2.4), primary lung tumors [41], oropharyngeal carcinomas [42], and hepatocellular carcinoma [43], and have shown performance similar to that of a radiation oncologist.

While AI auto contouring tools offer significant time savings to render the RT clinical workflow more efficient and improve reproducibility and standardization in contouring, the accuracy of these contours are ultimately responsible to the radiation oncologist. Therefore, these auto generated contours still need to be reviewed by the clinical staff and radiation oncologist for accuracy and completeness and, currently, still require some manual editing.

2.2.4 Treatment planning

The iterative manual process of treatment planning by dosimetrists can be intensely time consuming and result in large variations in the quality of treatment plans [44]. There have been many approaches to automate the treatment planning process, such as knowledge-based planning [45–47] and predicting objective function weights [48], however, these approaches are usually designed for a specific disease site and are limited in their ability to accommodate patient-specific challenges such as geometry or previous treatment. As a result, the quality of the resulting plans often needs further refinement by a dosimetrist.

Automating the treatment planning process with AI tools is of considerable interest in the field of radiation oncology, and two general processes are involved.

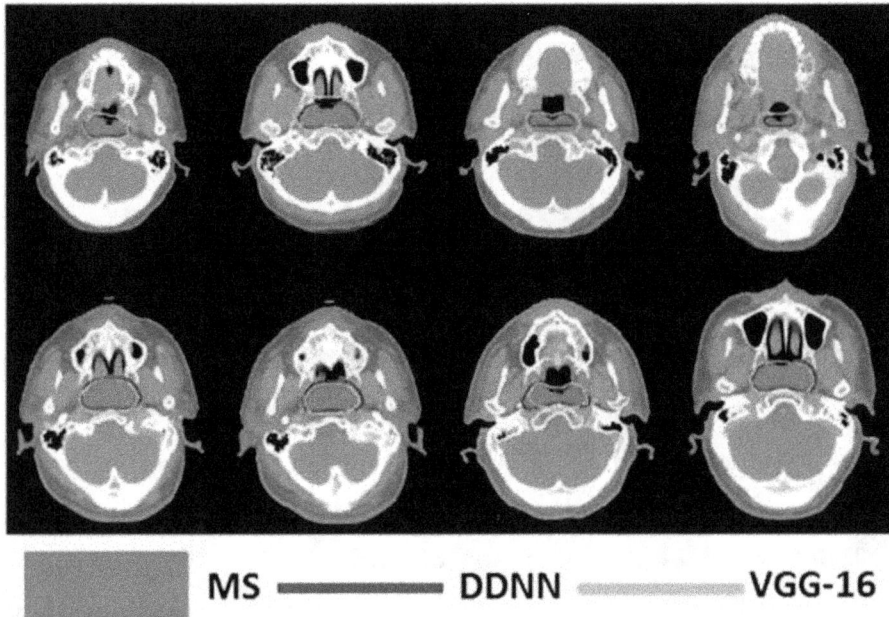

Figure 2.4. Segmentation of a nasopharynx gross tumor volume shown on axial CT slices displaying the manual segmentation (MS) by a radiation oncologist (fuchsia), and two AI algorithms: deep deconvolutional neural network (DDNN, blue) and a very deep convolutional network (VGG-16, green). The DDNN algorithm outperformed the VGG-16 in segmenting the gross tumor volume. (Reproduced from [40]. CC BY 4.0.)

First, given the patient image (e.g. CT) and contours, an optimal dose distribution is predicted, then the appropriate linac parameters to achieve that dose distribution are identified. These AI tools use algorithms that have been trained with previous treatment plans, learning the relationship between patient geometry and achievable dose distributions with trade-offs. AI tools for automated treatment planning have been developed for various disease sites such as prostate [14, 49], pancreas [50, 51] (figure 2.5), and head and neck [52, 53] cancers. The machine learning treatment planning module in the RayStation Treatment Planning System (RaySearch Laboratories, Stockholm, Sweden) was the first commercially available treatment planning system to have an AI tool available for automating treatment planning with a model for head and neck cancer [54]. This AI tool comes with pre-trained models from other institutions as well as the ability for a particular clinic to train their own model using their own data.

In addition to the manual treatment planning process by dosimetrists, the dose calculation in the treatment planning software can be time consuming. Typically, dose calculation algorithms have a tradeoff between efficiency and accuracy, where the more efficient algorithms are less accurate. AI tools have also been developed to increase the speed of dose calculation algorithms without sacrificing accuracy [55].

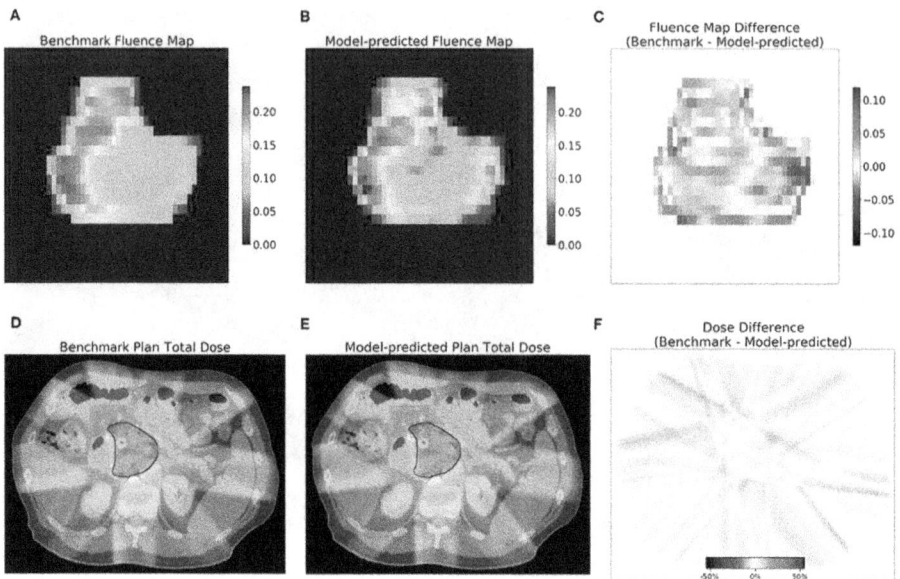

Figure 2.5. Example of a fluence map benchmark plan (A) and model-predicted (B) for pancreas SBRT using an AI algorithm, with the difference between the benchmark and model-predicted fluence shown in (C), and the corresponding treatment plans (D), (E), and difference in dose (F). (Reproduced from [51]. CC BY 4.0.)

2.2.5 Quality assurance

A significant portion of a medical physicist's time is spent performing and overseeing QA tasks. These tasks exist to ensure patients are receiving the intended treatment, identify mistakes that may have been made, and ensure that the technology involved in RT is performing as expected. These QA tasks are often very time-consuming manual repetitive processes. Every treatment plan has a secondary dose measurement performed on the plan, either through a secondary dose calculator, or through a physical dose measurement delivered by the linac to a phantom, or sometimes both. The physical dose measurements for every patient plan can be intensely time consuming, and the majority of plans pass dose measurement. When a plan fails this QA step, a physicist will investigate the cause of failure, whether it be the plan itself, the performance of the linac, detector malfunction or user error. AI tools have been developed to analyze treatment plans, and predict QA passing rates and possible sources of failure [56–59]. This approach potentially eliminates the need for physical dose measurements of individual plans, increasing efficiency and decreasing the resources necessary to measure these plans.

While this approach of reducing patient-specific QA measurements by using AI tools eliminates the additional QA of the linac that is provided by physical dose measurements, routine machine QA is performed at regular intervals (e.g. daily, monthly, annually) to assess linac performance. These routine machine QA measurements also require significant effort and time, where often the QA tests pass. AI tools have been developed using longitudinal data to predict trends in the linac output as a tool to alert the need for preventative action [60]. AI tools have also been developed to potentially improve TPS modeling of the linac, such as assisting in reducing MLC positional errors [61] found between the treatment plan and delivery by incorporating predicted MLC positions into the TPS. In addition, beam modeling in the TPS can have adjustable parameters, for example, in the Eclipse TPS (Varian Medical Systems, Palo Alto, CA), the transmission factor and dosimetric leaf gap are adjustable MLCs parameters. Inaccuracies in these parameters will impact the dose distribution and contribution to disagreement between the TPS and delivered dose. AI tools have been developed to detect and classify errors in these MLC modeling parameters to improve the accuracy of beam modeling in the TPS [62].

2.2.6 Treatment delivery

Modern linacs are equipped with kV imaging and CBCT for image guidance. Compared to conventional CT, CBCTs often have more severe imaging artifacts which can obscure the region of interest for patient set-up and potential use of CBCT for adaptive RT. AI algorithms have been developed to improve the image quality of CBCT to ultimately improve the accuracy of patient set-up [63] and enable adaptive RT [64]. Acquisition of CBCTs can take tens of seconds, and be subject to motion such as respiratory and internal motion. AI tools have been developed for CBCT to reduce scan time and exposure dose by using high-speed CBCTs with the AI tools to generate images with image quality suitable for image-guided RT [65].

Respiratory motion is one type of motion that is of concern in RT, particularly for thoracic and abdominal cancers. While many different motion management strategies exist, one strategy utilizes an external surrogate placed on the patient's chest, such as the Varian RPM system. This system follows the motion of the surrogate throughout the patient's breathing cycle to indicate when the patient is in the correct breathing phase and indicate when the radiation treatment should be delivered. There is an underlying assumption that the position of the surrogate correlates directly with the movement of the tumor, however, this assumption fails to capture the intricacies of tumor motion with respiration. AI tools have been developed to correlate tumor position with the motion of external surrogates and also predict tumor position for irregular breathing patterns and complex tumor motion [66] and address latency between the external surrogate and radiation delivery by the linac [67, 68].

2.2.7 Response assessment and toxicity management

Response to RT is typically assessed by evaluating the response of the tumor in terms of the change in size based on the response evaluation criteria in solid tumors [69] in medical images. AI algorithms have the potential to evaluate additional imaging features such as texture and intensity, potentially providing greater predictive power to cancer-specific outcomes. Studies have investigated the use of AI algorithms on pre-, on- and post-treatment medical images to predict patient outcomes such as overall survival and development of distant metastasis and locoregional recurrence for various cancers such as bladder [70, 71], lung [72–74], and pancreatic [75] cancer. The overall goal of these applications of AI in response to assessment of RT is to provide more information to the physician to enable personalized treatment and earlier interventions to improve outcomes for cancer patients.

Evaluation of a patient's response to RT is not only the response of the tumor but also the response of the surrounding critical OARs. One challenge that can be encountered is the presence of radiation-induced toxicities, which can make the detection of disease recurrence challenging. For example, in lung cancer patients, the presence of radiation-induced fibrosis and local tumor recurrence can look similar on CT scans and be overlooked. AI algorithms have been developed to analyze imaging features in medical images to assist physicians in distinguishing between radiation-induced tissue damage and cancer-specific outcomes [76]. Furthermore, studies have investigated the potential of AI tools to predict the severity of toxicities associated with RT such as acute dysphagia [77], xerostomia [78], pneumonitis [79, 80] and rectal toxicities [81]. These tools could enable physicians to predict toxicities prior to RT and lead to anticipatory management before treatment and/or secondary prevention of toxicities after treatment has been delivered.

2.3 Summary

Overall, the incorporation of AI tools in RT has the potential to improve efficiency in the clinical workflow, which has already begun with the use of AI-based auto contouring tools. Further incorporation of these tools will increase the standardization of clinical care and also has the potential to improve clinical care by assisting clinicians as decision-support tools by potentially providing more insight and ability to comprehend the large amounts of patient data available to guide treatment decisions. The increase in the use of AI tools in the clinic has the potential to ultimately change the scope and workload of the role groups involved, by reducing workloads to focus on and identify the most important and clinically relevant issues in improving patient care.

References

[1] Cuculich P S *et al* 2017 Noninvasive cardiac radiation for ablation of ventricular tachycardia *N. Engl. J. Med.* **377** 2325–36

[2] Petit J H, Herman J M, Nagda S, DiBiase S J and Chin L S 2003 Radiosurgical treatment of trigeminal neuralgia: evaluating quality of life and treatment outcomes *Int. J. Radiat. Oncol. Biol. Phys.* **56** 1147–53

[3] Ogilvy C S 1990 Radiation therapy for arteriovenous malformations: a review *Neurosurgery* **26** 725–35

[4] Huynh E *et al* 2020 Artificial intelligence in radiation oncology *Nat. Rev. Clin. Oncol.* **17** 771–81

[5] Hoisak J D P, Paxton A B, Waghorn B J and Pawlicki T 2020 *Surface Guided Radiation Therapy* (Boca Raton, FL: CRC Press)

[6] Saw C B, Brandner E, Selvaraj R, Chen H, Saiful Huq M and Heron D E 2007 A review on the clinical implementation of respiratory-gated radiation therapy *Biomed. Imaging Interv. J.* **3** e40

[7] Kann B H *et al* 2018 Pretreatment identification of head and neck cancer nodal metastasis and extranodal extension using deep learning neural networks *Sci. Rep.* **8** 14036

[8] Hong J C, Niedzwiecki D, Palta M and Tenenbaum J D 2018 Predicting emergency visits and hospital admissions during radiation and chemoradiation: an internally validated pretreatment machine learning algorithm *JCO Clin. Cancer Inform.* **2** 1–11

[9] Savova G K *et al* 2017 DeepPhe: a natural language processing system for extracting cancer phenotypes from clinical records *Cancer Res.* **77** e115–8

[10] Narayan V M *et al* 2023 Evaluation of a natural language processing model to identify and characterize patients in the United States with high-risk non-muscle-invasive bladder cancer *JCO Clin. Cancer Inform.* **7** e2300096

[11] Jochems A *et al* 2017 Developing and validating a survival prediction model for NSCLC patients through distributed learning across 3 countries *Int. J. Radiat. Oncol. Biol. Phys.* **99** 344–52

[12] Deist T M *et al* 2018 Machine learning algorithms for outcome prediction in (chemo) radiotherapy: an empirical comparison of classifiers *Med. Phys.* **45** 3449–59

[13] Janssen B V *et al* 2022 Imaging-based machine-learning models to predict clinical outcomes and identify biomarkers in pancreatic cancer: a scoping review *Ann. Surg.* **275** 560–7

[14] Ma J *et al* 2021 A feasibility study on deep learning-based individualized 3D dose distribution prediction *Med. Phys.* **48** 4438–47

[15] Sonoda A *et al* 2015 Erratum to: Evaluation of the quality of CT images acquired with the single energy metal artifact reduction (SEMAR) algorithm in patients with hip and dental prostheses and aneurysm embolization coils *Jpn. J. Radiol.* **33** 717

[16] Yu L, Zhang Z, Li X and Xing L 2021 Deep sinogram completion with image prior for metal artifact reduction in CT images *IEEE Trans. Med. Imaging* **40** 228–38

[17] Kim H *et al* 2022 Metal artifact reduction in kV CT images throughout two-step sequential deep convolutional neural networks by combining multi-modal imaging (MARTIAN) *Sci. Rep.* **12** 20823

[18] Arabi H and Zaidi H 2021 Deep learning-based metal artefact reduction in PET/CT imaging *Eur. Radiol.* **31** 6384–96

[19] Latifi K, Caudell J, Zhang G, Hunt D, Moros E G and Feygelman V 2018 Practical quantification of image registration accuracy following the AAPM TG-132 report framework *J. Appl. Clin. Med. Phys.* **19** 125–33

[20] Wu G, Kim M, Wang Q, Munsell B C and Shen D 2016 Scalable high-performance image registration framework by unsupervised deep feature representations learning *IEEE Trans. Biomed. Eng.* **63** 1505–16

[21] Fu Y, Lei Y, Wang T, Curran W J, Liu T and Yang X 2020 Deep learning in medical image registration: a review *Phys. Med. Biol.* **65** 20TR01

[22] Johnstone E *et al* 2018 Systematic review of synthetic computed tomography generation methodologies for use in magnetic resonance imaging—only radiation therapy *Int. J. Radiat. Oncol. Biol. Phys.* **100** 199–217

[23] Thorwarth D *et al* 2019 Synthetic CT generation for the pelvic region based on dixon-MR sequences: workflow, dosimetric quality and daily patient positioning *Siemens MAGNETOM Flash* **73** 23–7

[24] Hoesl M, Corral N E and Mistry N MR-based Synthetic CT reimagined. *An AI-based algorithm for continuous Hounsfield units in the pelvis and brain–with syngo. via RT Image Suite (VB60)* https://www.siemens-healthineers.com/en-uk/magnetic-resonance-imaging/clinical-specialities/synthetic-ct

[25] Lerner M, Medin J, Jamtheim Gustafsson C, Alkner S, Siversson C and Olsson L E 2021 Clinical validation of a commercially available deep learning software for synthetic CT generation for brain *Radiat. Oncol.* **16** 66

[26] Nelms B E, Tomé W A, Robinson G and Wheeler J 2012 Variations in the contouring of organs at risk: test case from a patient with oropharyngeal cancer *Int. J. Radiat. Oncol. Biol. Phys.* **82** 368–78

[27] Tsang Y *et al* 2019 Assessment of contour variability in target volumes and organs at risk in lung cancer radiotherapy *Tech. Innov. Patient. Support. Radiat. Oncol.* **10** 8–12

[28] Henderson E G A, Vasquez Osorio E M, van Herk M and Green A F 2022 Optimising a 3D convolutional neural network for head and neck computed tomography segmentation with limited training data *Phys. Imaging. Radiat. Oncol.* **22** 44–50

[29] Henderson E G A, Vasquez Osorio E M, van Herk M, Brouwer C L, Steenbakkers R J H M and Green A F 2023 Accurate segmentation of head and neck radiotherapy CT scans with 3D CNNs: consistency is key *Phys. Med. Biol.* **68** 085003

[30] Peng Y *et al* 2023 Improved accuracy of auto-segmentation of organs at risk in radiotherapy planning for nasopharyngeal carcinoma based on fully convolutional neural network deep learning *Oral Oncol.* **136** 106261

[31] Lustberg T *et al* 2018 Clinical evaluation of atlas and deep learning based automatic contouring for lung cancer *Radiother. Oncol.* **126** 312–7

[32] Hu P, Wu F, Peng J, Liang P and Kong D 2016 Automatic 3D liver segmentation based on deep learning and globally optimized surface evolution *Phys. Med. Biol.* **61** 8676–98

[33] Chin V *et al* 2023 Validation of a fully automated hybrid deep learning cardiac substructure segmentation tool for contouring and dose evaluation in lung cancer radiotherapy *Clin. Oncol.* **35** 370–81

[34] Jin X *et al* 2021 Robustness of deep learning segmentation of cardiac substructures in noncontrast computed tomography for breast cancer radiotherapy *Med. Phys.* **48** 7172–88

[35] Doolan P J *et al* 2023 A clinical evaluation of the performance of five commercial artificial intelligence contouring systems for radiotherapy *Front. Oncol.* **13** 1213068

[36] Men K, Geng H, Biswas T, Liao Z and Xiao Y 2020 Automated quality assurance of OAR contouring for lung cancer based on segmentation with deep active learning *Front. Oncol.* **10** 986

[37] Peters L J *et al* 2010 Critical impact of radiotherapy protocol compliance and quality in the treatment of advanced head and neck cancer: results from TROG 02.02 *J. Clin. Oncol.* **28** 2996–3001

[38] Brade A M *et al* 2018 Radiation therapy quality ssurance (RTQA) of concurrent chemo-radiation therapy for locally advanced non-small cell lung cancer in the PROCLAIM phase 3 trial *Int. J. Radiat. Oncol. Biol. Phys.* **101** 927–34

[39] Ohri N, Shen X, Dicker A P, Doyle L A, Harrison A S and Showalter T N 2013 Radiotherapy protocol deviations and clinical outcomes: a meta-analysis of cooperative group clinical trials *J. Natl Cancer Inst.* **105** 387–93

[40] Men K *et al* 2017 Deep deconvolutional neural network for target segmentation of nasopharyngeal cancer in planning computed tomography images *Front. Oncol.* **7** 315

[41] Mak R H *et al* 2019 Use of crowd innovation to develop an artificial intelligence-based solution for radiation therapy targeting *JAMA Oncol.* **5** 654–61

[42] Cardenas C E *et al* 2018 Deep learning algorithm for auto-delineation of high-risk oropharyngeal clinical target volumes with built-in dice similarity coefficient parameter optimization function *Int. J. Radiat. Oncol. Biol. Phys.* **101** 468–78

[43] Yang Z *et al* 2024 Deep learning based automatic internal gross target volume delineation from 4D-CT of hepatocellular carcinoma patients *J. Appl. Clin. Med. Phys.* **25** e14211

[44] Berry S L, Boczkowski A, Ma R, Mechalakos J and Hunt M 2016 Interobserver variability in radiation therapy plan output: results of a single-institution study *Pract. Radiat. Oncol.* **6** 442–9

[45] Shao Y *et al* 2023 Novel in-house knowledge-based automated planning system for lung cancer treated with intensity-modulated radiotherapy *Strahlenther Onkol.* **200** 967–82

[46] Adams J *et al* 2023 Plan quality analysis of automated treatment planning workflow with commercial auto-segmentation tools and clinical knowledge-based planning models for prostate cancer *Cureus* **15** e41260

[47] Harms J, Pogue J A, Cardenas C E, Stanley D N, Cardan R and Popple R 2023 Automated evaluation for rapid implementation of knowledge-based radiotherapy planning models *J. Appl. Clin. Med. Phys.* **24** e14152

[48] Boutilier J J, Lee T, Craig T, Sharpe M B and Chan T C Y 2015 Models for predicting objective function weights in prostate cancer IMRT *Med. Phys.* **42** 1586–95

[49] Nguyen D *et al* 2019 A feasibility study for predicting optimal radiation therapy dose distributions of prostate cancer patients from patient anatomy using deep learning *Sci. Rep.* **9** 1076

[50] Campbell W G *et al* 2017 Neural network dose models for knowledge-based planning in pancreatic SBRT *Med. Phys.* **44** 6148–58

[51] Wang W *et al* 2020 Fluence map prediction using deep learning models—direct plan generation for pancreas stereotactic body radiation therapy *Front. Artif. Intell.* **3** 68

[52] Gronberg M P, Gay S S, Netherton T J, Rhee D J, Court L E and Cardenas C E 2021 Technical note: dose prediction for head and neck radiotherapy using a three-dimensional dense dilated U-net architecture *Med. Phys.* **48** 5567–73

[53] McIntosh C, Welch M, McNiven A, Jaffray D A and Purdie T G 2017 Fully automated treatment planning for head and neck radiotherapy using a voxel-based dose prediction and dose mimicking method *Phys. Med. Biol.* **62** 5926

[54] RaySearch Laboratories 2019 Machine learning automated treatment planning *Raystation* https://raysearchlabs.com/siteassets/about-overview/media-center/wp-re-ev-n-pdfs/white-papers/whitepaper_ml_automatedplanning_raystation.pdf

[55] Xing Y, Nguyen D, Lu W, Yang M and Jiang S 2020 Technical note: a feasibility study on deep learning-based radiotherapy dose calculation *Med. Phys.* **47** 753–8

[56] Valdes G, Scheuermann R, Hung C Y, Olszanski A, Bellerive M and Solberg T D 2016 A mathematical framework for virtual IMRT QA using machine learning *Med. Phys.* **43** 4323

[57] Valdes G, Chan M F, Lim S B, Scheuermann R, Deasy J O and Solberg T D 2017 IMRT QA using machine learning: a multi-institutional validation *J. Appl. Clin. Med. Phys.* **18** 279–84

[58] Zhu H, Zhu Q, Wang Z, Yang B, Zhang W and Qiu J 2023 Patient-specific quality assurance prediction models based on machine learning for novel dual-layered MLC linac *Med. Phys.* **50** 1205–14

[59] Tozuka R *et al* 2023 Improvement of deep learning prediction model in patient-specific QA for VMAT with MLC leaf position map and patient's dose distribution *J. Appl. Clin. Med. Phys.* **24** e14055

[60] Li Q and Chan M F 2017 Predictive time-series modeling using artificial neural networks for linac beam symmetry: an empirical study *Ann. N. Y. Acad. Sci.* **1387** 84–94

[61] Carlson J N K, Park J M, Park S Y, Park J I, Choi Y and Ye S J 2016 A machine learning approach to the accurate prediction of multi-leaf collimator positional errors *Phys. Med. Biol.* **61** 2514–31

[62] Nakamura S *et al* 2023 Deep learning-based detection and classification of multi-leaf collimator modeling errors in volumetric modulated radiation therapy *J. Appl. Clin. Med. Phys.* **24** e14136

[63] Kida S *et al* 2018 Cone beam computed tomography image quality improvement using a deep convolutional neural network *Cureus* **10** e2548

[64] Yang B, Liu Y, Zhu J, Dai J and Men K 2023 Deep learning framework to improve the quality of cone-beam computed tomography for radiotherapy scenarios *Med. Phys.* **50** 7641–53

[65] Kurosawa T, Nishio T, Moriya S, Tsuneda M and Karasawa K 2020 Feasibility of image quality improvement for high-speed CBCT imaging using deep convolutional neural network for image-guided radiotherapy in prostate cancer *Phys. Med.* **80** 84–91

[66] Isaksson M, Jalden J and Murphy M J 2005 On using an adaptive neural network to predict lung tumor motion during respiration for radiotherapy applications *Med. Phys.* **32** 3801–9

[67] Pohl M, Uesaka M, Takahashi H, Demachi K and Bhusal Chhatkuli R 2022 Prediction of the position of external markers using a recurrent neural network trained with unbiased online recurrent optimization for safe lung cancer radiotherapy *Comput. Methods Programs Biomed.* **222** 106908

[68] Bukovsky I *et al* 2015 A fast neural network approach to predict lung tumor motion during respiration for radiation therapy applications *BioMed Res. Int.* **2015** 489679

[69] Eisenhauer E A *et al* 2009 New response evaluation criteria in solid tumours: revised RECIST guideline (version 1.1) *Eur. J. Cancer* **45** 228–47

[70] Cha K H *et al* 2017 Bladder cancer treatment response assessment in CT using radiomics with deep-learning *Sci. Rep.* **7** 8738

[71] Choi S J, Park K J, Heo C, Park B W, Kim M and Kim J K 2021 Radiomics-based model for predicting pathological complete response to neoadjuvant chemotherapy in muscle-invasive bladder cancer *Clin. Radiol.* **76** 627.e13–621

[72] Xu Y *et al* 2019 Deep learning predicts lung cancer treatment response from serial medical imaging *Clin. Cancer Res.* **25** 3266–75

[73] Liu K *et al* 2024 Development and validation of a deep learning signature for predicting lymphovascular invasion and survival outcomes in clinical stage IA lung adenocarcinoma: a multicenter retrospective cohort study *Transl. Oncol.* **42** 101894

[74] Zhang X *et al* 2024 Exploring non-invasive precision treatment in non-small cell lung cancer patients through deep learning radiomics across imaging features and molecular phenotypes *Biomark Res.* **12** 12

[75] Chen X *et al* 2017 Assessment of treatment response during chemoradiation therapy for pancreatic cancer based on quantitative radiomic analysis of daily CTs: an exploratory study *PLoS One* **12** e0178961

[76] Kunkyab T *et al* 2023 Radiomic analysis for early differentiation of lung cancer recurrence from fibrosis in patients treated with lung stereotactic ablative radiotherapy *Phys. Med. Biol.* **68** 165015

[77] Dean J *et al* 2018 Incorporating spatial dose metrics in machine learning-based normal tissue complication probability (NTCP) models of severe acute dysphagia resulting from head and neck radiotherapy *Clin. Transl. Radiat. Oncol.* **8** 27–39

[78] Gabryś H S, Buettner F, Sterzing F, Hauswald H and Bangert M 2018 Design and selection of machine learning methods using radiomics and dosiomics for normal tissue complication probability modeling of xerostomia *Front. Oncol.* **8** 35

[79] Cunliffe A, Armato S G 3rd, Castillo R, Pham N, Guerrero T and Al-Hallaq H A 2015 Lung texture in serial thoracic computed tomography scans: correlation of radiomics-based features with radiation therapy dose and radiation pneumonitis development *Int. J. Radiat. Oncol. Biol. Phys.* **91** 1048–56

[80] Chen S, Zhou S, Yin F F, Marks L B and Das S K 2007 Investigation of the support vector machine algorithm to predict lung radiation-induced pneumonitis *Med. Phys.* **34** 3808–14

[81] Zhen X *et al* 2017 Deep convolutional neural network with transfer learning for rectum toxicity prediction in cervical cancer radiotherapy: a feasibility study *Phys. Med. Biol.* **62** 8246–63

Chapter 3

Artificial intelligence in clinical decision making

Xinyu Zhang, Jiang Zhang, Xinzhi Teng, Yuanpeng Zhang and Jing Cai

With the fast development of artificial intelligence (AI) technologies, their application in clinical decision making has been broadly explored. This chapter provides an overview and fundamental understanding of AI in clinical decision making. It starts with a brief introduction of clinical decision making and medical AI, followed by the development of medical AI and its algorithms designed to handle various clinical data. Specifically, radiomics, a common method to develop models from medical images, and the algorithms to integrate diverse clinical data types and improve interpretability of medical AI are introduced. Then, the applications of AI in various clinical scenarios are listed, encompassing diagnosis and disease phenotyping, personalized treatment, as well as treatment outcome and prognosis prediction. In the end, the existing challenges and potential future directions for further developments of medical AI are discussed. Overall, this chapter provides insights into the current state, major applications, and future prospects of AI in clinical decision making.

3.1 Introduction

3.1.1 Introduction of clinical decision making and AI

Clinical decision making refers to the process in which the healthcare providers make decisions when they are diagnosing and treating patients, aiming to provide accurate diagnosis and optimal treatment to maximize benefits for patients. It happens in the entire process of disease management involving several aspects:

> **Information acquisition:** Enquire into the disease history of the patient, conduct physical and laboratory examinations, and gather other related information to understand the patient's condition.
>
> **Problem identification and diagnosis:** Identify potential health problems by analysing the obtained information and make a diagnosis.
>
> **Treatment planning:** Recommend appropriate treatment schemes according to diagnosis, disease progress, the healthcare provider's experience and knowledge, and other conditions (economic, patient's preference, etc).

Follow-up: Monitor disease progress and treatment effect and make adjustments if needed.

Traditional clinical decision making is an exhaustive, comparative, and selective process. After considering the basic conditions of patients, healthcare providers will: '(1) list all possible actions, (2) list all possible outcomes, (3) predict the probability of each outcome from each action, and then (4) select the best action based on outcome likelihood and outcome utility' [1]. In practice, this process mostly relies on the subjective experience and professional knowledge of healthcare providers, leading to various and suboptimal decisions. Furthermore, owing to the development of modern technology, there is an explosively increasing volume and types of medical information, encompassing high-resolution images, continuous physiological records, genome sequencing data, and so on. Effective interpretation of such medical big data surpasses the capability of humans alone but can be achieved by artificial intelligence (AI) using advanced machine learning or deep learning algorithms, thereby making more personalized and accurate clinical decisions.

In recent decades, the application of AI in medicine has been explored broadly. The topics vary from diagnostic support systems [2] and risk prediction models [3] to personalized medicine [4] and outcome prediction [5]. They aim to harness the potential of AI to facilitate accurate, effective, and personalized clinical decision making using various AI techniques. In health data analytics, AI has inherent advantages in the efficient processing of data with large amounts and variety, and in objective decision making. Previous research also highlighted multiple benefits of AI applications in healthcare, including accelerating the decision-making process [6, 7], enhancing clinical decision-making capacity [8, 9], improving patient outcomes [10, 11], and so on. In all, AI has shown great potential in the medical field. As recognized by healthcare providers, AI could serve as a powerful tool in clinical practice and dramatically change the overall workflow of clinical decision making in the future.

3.1.2 The role of AI in clinical decision making

3.1.2.1 Diagnostic decision support

Diagnosis is the first critical decision healthcare providers make during the process of disease management. In 1998, the first commercial computer-aided diagnosis (CAD) system was approved by the United States Food and Drug Administration (FDA) for mammography. Subsequently, more commercial CAD systems for other medical images, such as computer tomography (CT) and magnetic resonance imaging (MRI), received FDA approval. To date, CAD is the most widely used application of AI in real-world clinical settings, particularly in the departments relying highly on images (radiology, pathology, gastroscopy, etc). Unlike computer diagnosis that aims at replacing humans, CAD provides recommendations or potential diagnoses to healthcare providers who make the final diagnosis. The usefulness of CAD in disease detection and diagnosis has been confirmed by previous research including for lung nodules [12, 13], calcifications [14, 15], intra-cranial aneurysms [16], fractures [17, 18], and so on. In addition, CAD can largely accelerate the diagnosis process from minutes to seconds, which is critical for some acute events, such as stroke and hemorrhage [6].

3.1.2.2 Patient profiling and precise medicine

Patient profiling involves gathering and analysing a variety of information on patients to discover the characteristics that are relevant to disease conditions and treatment response. Patient profiles include all the clinical, pathological, biological, and other information, allowing AI to extract insights associated with disease severity and classification. Many diseases, such as cancer, are heterogeneous and contain subtypes yet to be discovered. In this regard, AI has been used in genomic profiling and multi-omics integration for the discovery of new subtypes, contributing to a deeper understanding of disease mechanisms and characteristics [19]. Furthermore, the capability of AI-based patient profiling in facilitating precise medicine was also evaluated [20]. In addition, AI also plays an important role in new drug development based on precise patient profiling [21].

3.1.2.3 Treatment assessment and prognosis prediction

The ultimate goal of clinical decision making is to improve the treatment outcome of patients. With AI assessing treatment response and predicting prognosis, healthcare providers are able to choose the appropriate therapeutics for patients and prevent them from unnecessary toxicity. One current method to evaluate treatment response is the response evaluation criteria in solid tumors (RECIST) based on tumor size change. However, some studies noticed that tumors may change in density or vascularization without obvious change in size [22]. For such changes that are less perceptible to human eyes, radiomics has shown great potential by detecting the texture changes of tumors on medical images for the prediction of treatment toxicity [23], survival [24], metastasis [25], and recurrence [26].

3.2 AI algorithms for clinical decision making

3.2.1 Workflow of AI development in clinical decision making

The AI algorithms for clinical decision making are mostly developed by the data-driven approach where the associations between a particular clinical endpoint and patient demographics are established in a quantitative manner. Personalized clinical decisions can be made based on accurate predictions of individual clinical outcomes. Several steps are generally involved during the development of AI algorithms, including data acquisition, feature engineering, and model construction and evaluation.

3.2.1.1 Data acquisition

The acquisition of data for the development of medical AI typically involves various components. Routinely produced clinical data can be retrospectively exported from the electronic medical record system (EMRS) as texts or tables. Imaging and structured data are mostly exported from imaging consoles or radiotherapy treatment planning systems following the digital imaging and communications in medicine (DICOM) standard. Some non-routine data, such as region-of-interest (ROI), that are not used for treatment plan evaluation (e.g. peritumoral region [27]), can be either manually drawn or automatically generated. Deep-learning-based auto-segmentation can also be used to accelerate the ROI generation, with optional manual adjustments.

3.2.1.2 Feature engineering
Feature engineering plays a crucial role in the workflow of AI, encompassing feature extraction, removal of non-repeatable features, and selection of relevant and independent features.

Feature extraction involves extracting reliable and meaningful quantitative features from multi-level data. In the context of medical images, features are extracted to capture intensity and texture characteristics, either by predefined mathematical formulas within a defined volume of interest or deep learning algorithms [28]. Additionally, geometric features can be utilized to quantify the relative positions and shape of tumors in relation to surrounding organs [10]. For radiation dose maps, quantitative features could include dose–volume-histogram (DVH) features and dosiomics features, which encompass radiomic-based features, and momentum-based features [29].

The removal of non-repeatable features eliminates features that cannot be reproduced under the same settings. Assessment of feature repeatability often involves utilizing test–retest cohorts or introducing perturbations to generate pseudo-test–retest cohorts [30]. By removing non-repeatable features, the generalizability of the model is enhanced, ensuring more reliable and consistent performance [31].

Feature selection focuses on identifying independent features that significantly contribute to the desired outcome for subsequent model construction. Accurate selection of features plays a vital role in enhancing model performance by incorporating only the most informative and discriminative features with a minimum risk of overfitting.

3.2.1.3 Model construction and evaluation
Constructing models involves selecting appropriate algorithms based on the selected features and the specific clinical task. Common machine learning algorithms include support vector machines, logistic regression, k-nearest neighbors, decision trees, random forests, and extreme gradient boosting. Area under the receiver operating characteristic curve (AUC), accuracy, F1 score, sensitivity, specificity, precision, positive predictive value (PPV), and negative predictive value (NPV) are commonly used to evaluate the performance of the model. Generalizability and imbalanced data are two factors significantly impacting model performance. Generalizability

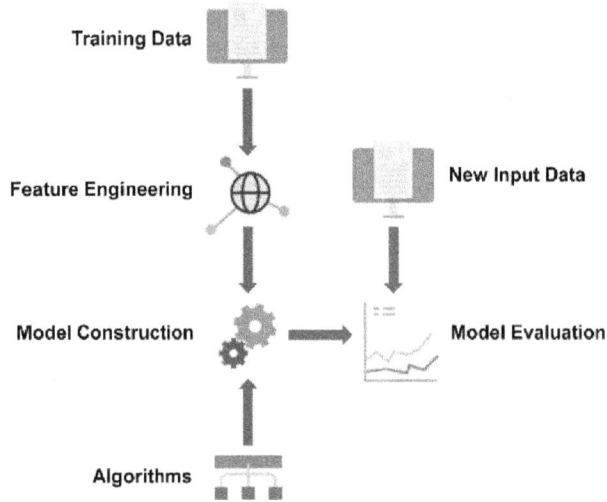

Figure 3.1. The process of model construction and evaluation.

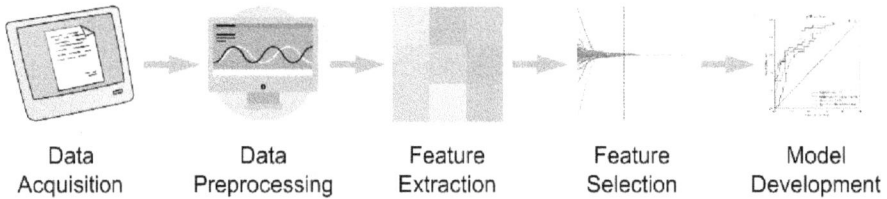

| Data | Data | Feature | Feature | Model |
| Acquisition | Preprocessing | Extraction | Selection | Development |

Figure 3.2. Common workflow of radiomics.

refers to how well a model trained on certain clinical data performs on unseen data. Techniques such as small-sample learning, manifold learning, and transfer learning can improve the generalizability of models. On the other hand, imbalanced datasets can be addressed through methods such as resampling or ensemble algorithms [32]. Figure 3.1 briefly illustrates the model construction and evaluation process.

3.2.2 Radiomics

Similar to general AI development, a typical workflow of radiomics involves data acquisition, data preprocessing, feature extraction, and model development. The process of data acquisition has been demonstrated in the previous section. Data preprocessing involves enhancing data quality by harmonization and removing irrelevant information, which can minimize bias and improve sensitivity. A large number of quantitative handcrafted or deep learning features can then be extracted from medical images. Finally, machine learning or deep learning models can be constructed from the extracted radiomics features. To reduce the risk of overfitting and enhance the model stability, several procedures can be adopted to reduce the number of features based on variance, collinearity, and relevance to clinical before model development. Figure 3.2 shows the common workflow of radiomics.

Radiomics feature mapping is a high-dimensional representation that visualizes radiomics feature distribution at different locations of the image. It can facilitate the explanations of the selected radiomics features and the final developed models by identifying the regions that contribute significantly to the positive and negative predictions. They can be further utilized for more intuitive clinical decision making. For example, the size of the highlighted tumor subregion based on the mapping of the radiomics feature discovered from the global value retains the predictive value of treatment efficacy for adjuvant chemotherapy on patients with locoregionally advanced nasopharyngeal carcinoma (NPC) [33]. It can also be directly applied to image mapping tasks, such as lung functional map generation from static CT images [34].

3.2.3 Data integration by AI

The individual clinical data of a patient is composed of various aspects of clinical information including the following categories. (i) Electronic medical record (EMR) data: patients' basic information, medical history, diagnostic records, treatment plans, etc. (ii) Medical imaging data: such as x-ray images, CT scans, MRI scans, etc. (iii) Laboratory test data: laboratory test results of blood, urine, tissue samples, etc. (iv) Vital signs data: physiological parameters of the patient such as heart rate, body temperature, blood pressure, etc. Data integration aims to analyse data from various sources, enabling more comprehensive personalized medical recommendations for clinical decision making. AI, through automating data extraction and transformation as well as various advanced techniques, can enhance the process of data integration.

Multi-omics involves the comprehensive analysis of two or more individual omics disciplines, such as genomics, transcriptomics, proteomics, metabolomics, and radiomics. It combines biological information from various levels and scales to obtain more accurate prediction. On the other hand, multi-view in machine learning refers to the fusion of data represented by multiple different feature sets [35]. For example, each type of electroencephalogram signal features extracted using different methods, such as wavelet packet decomposition (WPD), short-time Fourier transform (STFT), kernel principal component analysis (kernel PCA), can be considered as a view. In comparison to the previous two methods, multi-modal machine learning has a broader scope as it encompasses a wider range of data types. In the clinical context, each source or form of information can be referred to as a modality [36]. It can be diverse data describing the same patient (such as patient records, medical images, lab reports, etc), or it can be imaging data generated by different imaging devices (such as x-ray, CT, MRI, etc). Multi-modal machine learning aims to build models that can handle and correlate multi-modal data, thereby leveraging the complementary nature of different modalities. While the three concepts are not exactly the same, they share similarities in terms of integrating diverse information. Whether multi-omics, multi-view, or multi-modal integration is used, it goes beyond simply stitching together different types of data, aiming to overcome the limitations of individual data sources and modalities.

3.2.4 Interpretability of AI models

Model interpretability is the ability to explain and understand the internal mechanisms and predictions of an AI model. The absence of interpretability of AI model predictions hinders the understanding of its underlying mechanisms, thereby the practical applications of medical AI. There are two major approaches to achieve interpretability. The first approach involves reducing the intrinsic complexity of machine learning models to enhance interpretability. Intrinsic interpretable machine learning models can display the relationship between model inputs and outputs, such as the explainable boosting machine (EBM) model. The second approach is post-hoc interpretability, which involves conducting interpretability analysis after model construction. Methods such as SHapley Additive exPlanations (SHAP) and local interpretable model-agnostic explanations (LIME) fall into this category. The scope of interpretability includes both global interpretability and local interpretability. Global interpretability provides an overall view of the model's features, weights, parameters, or structure. Local interpretability explains the prediction results of individual instances [37].

Instead of the interpretability of AI models, clinical practitioners often place more emphasis on the interpretability of features, particularly on how features are related to clinical objectives. The interpretability of individual features can provide meaningful explanations for the predicted results. Certain features of AI models may have biological significance themselves. For example, the interpretability of radiomics features can be enhanced by exploring their associations with tumor heterogeneity. Feature importance is a common method to interpret features by revealing the weights and magnitudes of features that are globally or locally interpretable in complex models [38]. A widely adopted and intuitive approach is correlation analysis, which assesses the significance of features by calculating the correlation coefficients between the features and the target. In addition, post-hoc interpretability methods such as SHAP can also analyse the importance of features by calculating their contributions to the model predictions, as shown in figure 3.3.

A fuzzy rule describes a fuzzy logical relationship. It consists of fuzzy conditions and a fuzzy conclusion and is typically structured in an 'IF–THEN' form. The fuzzy conditions describe the state of the input variables, while the fuzzy conclusion describes the state of the output variable. Fuzzy rules are interpretable because they use natural language terms (e.g. 'high', 'medium', 'low') and have intuitive logical reasoning relationships. The fuzzy model conducts fuzzy reasoning based on fuzzy rules, and then transforms fuzzy output into specific operations. The classical Takagi–Sugeuo–Kang (TSK) fuzzy model determines the parameters of the conclusion part of the fuzzy rule by parameter estimation [39]. The TSK fuzzy model is widely used in the field of AI due to its good nonlinear approximation ability and strong interpretability.

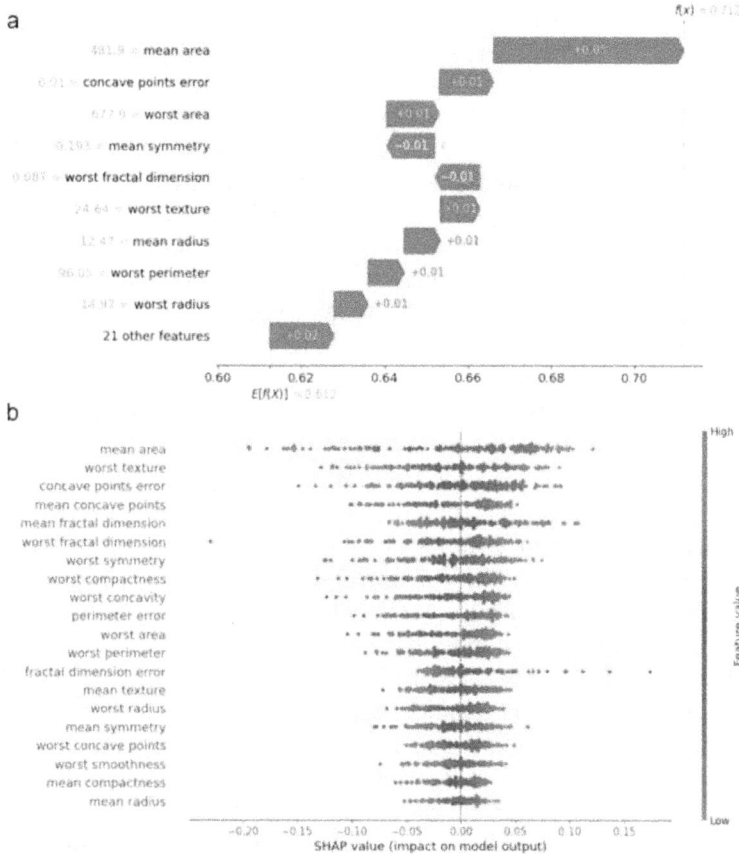

Figure 3.3. Example of SHAP plots based on the breast cancer dataset (an open-source dataset in Python's scikit-learn library). (a) Waterfall plot for local interpretation. The x-axis represents SHAP values and the y-axis represents feature names and their corresponding values in an individual sample. (b) Summary plot for global interpretation. The x-axis represents SHAP values and the y-axis represents feature names. The importance of features decreases sequentially from top to bottom.

3.3 Application of AI in clinical decision making

3.3.1 Diagnosis and disease phenotyping

Early disease detection aims to promptly identify diseases, enabling timely intervention and management. AI, particularly in conjunction with medical imaging, has demonstrated substantial potential in disease detection. In recent years, COVID-19 has had a profound impact on global public health, for which medical imaging is frequently employed to detect suspected COVID-19 cases. Numerous AI models based on chest x-ray images have been developed for automated diagnosis and enhanced accuracy in lung disease classification. For instance, an interpretable TSK fuzzy system has been developed to leverage radiomics features extracted from chest x-ray images to detect COVID-19, which achieved a high level of classification accuracy while preserving interpretability [40]. Additionally, a two-step feature merging method has been proposed to leverage the attention mechanism of deep learning neural networks to integrate both deep learning features and radiomics features, achieving enhanced classification accuracy [41].

Disease staging is part of diagnosis assessing the severity and progression of disease. Specifically, cancer staging determines the extent of tumor growth and spread within the body, for example using the TNM staging system. It helps predict patient prognosis and guide treatment decisions. AI has been actively explored in quantitative analysis of imaging and anatomical information for improved staging. For example, an improved N staging system with better survival stratification was proposed using quantitative spatial characterizations of lymph node tumor anatomy for NPC patients [10]. In this study, new angle and distance descriptors were designed for precise geometric localizations of the lymph node tumor relative to the surrounding organs and selected using machine learning techniques for targeted prediction of patient survival.

Disease phenotyping refers to the process of identifying and characterizing the observable characteristics or traits of a disease, which is crucial in understanding the manifestation and progression of diseases, as well as their susceptibility to treatment. AI can be applied to predict the existing disease phenotypes from the routinely generated medical data with major contributions in efficiency, low-cost, and non-invasiveness. For example, radiomics has been successfully applied in predicting the status of HER2 and HR using ADC in invasive breast cancer [42]. The developed radiomics signatures retained similar predictive values in treatment response evaluation and therefore could serve as non-invasive surrogates of existing bio-markers. Another study discovered a high correlation between the inherent lung texture information extracted by radiomics from CT images with pulmonary function measurements, suggesting a potential fast and low-cost approach to generate pulmonary function phenotyping for diagnosis and treatment guidance [34, 43].

3.3.2 Personalized treatment

Personalized treatment has emerged as a promising approach to improve patient outcomes in various cancers. It aims to tailor therapy based on specific patient characteristics to achieve optimal results. The current progress in personalized treatment has been driven by advancements in imaging analysis, such as radiomics that provides valuable information about tumor characteristics, such as size and texture, aiding in treatment planning and response assessment. One example of the use of radiomics in NPC is the identification of patients who might benefit from adjuvant chemotherapy for local-regionally advanced disease [33]. Radiomic-based features extracted from pre-treatment imaging scans can be used to develop predictive models and stratify patients based on their likelihood of treatment response. This approach holds promise in optimizing treatment selection, minimizing unnecessary interventions, and improving outcomes for patients with NPC.

Adaptive radiation therapy (ART) is a dynamic treatment approach that enables real-time adjustments to radiation therapy plans based on changes in a patient's anatomy, or other relevant factors during treatment. It takes into account the dynamic nature of tumors and surrounding tissues, enhancing treatment accuracy and improving patient outcomes. An integral component of ART involves the integration of imaging techniques, such as cone-beam CT, throughout treatment to provide information on changes in tumor size and location. The acquired imaging data are then utilized to redefine treatment plans. Recent advancements in AI, particularly in the field of radiomics, have shown promise in identifying patients who may require ART prior to the initiation of RT. Radiomics features extracted from pre-treatment T1-weighted (T1-w) and T2-weighted (T2-w) MR images within the primary target for RT, along with a logistic regression model, can help identify potential patients who may benefit from ART during radical concurrent chemo-radiation therapy [44]. Additionally, radiomics features extracted from radiation dose maps and contours depicting the relative position between the target and organs at risk (OARs) have further confirmed the pivotal role of radiomics in determining the need for ART [45]. Furthermore, studies have been conducted to predict the suitability of thermoplastic masks, which may become ill-fitted due to lymph node shrinkage [46]. Radiomics provides clinicians with an opportunity to identify patients at risk of requiring ART due to tumor shrinkage, allowing for increased attention and appropriate intervention. And the developed model can benefit low-risk patients by potentially omitting weekly cone-beam CT scans, thereby minimizing unnecessary radiation exposure.

3.3.3 Treatment outcome and prognosis prediction

Treatment response, as an important measure of the effectiveness of a given treatment, helps clinicians determine whether a particular therapy is working and whether any adjustments need to be made to the treatment plan. Common treatment response indicators are tumor shrinkage, pathological response, and survival. Pathological response to the novel sequential trans-arterial chemoembolization (TACE)–stereotactic body radiotherapy (SBRT)–immunotherapy for unresectable hepatocellular carcinoma patients were successfully predicted by the individual pre-treatment radiomics and delta-radiomics features from multi-phase contrast-enhanced MRI [47]. A recent study fused multi-modal data fusion with label-softening technique alongside a multi-kernel-based radial basis function (RBF) neural network, to mitigate the inherent disparity of different data modalities for effective predictions of distant metastasis of NPC patients [48]. Treatment outcome prediction often encounters the challenge of sample imbalance. Zhang *et al* addressed the challenge in survival prediction by a high-generalizable classifier, multi-kernel regression with graph embedding (MERGE), and an imbalance framework, sensitivity-based under-sampling (SUS), and achieved a promising performance in similar tasks [49].

Treatment side effects are another important consideration during treatment planning and disease management. By leveraging diverse quantitative medical data, AI models have shown great potential in predicting various side effects for radiation oncology. Radiotherapy-induced acute oral mucositis is the most prevalent side effect among NPC patients, which may compromise the quality of life or even survival of NPC patients. Various factors have been discovered to be correlated with the incidence and severity of oral mucositis, such as pre-treatment body mass index (BMI) [50], nutrition status [51], and mean oral cavity dose [52]. One recent study attempted the integration of radiomics features and dosiomics features and achieved the best validation performance (mean AUC = 0.81) among the existing models [29].

Esophageal fistula (EF) is a severe complication that occurs in 4%–25% of patients undergoing radiotherapy treatment for esophageal cancer, which is correlated with clinical factors such as age and tumor grade [53, 54]. Recently, AI models based on radiomics, and deep learning analysis of medical images have been applied for personalized prediction of EF [55, 56]. The integration of dosiomics and radiomics features from both the esophagus and gross tumor volume further improved EF prediction [57].

Radiation pneumonitis is a type of lung injury caused by radiation and acute radiation pneumonitis is one of the most severe complications that can occur within six months after commencing radiotherapy treatment [58]. Dose–volume statistics have been investigated but contain limited predictability, possibly due to the inter-patient and intra-patient heterogeneity in response to radiation. One novel study by Li *et al* attempted to integrate the dosimetric and radiomic information by extracting radiomics-based lung texture information from different dose-interval subregions and built a model with better performance than the whole lung model [59]. Further integration of lung function information with a radiomics–dosiomics model established from different lung function subregions demonstrated enhanced performance in predicting radiation pneumonitis [60]. Acute radiation esophagitis is another common complication during and after lung cancer treatment. One previous study discovered that radiomics features from the CT images resulted in an AI model with satisfactory performance in acute radiation esophagitis prediction [61].

3.4 Challenges and future directions of AI in clinical decision making

3.4.1 Challenges and concerns

3.4.1.1 Data quality and privacy

One of the prerequisites of training an accurate and generalizable model is the use of high-quality data. Data with too much noise from either poor image quality or mislabeled clinical outcomes often contain minimum information to be learnt by the AI models. Highly biased data due to poorly standardized data acquisition protocols will significantly degrade model generalizability. In addition to purposely generating and acquiring high-quality data from a carefully designed experiment, such as a clinical trial, several techniques have been proposed and applied to identify poor-quality data. The direct uncertainty prediction model and Bayesian technique can be used to evaluate the uncertainty of the prediction by training on samples with multiple labels [62, 63]. Another technique called untrainable data cleansing can identify potentially incorrect and noisy samples by inferencing the existing single-label samples, which is more practical for datasets with limited annotations [64].

Concerns regarding patient data privacy have long been raised throughout the development of medical AI. Patient data are originally produced and managed by healthcare institutions under the supervision of government or other public bodies. However, collaborations between public and private sectors are often encouraged for healthcare innovations, which may compromise patient privacy due to poor data management on the private side or data leakage from the black-box models [65]. Regulations for the responsible use and management of patient data for medical AI development are crucial for data privacy protection, but a balance should be maintained so as not to slow down medical AI development.

3.4.1.2 Integration with existing healthcare systems

While many studies focus on using AI alone to perform a specific task, in reality, it is more feasible for humans and AI to collaborate for improved efficiency while minimizing risk. The impact of AI on the behavior and decision making of healthcare providers still remains unclear, as it can vary according to their experience and specific tasks [66]. On the other hand, integrating medical AI into existing clinical routines poses significant challenges. Clinical professionals have established a routine workflow without AI through decades of clinical practice, leaving no room for AI to play its role without changing the current protocol. The existing picture archiving and communication system (PACS) is mostly a closed system, which forces many commercial medical AI applications to be developed as separate systems such as web applications or widgets to interact with radiologists and show interpretation results [67]. This makes the use of AI assistance a tedious and repetitive process from the perspective of manual data transmission and results input. Standards for data transition and the framework of integrated workflow are needed to realize seamless AI integration.

3.4.2 Future directions

3.4.2.1 Emerging trends and technologies

The cross-disciplinary integration is a hot research topic in the current application of AI in clinical settings. However, challenges related to data integration and feature selection must be overcome to effectively merge multiple domains. Moreover, AI is driving the transformation of the traditional healthcare model. Intelligent wearable devices and the medical Internet of Things are advancing rapidly, allowing for real-time monitoring of patients' physiological indicators. This progress is paving the way for personalized healthcare decision making in the near future.

3.4.2.2 Reliability and interpretability

The development of trustworthy and reliable AI models is of paramount importance for successful and responsible clinical deployment. Efforts should be made at different stages of the AI model development to improve reliability, including data preprocessing, feature selection, and model development. Proper data processing could reduce data bias and enhance the signal-to-noise ratio, thus helping with model convergence and avoiding overfitting. Feature repeatability based on perturbation or test–retest should be considered during feature selection to ensure reliable predictions. A more rigorous and standardized process is warranted for reliable AI model development.

Model interpretability is another important aspect of model reliability as it can help identify and correct biases, errors, or unwanted behaviors in the model, as well as provide insights into the data and the problem domain. However, there is currently no single best way to interpret a model, and different methods may have different advantages and limitations depending on the context and the goal of the interpretation. Section 3.2 has mentioned several interpretable methods that can be explored further.

3.4.2.3 *Closing the gap between research and practice*

Despite the boom in medical AI, most of the approaches have been developed and evaluated in a laboratory setting. Only less than one hundred of over 17 000 medical AI studies were implemented in a real-life clinical setting [66]. While the research setting is homogeneous, real clinical practice often encounters various situations. AI models trained in a specific patient cohort or under a specific scenario may not be adaptive to the diverse conditions in clinical practice. Continuous efforts in validating the effectiveness of AI and promoting better study design will contribute to bridging the gap between laboratory research and real clinical practice.

In addition, there remains the problem of how AI can be seamlessly integrated into current clinical workflow. At the RSNA 2020 Annual Meeting, an Imaging AI in Practice (IAIP) demonstration showed an AI-integrated workflow in a simulated clinical environment, where AI functioned in several critical clinical decision-making steps including imaging examination ordering, protocoling, acquisition, display, interpretation, reporting, and follow-up [68]. It highlights the crucial role of consistent interoperability standards and effective human–AI interaction in an integrated circumstance. The demonstration shows a successful integration where AI is no longer working as an additional unit in disease detection or treatment selection only, but rather is fully integrated into and dramatically changes the overall workflow of current clinical practice.

3.5 Summary

In this chapter, we introduced the major techniques and applications of AI in clinical decision making. Clinical decision making happens in the entire spectrum of health management, including disease diagnosis, treatment planning, and prognosis. Making fast and accurate clinical decisions is critical for effective disease management and thus improving patients' quality of life. In the era of AI, clinical decisions can be more intelligent with more accurate information of patients' conditions and predictions of treatment outcomes. Numerous efforts have been made to cope with the special characteristics of clinical data and develop advanced AI techniques for model construction. Some well-developed AI models have been applied to different clinical decision-making scenarios and obtained promising achievements, which demonstrates AI's ability to guide clinical practice and assist in clinical decision making. In summary, it is believed that AI has the potential to be an efficient and reliable assistant for healthcare providers in making clinical decisions. Further research is needed to address the existing challenges and concerns. Only after that can we harness the full potential of AI in clinical decision making and pave the way for better healthcare outcome and personalized patient care.

References

[1] Patton D D 1978 Introduction to clinical decision making *Semin. Nucl. Med.* **8** 273–82

[2] Chamberlin J *et al* 2021 Automated detection of lung nodules and coronary artery calcium using artificial intelligence on low-dose CT scans for lung cancer screening: accuracy and prognostic value *BMC Med.* **19** 55

[3] Bhuiyan A, Wong T Y, Ting D S W, Govindaiah A, Souied E H and Smith R T 2020 Artificial intelligence to stratify severity of age-related macular degeneration (AMD) and predict risk of progression to late AMD *Transl. Vis. Sci. Technol.* **9** 25

[4] Schork N J 2019 Artificial intelligence and personalized medicine *Precision Medicine in Cancer Therapy* ed D D Von Hoff and H Han (Cham: Springer International) pp 265–83

[5] Huang S, Yang J, Fong S and Zhao Q 2020 Artificial intelligence in cancer diagnosis and prognosis: opportunities and challenges *Cancer Lett.* **471** 61–71

[6] Titano J J *et al* 2018 Automated deep-neural-network surveillance of cranial images for acute neurologic events *Nat. Med.* **24** 1337–41

[7] Nicolae A *et al* 2020 Conventional vs machine learning-based treatment planning in prostate brachytherapy: results of a phase I randomized controlled trial *Brachytherapy* **19** 470–6

[8] Dembrower K *et al* 2020 Effect of artificial intelligence-based triaging of breast cancer screening mammograms on cancer detection and radiologist workload: a retrospective simulation study *Lancet Digit. Health* **2** e468–74

[9] Yoo Y J, Ha E J, Cho Y J, Kim H L, Han M and Kang S Y 2018 Computer-aided diagnosis of thyroid nodules via ultrasonography: initial clinical experience *Korean J. Radiol.* **19** 665

[10] Zhang J *et al* 2023 Quantitative spatial characterization of lymph node tumor for N stage improvement of nasopharyngeal carcinoma patients *Cancers* **15** 230

[11] Sevakula R K, Au-Yeung W M, Singh J P, Heist E K, Isselbacher E M and Armoundas A A 2020 State-of-the-art machine learning techniques aiming to improve patient outcomes pertaining to the cardiovascular system *J. Am. Heart Assoc.* **9** e013924

[12] Nam J G *et al* 2019 Development and validation of deep learning-based automatic detection algorithm for malignant pulmonary nodules on chest radiographs *Radiology* **290** 218–28

[13] Cheng J Z *et al* 2016 Computer-aided diagnosis with deep learning architecture: applications to breast lesions in US images and pulmonary nodules in CT scans *Sci. Rep.* **6** 24454

[14] Liu H *et al* 2021 A deep learning model integrating mammography and clinical factors facilitates the malignancy prediction of BI-RADS 4 microcalcifications in breast cancer screening *Eur. Radiol.* **31** 5902–12

[15] Graffy P M, Liu J, O'Connor S, Summers R M and Pickhardt P J 2019 Automated segmentation and quantification of aortic calcification at abdominal CT: application of a deep learning-based algorithm to a longitudinal screening cohort *Abdom. Radiol.* **44** 2921–8

[16] Joo B *et al* 2020 A deep learning algorithm may automate intracranial aneurysm detection on MR angiography with high diagnostic performance *Eur. Radiol.* **30** 5785–93

[17] Jin L *et al* 2020 Deep-learning-assisted detection and segmentation of rib fractures from CT scans: development and validation of FracNet *eBioMedicine* **62** 103106

[18] Yoon A P, Lee Y L, Kane R L, Kuo C F, Lin C and Chung K C 2021 Development and validation of a deep learning model using convolutional neural networks to identify scaphoid fractures in radiographs *JAMA Netw. Open* **4** e216096

[19] Wolf D M *et al* 2022 Redefining breast cancer subtypes to guide treatment prioritization and maximize response: predictive biomarkers across 10 cancer therapies *Cancer Cell.* **40** 609–623.e6

[20] Baxi V, Edwards R, Montalto M and Saha S 2022 Digital pathology and artificial intelligence in translational medicine and clinical practice *Mod. Pathol.* **35** 23–32

[21] Lamberti M J *et al* 2019 A study on the application and use of artificial intelligence to support drug development *Clin. Ther.* **41** 1414–26

[22] Geady C, Shultz D B, Razak A R A, Schuetze S and Haibe-Kains B 2022 Radiomics in sarcoma trials: a complement to RECIST for patient assessment *J. Cancer Metastasis Treat.* **8** 45

[23] Tan D, Mohamad Salleh S A, Manan H A and Yahya N 2023 Delta-radiomics-based models for toxicity prediction in radiotherapy: a systematic review and meta-analysis *J. Med. Imaging. Radiat. Oncol.* **67** 564–79

[24] Cousin F *et al* 2023 Radiomics and delta-radiomics signatures to predict response and survival in patients with non-small-cell lung cancer treated with immune checkpoint inhibitors *Cancers* **15** 1968

[25] Jeon S H *et al* 2019 Delta-radiomics signature predicts treatment outcomes after preoperative chemoradiotherapy and surgery in rectal cancer *Radiat. Oncol.* **14** 43

[26] Fave X, Zhang L, Yang J *et al* 2017 Using pretreatment radiomics and delta-radiomics features to predict non-small cell lung cancer patient outcomes *Int. J. Radiat. Oncol. Biol. Phys.* **98** 249

[27] Braman N M *et al* 2017 Intratumoral and peritumoral radiomics for the pretreatment prediction of pathological complete response to neoadjuvant chemotherapy based on breast DCE-MRI *Breast Cancer Res.* **19** 57

[28] van Griethuysen J J M *et al* 2017 Computational radiomics system to decode the radiographic phenotype *Cancer Res.* **77** e104–7

[29] Dong Y *et al* 2023 Multimodal data integration to predict severe acute oral mucositis of nasopharyngeal carcinoma patients following radiation therapy *Cancers* **15** 2032

[30] Teng X *et al* 2022 Building reliable radiomic models using image perturbation *Sci. Rep.* **12** 10035

[31] Teng X *et al* 2022 Improving radiomic model reliability using robust features from perturbations for head-and-neck carcinoma *Front. Oncol.* **12** 974467

[32] Zhang Y P *et al* 2023 Artificial intelligence-driven radiomics study in cancer: the role of feature engineering and modeling *Mil. Med. Res.* **10** 22

[33] Teng X *et al* 2023 Explainable machine learning via intra-tumoral radiomics feature mapping for patient stratification in adjuvant chemotherapy for locoregionally advanced nasopharyngeal carcinoma *Radiol. Med.* **128** 828–38

[34] Huang Y H *et al* 2023 Respiratory invariant textures from static computed tomography scans for explainable lung function characterization *J. Thorac. Imaging* **38** 286–96

[35] Xu C, Tao D and Xu C 2013 A survey on multi-view learning arXiv: 1304.5634v1

[36] Baltrušaitis T, Ahuja C and Morency L P 2019 Multimodal machine learning: a survey and taxonomy *IEEE Trans. Pattern Anal. Mach. Intell.* **41** 423–43

[37] Molnar, C., 2020. *Interpretable Machine Learning* (Victoria: LeanPub)

[38] Hanif A, Zhang X and Wood S 2021 A survey on explainable artificial intelligence techniques and challenges *2021 IEEE 25th Int. Enterprise Distributed Object Computing Workshop (EDOCW)* pp 81–9

[39] Takagi T and Sugeno M 1985 Fuzzy identification of systems and its applications to modeling and control *IEEE Trans. Syst. Man Cybern.* **SMC-15** 116–32

[40] Zhang Y *et al* 2022 Radiomics-based detection of COVID-19 from chest x-ray using interpretable soft label-driven TSK fuzzy classifier *Diagnostics* **12** 2613

[41] Yang D *et al* 2023 Deep learning attention-guided radiomics for COVID-19 chest radiograph classification *Quant. Imaging. Med. Surg.* **13** 572–84

[42] Teng X *et al* 2023 Noninvasive imaging signatures of HER2 and HR using ADC in invasive breast cancer: repeatability, reproducibility, and association with pathological complete response to neoadjuvant chemotherapy *Breast. Cancer. Res.* **25** 77

[43] Faught A M *et al* 2017 Evaluating the toxicity reduction with computed tomographic ventilation functional avoidance radiation therapy *Int. J. Radiat. Oncol.* **99** 325–33

[44] Yu T T *et al* 2019 Pretreatment prediction of adaptive radiation therapy eligibility using MRI-based radiomics for advanced nasopharyngeal carcinoma patients *Front. Oncol.* **9** 1050

[45] Lam S K *et al* 2021 Multi-organ omics-based prediction for adaptive radiation therapy eligibility in nasopharyngeal carcinoma patients undergoing concurrent chemoradiotherapy *Front. Oncol.* **11** 792024

[46] Lam S K *et al* 2022 A multi-center study of CT-based neck nodal radiomics for predicting an adaptive radiotherapy trigger of ill-fitted thermoplastic masks in patients with nasopharyngeal carcinoma *Life* **12** 241

[47] Ho L M, Lam S K, Zhang J, Chiang C L, Chan A C Y and Cai J 2023 Association of multiphasic MR-based radiomic and dosimetric features with treatment response in unresectable hepatocellular carcinoma patients following novel sequential TACE-SBRT-immunotherapy *Cancers* **15** 1105

[48] Sheng J, Lam S, Zhang J, Zhang Y and Cai J 2023 Multi-omics fusion with soft labeling for enhanced prediction of distant metastasis in nasopharyngeal carcinoma patients after radiotherapy *Comput. Biol. Med.* **168** 107684

[49] Zhang Y *et al* 2022 Integration of an imbalance framework with novel high-generalizable classifiers for radiomics-based distant metastases prediction of advanced nasopharyngeal carcinoma *Knowl.-Based Syst.* **235** 107649

[50] Saito N, Imai Y, Muto T and Sairenchi T 2012 Low body mass index as a risk factor of moderate to severe oral mucositis in oral cancer patients with radiotherapy *Support Care Cancer Off. J. Multinatl. Assoc. Support Care Cancer* **20** 3373–7

[51] Shu Z *et al* 2020 Nutritional status and its association with radiation-induced oral mucositis in patients with nasopharyngeal carcinoma during radiotherapy: a prospective study *Front. Oncol.* **10** 594687

[52] Orlandi E *et al* 2018 Multivariable model for predicting acute oral mucositis during combined IMRT and chemotherapy for locally advanced nasopharyngeal cancer patients *Oral Oncol.* **86** 266–72

[53] Wang X *et al* 2022 Risk factors of esophageal fistula induced by re-radiotherapy for recurrent esophageal cancer with local primary site *BMC Cancer* **22** 207

[54] Zhu C, Wang S, You Y, Nie K and Ji Y 2019 Risk factors for esophageal fistula in esophageal cancer patients treated with radiotherapy: a systematic review and meta-analysis *Oncol. Res. Treat.* **43** 34–41

[55] Xu Y *et al* 2021 Integrating clinical data and attentional CT imaging features for esophageal fistula prediction in esophageal cancer *Front. Oncol.* **11** 688706

[56] Li Z, Gong J, Shi L, Li J, Yang Z, Chai G, Lv B, Xiang G, Wang B, Carr S R and Fiorelli A 2024 Clinical-radiomics nomogram for the risk prediction of esophageal fistula in patients with esophageal squamous cell carcinoma treated with intensity-modulated radiation therapy or volumetric-modulated arc therapy *J. Thorac. Dis.* **16** 2032–48

[57] Guo W, Li B, Xu W, Cheng C, Qiu C, Sam S K, Zhang J, Teng X, Meng L, Zheng X and Wang Y 2024 Multi-omics and multi-VOIs to predict esophageal fistula in esophageal cancer patients treated with radiotherapy *J. Cancer Res. Clin. Oncol.* **150** 39

[58] Zander D S and Rassaei N 2018 Drug reactions and other iatrogenic pulmonary diseases *Pulmonary Pathology* Foundations in Diagnostic Pathology 2nd edn ed D S Zander and C F Farver (Amsterdam: Elsevier) pp 396–408

[59] Li B *et al* 2022 Lung subregion partitioning by incremental dose intervals improves omics-based prediction for acute radiation pneumonitis in non-small-cell lung cancer patients *Cancers* **14** 4889

[60] Li B *et al* 2022 Function-wise dual-omics analysis for radiation pneumonitis prediction in lung cancer patients *Front. Pharmacol.* **13** 971849

[61] Zheng X *et al* 2023 Multi-omics to predict acute radiation esophagitis in patients with lung cancer treated with intensity-modulated radiation therapy *Eur. J. Med. Res* **28** 126

[62] Raghu M *et al* 2019 Direct uncertainty prediction for medical second opinions *Proc. Mach. Learn. Res.* **97** 5281–90 https://proceedings.mlr.press/v97/raghu19a.html

[63] Kendall A and Gal Y 2017 What uncertainties do we need in Bayesian deep learning for computer vision? *Advances in Neural Information Processing Systems* vol 30 (Red Hook, NY: Curran Associates)

[64] Dakka M A *et al* 2021 Automated detection of poor-quality data: case studies in healthcare *Sci. Rep.* **11** 18005

[65] Murdoch B 2021 Privacy and artificial intelligence: challenges for protecting health information in a new era *BMC Med. Ethics* **22** 122

[66] Yin J, Ngiam K Y and Teo H H 2021 Role of artificial intelligence applications in real-life clinical practice: systematic review *J. Med. Internet Res.* **23** e25759

[67] Blezek D J, Olson-Williams L, Missert A and Korfiatis P 2021 AI integration in the clinical workflow *J. Digit. Imaging* **34** 1435–46

[68] Wiggins W F *et al* 2021 Imaging AI in practice: a demonstration of future workflow using integration standards *Radiol. Artif. Intell.* **3** e210152

Chapter 4

Imaging technologies in radiation therapy

Xinru Chen, Cenji Yu, Gregory Sharp and Jinzhong Yang

Imaging technologies play a pivotal role in the evolution of radiation therapy, enabling the precise delivery of treatment while minimizing damage to surrounding healthy tissues. In adaptive radiotherapy, the integration of advanced imaging modalities is essential for treatment adjustments based on changes in tumor size, position, and biological characteristics. The ability to dynamically assess and respond to these changes enhances treatment accuracy, ensuring that radiation is delivered optimally throughout the course of therapy. A variety of imaging techniques, each with distinct capabilities, are currently available for use in radiation therapy. These include computed tomography (CT) and magnetic resonance imaging (MRI), positron emission tomography (PET), four-dimensional (4D)-CT and 4D-MRI, and so on. This chapter focuses on the unique contribution of each imaging modality to different stages of radiation therapy, from treatment planning to treatment guidance, motion management, and post-treatment assessment. The advancement of imaging technologies supports the growing need for personalized and precise radiation therapy.

4.1 Introduction

Imaging is a central component of adaptive radiotherapy (ART), because it defines the anatomic and functional changes to be addressed. The earliest proposal for ART in 1997 already provided for the use of imaging to measure and inform geometric changes in anatomy [1], and included a phase II study on off-line ART for prostate cancer [2]. Off-line ART using cone beam computed tomography (CBCT), magnetic resonance imaging (MRI), and functional imaging have been conducted as early as the late 2000s [3, 4]. Pre-treatment online adaptive radiotherapy using MRI has been used since 2014 [5], and using CBCT since at least 2020 [6].

In this chapter, we present the current state-of-the-art in imaging for radiation therapy, with a focus on the technologies and methods used in adaptive therapy. Off-line adaptive therapy is commonly performed when pre-treatment imaging using

doi:10.1088/978-0-7503-6119-4ch4

CBCT shows anatomic change but can also be determined from computed tomography (CT), positron emission tomography (PET), or MRI. Online adaptive therapy is generally based on CBCT or MRI, with PET being a recent addition. In principle, the use of MRI or PET can provide important functional information about changes in the tumor, in addition to anatomic changes. However, adaptation that shrinks the target volume based on either anatomic or functional imaging risks undertreatment of the disease.

4.2 Imaging for treatment planning

Tumor delineation stands as a pivotal process in radiotherapy, influencing treatment accuracy and patient outcomes. Medical imaging plays a crucial role in this regard by facilitating the precise localization of tumor targets for radiation delivery. Historically, planar x-ray imaging served as the primary modality for this purpose. However, the advent of CT revolutionized the field by enabling three-dimensional visualization of both the tumor and surrounding normal tissues within the patient anatomy. CT integration into radiotherapy treatment planning ushered in a new era of three-dimensional dose optimization and enhanced patient positioning accuracy. Despite these advancements, CT exhibits limitations in tissue contrast and lacks functional insights.

The emergence of linear accelerators (linacs) and advanced dose delivery techniques underscores the importance of achieving higher precision in radiotherapy. The accuracy of manual tumor delineation on CT now dictates the level of treatment precision attainable. Consequently, there is a growing demand for more refined tumor definition techniques to optimize patient outcomes. Integrating complementary imaging modalities such as MRI and PET offers a promising avenue for enhancing tumor delineation. MRI excels in providing superior soft tissue contrast, thereby facilitating more accurate tumor delineation compared to CT. PET imaging, on the other hand, offers valuable metabolic and functional information critical for tumor grading and delineation. By combining the strengths of CT with these modalities, clinicians can access a comprehensive dataset that improves tumor definition and, ultimately, treatment efficacy in radiotherapy.

4.2.1 CT simulation

CT provides volumetric imaging for both diagnostic imaging and radiation oncology. CT uses a gantry-mounted x-ray source and detectors to record x-ray transmission of an object. The x-ray source consists of a cathode and an anode. Electrons are produced by the cathode and then accelerated towards a rotating tungsten anode to create x-ray via Bremsstrahlung. The detectors are usually made of a scintillating material, converting x-ray to visible light, which is then collected by a photodiode. During image acquisition, the x-ray and detectors rotate simultaneously. The raw x-ray projection data form a sinogram. The CT image is reconstructed from the sinogram using filtered-back-projection (FBP) techniques. The output of FBP is the linear attenuation coefficient (μ) for each voxel. CT images are displayed with Hounsfield units (HU):

$$HU = 1000 \times \frac{\mu_{material} - \mu_{water}}{\mu_{water}}.$$

CT is commonly used in radiation oncology for patient simulation. It provides planning CT volumes for patient positioning and dose calculation. The CT simulator has a flat couch to mimic the treatment couch of a linac so that the patient pose is similar during treatment. They also have lasers to help reproduce the patient position when aligning for treatment. Unlike CTs in diagnostic imaging, HU accuracy is crucial for CT simulators. The HU is converted to electron density and serves as the basis for dose calculation. The electron density derived from the CT simulator is the gold standard for dose calculation. Therefore, an accurate calibration curve is required during the commissioning of the scanner to ensure accurate dose calculation.

Technological advances in CT have been applied to radiation oncology. Coolens *et al* implemented a 320-slice volumetric scanner for CT simulation [7]. By using volume scanning instead of helical scanning, the scanner can capture the entire treatment site within a single gantry rotation. The scan time is thus reduced, and motion artifacts are minimized. Most centers, however, still use the larger bore helical scanners. Dual-energy CT (DECT) was investigated as a candidate for simulation in proton therapy. By capturing CT images under two energies, DECT can differentiate x-ray attenuation change in density or chemical composition [8]. It can then calculate stopping power ratio and improve proton radiotherapy planning by reducing range uncertainties. Currently, the high level of noise still hinders the wider adoption of DECT in proton therapy simulation [9]. More recently, clinical deployment of photon counting CT (PCCT) also provides opportunities in the improvement of radiation simulation. The photon counting detector can resolve energy by counting photons in selected energy bins. It has the potential to directly calculate the stopping power ratio using the Bethe–Bloch equation. The scanner achieved stopping power ratio estimates that are comparable to DECT scanners [10]. PCCT is also capable of generating quantitative contrast enhanced CT scans. It can leverage the photon counting detector's energy resolution to provide increased tissue and contrast agent discrimination. This capability helps PCCT generate virtual non-contrast electron density and stopping power [11]. Patients can potentially avoid a non-contrast scan as well as its dose during simulation.

4.2.2 4D-CT

Four-dimensional CT (4D-CT) is often used for motion management during patient simulation. Patient breathing motion can often introduce uncertainty and blurring in simulation CT scans. 4D-CT captures multiple CT volumes at different phases of a patient's breathing motion. This acquisition protocol oversamples at every position of interest in the superior–inferior direction by using the axial cine mode. Multiple CT images are reconstructed per slice and each of them represents a different anatomical state during a respiratory cycle. These CT images are sorted based on the phase of breathing measured by a breathing monitoring device such as respiratory gating system or abdominal belt [12]. The entire 4D-CT volume captures the patient motion throughout the entire breathing cycle. Maximum intensity projection and average CT are often compiled from the 4D-CT volume to account for patient motion. Clinicians can then define the treatment target based on the tumor and organs-at-risk (OARs) motion throughout the treatment.

4.2.3 PET/CT

PET serves as a valuable tool for investigating the biodistribution of radio-labeled tracers, thereby enabling crucial metabolic and functional insights based on the biochemical pathways of these tracers. Among the commonly utilized tracers, fluorine-18 fludeoxyglucose (^{18}F-FDG) stands out as a glucose analog that undergoes cellular uptake and subsequent intracellular entrapment. Through this mechanism, FDG-PET identifies metabolically active tissue within the body. PET/CT imaging combines anatomical and metabolic information, with CT images providing anatomical reference points and aiding in attenuation correction for PET data. The integration of PET and CT functionalities within a hybrid device mitigates the risk of misalignment associated with patient repositioning [13]. PET/CT plays a pivotal role in identifying primary tumors and associated regional lymph nodes based on the increased uptake of ^{18}F-FDG [14]. Its utility becomes particularly evident in scenarios where tumor volumes are poorly defined or when dose escalation is warranted, necessitating precise delineation of tumor volumes and distinct boundaries from surrounding tissues.

Studies have underscored the efficacy of PET/CT in tumor delineation for various cancers, including lung, head and neck, esophageal, and cervical malignancies [15]. In lung cancer, PET/CT facilitates more accurate lymph node staging [16], reduces inter-observer variability during tumor delineation [17], and refines the delineation of tumor borders in conjunction with atelectasis [18]. Notably, PET/CT-derived gross tumor volumes (GTVs) have demonstrated superior accuracy when comparing with surgical specimens in a head and neck cancer study [19]. Prospective investigations in esophageal and cervical cancers have corroborated the positive impact of PET/CT on tumor delineation and the significant reduction in late radiation toxicity [20–22]. The evolution of PET/CT-guided radiotherapy has gained interest in dose painting strategies targeting specific tumor sub-volumes based on biological imaging [23]. Escalated doses can be prescribed to radio-resistant tumor regions to enhance local tumor control [24].

Despite the widespread use of ^{18}F-FDG, other PET tracers such as fluorine-18 fluoromisonidazole (FMISO) and fluorine-18 fluoroazomycin arabinoside (FAZA) provide non-invasive and quantitative assessments of tumor hypoxia—a critical determinant of radiation treatment resistance. Hypoxia volumes measured via FMISO-PET serve as predictive factors for patient survival in head and neck cancer [25]. Targeting hypoxic tumor volumes with escalated doses represents a promising strategy to improve tumor control. Additionally, the active cellular proliferation characteristic of tumors can be assessed using fluorine-18 fluorothymidine (^{18}F-FLT), a thymidine analogue that monitors thymidine kinase activity—a surrogate marker for cell proliferation [26]. Given its low uptake in inflammatory tissues, ^{18}F-FLT is preferred in highly inflammatory cancers such as head and neck cancer, where false-positive results from FDG-PET could lead to the enlargement of GTVs [27].

While PET imaging aids in avoiding tumor misses and minimizing unnecessary radiation exposure to healthy tissues, its spatial resolution remains a limitation compared to modern CT scanners [28]. The spatial resolution of current PET scanners typically ranges from 5 to 8 mm, which may result in the oversight of small lesions, particularly in cases of significant patient motion [29]. Furthermore, there is a risk of including non-malignant FDG-avid tissue within the target volume, potentially increasing the likelihood of long-term complications. The delineation method employed significantly impacts the quality assessment of GTVs. While thresholding based on a percentage of the maximum tumor standardized uptake value (SUV_{max}) is a common approach [30], alternative methods such as contrast-based [31], gradient-based [32], and statistically stochastic algorithms [33] are also utilized, with their efficacy dependent on imaging parameters and tumor characteristics [30].

4.2.4 MRI

Despite its established role in diagnostic imaging, MRI has emerged as a valuable complement to CT imaging in radiotherapy treatment planning. MRI offers several advantages over CT, notably superior soft tissue contrast and its intrinsic three-dimensional imaging capability. However, limitations include the absence of electron density information, geometric distortion, and a restricted field-of-view (FOV). Nonetheless, advancements in MRI technology have facilitated its integration into the radiotherapy workflow. Initially, disparities in patient positioning between diagnostic MR scans and radiotherapy simulation CT scans posed challenges due to the differences between curved cushion-lined MR systems with flat-bed couches in CT scanners. Subsequent availability of commercial MRI-simulators featuring flat-bed couches has mitigated this issue. Nevertheless, image co-registration remains essential to align the two modalities within the same coordinate system. Image registration introduces systematic geometrical uncertainties of 2–3 mm throughout the treatment process, potentially compromising tumor control [34]. The integration of MRI into treatment planning has yielded significant improvements in target delineation quality and reduced inter-observer variability, particularly in tumors of the brain, head and neck, and pelvis [35].

As a multi-parametric modality, MR systems offer both anatomical and functional information through diverse techniques and sequences. The concept of MR-only treatment planning has recently gained traction [34]. While MRI inherently lacks direct electron density information, various methods have been proposed to generate synthetic CT images based on MRI data [36, 37]. However, challenges such as image distortion and artifacts have hindered the widespread adoption of MRI as a primary imaging modality in radiotherapy planning. Despite these challenges, ongoing research aims to address these limitations and further optimize the integration of MRI into radiotherapy planning workflows [38 41].

4.2.4.1 Anatomical MRI

MRI relies on the detection of nuclear magnetic moments, primarily originating from hydrogen nuclei (protons) that are predominantly found in water and lipids within the body. These protons undergo precession at the Larmor frequency ($\omega_0 = \gamma B_0$) when subjected to a strong main magnetic field (B_0), where γ represents the gyromagnetic ratio. MR images can be acquired to visualize the distribution of protons in the body, commonly referred to as proton density images. However, proton density images typically exhibit limited tissue contrast, although they prove valuable in diagnosing conditions such as edema and inflammatory diseases [42]. The most frequently employed anatomical MRI sequences include T1-weighted (T1w) and T2-weighted (T2w) scans, which rely on the manipulation of longitudinal (T1) and transverse (T2) relaxation times. These relaxation times are influenced by molecular motion and interactions within tissues, resulting in varying signal characteristics across different tissue types. Contrast in MRI is achieved by weighting signals based on T1 and T2 relaxation times. T1w images are generated using short echo time (TE) and relaxation time (TR), whereas T2w images are produced using relatively longer TE and TR parameters. Various techniques, such as fat saturation, inversion-recovery imaging, and opposed-phase imaging, can be employed to suppress fat signal, enhancing tissue contrast [43]. T1w and T2w images find extensive utility in MR-guided adaptive radiotherapy, facilitating improved visualization and delineation of target volumes [44].

4.2.4.2 Post-contrasted MRI

Paramagnetic or superparamagnetic agents capable of significantly altering the relaxation times (T1 and/or T2) of nearby protons serve as crucial MRI contrast agents. Among the most employed agents is gadolinium-based contrast agent, which effectively shortens T1 relaxation times. Tissues enhanced with gadolinium-based agents exhibit increased signals in T1w images. Studies indicate that gadolinium-contrasted MRI yields better concordance with biopsy findings compared to T2w MRI [45]. Another prevalent contrast agent is superparamagnetic iron oxide (SPIO) particles, which attenuate T2 signals in tissues where they accumulate, and are commonly employed in imaging of kidneys and spleens [46]. Additionally, manganese-based and iron platinum-based agents are currently under investigation [47].

Dynamic contrast enhanced MRI (DCE-MRI) involves the acquisition of T1w images before and after the administration of contrast agents. DCE-MRI enables the measurement of multiple parameters related to tissue perfusion and micro-vascular status. Integration of DCE-MRI into tumor delineation protocols has been shown to reduce inter-observer variability [48]. Dynamic susceptibility contrast MRI (DSC-MRI) captures local magnetic inhomogeneities between extra- and intra-vascular volumes, generating attenuated T2 signals due to the presence of contrast agents within the vasculature [49]. Moreover, blood oxygen level-dependent (BOLD) imaging exploits differences in magnetic susceptibility between oxyhemo-globin and deoxyhemoglobin, while diffusion-weighted imaging (DWI) quantifies molecular diffusion properties within tissues. These modalities have demonstrated efficacy in delineating tumor boundaries [50–54]. However, considerable variation exists in the consistency of target volumes delineated using these protocols [55, 56].

4.3 Imaging for treatment guidance

4.3.1 Portal imaging

Modern image-guided radiation therapy (IGRT) systems are typically equipped with two imaging panels, the electric portal imaging device (EPID) and kV imaging panel. The EPID is used to capture 2D-MV planar images. It is typically an amorphous-silicon (a-Si) flat-panel imaging device mounted on a robotic arm directly under the linac head. The Varian Truebeam equipped with the latest aS1200 panel has a 40 × 40 cm^2 active imaging area and a pixel size of 0.0336 cm. The robotic arm allows a source to EPID distance from 95 to 180 cm. Improvements have been made on the panel so that it can handle a flattening filter free (FFF) dose rate without saturation at any source to detector distance [57]. Elekta linacs are equipped with iViewGT EPID. The active imaging area is 41 × 41 cm^2. The image matrix is created from an array of 1024 × 1024 diodes with a pitch of 400 μm [58]. Both the Varian and Elekta IGRT systems are also capable of capturing kV planar images. The Varian On-Board Imager (OBI) has two robotic arms that are mounted perpendicular to the radiation beam. One holds the x-ray source and the other holds the a-Si flat-panel detector. The active imaging area is 40 × 30 cm^2 for the OBI system. The user can adjust the source to imager distance from 100 to 182.5 cm depending on the imaging protocol. The Elekta X-ray Volume Imaging (XVI) system has a similar layout with two robotic arms. The active imaging is 42.5 × 42.5 cm^2. The high contrast spatial resolutions of the two systems are comparable [58, 59]. Both kV and MV planar imaging techniques are quick to acquire and deliver less dose to the patient. While soft tissue might be difficult to visualize on planar images, bony structures or fiducials are visible. This makes planar x-ray imaging ideal for treatment set-up verification.

4.3.2 CBCT

4.3.2.1 kV-CBCT
For modern IGRT systems, gantry-mounted kV imaging is an important component. Elekta's XVI and Varian's OBI provide imaging at the same isocenter of the linear accelerator. With kV-CBCT, volumetric imaging is available for therapists to align patient to the reference CT simulation image before each fraction. This allows the localization of patient anatomy at each treatment fraction and improves the accuracy of treatment delivery.

The developments in flat-panel detectors made gantry-mounted kV-CBCT possible. The a-Si flat-panel detector used in gantry-mounted kV imaging systems is made up of a CsI plastic scintillator which converts the x-ray photons into visible light which is then detected by a-Si thin film transistor (TFT) and read out as an electrical signal [60]. This indirect detector is ideal for the orthogonal configuration proposed by Jaffray *et al* [61] due to its compact size and potential for high resolution imaging. Cone beam reconstruction was applied to reconstruct a volumetric image from the flat panel. Compared to multi-slice detectors in fan beam CTs, the a-Si flat panel has a lower x-ray cross section, higher noise, longer readout, and longer time to reset. These properties are important factors to consider when it is used as image guidance for adaptive radiation therapy. In addition, the on-board CBCT's FOV is limited by the size of the flat-panel detector. Cone beam reconstruction only requires a 180° rotation under full-fan mode to acquire a sonogram for a volumetric image. A half fan technique was proposed to increase the FOV to up to 50 cm. The detector and the kV source are offset in this configuration. A 360° rotation is required to acquire two separate sonograms that are stitched together for a full view of the patient.

Accurate characterization of the HU is crucial for CBCT used in adaptive therapy settings. Calibration of the flat panel is thus essential for an adaptive program. The pixel array of the flat-panel detector is made of groups of a-Si units. Each pixel has different calibration curve. Dark field calibration is used to characterize the dark signal of the pixel. Flood field calibration is used to characterize the slope of the calibration curve. Individual calibration curves are applied to each pixel so that the response of the flat panel remains uniform despite variances within readout electronics. However, cone beam geometry introduces non-uniformity in HU characterization for CBCT. The x-ray scatter is more pronounced at the center of the CBCT image for large FOV scans. This leads to cupping artifacts and introduces non-uniformity into the volumetric image. CBCT is also susceptible to motion artifacts. Since the on-board imager takes around 60s to complete the acquisition, CBCT is more susceptible to motion artifacts compared to fan beam CT. Metal artifacts in CBCT are also more pronounced due to the lack of metal artifact reduction common in diagnostic CT. These artifacts contribute to uncertainties in HU characterization and should be noted for CBCT-based adaptive therapy programs.

4.3.2.2 Hypersight kV-CBCT

The new Hypersight kV-CBCT system integrated in the Halcyon/Ethos ring style linac was introduced recently. The new system applied iterative CBCT image reconstruction (iCBCT) techniques to reconstruct the volumetric image. Compared to the filter back projection-based Feldkamp–Davis–Kress (FDK) algorithm, iCBCT exhibited increased accuracy in CT number accuracy and reduced noise. In addition, a larger kV imaging panel (86×43 cm^2 versus 43×43 cm^2) made of cesium iodide scintillator (higher efficiency) was added. With the larger panel, the imager operates in full-fan mode. The detector with a high frame rate also enabled a faster scan time down to 5.9 s. A new anti-scatter grid was introduced. A more robust scatter correction algorithm incorporating Acuros CTS based scatter model and Monte Carlo based hardware scatter was incorporated in the iCBCT software [62]. It also incorporated an extended FOV (eFOV) up to 70 cm and metal artifact reduction (MAR).

The new CBCT addressed many existing concerns with CBCT regarding scatter correction, metal artifacts, and motion artifacts for image quality. For adaptive therapy purposes, the CBCT system generated encouraging results. The new imaging system achieved more realistic CT numbers under the CBCT mode. In a recent study by Bogowicz *et al* [63], the CBCT-based planning dose distributions showed an agreement above 97% and 93% for gamma analysis with criteria of 3%/1 mm and 2%/1 mm, respectively, compared with the simulation CT dose distribution. All dose–volume histogram (DVH) differences between CT and CBCT were below 2%. The CBCT images provided by the Hypersight kV-CBCT system would be suitable for online adaptive radiotherapy workflow.

4.3.3 CT-on-rail and CT-linac

In modern radiotherapy, the minimization of treatment margins holds significant importance as these margins directly correlate with excessive tissue toxicity and impose constraints on the dose escalation necessary for improved tumor control. Enhancing the accuracy of daily patient set-up and tumor localization represents a pivotal approach to address this challenge. The integration of in-room CT scanners has significantly contributed to the implementation of imaging-guided techniques [64]. Siemens introduced the PRIMATOM system, featuring a fixed couch and diagnostic CT scanners mounted on rails, commonly referred to as 'CT-on-rail' systems. In this set-up, the linac gantry and CT gantry can be positioned on opposite ends of the treatment couch. Pre-treatment 3D CT localization of the tumor is achieved by rotating the couch 180°. The reported positional accuracy of the couch in CT-on-rail systems is within 0.4 mm in all three directions [65]. Systematic investigations have been conducted to assess the mechanical uncertainties of CT-on-rail systems [66]. Given the superior image quality and the ability to visualize real-time anatomy while the patient is immobilized, CT-on-rail systems have found extensive application in clinical studies, particularly in prostate cancer treatment. Various institutions have reported the feasibility and dosimetric advantages of CT-on-rail for daily prostate alignment [67–69]. Moreover, the system has demonstrated utility in other treatment sites characterized by significant target position variability, such as the lungs and liver [70, 71].

Another innovative solution incorporating in-room CT scanning is the CT-linac system, which integrates a C-arm linear accelerator with a CT scanner coaxially attached behind the linear accelerator. Unlike the CT-on-rail approach, the CT-linac system eliminates the need for 180 ° couch rotation, thereby reducing the uncertainties associated with rotation. Investigations have demonstrated that the CT-linac system offers clinically acceptable plan quality and dose delivery efficiency [72–74].

4.3.4 MR-linac

The MR-linac represents one of the latest developments of image-guided adaptive radiotherapy. It utilizes real-time on-board MRI during treatment sessions to guide and adapt the delivery of radiation. A unique advantage of MR-guided radiotherapy (MRgRT) is the superior visualization of tumors and soft tissues provided by the real-time MRI [75]. The crispy target visualization and online adaptive platform offered by MR-linac enables precise targeting while minimizing radiation exposure to healthy tissues, leading to improved therapeutic outcomes. In addition, MRgRT has the advantage of real-time imaging while the treatment beam is on, enabling real-time target motion monitoring and tracking, further improving the precision of radiation treatment. The currently most popular MR-linac systems are summarized below. Details of the MRgRT can be found in chapter 16.

4.3.4.1 Low field MR-linac

The ViewRay MRIdian system is a representative of low field MR-linac systems. The ViewRay system integrates a 0.35 tesla low field MRI scanner with a linear accelerator for MRI-guided treatment. This system is the first MR-linac device used for clinical MRgRT and received Food and Drug Administration (FDA) approval in 2017 [5]. The MRIdian system consists of a split-bore superconducting magnet with a bore diameter of 70 cm perpendicular to a 6 MV FFF linear accelerator system. The linear accelerator produces coplanar static intensity-modulated radiation therapy (IMRT) fields and delivers dose at 650 MU/min with a 0.5 revolutions per minute (rpm) gantry rotation. The MRI system uses a balanced steady state free precession pulse sequence for MR imaging that can be used for treatment planning and set-up verification. The MRIdian system also allows for real-time imaging during treatment beam-on, enabling intrafraction motion monitoring during treatment. This feature allows for real-time tumor tracking and automatic beam gating based on user defined gating boundaries on a sagittal cine image [76]. Another low field MR-linac system is the MagnetTx Aurora-RT, which is a 0.5 tesla MR-linac utilizing an open bore in-line design to mitigate the electron return effect [77]. The Aurora-RT received FDA premarket clearance in 2022 and treated its first patient in 2023.

4.3.4.2 High field MR-linac

The Elekta Unity system (Elekta AB, Stockholm, Sweden) is the first high field MR-linac that integrates a 7 MV FFF linac system and a 1.5 tesla Philips (Philips Healthcare, Best, the Netherlands) MRI system [78]. The Unity system is designed as a bore-type machine with a linac system rotating around the MRI system, which has an inner bore diameter of 70 cm [79]. The radiation beam is perpendicular to the magnetic field orientation. The treatment couch moves in the longitudinal direction only; however, during treatment the couch is not designed to move to adjust treatment isocenter location. Instead, online adaptive planning is utilized to account for isocenter shifts. The system offers an integrated online adaptive planning workflow and every fraction treated with Elekta Unity requires an online adaptive planning. The system also allows for simultaneous MR imagining and treatment delivery. In its first version, the Unity system offered only tumor motion monitoring [80]. In late 2023, Elekta released the comprehensive motion management (CMM) system, allowing for different levels of motion management for better control of respiratory motion and other motion uncertainty during treatment delivery [81]. It is also worth noting that due to the high strength of the magnetic field, the beam profile is inherently off-center and asymmetric, and the electron return effect can cause electrons to change trajectory to 'return' to a higher density material at the interface of exiting a higher density material into a lower density material [82].

4.3.5 PET-linac

The advent of PET-linac systems, exemplified by the Reflexion system, has introduced the concept of biology-guided radiotherapy (BgRT) [83]. Integrating both kV CT and PET scanners within a ring gantry linear accelerator, the Reflexion system enables real-time beamlet conformation based on PET signals acquired from the tumor, with sub-second latency. This swift response capability allows the system to manage patient motion without the need for motion trackers or breath-holding techniques. Moreover, PET images generated by the Reflexion system exhibit comparability to those obtained from traditional PET/CT scanners [84]. PET images hold significant potential in the realm of biologically adaptive radiation therapy (BART), which integrates tumor or OAR function into adaptive planning strategies. Prior trials have demonstrated the advantages of intra-treatment FDG and hypoxia PET images in facilitating dose escalation and enhancing local tumor control [85, 86]. The evolution of PET-linac technology is expected to facilitate clinical trials aimed at investigating the efficacy of daily PET-guided plan adaptation.

4.4 Imaging for motion management

4.4.1 ExacTrac

Novalis ExacTrac system is an x-ray system designed for stereotactic radiosurgery (SRS) and stereotactic body radiotherapy (SBRT). The system consists of two components: a real-time infrared (IR) tracking system and a kV imaging system. The IR system detects motion in real time using the IR reflecting markers. These markers can be placed on the reference frame mounted on the treatment couch, or on the patient's skin. The camera combined with the IR system confirms patient positioning and monitors patient movement. The x-ray system has two x-ray tubes installed in the floor and two flat-panel detectors mounted on the ceiling. The system is mounted obliquely to the mid-sagittal plane of the accelerator. The x-ray system acquires projection images and localizes the patient by registering bony landmarks or implanted markers with the corresponding digitally reconstructed radiograph (DRR) from the planning CT.

4.4.2 Varian triggered imaging

Triggered imaging is a kV imaging technique included in the Varian advanced imaging package. Triggered imaging uses the OBI of the Varian Truebeam to monitor high contrast regions during treatment delivery. The high contrast regions are typically implanted fiducial markers, endogenous patient anatomy (vertebral body and spinous process), or endogenous orthopedic hardware [87]. The kV images are typically taken with an intrafraction motion review application at specific gantry intervals to ensure accurate delivery. The system is capable of auto beam hold (ABH), pausing the beam delivery when the tracking region falls outside of tolerance. Varian triggered imaging enables intrafraction IGRT. There have been studies to conduct spine SBRT using spinal fixation hardware with Varian triggered imaging [88].

4.4.3 4D-CBCT

Four-dimensional CBCT (4D-CBCT) was developed to address respiratory motion artifacts from CBCT. Under a 4D acquisition mode, the CBCT sorts projections into different respiratory phase bins according to the patient's breathing cycle. Just like 4D-CT, it provides a set of phase-resolved volumetric images and minimizes motion blurring artifacts [89]. 4D-CBCT images can also be aligned with 4D-CT images to correct set-up errors or monitor motion prior to treatment. The application of 4D-CBCT in the clinic, however, is limited due to its long acquisition time. The total acquisition time for an Elekta XVI system is around 4 min. Recent developments in deep learning-driven reconstruction in 4D-CBCT have the potential to expedite the deployment of 4D-CBCT in clinics [90].

4.4.4 Cine MRI

The rapid acquisition of 2D cine MRI presents a valuable opportunity for real-time target position verification in MRgRT settings. Utilizing single or orthogonal 2D cine MRI images at a frequency of approximately 5 frames per second (fps) within modern MR-linac systems enables dynamic motion monitoring [91, 92]. Real-time cine MRI serves multiple purposes, including motion tracking [92, 93] and beam gating techniques [94, 95] to mitigate uncertainties stemming from intrafraction motion. Motion tracking algorithms utilize image registration to continuously assess target location, allowing for real-time adjustments of multi-leaf collimator (MLC) leaf positions to accommodate changes in the target position [96]. Beam gating relies on comparing real-time 2D cine MRI with pre-treatment reference MRI to calculate target contour shifts, gating off the beam when the target exceeds predefined boundaries [97]. Additionally, investigations into dynamic slice selection or multi-slice cine acquisition techniques aim to extend real-time motion monitoring to multiple targets or OARs [98, 99]. Moreover, the availability of cine MRI facilitates the evaluation of the relationship between tumors and surrogate markers used for motion management, such as the skin surface. Retrospective studies have raised concerns regarding the weak correlation between vertical belly motion and longitudinal tumor motion [100].

4.4.5 4D-MRI

Respiratory-correlated four-dimensional MRI (RC-4D-MRI) serves as a valuable tool for characterizing respiratory motion throughout the thorax and abdomen, offering improved visualization of OARs and enhanced flexibility in image orientation compared to 4D-CT [101]. Various strategies are employed to gather volumetric data in RC-4D-MRI. 2D retrospective algorithms capture signals repeatedly from the same volume and subsequently sort them according to the respiratory cycle [102, 103]. However, retrospective algorithms are susceptible to unstable respiratory motion, leading to missing slices. In contrast, 2D prospective algorithms acquire slices based on real-time respiratory signals, thus avoiding missing slices and enhancing acquisition efficiency [104, 105]. Recently, algorithms utilizing 3D read-outs have emerged, offering improved signal-to-noise ratio (SNR), enhanced geometric correction, motion averaging effects, and increased flexibility in image dimensions [106–108]. Unlike RC-4D-MRI, which employs respiratory phase as the fourth dimension, time-resolved four-dimensional MRI (TR-4D-MRI) does not assume periodic respiratory motion, representing real-time data in the fourth dimension. Consequently, TR-4D-MRI offers advantages in assessing irregular respiratory motion or joint organ motion resulting from cardiac or digestive motion [109]. 4D-MRI serves to provide valuable reference images for treatment planning and the derivation of target and OAR motion models. A common motion management strategy involves delineating the internal target volume (ITV) by propagating gross tumor volume contours across different phases to encompass the dynamic target motion range [110].

4.4.6 Surface imaging

VisionRT is a surface imaging system for patient motion monitoring and tracking. The system uses a pair of 3D cameras to project a speckled light pattern onto the patient surface. The distortions and changes in the pattern are used for 3D reconstruction. VisionRT's software then constructs a 3D surface model by rendering points into wireframe. This surface was then rigidly registered to a reference surface in six degree of freedom (6DOF) to account for translational and rotational shifts [111]. The reference surface can be the recorded surface of the patient or derived from the body contours from CT volumetric data. The VisionRT system can then display the 6DOF shift within the region-of-interest in real time to help monitor or align the patient surface. These shifts can also be used to trigger beam hold during treatment when the shift exceeded the preset threshold.

4.5 Imaging for treatment assessment

Treatment assessment plays a crucial role in evaluating the efficacy of interventions and guiding clinical decision-making for healthcare providers. Medical imaging techniques enable comprehensive, three-dimensional, and non-invasive assessment of tumors throughout the body. Traditionally, changes in tumor size observed in anatomical imaging have served as the primary criterion for treatment response assessment, as outlined in guidelines such as those established by the World Health Organization (WHO) and the response evaluation criteria in solid tumors (RECIST) [112–114]. However, tumor size changes in many cases are slow to manifest and occasionally challenging to discern, potentially leading to delays in therapeutic decision-making [115]. In contrast, functional imaging methodologies offer the capability to detect changes in biological and metabolic activities within tumors, providing insights into cellular-level changes and facilitating earlier tumor assessments.

4.5.1 Contrasted CT

Contrast-enhanced CT serves as a prominent modality for evaluating treatment response in clinical practice. Upon intravenous administration of iodinated contrast agents, CT signals undergo enhancement due to increased attenuation, directly proportional to the concentration of the administered agents. This enhancement pattern is influenced by factors including blood flow, capillary permeability, diffusion rate, and the volume of the extravascular extracellular space. Dynamic contrast enhanced CT (DCE-CT) involves acquiring a temporal series of images during contrast agent administration, enabling assessment of tumor vascular support [116]. The inherent quantitative relationship between signal enhancement and contrast concentration facilitates precise perfusion assessment, as a notable advantage over DCE-MRI [117]. Moreover, DCE-CT demonstrates high reproducibility. Changes in vascular volume observed in DCE-CT can serve as valuable biomarkers for treatment response assessment, as microvascular damage constitutes a critical mechanism underlying tumor response to radiation therapy [118]. Numerous studies have documented reductions in parameters such as blood flow, blood volume, mean transit time, and permeability–surface-area product following radiochemotherapy in patients with diverse malignancies, underscoring the utility of DCE-CT in monitoring treatment response and guiding therapeutic decisions [119–125].

4.5.2 PET/CT

As depicted in section 4.2.2, PET/CT enables the monitoring of biological and metabolic functions within the body using diverse tracers. Given that tumor response is linked to tumor biology and microenvironmental characteristics, PET/CT emerges as a potent modality for assessing early tumor response following radiotherapy, thereby facilitating personalized treatment management [126]. FDG-PET is widely utilized in the treatment assessment of progressive tumors with high FDG avidity, including lymphoma [127–129], breast cancer [130–132], non-small cell lung cancer [133–135], esophageal cancer [136–138], colorectal cancer [139, 140], and various other malignancies [141–145]. The post-treatment SUV_{max} has been reported to be predictive of complete response and patient survival [146–148]. Studies have shown that FDG-PET achieves higher sensitivity and specificity compared to DCE-CT in lymphoma and ovarian malignancy [149–151]. Moreover, PET/CT can be employed to image cell proliferation using ^{18}F-FLT. Unlike FDG, FLT is exclusively taken up by actively dividing cells. Changes in FLT uptake serve as indicators of cellular response to treatment even before visible alterations in tumor volume manifest, providing early decision support for patients [152, 153].

4.5.3 Functional MRI

Pathophysiological and microstructural changes in metabolic tissue profile, tissue blood perfusion, microvessel permeability, and water mobility can be evaluated using functional MRI techniques such as DCE-MRI, DWI, and magnetic resonance spectroscopy (MRS) [154]. Similar to DCE-CT, DCE-MRI enables the assessment of perfusion and permeability for studying tumor vascular physiology. Estimated DCE-MRI parameters have been correlated with treatment response in various cancers including brain tumor, head and neck cancer, breast cancer, rectal cancer, and prostate cancer [155–159]. DWI is sensitive to the Brownian motion of microscopic water molecules. Tumor necrosis in response to therapy typically exhibits decreased cellularity, resulting in reduced signal on DWI and increased apparent diffusion coefficient (ADC) [160]. Changes in diffusion signal and ADC have proven valuable in predicting tumor response in numerous studies [161–163]. MRS offers insight into the metabolic composition of tissue, including metabolism, membrane turnover, necrosis, energy homeostasis, and proliferation [154]. Tumor response is often associated with increased signals from lactate, lipid, or choline concentrations [164–168].

4.6 Summary

Imaging is playing an increasingly important role in radiation oncology, from pre-treatment tumor staging, treatment planning, target delineation, to in-treatment image-guidance and post-treatment response monitoring. Traditionally, CT plays the most important role in the pre-treatment stage. A well calibrated CT image provides accurate electron density for dose calculation and clear anatomical information for treatment target and OAR delineation in modern treatment planning. In recent years, MR has played a more and more important role in pre-treatment, given the sophisticated technological advancements in synthetic CT creation [169, 170] and crispy soft tissue visualization. In-treatment guidance, from traditional portal imaging to CBCT and CT-on-rail, and most recent MR guidance (MR-linac) and biological guidance (PET-linac), the technological advancement has enabled high-precision radiation oncology with real-time adaptive planning. In post-treatment, functional MRI and PET have been widely used as an effective non-invasive tool to monitor treatment response [171]. They are often used as informative tools to decide whether further invasive operation is needed or not to achieve optimal cancer management. Finally, it is also worth mentioning that artificial intelligence (AI) has greatly reshaped the future of imaging in radiation oncology. AI technologies have been widely used in image reconstruction, post-reconstruction image processing, treatment planning, treatment guidance, and predictive modeling for treatment outcome monitoring [172]. In future research, a deeper integration of AI technologies with all aspects of imaging in radiation oncology should be a focus. Particularly, the exploration of pre-treatment and in-treatment quantitative imaging biomarkers for treatment outcome prediction, patient stratification, and personalized treatment would be an important research area.

References

[1] Yan D, Vicini F, Wong J and Martinez A 1997 Adaptive radiation therapy *Phys. Med. Biol.* **42** 123–32
[2] Martinez A A *et al* 2001 Improvement in dose escalation using the process of adaptive radiotherapy combined with three-dimensional conformal or intensity-modulated beams for prostate cancer *Int. J. Radiat. Oncol.* **50** 1226–34

[3] Nijkamp J *et al* 2008 Adaptive radiotherapy for prostate cancer using kilovoltage cone-beam computed tomography: first clinical results *Int. J. Radiat. Oncol.* **70** 75–82

[4] Geets X *et al* 2007 Adaptive biological image-guided IMRT with anatomic and functional imaging in pharyngo-laryngeal tumors: impact on target volume delineation and dose distribution using helical tomotherapy *Radiother. Oncol.* **85** 105–15

[5] Mutic S and Dempsey J F 2014 The ViewRay system: magnetic resonance-guided and controlled radiotherapy *Semin. Radiat. Oncol.* **24** 196–9

[6] Andersson L *et al* 2020 PO-1939: training of RTT on CBCT online adaptive radiotherapy—first step finding the future 'adapters' *Radiother. Oncol.* **152** S1079

[7] Coolens C *et al* 2009 Implementation and characterization of a 320-slice volumetric CT scanner for simulation in radiation oncology *Med. Phys.* **36** 5120–7

[8] Zhu J and Penfold S N 2016 Dosimetric comparison of stopping power calibration with dual-energy CT and single-energy CT in proton therapy treatment planning *Med. Phys.* **43** 2845–54

[9] Bär E, Lalonde A, Royle G, Lu H-M and Bouchard H 2017 The potential of dual-energy CT to reduce proton beam range uncertainties *Med. Phys.* **44** 2332–44

[10] Hu G *et al* 2022 Assessment of quantitative information for radiation therapy at a first-generation clinical photon-counting computed tomography scanner *Front. Oncol.* **12** 970299

[11] Simard M, Lapointe A, Lalonde A, Bahig H and Bouchard H 2019 The potential of photon-counting CT for quantitative contrast-enhanced imaging in radiotherapy *Phys. Med. Biol.* **64** 115020

[12] Rietzel E, Pan T and Chen G T Y 2005 Four-dimensional computed tomography: image formation and clinical protocol *Med. Phys.* **32** 874–89

[13] Senan S and De Ruysscher D 2005 Critical review of PET-CT for radiotherapy planning in lung cancer *Crit. Rev. Oncol. Hematol.* **56** 345–51

[14] Fonti R, Conson M and Del Vecchio S 2019 PET/CT in radiation oncology *Semin. Oncol.* **46** 202–9

[15] Jelercic S and Rajer M 2015 The role of PET-CT in radiotherapy planning of solid tumours *Radiol. Oncol.* **49** 1–9

[16] De Ruysscher D *et al* 2005 Selective mediastinal node irradiation based on FDG-PET scan data in patients with non-small-cell lung cancer: a prospective clinical study *Int. J. Radiat. Oncol.* **62** 988–94

[17] Steenbakkers R J H M *et al* 2006 Reduction of observer variation using matched CT-PET for lung cancer delineation: a three-dimensional analysis *Int. J. Radiat. Oncol.* **64** 435–48

[18] Nestle U, Kremp S and Grosu A-L 2006 Practical integration of [^{18}F]-FDG-PET and PET-CT in the planning of radiotherapy for non-small cell lung cancer (NSCLC): the technical basis, ICRU-target volumes, problems, perspectives *Radiother. Oncol.* **81** 209–25

[19] Daisne J-F *et al* 2004 Tumor volume in pharyngolaryngeal squamous cell carcinoma: comparison at CT, MR imaging, and FDG PET and validation with surgical specimen *Radiology* **233** 93–100

[20] Leong T *et al* 2006 A prospective study to evaluate the impact of FDG-PET on CT-based radiotherapy treatment planning for oesophageal cancer *Radiother. Oncol.* **78** 254–61

[21] Kidd E A *et al* 2010 Clinical outcomes of definitive intensity-modulated radiation therapy with fluorodeoxyglucose–positron emission tomography simulation in patients with locally advanced cervical cancer *Int. J. Radiat. Oncol.* **77** 1085–91

[22] Schreurs L M A *et al* 2010 Impact of 18-fluorodeoxyglucose positron emission tomography on computed tomography defined target volumes in radiation treatment planning of esophageal cancer: reduction in geographic misses with equal inter-observer variability: PET/CT improves esophageal target definition *Dis. Esoph.* **23** 493–501

[23] Bradley J *et al* 2004 Impact of FDG-PET on radiation therapy volume delineation in non-small-cell lung cancer *Int. J. Radiat. Oncol.* **59** 78–86

[24] Aerts H J W L *et al* 2009 Identification of residual metabolic-active areas within individual NSCLC tumours using a pre-radiotherapy ^{18}fluorodeoxyglucose-PET-CT scan *Radiother. Oncol.* **91** 386–92

[25] Rajendran J G *et al* 2006 Tumor hypoxia imaging with [F-18] fluoromisonidazole positron emission tomography in head and neck cancer *Clin. Cancer Res.* **12** 5435–41

[26] Iommelli F *et al* 2014 Monitoring reversal of MET-mediated resistance to EGFR tyrosine kinase inhibitors in non-small cell lung cancer using 3′-deoxy-3′-[^{18}F]-fluorothymidine positron emission tomography *Clin. Cancer Res.* **20** 4806–15

[27] McKay M J, Taubman K L, Foroudi F, Lee S T and Scott A M 2018 Molecular imaging using PET/CT for radiation therapy planning for adult cancers: current status and expanding applications *Int. J. Radiat. Oncol.* **102** 783–91

[28] Soret M, Bacharach S L and Buvat I 2007 Partial-volume effect in PET tumor imaging *J. Nucl. Med.* **48** 932–45

[29] Specht L and Berthelsen A K 2018 PET/CT in radiation therapy planning *Semin. Nucl. Med.* **48** 67–75

[30] Firouzian A, Kelly M D and Declerck J M 2014 Insight on automated lesion delineation methods for PET data *EJNMMI Res.* **4** 69

[31] Schaefer A, Kremp S, Hellwig D, Rübe C, Kirsch C-M and Nestle U 2008 A contrast-oriented algorithm for FDG-PET-based delineation of tumour volumes for the radiotherapy of lung cancer: derivation from phantom measurements and validation in patient data *Eur. J. Nucl. Med. Mol. Imaging* **35** 1989–99

[32] Geets X, Lee J A, Bol A, Lonneux M and Grégoire V 2007 A gradient-based method for segmenting FDG-PET images: methodology and validation *Eur. J. Nucl. Med. Mol. Imaging* **34** 1427–38

[33] Hatt M, Cheze Le Rest C, Turzo A, Roux C and Visvikis D 2009 A fuzzy locally adaptive Bayesian segmentation approach for volume determination in PET *IEEE Trans. Med. Imaging* **28** 881–93

[34] Owrangi A M, Greer P B and Glide-Hurst C K 2018 MRI-only treatment planning: benefits and challenges *Phys. Med. Biol.* **63** 05TR01

[35] Devic S 2012 MRI simulation for radiotherapy treatment planning *Med. Phys.* **39** 6701

[36] Edmund J M and Nyholm T 2017 A review of substitute CT generation for MRI-only radiation therapy *Radiat. Oncol.* **12** 28

[37] Johnstone E *et al* 2018 Systematic review of synthetic computed tomography generation methodologies for use in magnetic resonance imaging-only radiation therapy *Int. J. Radiat. Oncol.* **100** 199–217

[38] Reichert M, Ai T, Morelli J N, Nittka M, Attenberger U and Runge V M 2015 Metal artefact reduction in MRI at both 1.5 and 3.0 T using slice encoding for metal artefact correction and view angle tilting *Br. J. Radiol.* **88** 20140601

[39] Koch K M *et al* 2011 Imaging near metal with a MAVRIC-SEMAC hybrid *Magn. Reson. Med.* **65** 71–82

[40] Maikusa N *et al* 2013 Improved volumetric measurement of brain structure with a distortion correction procedure using an ADNI phantom *Med. Phys.* **40** 062303

[41] Price R G, Knight R A, Hwang K, Bayram E, Nejad-Davarani S P and Glide-Hurst C K 2017 Optimization of a novel large field of view distortion phantom for MR-only treatment planning *J. Appl. Clin. Med. Phys.* **18** 51–61

[42] Grande F D, Guggenberger R and Fritz J 2021 Rapid musculoskeletal MRI in 2021: value and optimized use of widely accessible techniques *Am. J. Roentgenol.* **216** 704–17

[43] Delfaut E M, Beltran J, Johnson G, Rousseau J, Marchandise X and Cotten A 1999 Fat suppression in MR imaging: techniques and pitfalls *RadioGraphics* **19** 373–82

[44] Van Houdt P J, Li S, Yang Y and Van Der Heide U A 2024 Quantitative MRI on MR-linacs: towards biological image-guided adaptive radiotherapy *Semin. Radiat. Oncol.* **34** 107–19

[45] Rouvière O *et al* 2004 Recurrent prostate cancer after external beam radiotherapy: value of contrast-enhanced dynamic MRI in localizing intraprostatic tumor—correlation with biopsy findings *Urology* **63** 922–7

[46] Na H B, Song I C and Hyeon T 2009 Inorganic nanoparticles for MRI contrast agents *Adv. Mater.* **21** 2133–48

[47] Xiao Y-D, Paudel R, Liu J, Ma C, Zhang Z-S and Zhou S-K 2016 MRI contrast agents: classification and application (review) *Int. J. Mol. Med.* **38** 1319–26

[48] Han K *et al* 2016 A prospective study of DWI, DCE-MRI and FDG PET imaging for target delineation in brachytherapy for cervical cancer *Radiother. Oncol.* **120** 519–25

[49] Skinner J T, Moots P L, Ayers G D and Quarles C C 2016 On the use of DSC-MRI for measuring vascular permeability *Am. J. Neuroradiol.* **37** 80–7

[50] Lagendijk J J W, Raaymakers B W, Van Den Berg C A T, Moerland M A, Philippens M E and Van Vulpen M 2014 MR guidance in radiotherapy *Phys. Med. Biol.* **59** R349–69

[51] Metcalfe P *et al* 2013 The potential for an enhanced role for MRI in radiation-therapy treatment planning *Technol. Cancer Res. Treat.* **12** 429–46

[52] Schmainda K M *et al* 2018 Multisite concordance of DSC-MRI analysis for brain tumors: results of a national cancer institute quantitative imaging network collaborative project *Am. J. Neuroradiol.* **39** 1008–16

[53] Van Der Heide U A, Houweling A C, Groenendaal G, Beets-Tan R G H and Lambin P 2012 Functional MRI for radiotherapy dose painting *Magn. Reson. Imaging* **30** 1216–23

[54] Lagendijk J J W, Raaymakers B W and Van Vulpen M 2014 The magnetic resonance imaging–linac system *Semin. Radiat. Oncol.* **24** 207–9

[55] Dalah E, Moraru I, Paulson E, Erickson B and Li X A 2014 Variability of target and normal structure delineation using multimodality imaging for radiation therapy of pancreatic cancer *Int. J. Radiat. Oncol.* **89** 633–40

[56] Groenendaal G *et al* 2010 Simultaneous MRI diffusion and perfusion imaging for tumor delineation in prostate cancer patients *Radiother. Oncol.* **95** 185–90

[57] Miri N, Keller P, Zwan B J and Greer P 2016 EPID-based dosimetry to verify IMRT planar dose distribution for the aS1200 EPID and FFF beams *J. Appl. Clin. Med. Phys.* **17** 292–304

[58] Stanley D N, Rasmussen K, Kirby N, Papanikolaou N and Gutiérrez A N 2018 An evaluation of the stability of image quality parameters of Elekta x-ray volume imager and iViewGT imaging systems *J. Appl. Clin. Med. Phys.* **19** 64–70

[59] Stanley D N, Papanikolaou N and Gutiérrez A N 2015 An evaluation of the stability of image-quality parameters of varian on-board imaging (OBI) and EPID imaging systems *J. Appl. Clin. Med. Phys.* **16** 87–98

[60] Kroening P 2012 Reducing dose while maintaining image quality for cone beam computed tomography *BSc Thesis* Houghton College, NY

[61] Jaffray D A, Drake D G, Moreau M, Martinez A A and Wong J W 1999 A radiographic and tomographic imaging system integrated into a medical linear accelerator for localization of bone and soft-tissue targets *Int. J. Radiat. Oncol. Biol. Phys.* **45** 773–89

[62] Wang A *et al* 2018 Acuros CTS: a fast, linear Boltzmann transport equation solver for computed tomography scatter—part II: system modeling, scatter correction, and optimization *Med. Phys.* **45** 1914–25

[63] Bogowicz M *et al* 2024 Evaluation of a cone-beam computed tomography system calibrated for accurate radiotherapy dose calculation *Phys. Imaging. Radiat. Oncol.* **29** 100566

[64] Ma C-M C and Paskalev K 2006 In-room CT techniques for image-guided radiation therapy *Med. Dosim.* **31** 30–9

[65] Kuriyama K *et al* 2003 A new irradiation unit constructed of self-moving gantry-CT and linac *Int. J. Radiat. Oncol.* **55** 428–35

[66] Court L, Rosen I, Mohan R and Dong L 2003 Evaluation of mechanical precision and alignment uncertainties for an integrated CT/LINAC system *Med. Phys.* **30** 1198–210

[67] Knight K, Touma N, Zhu L, Duchesne G and Cox J 2009 Implementation of daily image-guided radiation therapy using an in-room CT scanner for prostate cancer isocentre localization *J. Med. Imaging Radiat. Oncol.* **53** 132–8

[68] Peng C, Ahunbay E, Chen G, Anderson S, Lawton C and Li X A 2011 Characterizing interfraction variations and their dosimetric effects in prostate cancer radiotherapy *Int. J. Radiat. Oncol.* **79** 909–14

[69] Kumabe A *et al* 2015 Three-dimensional conformal arc radiotherapy using a C-arm linear accelerator with a computed tomography on-rail system for prostate cancer: clinical outcomes *Radiat. Oncol.* **10** 208

[70] Ikushima H *et al* 2011 Daily alignment results of in-room computed tomography-guided stereotactic body radiation therapy for lung cancer *Int. J. Radiat. Oncol.* **79** 473–80

[71] Yang Z *et al* 2019 Effect of setup and inter-fraction anatomical changes on the accumulated dose in CT-guided breath-hold intensity modulated proton therapy of liver malignancies *Radiother. Oncol.* **134** 101–9

[72] Jiang D *et al* 2023 Total marrow lymphoid irradiation IMRT treatment using a novel CT-linac *Eur. J. Med. Res.* **28** 463

[73] Yu L, Zhao J, Zhang Z, Wang J and Hu W 2021 Commissioning of and preliminary experience with a new fully integrated computed tomography Linac *J. Appl. Clin. Med. Phys.* **22** 208–23

[74] Sun W *et al* 2024 The performance of a new type accelerator uRT-linac 506c evaluated by a quality assurance automation system *J. Appl. Clin. Med. Phys.* **25** e14226

[75] Keall P J *et al* 2022 Integrated MRI-guided radiotherapy—opportunities and challenges *Nat. Rev. Clin. Oncol.* **19** 458–70

[76] Ng J *et al* 2023 MRI-LINAC: a transformative technology in radiation oncology *Front. Oncol.* **13** 1117874

[77] Huang C-Y, Yang B, Lam W W, Geng H, Cheung K Y and Yu S K 2023 Magnetic field induced dose effects in radiation therapy using MR-linacs *Med. Phys.* **50** 3623–36

[78] Raaymakers B W *et al* 2009 Integrating a 1.5 T MRI scanner with a 6 MV accelerator: proof of concept *Phys. Med. Biol.* **54** N229–237

[79] Roberts D A *et al* 2021 Machine QA for the Elekta Unity system: a report from the Elekta MR-linac consortium *Med. Phys.* **48** e67–85

[80] Jassar H *et al* 2023 Real-time motion monitoring using orthogonal cine MRI during MR-guided adaptive radiation therapy for abdominal tumors on 1.5T MR-linac *Med. Phys.* **50** 3103–16

[81] Grimbergen *et al* 2023 Gating and intrafraction drift correction on a 1.5 T MR-linac: clinical dosimetric benefits for upper abdominal tumors *Radiother. Oncol. J. Eur. Soc. Ther. Radiol. Oncol.* **189** 109932

[82] Raaijmakers A J E, Raaymakers B W and Lagendijk J J W 2008 Magnetic-field-induced dose effects in MR-guided radiotherapy systems: dependence on the magnetic field strength *Phys. Med. Biol.* **53** 909–23

[83] Oderinde O M, Shirvani S M, Olcott P D, Kuduvalli G, Mazin S and Larkin D 2021 The technical design and concept of a PET/CT linac for biology-guided radiotherapy *Clin. Transl. Radiat. Oncol.* **29** 106–12

[84] Surucu M *et al* 2021 Comparison of a first-in-class LINAC-integrated PET system and a diagnostic PET/CT scanner *Int. J. Radiat. Oncol.* **111** e515–6

[85] Lee N *et al* 2016 Strategy of using intratreatment hypoxia imaging to selectively and safely guide radiation dose de-escalation concurrent with chemotherapy for locoregionally advanced human papillomavirus-related oropharyngeal carcinoma *Int. J. Radiat. Oncol.* **96** 9–17

[86] Kong F-M *et al* 2017 Effect of midtreatment PET/CT-adapted radiation therapy with concurrent chemotherapy in patients with locally advanced non-small-cell lung cancer: a phase 2 clinical trial *JAMA Oncol.* **3** 1358

[87] Koo J *et al* 2021 Triggered kV imaging during spine SBRT for intrafraction motion management *Technol. Cancer Res. Treat.* **20**

[88] Cetnar A J *et al* 2023 Implementation of triggered kilovoltage imaging for stereotactic radiotherapy of the spine for patients with spinal fixation hardware *Phys. Imaging. Radiat. Oncol.* **25** 100422

[89] Jia X, Tian Z, Lou Y, Sonke J and Jiang S B 2012 Four-dimensional cone beam CT reconstruction and enhancement using a temporal nonlocal means method *Med. Phys.* **39** 5592–602

[90] Zhang Y, Huang X and Wang J 2019 Advanced 4-dimensional cone-beam computed tomography reconstruction by combining motion estimation, motion-compensated reconstruction, biomechanical modeling and deep learning *Vis. Comput. Ind. Biomed. Art.* **2** 23

[91] Sawant A *et al* 2014 Investigating the feasibility of rapid MRI for image-guided motion management in lung cancer radiotherapy *BioMed. Res. Int.* **2014** 1–6

[92] Keiper T D *et al* 2020 Feasibility of real-time motion tracking using cine MRI during MR-guided radiation therapy for abdominal targets *Med. Phys.* **47** 3554–66

[93] Jassar H *et al* 2023 Real-time motion monitoring using orthogonal cine MRI during MR-guided adaptive radiation therapy for abdominal tumors on 1.5T MR-linac *Med. Phys.* **50** 3103–16

[94] Cunningham J M *et al* 2022 On-line adaptive and real-time intrafraction motion management of spine-SBRT on an MR-linac *Front. Phys.* **10** 882564

[95] Akdag O *et al* 2022 First experimental exploration of real-time cardiorespiratory motion management for future stereotactic arrhythmia radioablation treatments on the MR-linac *Phys. Med. Biol.* **67** 065003

[96] Sawant A *et al* 2008 Management of three-dimensional intrafraction motion through real-time DMLC tracking *Med. Phys.* **35** 2050–61

[97] Ehrbar S *et al* 2022 MR-guided beam gating: residual motion, gating efficiency and dose reconstruction for stereotactic treatments of the liver and lung *Radiother. Oncol.* **174** 101–8

[98] Mickevicius N J, Chen X, Boyd Z, Lee H J, Ibbott G S and Paulson E S 2018 Simultaneous motion monitoring and truth-in-delivery analysis imaging framework for MR-guided radiotherapy *Phys. Med. Biol.* **63** 235014

[99] Keijnemans K, Borman P T S, Uijtewaal P, Woodhead P L, Raaymakers B W and Fast M F 2022 A hybrid 2D/4D-MRI methodology using simultaneous multislice imaging for radiotherapy guidance *Med. Phys.* **49** 6068–81

[100] Mao W, Kim J and Chetty I J 2022 Association between internal organ/liver tumor and external surface motion from cine MR images on an MRI-linac *Front. Oncol.* **12** 868076

[101] Stemkens B, Paulson E S and Tijssen R H N 2018 Nuts and bolts of 4D-MRI for radiotherapy *Phys. Med. Biol.* **63** 21TR01

[102] Liu Y *et al* 2014 Investigation of sagittal image acquisition for 4D-MRI with body area as respiratory surrogate *Med. Phys.* **41** 101902

[103] Cai J, Chang Z, Wang Z, Paul Segars W and Yin F 2011 Four-dimensional magnetic resonance imaging (4D-MRI) using image-based respiratory surrogate: a feasibility study *Med. Phys.* **38** 6384–94

[104] Du D *et al* 2015 High-quality T2-weighted 4-dimensional magnetic resonance imaging for radiation therapy applications *Int. J. Radiat. Oncol.* **92** 430–7

[105] Glide-Hurst C K *et al* 2015 Four dimensional magnetic resonance imaging optimization and implementation for magnetic resonance imaging simulation *Pract. Radiat. Oncol.* **5** 433–42

[106] Han F, Zhou Z, Cao M, Yang Y, Sheng K and Hu P 2017 Respiratory motion-resolved, self-gated 4D-MRI using rotating Cartesian k-space (ROCK) *Med. Phys.* **44** 1359–68

[107] Stemkens B *et al* 2015 Optimizing 4-dimensional magnetic resonance imaging data sampling for respiratory motion analysis of pancreatic tumors *Int. J. Radiat. Oncol.* **91** 571–8

[108] Deng Z *et al* 2017 Improved vessel–tissue contrast and image quality in 3D radial sampling-based 4D-MRI *J. Appl. Clin. Med. Phys.* **18** 250–7

[109] Li G, Liu Y and Nie X 2019 Respiratory-correlated (RC) vs time-resolved (TR) four-dimensional magnetic resonance imaging (4DMRI) for radiotherapy of thoracic and abdominal cancer *Front. Oncol.* **9** 1024

[110] Paulson E S and Tijssen R H N 2019 Motion management *MRI Radiotheraphy* ed G Liney and U Van Der Heide (Cham: Springer International) pp 107–16

[111] Al-Hallaq H A *et al* 2022 AAPM task group report 302: surface-guided radiotherapy *Med. Phys.* **49** e82–e112

[112] Kang H, Lee H Y, Lee K S and Kim J-H 2012 Imaging-based tumor treatment response evaluation: review of conventional, new, and emerging concepts *Korean J. Radiol.* **13** 371

[113] Eisenhauer E A *et al* 2009 New response evaluation criteria in solid tumours: revised RECIST guideline (version 1.1) *Eur. J. Cancer* **45** 228–47

[114] Therasse P *et al* 2000 New guidelines to evaluate the response to treatment in solid tumors *JNCI J. Natl Cancer Inst.* **92** 205–16

[115] Campbell A, Davis L M, Wilkinson S K and Hesketh R L 2019 Emerging functional imaging biomarkers of tumour responses to radiotherapy *Cancers* **11** 131

[116] Miles K A 1999 Tumour angiogenesis and its relation to contrast enhancement on computed tomography: a review *Eur. J. Radiol.* **30** 198–205

[117] Marcus C D, Ladam-Marcus V, Cucu C, Bouché O, Lucas L and Hoeffel C 2009 Imaging techniques to evaluate the response to treatment in oncology: current standards and perspectives *Crit. Rev. Oncol. Hematol.* **72** 217–38

[118] Garcia-Barros M *et al* 2003 Tumor response to radiotherapy regulated by endothelial cell apoptosis *Science* **300** 1155–9

[119] Bellomi M, Petralia G, Sonzogni A, Zampino M G and Rocca A 2007 CT perfusion for the monitoring of neoadjuvant chemotherapy and radiation therapy in rectal carcinoma: initial experience *Radiology* **244** 486–93

[120] Sahani D V *et al* 2005 Assessing tumor perfusion and treatment response in rectal cancer with multisection CT: initial observations *Radiology* **234** 785–92

[121] Ursino S *et al* 2016 Role of perfusion CT in the evaluation of functional primary tumour response after radiochemotherapy in head and neck cancer: preliminary findings *Br. J. Radiol.* **89** 20151070

[122] Coolens C, Driscoll B, Foltz W D, Jaffray D A and Chung C 2015 Early detection of tumor response using volumetric DCE-CT and DCE-MRI in metastatic brain patients treated with radiosurgery *Int. J. Radiat. Oncol.* **93** S7

[123] Šurlan-Popovič K, Bisdas S, Rumboldt Z, Koh T S and Strojan P 2010 Changes in perfusion CT of advanced squamous cell carcinoma of the head and neck treated during the course of concomitant chemoradiotherapy *Am. J. Neuroradiol.* **31** 570–5

[124] Kino A *et al* 2017 Perfusion CT measurements predict tumor response in rectal carcinoma *Abdom. Radiol.* **42** 1132–40

[125] Patchett N, Furlan A and Marsh J W 2016 Decrease in tumor enhancement on contrast-enhanced CT is associated with improved survival in patients with hepatocellular carcinoma treated with Sorafenib *Jpn. J. Clin. Oncol.* **46** 839–44

[126] Bussink J, Van Herpen C M, Kaanders J H and Oyen W J 2010 PET-CT for response assessment and treatment adaptation in head and neck cancer *Lancet Oncol.* **11** 661–9

[127] Juweid M E *et al* 2007 Use of positron emission tomography for response assessment of lymphoma: consensus of the imaging subcommittee of International Harmonization Project in lymphoma *J. Clin. Oncol.* **25** 571–8

[128] Cheson B D *et al* 2007 Revised response criteria for malignant lymphoma *J. Clin. Oncol.* **25** 579–86

[129] Lin C *et al* 2007 Early ^{18}F-FDG PET for prediction of prognosis in patients with diffuse large B-cell lymphoma: SUV-based assessment versus visual analysis *J. Nucl. Med.* **48** 1626–32

[130] Fueger B J *et al* 2005 Performance of 2-deoxy-2-[F-18]fluoro-d-glucose positron emission tomography and integrated PET/CT in restaged breast cancer patients *Mol. Imaging Biol.* **7** 369–76

[131] Radan L, Ben-Haim S, Bar-Shalom R, Guralnik L and Israel O 2006 The role of FDG-PET/CT in suspected recurrence of breast cancer *Cancer* **107** 2545–51

[132] Kostakoglu L and Goldsmith S J 2003 ^{18}F-FDG PET evaluation of the response to therapy for lymphoma and for breast, lung, and colorectal carcinoma *J. Nucl. Med.* **44** 224–39

[133] Eschmann S M *et al* 2007 ^{18}F-FDG PET for assessment of therapy response and preoperative re-evaluation after neoadjuvant radio-chemotherapy in stage III non-small cell lung cancer *Eur. J. Nucl. Med. Mol. Imaging* **34** 463–71

[134] Weber W A *et al* 2003 Positron emission tomography in non-small-cell lung cancer: prediction of response to chemotherapy by quantitative assessment of glucose use *J. Clin. Oncol.* **21** 2651–7

[135] Hoekstra C J *et al* 2005 Prognostic relevance of response evaluation using [^{18}F]–2-fluoro-2-deoxy-D-glucose positron emission tomography in patients with locally advanced non-small-cell lung cancer *J. Clin. Oncol.* **23** 8362–70

[136] Wieder H A *et al* 2004 Time course of tumor metabolic activity during chemoradiotherapy of esophageal squamous cell carcinoma and response to treatment *J. Clin. Oncol.* **22** 900–8

[137] Wieder H and Weber W 2009 Prediction of tumour response by FDG-PET in patients with adenocarcinomas of the oesophagogastric junction *Eur. J. Nucl. Med. Mol. Imaging* **36** 158–9

[138] Lordick F *et al* 2007 PET to assess early metabolic response and to guide treatment of adenocarcinoma of the oesophagogastric junction: the MUNICON phase II trial *Lancet. Oncol.* **8** 797–805

[139] De Geus-Oei L F *et al* 2008 Chemotherapy response evaluation with FDG–PET in patients with colorectal cancer *Ann. Oncol.* **19** 348–52

[140] Cascini G L *et al* 2006 ^{18}F-FDG PET is an early predictor of pathologic tumor response to preoperative radiochemotherapy in locally advanced rectal cancer *J. Nucl. Med.* **47** 1241–8

[141] Avril N *et al* 2005 Prediction of response to neoadjuvant chemotherapy by sequential F-18-fluorodeoxyglucose positron emission tomography in patients with advanced-stage ovarian cancer *J. Clin. Oncol.* **23** 7445–53

[142] Brun E *et al* 2002 FDG PET studies during treatment: prediction of therapy outcome in head and neck squamous cell carcinoma *Head Neck* **24** 127–35

[143] McCollum A D *et al* 2004 Positron emission tomography with ^{18}F-fluorodeoxyglucose to predict pathologic response after induction chemotherapy and definitive chemoradiotherapy in head and neck cancer *Head Neck* **26** 890–6

[144] Benz M R *et al* 2008 Treatment monitoring by ^{18}F-FDG PET/CT in patients with sarcomas: interobserver variability of quantitative parameters in treatment-induced changes in histopathologically responding and nonresponding tumors *J. Nucl. Med.* **49** 1038–46

[145] Steinert H C, Dellea M M S, Burger C and Stahel R 2005 Therapy response evaluation in malignant pleural mesothelioma with integrated PET–CT imaging *Lung Cancer* **49** S33–5

[146] Sheikhbahaei S, Mena E, Marcus C, Wray R, Taghipour M and Subramaniam R M 2016 ^{18}F-FDG PET/CT: therapy response assessment interpretation (Hopkins criteria) and survival outcomes in lung cancer patients *J. Nucl. Med.* **57** 855–60

[147] Kremer R *et al* 2016 FDG PET/CT for assessing the resectability of NSCLC patients with N2 disease after neoadjuvant therapy *Ann. Nucl. Med.* **30** 114–21

[148] De Leyn P *et al* 2006 Prospective comparative study of integrated positron emission tomography-computed tomography scan compared with remediastinoscopy in the assessment of residual mediastinal lymph node disease after induction chemotherapy for mediastinoscopy-proven stage IIIA-N2 non-small-cell lung cancer: a Leuven Lung Cancer Group Study *J. Clin. Oncol.* **24** 3333–9

[149] Marchetti L *et al* 2021 Diagnostic contribution of contrast-enhanced CT as compared with unenhanced low-dose CT in PET/CT staging and treatment response assessment of ^{18}F-FDG–avid lymphomas: a prospective study *J. Nucl. Med.* **62** 1372–9

[150] Yassin A, El Sheikh R H and Ali M M 2020 PET/CT vs CECT in assessment of therapeutic response in lymphoma *Egypt J. Radiol. Nucl. Med.* **51** 238

[151] Tawakol A, Abdelhafez Y G, Osama A, Hamada E and El Refaei S 2016 Diagnostic performance of ^{18}F-FDG PET/contrast-enhanced CT versus contrast-enhanced CT alone for post-treatment detection of ovarian malignancy *Nucl. Med. Commun.* **37** 453–60

[152] Bollineni V R, Kramer G M, Jansma E P, Liu Y and Oyen W J G 2016 A systematic review on [^{18}F]FLT-PET uptake as a measure of treatment response in cancer patients *Eur. J. Cancer* **55** 81–97

[153] Bhatnagar P, Subesinghe M, Patel C, Prestwich R and Scarsbrook A F 2013 Functional imaging for radiation treatment planning, response assessment, and adaptive therapy in head and neck cancer *RadioGraphics* **33** 1909–29

[154] Dhermain F G, Hau P, Lanfermann H, Jacobs A H and Van Den Bent M J 2010 Advanced MRI and PET imaging for assessment of treatment response in patients with gliomas *Lancet Neurol.* **9** 906–20

[155] Yankeelov T E *et al* 2007 Integration of quantitative DCE-MRI and ADC mapping to monitor treatment response in human breast cancer: initial results *Magn. Reson. Imaging* **25** 1–13

[156] Haider M A *et al* 2008 Dynamic contrast-enhanced magnetic resonance imaging for localization of recurrent prostate cancer after external beam radiotherapy *Int. J. Radiat. Oncol.* **70** 425–30

[157] King A D *et al* 2015 DCE-MRI for pre-treatment prediction and post-treatment assessment of treatment response in sites of squamous cell carcinoma in the head and neck *PLoS One* **10** e0144770

[158] Dijkhoff R A P, Beets-Tan R G H, Lambregts D M J, Beets G L and Maas M 2017 Value of DCE-MRI for staging and response evaluation in rectal cancer: a systematic review *Eur. J. Radiol.* **95** 155–68

[159] Nelson S J 2011 Assessment of therapeutic response and treatment planning for brain tumors using metabolic and physiological MRI *NMR Biomed.* **24** 734–49

[160] Chandarana H, Wang H, Tijssen R H N and Das I J 2018 Emerging role of MRI in radiation therapy *J. Magn. Reson. Imaging* **48** 1468–78

[161] Bains L J, Zweifel M and Thoeny H C 2012 Therapy response with diffusion MRI: an update *Cancer Imaging* **12** 395–402

[162] Hamstra D A, Rehemtulla A and Ross B D 2007 Diffusion magnetic resonance imaging: a biomarker for treatment response in oncology *J. Clin. Oncol.* **25** 4104–9

[163] Padhani A R and Koh D-M 2011 Diffusion MR imaging for monitoring of treatment response *Magn. Reson. Imaging Clin. N. Am.* **19** 181–209

[164] Yoshino E *et al* 1996 Irradiation effects on the metabolism of metastatic brain tumors: analysis by positron emission tomography and ^{1}H-magnetic resonance spectroscopy *Stereotact. Funct. Neurosurg.* **66** 240–59

[165] Zeng Q-S, Li C-F, Zhang K, Liu H, Kang X-S and Zhen J-H 2007 Multivoxel 3D proton MR spectroscopy in the distinction of recurrent glioma from radiation injury *J. Neurooncol.* **84** 63–9

[166] Prat R *et al* 2010 Relative value of magnetic resonance spectroscopy, magnetic resonance perfusion, and 2-(^{18}F) fluoro-2-deoxy-D-glucose positron emission tomography for detection of recurrence or grade increase in gliomas *J. Clin. Neurosci.* **17** 50–3

[167] Weybright P *et al* 2005 Differentiation between brain tumor recurrence and radiation injury using MR spectroscopy *Am. J. Roentgenol.* **185** 1471

[168] Rock J P *et al* 2002 Correlations between magnetic resonance spectroscopy and image-guided histopathology, with special attention to radiation necrosis *Neurosurgery* **51** 912–20

[169] Chen X *et al* 2024 SC-GAN: Structure-completion generative adversarial network for synthetic CT generation from MR images with truncated anatomy *Comput. Med. Imaging Graph.* **113** 102353

[170] Zhao Y *et al* 2023 Compensation cycle consistent generative adversarial networks (Comp-GAN) for synthetic CT generation from MR scans with truncated anatomy *Med. Phys.* **50** 4399–414

[171] Zhang Z *et al* 2018 A predictive model for distinguishing radiation necrosis from tumour progression after gamma knife radiosurgery based on radiomic features from MR images *Eur. Radiol.* **28** 2255–63

[172] Beaton L, Bandula S, Gaze M N and Sharma R A 2019 How rapid advances in imaging are defining the future of precision radiation oncology *Br. J. Cancer* **120** 779–90

Chapter 5

Big data for artificial intelligence in radiation oncology

Jie Fu*, Sunan Cui* and X. Sharon Qi

This chapter explores the role of big data in advancing artificial intelligence (AI) applications within radiation oncology. With the increasing volume, variety, and velocity of data in healthcare, radiation oncology has embraced big data to enhance patient care, streamline workflows, and drive innovations in precision oncology. The chapter begins by introducing the foundational concept of big data and identifying common data sources in radiation oncology. It then describes a typical big data lifecycle and illustrates how AI is normally used for big data analysis. Examples are presented to demonstrate the use of big data in AI-driven medical image segmentation, treatment planning, treatment response prediction, quality assurance (QA), and clinical decision support. These applications have demonstrated the potential to improve accuracy, efficiency, and personalized treatment in radiation oncology. The chapter concludes with discussion of the challenges and future perspectives of big data in radiation oncology.

5.1 Introduction to big data in radiation oncology

5.1.1 Overview of big data

With the rapid advancement of digital technologies, more people worldwide are gaining easier access to the Internet. This expanded connectivity generates vast amounts of data daily across our digitalized society. The term 'big data' refers to datasets that are too large and complex to be managed using conventional data management systems and techniques [1].

Big data is often characterized by several critical dimensions, commonly known as the 'Vs' shown in figure 5.1. Initially conceptualized by Doug Laney in 2001, the three primary characteristics were encapsulated by the terms: volume, velocity, and variety [1, 2]. Volume refers to the enormous amount of data produced. Velocity

---

* Both authors contributed equally to this book chapter.

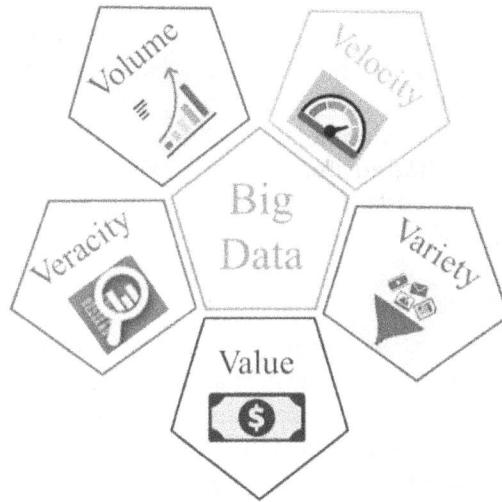

Figure 5.1. The 5 Vs (volume, velocity, variety, veracity, and value) of big data.

describes the rapid rate at which data are generated and need to be processed, often in real-time. Additionally, variety addresses the myriad forms of data, such as text, images, and videos, adding to the complexity of data management and analysis. As the field of big data has evolved, additional dimensions have been introduced to address the broader challenges. Veracity focuses on the reliability and accuracy of data, recognizing that data can be affected by inconsistencies, biases, and anomalies [3]. The goal of big data collection and analysis is to derive value, i.e., to distill meaningful and actionable insights from large and complex datasets [4, 5]. This expanded framework of the Vs offers a comprehensive understanding of big data.

Addressing the challenges of big data necessitates the advancement and adoption of innovative technologies. The key elements of big data analysis include parallel and distributed computing, which enable data processing across multiple computing nodes, and scalable AI models that can maintain or improve performance as data volume expands [6, 7]. Additionally, the capability for real-time querying allows the instantaneous retrieval and analysis of data, which is particularly important when time-sensitive decisions are required [8]. The infrastructures supporting the processing of big data include distributed file systems that allow for data to be stored across multiple locations, computing clusters that aggregate the processing power of numerous computers, and cloud computing that offers scalable and on-demand computing resources [9, 10]. Furthermore, it is essential to design scalable and user-friendly workflows that process data consistently and enable the application of analytical methods across different datasets.

The advent of big data has not only transformed the landscape of data analytics but also revolutionized how we use information in the twenty-first century. Analysing big data holds the potential to unlock insights that were previously unattainable and facilitate people to make data-driven decisions [11, 12]. Within the healthcare sector, big data has the potential to help physicians personalize treatment for patients through the integration of patient-specific data such as genomics, medical history, etc [13]. It also drives innovation by uncovering new treatment regimens and guiding adaptive therapy. Furthermore, it can optimize hospital operations by streamlining workflows, staff allocation, and resource utilization. Big data also enhances patient engagement through customized communication, educational materials, and treatment plans, thereby increasing adherence to medical advice. Ultimately, big data could revolutionize cancer care by enhancing precision, fostering innovation, improving efficiency, and increasing patient involvement [14–16].

5.1.2 Sources of big data in radiation oncology

Radiation oncology stands at the forefront of accumulating digital patient data, pivotal for enhancing patient care through novel big data initiatives [16]. The discipline's long-standing tradition of data collection makes it an ideal landscape for exploring big data. Collecting and analyzing data from large cohorts of patients could open new avenues for improved safety, more efficient workflow, and precision oncology [17–19].

Radiation oncology uniquely amalgamates various types of data from patients and relies heavily on various computer systems to operate [20]. In the conventional workflow shown in figure 5.2, physicians would retrieve patient data from electronic health records (EHRs) to assist in disease diagnosis and clinical decision-making. These data include patient demographics, medical notes, diagnostic images, lab and test results, drug prescriptions, etc. For example, pathology and genetic tests are sometimes requested for cancer diagnosis and tailoring radiation treatments. Once physicians decide to treat patients with radiation therapy, medical images such as CT, MRI, PET, or other modalities are acquired using the imaging device software. These images are then sent to the picture archiving and communication system

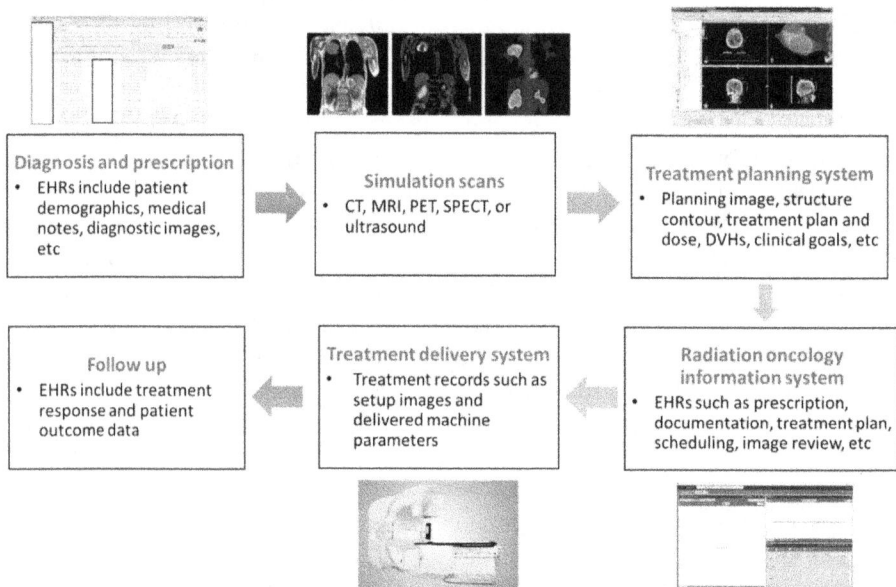

Figure 5.2. Typical workflow for radiation therapy along with the acquired data. Abbreviations: EHRs = electronic health records; DVHs = dose-volume histograms.

(PACS) using digital imaging and communications in medicine (DICOM) formats for data storage and image review. The acquired images are transferred from PACS to the treatment planning system (TPS), where the contours of treatment targets and organs-at-risk (OARs) are delineated, and radiation treatment plans are created based on the contours and clinical goals. Dose distributions of the generated plans are calculated for plan evaluation.

After the plan is approved and reviewed, its machine parameters are transferred from TPS to the radiation oncology information system (ROIS), which records and verifies every treatment fraction. ROIS also supports patient scheduling, charting, image review, etc. Treatment plans also require patient-specific QA before treatment delivery. The whole treatment may be delivered via a single fraction in one day or tens of fractions across several weeks. Before each treatment fraction, the treatment delivery system (TDS) retrieves the plan parameters from ROIS to treat patients. Daily set-up images, such as x-rays, CBCT, or MRI, are acquired to assist in patient positioning. These daily images and the delivered treatment data, such as machine parameters, are sent from TDS to ROIS for recording and verification. Additionally, follow-up exams could be conducted between treatment fractions or months after the treatment completion to evaluate treatment response and patient outcome. All of these acquired data contribute to radiation oncology big data that can be characterized using the aforementioned five Vs.

Big data in radiation oncology can be categorized into three types. First, structured data refers to any data that can be stored in a relational database in table format with rows and columns. These include patient information such as gender and age, prescriptions, plan parameters, delivery records, billing codes, etc. Second, semi-structured data have a structure but do not fit into the relational database. These consist of clinical notes, diagnosis reports, patient feedback, etc. JSON and XML are common types of semi-structured data. Lastly, unstructured data are unorganized and do not fit into the relational database system. Examples include medical images, text files, audio, video, etc. Integrating these various data types into a cohesive analytical framework presents significant challenges, necessitating advanced computational technologies and sophisticated data management systems.

5.1.3 Big data and AI in radiation oncology

The relationship between big data and AI is both symbiotic and integral for advancing radiation oncology. Big data serves as essential fuel for AI models, in particular those based on deep learning, to learn and evolve. The more diverse data these algorithms are exposed to, the more accurate and effective they become. On the other hand, big data is often too complex for traditional data processing methods. AI models can process, analyse, and extract meaningful insights from big data efficiently. For example, natural language processing (NLP) can be leveraged to extract relevant information from medical notes [21], and AI models can be trained to identify anomalies and correlations within big data that would be difficult for humans to identify.

The integration of big data and AI allows us to improve clinical workflow and personalize treatment in radiation oncology. For example, AI models could be trained to improve the quality of diagnostic images and treatment set-up images [22, 23]. AI-based segmentation models could be used to minimize inter-observer variations and improve the contour delineation efficiency [24]. AI-based automatic planning also allows us to standardize and shorten the treatment planning workflow [25]. Furthermore, AI-based predictive modeling could forecast clinical outcomes, guiding informed clinical decision-making [26].

5.2 Big data lifecycle in radiation oncology

The big data lifecycle refers to the stages through which big data progresses, from its generation to its utilization and disposal. Figure 5.3 shows the typical big data lifecycle in radiation oncology, which includes five stages consisting of data aggregation and storage, data sharing and security, data visualization, knowledge creation and implementation, and data archive and deletion.

5.2.1 Data aggregation and storage

Data aggregation is a complex process involving the collection of diverse raw data from various sources, transforming these raw data into a format suitable for advanced statistical or machine learning analysis. In the realm of radiation oncology, data originate from multiple channels such as TPS, TDS, PACS, EMR, ROIS, QA software, simple CSV files, and spreadsheets [27]. Furthermore, breakthroughs in laboratory technology have amplified the availability of genomic and proteomic information, adding valuable resources to the field of radiation oncology. There are several

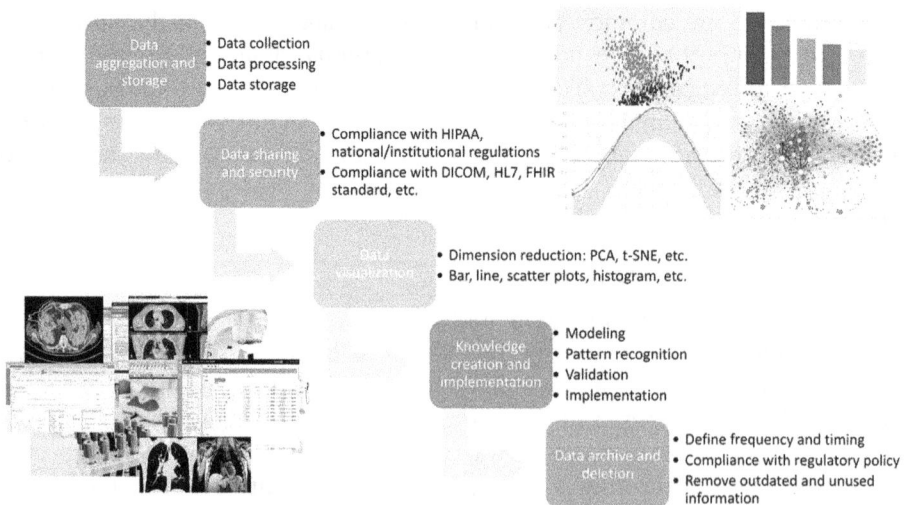

Figure 5.3. Big data lifecycle in radiation oncology: data aggregation and storage, data sharing and security, data visualization, knowledge creation and implementation, and data archive and deletion. Abbreviations: HIPAA = health insurance portability and accountability act; PCA = principal component analysis; t-SNE = t-distributed stochastic neighbor embedding.

considerations in the process of data collection. Many systems contain a mix of useful and irrelevant data. Filtering out pertinent information becomes crucial. For instance, among numerous plans in a TPS, only specific approved or delivered plans might be relevant for analysis. Data may not always be stored in convenient formats for analysis. For instance, images exported from PACS systems are often in DICOM format, necessitating additional processing to obtain 3D images suitable for analysis. Data from various sources require establishing unified identifiers. For example, to derive an OAR dose distribution, linking DICOM CT images, RT structure, and RT dose files becomes essential for future reference and analysis.

The selection of data to collect is tailored to each specific project. Ideally, a unified data infrastructure should cater to the diverse needs of projects, such as prospective/retrospective clinical trials, research documentation, and routine clinical record-keeping. It is crucial to find a balance between making data retrieval easy, ensuring storage efficiency, and maintaining a comprehensive dataset. This decision plays a pivotal role in the data collection process.

Once data are gathered, it is important for them undergo further processing to guarantee their integrity before saving them into the database. Key aspects to focus on include accuracy, consistency, and completeness. First, the extracted data should undergo a validation process to confirm their accuracy. Second, if the same variable exists in different sources, it is prudent to cross-verify for consistency and rectify any discrepancies encountered. Lastly, ensuring that all essential information is extracted is vital. In cases where missing data are encountered, exhaustive efforts should be made to locate them. If unsuccessful, they should be marked as missing data. This meticulous approach safeguards the reliability of the stored information, ensuring its usefulness and accuracy for future analyses.

Data storage serves critical functions for archival and future use. It is imperative to select a storage solution that boasts scalability, enabling seamless accommodation of escalating data volumes and ensuring efficient data retrieval even with extensive datasets. Equally vital is the presence of accurate documentation and metadata. This documentation acts as a guide, aiding in comprehending the stored information for future applications. Moreover, ensuring data reliability is paramount. This is achieved through implementing redundancies within the database and adopting reliable storage solutions. These redundancies serve as safeguards, protecting against unforeseen database corruption resulting from unexpected hardware failures. Additionally, regular archiving of the database reinforces these redundancies, providing an added layer of protection and ensuring data integrity over time.

5.2.2 Data sharing and security

Data sharing plays a pivotal role in maximizing the utility of existing data sources for several reasons. First, it ensures the verification and reproducibility of research, fostering transparency within the scientific community. Second, data sharing facilitates informed decision-making not only within the originating institution but also across various entities and systems. Additionally, making data accessible to a wider audience of researchers allows us to accelerate scientific progress and innovation, thereby contributing significantly to societal advancements. Including more diverse data from multiple institutions to train AI models also reduces biases and enhances model generalizability. This collaborative approach not only enriches the research landscape but also promotes the overall welfare of society.

Ensuring data security and privacy [28] is of utmost importance when it comes to storing, transmitting, and sharing medical information. Particularly concerning patients' sensitive health data, such as names, addresses, and medical records, stringent measures are in place to safeguard this information from any unauthorized access, use, or disclosure. Compliance with regulations such as health insurance portability and accountability act (HIPAA), national laws, and institutional policies is mandatory in this regard. To maintain the confidentiality of patient data during transmission, secure methods such as encrypted connections are employed, guaranteeing protection against interception or tampering. These measures serve to prevent unauthorized access and data breaches of health records. However, the process of data sharing is far from straightforward due to the intricate web of regulatory requirements and the imperative need to safeguard health data privacy. Addressing this challenge, a novel approach, federated learning [29], has gained traction in the field of radiation oncology. This paradigm eliminates the necessity of data leaving their originating institution. Instead, only the model derived from the data is transferred. While this method partially resolves the issue, it does not always prove as effective as direct data sharing, which continues to be a complex and evolving endeavor in the realm of healthcare data management.

It is important to highlight that integrating certain standards into big data sharing and storing, particularly in the healthcare sector, can be highly advantageous. Standards such as DICOM, Health Level Seven (HL7), and the Fast Healthcare Interoperability Resource (FHIR) not only enhance interoperability but also drive cost efficiency, ensure compliance with regulations, and bolster data security within the healthcare industry.

5.2.3 Data visualization

Data visualization [30] is the art of representing complex datasets using visual aids such as charts, graphs, maps, and interactive dashboards. This visual representation serves as a powerful tool, enabling users to explore, comprehend, and communicate intricate data patterns effectively. When dealing with extensive datasets, visualization becomes especially crucial as it allows for quick exploration and identification of noteworthy patterns that might warrant further investigation. Additionally, it aids in error detection by highlighting outliers, ensuring data accuracy and reliability. Database tools integrated with visualization features offer users an interactive and exploratory approach to analyzing data. For instance, in the context of radiation oncology, visualizing OAR dose–volume histograms (DVHs) for an entire patient cohort can reveal how treatment plans align with clinical goals. Similarly, employing bar plots with dosimetric statistics grouped by outcome variables can unveil potential correlations. Another key advantage of data visualization is its ability to facilitate information sharing. By presenting data visually, it

becomes easier to convey insights to diverse audiences, fostering a better understanding of the underlying information.

Several common visualization tools are widely used, including bar plots, histograms, line charts, and scatter plots. These tools provide different perspectives on the
data, allowing users to gain insights into various aspects of their datasets. Moreover,
advanced techniques such as tree maps, principal component analysis (PCA),
clustering algorithms, and t-distributed stochastic neighbor embedding (t-SNE)
[31] further enhance the visualization process. PCA, for example, reduces data
dimensions, simplifying complex datasets and aiding in visualization. Clustering
algorithms group similar data points, revealing inherent patterns, while t-SNE helps
visualize high-dimensional data in low-dimensional space, preserving data
relationships.

In summary, data visualization, coupled with sophisticated algorithms and tools,
not only aids in exploring and understanding large datasets but also serves as a
valuable tool for users to make informed decisions and communicate findings
effectively.

5.2.4 Knowledge creation and implementation

Knowledge creation involves acquiring insights through rigorous data analysis. This
process entails building models, identifying patterns, and devising efficient strategies
using data-driven approaches. Extensive validation and testing are essential components of this process. Once the tools are developed, they must be seamlessly
integrated into real clinical settings, ensuring practical implementation and continuous refinement.

The implementation of data-driven tools in healthcare presents numerous
challenges [32, 33]. First, these tools ideally should be interpretable, offering insights
into their decision-making processes to establish trust among healthcare professionals. Second, they need to be user-friendly and seamlessly integrated into existing
workflows or systems. Rigorous validation through clinical trials is also essential to
ensure their effectiveness and safety before they can be widely adopted.
Furthermore, continuous QA programs are essential to monitor their performance
over time. Ethical concerns, such as biases in algorithms and accountability in cases
of failure, must be thoroughly investigated. Additionally, the regulatory approval
process is required to ensure both efficacy and safety.

5.2.5 Data archiving and deletion

Effectively managing the continuous influx of data is essential, with archiving and
deletion playing pivotal roles in this process [34]. Archiving involves preserving data
for the long term, typically governed by a well-defined data archiving policy that
outlines the frequency and timing of these activities. This strategic approach not
only facilitates efficient data management but also ensures alignment with organizational data retention policies and regulatory standards. Archiving data, often
transitioned from active databases to cost-effective cold storage, becomes an
efficient tool for achieving compliance while mitigating storage costs. Retrieval

mechanisms are in place, allowing organizations to access archived data when necessary. In sectors such as healthcare, archived data serve as a valuable resource for clinical trials and medical research.

Data deletion is a crucial step in optimizing storage resources and streamlining the management of expansive datasets. By eliminating outdated or inaccurate information, organizations can maintain high data quality, ensuring the accuracy and reliability of analytical processes. Additionally, the removal of unused or outdated data plays a pivotal role in mitigating security risks, reducing the potential surface area for breaches, and minimizing the impact in case of a security incident.

5.3 Big data analytics with AI

5.3.1 Data processing and integration

Data processing is a comprehensive procedure designed to transform raw data into a format suitable for analysis. This intricate process encompasses various essential stages. Data cleaning involves identifying and rectifying outliers, errors, inconsistencies, and inaccuracies. Data filtering allows the selection of specific data subsets based on predefined inclusion or exclusion criteria. The transformative phase involves several methods. Normalization, or standardization, scales numerical values to a standard range, eliminating biases. Discretization or binning converts continuous data into discrete variables, facilitating categorical analysis. Encoding transforms categorical data into numeric values, ensuring compatibility with analytical models. Data smoothing techniques, such as moving averages, reduce noise, aiding in the identification of underlying trends. Additionally, data imputation could be used to replace missing data with values computed using statistical methods or advanced machine learning techniques, ranging from basic mean or median imputation to more sophisticated regression-based approaches.

In the advanced stages of processing, an analytical component becomes integral. It aims to delve into patterns and relationships among data samples. Clustering, for instance, unveils inherent patterns by grouping similar samples, while regression forecasts relationships between variables, offering valuable insights for data transformation. Moreover, feature extraction methods such as PCA reveal essential features contributing to dataset variance. This wealth of information provides insights into processing and integrating the data for downstream modeling tasks.

In specific domains such as radiation oncology, additional processing steps are required for handling various data sources. For text data, NLP techniques such as tokenization, stemming, and sentiment analysis are applied to clinical notes, patient histories, radiology reports, pathology reports, and EHRs. In imaging data, processes such as image enhancement, registration, augmentation, and feature extraction are implemented for the meticulous processing of medical images, such as CT, MRI, and PET. These advanced processing steps not only ensure data integrity and quality but also unlock deeper insights, particularly in complex fields such as RO. Leveraging sophisticated methods becomes pivotal in extracting meaningful information from diverse datasets as technology continues to evolve.

Data integration serves as a pivotal process, bringing together information from diverse sources to enhance analysis, reporting, and decision-making. In specialized fields such as radiation oncology, there is a growing emphasis on integrating patient data from systems such as EHRs, ROIS, TPS, etc. By amalgamating patients' medical histories, lab results, imaging data, clinical information, and treatment plans, a comprehensive patient-specific view emerges, significantly supporting clinical decision-making, particularly in the context of precision medicine.

Various methods can be employed for effective data integration. Matching and linkage algorithms, alongside merge and join algorithms, play a crucial role in identifying and linking data related to the same entity. Transformation and clustering algorithms, as previously discussed, prove efficient when dealing with data from diverse sources, contributing to a more unified and coherent dataset. Additionally, the integration landscape benefits from the application of machine learning algorithms such as decision trees, random forest (RF) [35], k-nearest neighbors (kNN) [36], support vector machine (SVM) [37], and deep learning methods.

These AI techniques not only assist in integrating data but also bring additional advantages. They are adept at reducing dimensionality, extracting latent features, and uncovering intricate patterns within a diverse set of input data. This dimensionality reduction and feature extraction contribute significantly to the seamless integration of data from disparate sources, enhancing the overall efficacy of the data integration process. As technology advances, AI techniques further refine the ability to extract meaningful insights from complex datasets, making data integration an ever-evolving and powerful facet of modern data management.

5.3.2 AI modeling

AI modeling stands as a pivotal phase for unraveling inherent patterns in datasets and crafting tools essential for informed clinical decision-making. The standard approach involves constructing AI models and validating their performance on independent datasets. During model development, a subset of data is often earmarked as a validation dataset. This subset becomes instrumental in refining the training hyperparameters, such as tweaking the strength of penalization terms or optimizing the choice of activation functions based on the model's validation performance.

The process of partitioning datasets into distinct sets involves various strategies. Stratified sampling ensures an equitable distribution of target classes across subsets, while time-based splitting arranges data chronologically. k-fold cross-validation (CV) divides data into k folds, iteratively training the model on $k - 1$ folds and testing on the remaining one. There are variations such as leave-one-out CV and stratified CV. The nested cross-validation method employs an inner loop of CV to pinpoint optimal model parameters and an outer loop to rigorously test the refined model. In essence, the choice of dataset partitioning method should align with the dataset's characteristics and the nature (e.g. size) of the AI task at hand. These techniques collectively contribute to the development of models that not only

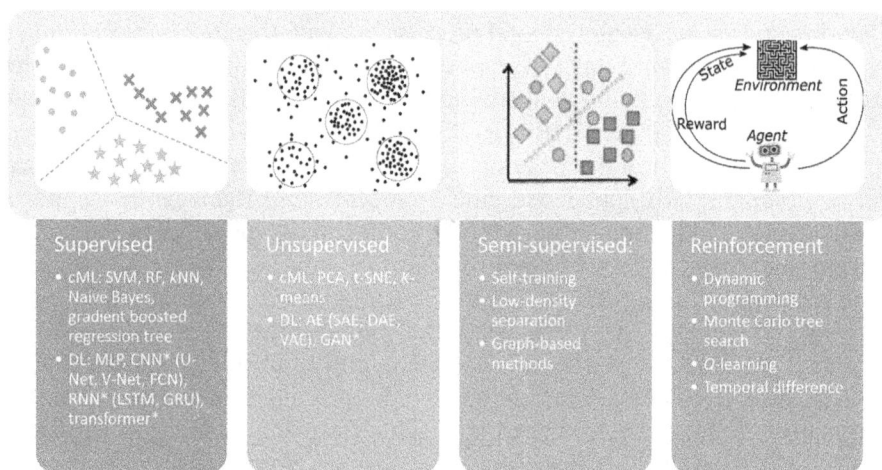

Figure 5.4. Overview of four machine learning paradigms and the example algorithms. . Abbreviations: cML = classical machine learning; DL = deep learning; SVM = support vector machine; RF = random forest; MLP = multi-layer perceptron; CNN = convolutional neural network; FCN = fully convolutional network; LSTM = long short-term memory; GRU = gated recurrent units; PCA = principal component analysis; t-SNE = t-distributed stochastic neighbor embedding; AE= autoencoder; SAE = sparse autoencoders; DAE = denoising autoencoders; VAE = variational autoencoders; GAN = generative adversarial networks. *These models could be trained using all three learning paradigms (supervised, unsupervised, and semi-supervised).

unravel intricate associations within data but also generalize effectively to new and unseen instances.

AI models encompass a wide array of categories, each tailored to the specific nature of the datasets they handle. Figure 5.4 shows different paradigms in machine learning along with the corresponding algorithms.

In supervised learning, which deals with labeled datasets, models are employed to address classification or regression challenges. Classical machine learning methods such as SVM, RF, kNN, and naive Bayes [38] are commonly utilized for these tasks. Furthermore, advanced deep learning architectures such as multi-layer perceptron (MLP), convolutional neural networks (CNNs) and their variants such as U-Net [39], V-Net [40], and the fully convolutional network (FCN) [41] demonstrate exceptional performance, particularly with tasks involving image inputs. Recurrent neural networks (RNNs) and their variants, including gated recurrent units (GRU) [42] and long short-term memory (LSTM) networks [43], play a pivotal role in analyzing sequential data such as time series data, natural language, DNA sequences, etc. However, RNNs struggle to capture long-term dependencies in sequences due to the vanishing gradient problem. It is also challenging to parallelize them due to the sequential processing manner. In contrast, transformer models [44] can process entire sequences simultaneously thanks to parallel computing and the self-attention mechanism.

Unsupervised learning deals with unlabeled datasets, focusing on tasks such as clustering and dimensionality reduction. Techniques such as PCA, k-means clustering, and t-SNE are commonly employed for these purposes. Additionally, sophisticated deep learning methods such as generative adversarial networks (GANs) [45] and autoencoders, including variants such as denoising autoencoders (DAEs) [46], sparse autoencoders (SAEs) [47], and variational autoencoders (VAEs) [48], offer powerful tools for unsupervised learning tasks.

Semi-supervised learning emerges as a crucial field, particularly in scenarios where labeled data are scarce or expensive to obtain. By leveraging both labeled and unlabeled data, semi-supervised learning approaches effectively learn from labeled examples while also capitalizing on the additional insights provided by unlabeled data. This approach proves particularly valuable when resource-intensive labeling processes pose constraints, enabling a more nuanced understanding of data patterns. Various training strategies, including self-training, low-density separation [49], and graph-based methods [50], contribute to the efficacy of semi-supervised learning algorithms. Notably, certain architectures such as CNNs, RNNs, and transformers exhibit versatility, allowing them to be applied across various learning paradigms, including supervised, semi-supervised, and unsupervised learning.

Reinforcement learning (RL) represents a distinct paradigm in machine learning, where intelligent agents learn to optimize their strategies by interacting with environments to maximize rewards. RL methods, such as dynamic programming, Monte Carlo tree search [51], Q-learning [52], and temporal difference learning, exemplify this approach, offering powerful techniques for solving complex decision-making problems in dynamic environments.

Recently, there have been remarkable advancements in foundation models and generative AI, signaling a pivotal breakthrough in the field of AI. A foundation model [53] is a large-scale AI model pre-trained on vast unlabeled data across various modalities such as text, images, audio, or video. It learns useful representations and patterns of data and can be adapted to perform a wide range of downstream tasks. Foundation models exhibit exceptional flexibility, adapting to supervised, semi-supervised, or unsupervised learning, depending on their training methodology. They can be classified based on the type of input data modalities they are designed to process. For example, large language models (LLMs) are text-based foundation models primarily used for NLP tasks. Examples of LLMs include generative pre-trained transformers (GPTs) [54] and bidirectional encoder representations from transformers (BERTs) [55]. Some LLMs are specifically tailored for medical applications, such as pubMedBERT [56], BioMedLM [57], and clinicalBERT [58]. Image-based models, consisting of self-distillation with no labels (DINO) [59] and masked autoencoders (MAEs) [60], are trained on image datasets and can be used for image recognition, object detection, and segmentation. Multimodal models are capable of handling multiple data types and are often trained to align different modalities for tasks that benefit from cross-modal understanding. Example models include contrastive language-image pretraining (CLIP) [61] and the large language and vision assistant (LLaVA) [62]. Generative AI refers to AI systems capable of generating new content akin to the data they were trained on. By modeling the underlying data distribution, these systems produce novel samples resembling the training data. Generative AI often builds upon foundation models. For instance, an LLM could be initially trained to understand and represent text data and be further fine-tuned or extended to perform generative tasks such as human language generation.

5.4 The application of big data in radiation oncology

5.4.1 Medical image segmentation

The applications of big data in medical image segmentation have shown great advancements in recent years [63]. In radiation oncology, contours of targets and OARs are required to generate treatment plans. However, manual segmentation is not only time-consuming but also prone to inter-observer variations. The slow segmentation process also decreases the efficiency of the online adaptive workflow and potentially affects the efficacy of adaptive plans. Therefore, it is critical to develop fast automatic segmentation methods that can help relieve clinical burden, standardize segmentation performance, and accelerate adaptive workflow.

Numerous pairs of images and contours in radiation oncology provide a rich source for training AI-based segmentation models, which have achieved state-of-the-art performance in medical image segmentation. Notably, the U-Net [39], introduced by Ronneberger *et al* in 2015, demonstrated the potential to generate accurate segmentations from input image slices. U-Net consists of an encoder and a decoder connected with skip connections. This encoder–decoder architecture has been incorporated as the backbone of many advanced AI-based medical image segmentation models such as AnatomyNet [64] and nn-U-Net [65].

AI-based models have been trained to generate OAR segmentation based on single- or multi-modal images. As a CT scan is routinely acquired for treatment planning in the conventional image-guided radiotherapy workflow, numerous models have been trained with pairs of CT images and OAR contours. For example, a WBNet proposed by Chen *et al* was trained using 505 CT scans of the head and neck, thorax, abdomen, and pelvis, and could accurately delineate 50 OARs [66]. Additionally, commercial AI-based segmentation tools such as Limbus Contour (Limbus AI, Canada) and Contour ProtégéAI (MIM Software Inc, USA) have been integrated into many hospitals worldwide for automatic OAR segmentation on CT scans [67, 68]. Many studies also focused on OAR segmentation based on MRI [67, 69] or ultrasound images [70] due to growing interest in using other image modalities for treatment guidance. The HaN-Seg dataset [71] contains both CT, MRI, and OAR contours of 56 head and neck cancer patients and could be trained to train a multi-modal segmentation model. However, CT and MRI scans of the same patients are not always available, which makes it challenging to acquire sufficient training data. Valindria *et al* demonstrated the benefits of multi-model learning for multi-organ segmentation based on unpaired CT and MRI scans acquired from different subjects [72].

The combination of big data and AI makes it possible to automatically generate accurate tumor and target contours. Many studies have shown that AI models, trained with pairs of clinical target volume (CTV) contours and CT scans, achieved promising performance in delineating CTV for patients with head and neck cancer [73], breast cancer [74], and cervical cancer [75]. Additionally, tumor segmentation sometimes involves multi-modal images. MRI provides superior soft tissue contrast compared with CT and has been increasingly used to delineate tumors in the brain, prostate, and abdomen. For instance, multi-modal MR images and manually drawn tumor contours from 180 glioblastoma patients were used to train a 3D multipath DenseNet that achieved accurate glioblastoma tumor segmentation [76]. Additionally, a commercial AI tool uses both CT and MRI scans to accurately detect and delineate metastatic brain tumors [77, 78]. On the other hand, PET images provide a functional assessment of a tumor and have become the modality of choice for delineating targets in patients with lung cancer, head and neck cancer, and esophageal cancer [77]. Groendahl *et al* showed that CNNs trained with multi-modal PET-CT images achieved better performance in delineating the gross tumor volume of head and neck images compared to the model trained with PET or CT images [79]. The modality-specific segmentation network (MoSNet) based on PET-CT images outperforms the state-of-the-art lung tumor segmentation models [80].

MedSAM, a foundation model trained with more than one million pairs of medical images and contours, demonstrates significant potential to enable universal medical image segmentation [81]. Public datasets for OAR segmentation include multi-organ abdominal CT reference standard segmentations [82], segmentation of thoracic organs-at-risk (SegTHOR) [83], and medical segmentation decathlon [84]. Public datasets for tumor segmentation include brain tumor segmentation (BraTS) [85], liver tumor segmentation (LiTS) [86], and DeepLesion [87]. More public datasets on image–contour pairs could be found in The Cancer Imaging Archive (TCIA) [88] and The Cancer Genome Atlas (TCGA) [89].

5.4.2 Automatic treatment planning

Intensity modulated radiation therapy (IMRT) and volumetric modulated arc therapy (VMAT) enable precise radiation delivery to tumors while sparing OARs. However, the manual treatment planning process normally involves multiple rounds of inverse optimization by trial and error to generate clinically acceptable plans. This manual workflow is very time-consuming, requires significant human expertise, and may not always yield optimal treatment plans. Online adaptive radiation therapy, which allows better inter-fraction organ motion management compared with non-adaptive treatment, has drawn significant clinical interest. However, this requires decreasing planning time to a few minutes.

Automatic treatment planning could be achieved by training AI models to predict 3D dose distribution, predict fluence maps, or automate the hyperparameter tuning process during inverse optimization. U-Net and its variants could be trained to predict clinical dose distributions based on the input of CT and/or contours of targets and OARs. Promising results have been achieved for cancer sites including the head and neck [90], breast [91], and prostate [92]. The predicted dose distributions or the corresponding DVHs could be fed into the dose optimization engine to generate deliverable plans. However, as historical plans used for model training may not always be optimal, plans generated using this method may be suboptimal. Instead of clinical dose distribution, these models can also be trained to predict Pareto optimal dose distributions based on the additional input of user-specified contour weights [93] or DVHs [94]. This allows the user to search for the optimal trade-off dose in real-time.

Fluence map prediction models could help skip the optimization step and potentially speed up the automatic treatment planning process. These models can be trained to take the AI-predicted dose distributions as their input and predict fluence maps [95], predict fluence maps directly based on contours [96], or simultaneously predict dose distribution and fluence maps based on CT and contours [97]. On the other hand, RL agents could be trained to observe intermediate plan DVHs and take action to adjust planning parameters for generating the plan with the maximized quality score [98].

5.4.3 Treatment response prediction

Precision oncology represents a paradigm shift in cancer treatment, leveraging the power of big data to tailor therapy to individual patients. This approach is grounded in the understanding that cancer is not a singular disease but rather a highly heterogeneous disease with unique genomic and phenotypic characteristics that vary among individual patients [99]. AI models, trained on extensive datasets such as patient demographics, genetic test results, medical images, and treatment plan dose distribution, can predict how individual patients will respond to specific treatment regimens. This could potentially allow us to improve patient outcomes and reduce the toxicity and burden of unnecessary treatments.

Many efforts have been made to utilize large-scale omics data to predict radiation therapy response. For example, genomic classifiers have been developed to stratify local recurrence risk after radiation therapy in breast cancer patients and identify those who would benefit from radiation therapy [100–102]. Radiomic features extracted from medical images have been found to correlate with genomic biomarkers and achieve promising performance in predicting treatment responses for patients with lung cancer, rectal cancer, etc [103]. Moreover, the integration of multi-omics data holds the potential to further enhance model prediction accuracy [104–106].

5.4.4 Quality assurance and patient safety

Ensuring QA and patient safety is a top priority in radiation oncology. The data relevant to this domain come from a variety of sources, including QA procedures and incident learning systems (ILSs) [107, 108]. Data generated from QA procedures include machine-specific data and patient-specific data. Machine-specific data can be from various categories, including dosimetric, mechanical, imaging, and respiratory gating. These data are normally obtained by measurements or checks during machine and TPS acceptance/commissioning/upgrading and routine daily/monthly/annual QA. Patient-specific data may include patient-specific QA conducted using either an array detector or electronic portal imaging device [109], treatment plan review [110], and machine delivery log files [119]. The ILS within radiation oncology [111] serves as a pivotal platform for healthcare professionals to both report and glean insights from incidents and near-misses tied to cancer treatment. Through meticulous data collection and analysis, ILS fosters a continuous drive toward enhancing quality within radiation oncology practices. It empowers healthcare providers to discern patterns, pinpoint root causes, and highlight areas ripe for improvement in patient safety and treatment delivery. Radiation Oncology ILS (RO-ILS) [112], jointly sponsored by ASTRO and AAPM, spearheads the establishment of a national database tasked with housing incidents, near-misses, and unsafe conditions reported across various institutions. Advocating for a collaborative approach, RO-ILS encourages sharing and learning from events submitted nationwide. This initiative promotes a culture of safety and collaboration within the radiation oncology community, ultimately culminating in elevated patient care outcomes.

With a wealth of data stemming from both QA and ILS, AI emerges as a powerful ally in several key areas. It can adeptly discern trends in QA task performance, identifying outliers that warrant closer examination. Furthermore, AI streamlines QA workflows by automating tasks such as plan review and imaging QA, thereby enhancing both efficiency and precision. By leveraging predictive analytics, AI forecasts which aspects are more prone to failure, allowing for proactive intervention and resource allocation [113].

5.4.5 Clinical decision support

Big data and AI tools hold significant promise in aiding healthcare professionals in decision-making processes by furnishing them with relevant, timely, and evidence-based information [114]. Clinical decision support systems, underpinned by big data and AI, can amalgamate patient-specific data and medical knowledge to offer recommendations for diagnosis, treatment, and patient care. In the realm of medicine, there is a burgeoning interest in leveraging foundation models across various data sources, including EHRs, clinical guidelines, medical literature, medical imaging, biological sequences, and molecular profiles [115, 116].

EHRs encompass both structured data—such as billing codes, demographics, and medications—and unstructured data, including medical notes, radiology reports, and lab reports. Challenges include irregularities such as ambiguous jargon and non-standard phrasal structure, necessitating domain expertise. Some example datasets include the deidentified clinical acronym sense inventory (CASI) [117] which contains snippets of clinical notes across specialties in four University of Minnesota-affiliated hospitals. The MIMIC-III critical care database contains approximately 2 million notes written between 2001 and 2012 in the ICU of Beth Israel Deaconess Medical Center [118, 119]. Foundation models have demonstrated capabilities such as extracting drug names from medical reports [120], responding to patient queries [121], summarizing clinical text [122], and predicting clinical needs based on clinical notes [123].

The wealth of information found in the scientific literature, clinical guidelines, and knowledge bases such as NCT guidelines and PubMed identifiers is invaluable for clinical decision-making. However, manually extracting predictive information from these sources can be time-consuming and requires extensive expertise. LLMs offer significant promise in this regard. For instance, a few-shot prediction model can leverage LLM representations, which encapsulate prior knowledge in scientific literature, to predict drug pair synergy in rare tissues with limited data [124].

Medical images, which include various modalities such as MRI, CT, and PET, play crucial roles in clinical decision-making throughout the diagnosis and treatment process. Foundation models hold immense potential to transform the utilization of medical images [115]. For instance, it is poised to revolutionize the field by introducing a new generation of versatile digital radiology assistants [125]. These assistants can support radiologists throughout their workflow, significantly reducing their workloads. Additionally, foundation models can integrate imaging with other multi-modal sources such as text, providing both model auditing and annotated images [126]. Text-to-image generative models, such as DALL-E [127], demonstrate promising performance in medical image generation and augmentation [128].

Biological data—including DNA and RNA sequences, genetic variations such as DNA copy number variations and DNA methylation patterns, and gene expression profiles from miRNA and single-cell RNA —hold significant potential for guiding decision-making in precision oncology. Public databases such as TCGA, Gene Expression Omnibus [129], and Protein Data Bank [130] serve as invaluable resources for researchers, enriching our understanding of cancer biology and guiding personalized treatment strategies to improve patient out-comes. Ongoing efforts to develop foundation models for biological sequences [131] facilitate various tasks, including multi-omic integration [132], RNA and protein function prediction [133], and genetic variant effect prediction [134]. Additionally, various foundation models have been utilized to assist in determin-ing treatment options based on molecular profiles and genetic alterations for cancer patients [135]. Looking ahead, foundation models hold tremendous potential for integrating multi-modal data, such as spatial transcriptome, DNA and RNA raw sequencing data, and accompanying EHRs and medical imaging, to transform traditional analytical approaches in cancer prognosis.

In summary, the integration of foundation models into clinical decision support systems holds great promise for advancing medical decision-making processes, although challenges remain in ensuring accuracy, privacy, and safety. Ongoing research and development efforts are critical in addressing these challenges and realizing the full potential of AI in healthcare.

5.5 Challenges and future perspectives

While the potential of big data in radiation oncology is enormous, its application is not without challenges. With data coming from various sources and in different formats, one of the foremost challenges is to ensure data quality and standardiza-tion. Robust model development and implementation require standardizing data analysis frameworks.

Most studies trained their AI models using a single-institutional dataset, which may lead to poor model generalizability in other institutions. This happens due to domain shifts arising from variations in patient populations, clinical protocols, imaging equipment, etc. Transfer learning [136] could help address domain shift issues and improve model robustness in real-word applications. Multi-institutional collaboration is another approach to reduce data biases, comply with regulatory guidelines that emphasize inclusivity and fairness, and enhance model performance. However, sharing data across institutions could potentially pose risks to data privacy and security. Given the sensitive nature of patient data, it is critical to ensure data confidentiality and protect against data breaches, which requires robust cybersecurity measures and adherence to regulations such as HIPAA. Federated learning is another essential technique to address the risks of data sharing across different institutions.

Translating the values from big data into clinical practice presents further challenges. For example, expensive prospective clinical trials may be required to test the safety and efficacy of the models for regulatory approval. Once approved, physicians must understand and trust AI models to be on board with clinical implementation. The decision-making process in many AI models' learning, particularly deep learning, is frequently perceived as a 'black box' due to their intricate and opaque decision-making processes. Explainable AI (XAI) [137] plays a crucial role in bringing transparency and building trust in the high-stakes clinical decision-making process that directly impacts patient lives. For clinicians, understanding and justifying AI-driven predictions is essential for patient safety and ethical care. By providing clear explanations, XAI can help prevent mistakes, support adherence to regulatory standards, and encourage responsible AI use in healthcare. Additionally, uncertainty quantification [138] could be applied to generate model predictions along with uncertainty estimation, which is critical for clinicians to evaluate the reliability of the predictions and identify challenging cases that need to be examined carefully. Moreover, there is an increasing demand for advanced computational infrastructures and skilled personnel to manage and analyse big data in radiation oncology. More efforts should be made to address these challenges.

Looking ahead, the evolving landscape of big data in radiation oncology is poised to revolutionize the field with more personalized, efficient, and effective treatment strategies. The emerging multi-omics data analysis is expected to provide deeper insights into the complexities of cancer biology and the varying responses of different cancers to treatments. By analyzing patterns and correlations using big data, researchers could identify new biomarkers and understand the molecular and genetic underpinnings of individual tumors. This could lead to a new era of radiation therapy, characterized by highly adaptive and personalized treatment regimens.

The integration of AI and big data is anticipated to enhance healthcare operational efficiency, facilitate more effective and cost-saving clinical workflows, streamline administrative processes, and optimize resource allocation. Big data applications also have the potential for remote patient monitoring, ensuring timely intervention during post-treatment follow-ups. Additionally, big data may empower patients with easy access to their health data, providing customized visualizations and enhancing patient engagement in treatment. This, in turn, could potentially improve patients' adherence to clinicians' instructions and ultimately enhance treatment outcomes.

5.6 Summary

In this chapter, we reviewed the transformative role of big data in advancing AI in radiation oncology. Diverse and large-scale datasets—spanning imaging, EMRs, biological sequences, and multi-omics—fuel increasingly powerful AI models that drive precision, efficiency, and personalization in cancer care. We outlined a typical big data lifecycle, emphasizing data aggregation, storage, sharing, visualization, and knowledge implementation. We then discussed AI techniques for big data processing, integration, and modeling, ranging from classical machine learning and deep learning to reinforcement learning and emerging foundation models. These approaches enable the applications in medical image segmentation, treatment planning, response prediction, quality assurance, and clinical decision support. Lastly, we identified the challenges including data heterogeneity, limited generalizability of institution-specific models, privacy concerns, and the opacity of AI models. Solutions such as transfer learning, multi-institutional collaboration, explainable AI, and uncertainty quantification are essential to ensure safe and trustworthy clinical integration.

The future of precision radiation oncology lies in analyzing big data using AI models. By harnessing these advances, the field is poised to deliver data-driven and personalized radiation therapy that could potentially improve outcomes and redefine standards of cancer care.

Reference

[1] Chen C L P and Zhang C Y 2014 Data-intensive applications, challenges, techniques and technologies: a survey on Big Data *Inf. Sci.* **275** 314–47

[2] Laney D 2001 3D data managment: controlling data volume, velocity and variety *Application Delivery Strategies, Technical Report* 494 META Group, Brussels 51

[3] Rubin V L 2014 Veracity roadmap: is big data objective, truthful and credible? *Adv. Class. Res. Online* **24** 4–15

[4] Roski J, Bo-Linn G W and Andrews T A 2014 Creating value in health care through big data: opportunities and policy implications *Health Aff.* **33** 1115–22

[5] Zeng J and Glaister K W 2018 Value creation from big data: looking inside the black box *Strateg. Organ.* **16** 105–40

[6] Dutta K 2017 Distributed computing technologies in big data analytics *Distributed Computing in Big Data Analytics* Scalable Computing and Communications S Mazumder, R Singh Bhadoria and G Deka (Cham: Springer)

[7] Desarkar A and Das A 2017 Big-data analytics, machine learning algorithms and scalable/parallel/distributed algorithms *Internet of Things and Big Data Technologies for Next Generation Healthcare* Studies in Big Data vol 23 (Cham: Springer) pp 159–97

[8] Liu X, Iftikhar N and Xie X 2014 Survey of real-time processing systems for big data *ACM Int. Conf. Proc. Ser.* (New York: Association for Computing Machinery) pp 356–61

[9] Rao T R, Mitra P, Bhatt R and Goswami A 2019 The big data system, components, tools, and technologies: a survey *Knowl. Inf. Syst.* **60** 1165–245

[10] Hashem I A T, Yaqoob I, Anuar N B, Mokhtar S, Gani A and Ullah Khan S 2015 The rise of 'big data' on cloud computing: review and open research issues *Inf. Syst.* **47** 98–115

[11] Anshari M, Almunawar M N, Lim S A and Al-Mudimigh A 2019 Customer relationship management and big data enabled: personalization and customization of services *Appl. Comput. Inform.* **15** 94–101

[12] Awan M J, Rahim M S M, Nobanee H, Munawar A, Yasin A and Zain A M 2021 Social media and stock market prediction: a big data approach *Comput. Mater. Contin.* **67** 2569–83

[13] Chen G *et al* 2022 Rapid progress in intelligent radiotherapy and future implementation *Cancer Invest.* **40** 425–36

[14] Lyu H G, Haider A H, Landman A B and Raut C P 2019 The opportunities and shortcomings of using big data and national databases for sarcoma research *Cancer* **125** 2926–34

[15] Mayo C S *et al* 2018 Treatment data and technical process challenges for practical big data efforts in radiation oncology *Med. Phys.* **45** e793–810

[16] Benedict S H, El Naqa I and Klein E E 2016 Introduction to big data in radiation oncology: exploring opportunities for research, quality assessment, and clinical care *Int. J. Radiat. Oncol. Biol. Phys.* **95** 871–2

[17] Potters L, Ford E, Evans S, Pawlicki T and Mutic S 2016 A systems approach using big data to improve safety and quality in radiation oncology *Int. J. Radiat. Oncol. Biol. Phys.* **95** 885–9

[18] McNutt T R *et al* 2018 Using big data analytics to advance precision radiation oncology *Int. J. Radiat. Oncol. Biol. Phys.* **101** 285–91

[19] Vogelius I R, Petersen J and Bentzen S M 2020 Harnessing data science to advance radiation oncology *Mol. Oncol.* **14** 1514–28

[20] Siochi R A *et al* 2009 Information technology resource management in radiation oncology *J. Appl. Clin. Med. Phys.* **10** 16–35

[21] Bitterman D S, Miller T A, Mak R H and Savova G K 2021 Clinical natural language processing for radiation oncology: a review and practical primer *Int. J. Radiat. Oncol. Biol. Phys.* **110** 641–55

[22] Higaki T, Nakamura Y, Tatsugami F, Nakaura T and Awai K 2019 Improvement of image quality at CT and MRI using deep learning *Jpn J. Radiol.* **37** 73–80

[23] Rusanov B *et al* 2022 Deep learning methods for enhancing cone-beam CT image quality toward adaptive radiation therapy: a systematic review *Med. Phys.* **49** 6019–54

[24] Wong J *et al* 2020 Comparing deep learning-based auto-segmentation of organs at risk and clinical target volumes to expert inter-observer variability in radiotherapy planning *Radiother. Oncol.* **144** 152–8

[25] Wang M, Zhang Q, Lam S, Cai J and Yang R 2020 A review on application of deep learning algorithms in external beam radiotherapy automated treatment planning *Front. Oncol.* **10** 580919

[26] Huynh E *et al* 2020 Artificial intelligence in radiation oncology *Nat. Rev. Clin. Oncol.* **17** 771–81

[27] Kessel K A and Combs S E 2015 Data management, documentation and analysis systems in radiation oncology: a multi-institutional survey *Radiat. Oncol.* **10** 230

[28] Abouelmehdi K, Beni-Hssane A, Khaloufi H and Saadi M 2017 Big data security and privacy in healthcare: a review *Procedia Comput. Sci.* **113** 73–80

[29] Pati S *et al* 2022 Federated learning enables big data for rare cancer boundary detection *Nat. Commun.* **13** 7346

[30] Park S, Bekemeier B, Flaxman A and Schultz M 2022 Impact of data visualization on decision-making and its implications for public health practice: a systematic literature review *Inform. Health Soc. Care.* **47** 175–93

[31] Van der Maaten L and Hinton G 2008 Visualizing data using t-SNE *J. Mach. Learn. Res.* **9** 2579–605

[32] McNutt T R, Moore K L and Quon H 2016 Big data needs and challenges for big data in radiation oncology *Int. J. Radiat. Oncol. Biol. Phys.* **95** 909–15

[33] Pastorino R *et al* 2019 Benefits and challenges of big data in healthcare: an overview of the European initiatives *Eur. J. Public. Health* **29** 23–7

[34] Li T, Vedula S S, Hadar N, Parkin C, Lau J and Dickersin K 2015 Innovations in data collection, management, and archiving for systematic reviews *Ann. Intern. Med.* **162** 287–94

[35] Breiman L 2001 Random forests *Mach. Learn.* **45** 5–32

[36] Guo G, Wang H, Bell D, Bi Y and Greer K 2003 KNN model-based approach in classification *On The Move to Meaningful Internet Systems 2003: CoopIS, DOA, and ODBASE. OTM 2003* Lecture Notes in Computer Science vol 2888 (Berlin: Springer) pp 986–96

[37] Noble W S 2006 What is a support vector machine? *Nat. Biotechnol.* **24** 1565–7

[38] Wickramasinghe I and Kalutarage H 2021 Naive Bayes: applications, variations and vulnerabilities: a review of literature with code snippets for implementation *Soft. Comput.* **25** 2277–93

[39] Ronneberger O, Fischer P and Brox T 2015 U-net: convolutional networks for biomedical image segmentation *Medical Image Computing and Computer-Assisted Intervention–MICCAI 2015* Lecture Notes in Computer Science vol 9351 (Berlin: Springer) pp 234–41

[40] Milletari F, Navab N and Ahmadi S-A 2016 V-Net: fully convolutional neural networks for volumetric medical image segmentation *2016 4th Int. Conf. on 3D Vision (3DV)* (Piscataway, NJ: IEEE) pp 565–71

[41] Long J, Shelhamer E and Darrell T 2015 Fully convolutional networks for semantic segmentation *Proc. of the IEEE Computer Society Conf. on Computer Vision and Pattern Recognition* vol 07–12*(June 2015)* (Piscataway, NJ: IEEE) pp 3431–40

[42] Dey R and Salemt F M 2017 Gate-variants of gated recurrent unit (GRU) neural networks *Midwest Symp. on Circuits and Systems* (Piscataway, NJ: IEEE) pp 1597–600

[43] Staudemeyer R C and Morris E R 2019 Understanding LSTM—a tutorial into long short-term memory recurrent neural networks arXiv: 1909.09586v1

[44] Vaswani A *et al* 2017 Attention is all you need *Advances in Neural Information Processing Systems* vol 30 (Red Hook, NY: Curran Associates)

[45] Goodfellow I *et al* 2020 Generative adversarial networks *Commun. ACM* **63** 139–44

[46] Gondara L 2016 Medical image denoising using convolutional denoising autoencoders *IEEE Int. Conf. on Data Mining Workshops, ICDMW* pp 241–6

[47] Meng L, Ding S and Xue Y 2017 Research on denoising sparse autoencoder *Int. J. Mach. Learn. Cybern.* **8** 1719–29

[48] Kingma D P and Welling M 2013 Auto-encoding variational Bayes arXiv: 1312.6114v11

[49] Chapelle O and Zien A 2005 Semi-supervised classification by low density separation *Proc. Mach. Learn. Res.* **R5** 57–64

[50] Chong Y, Ding Y, Yan Q and Pan S 2020 Graph-based semi-supervised learning: a review *Neurocomputing* **408** 216–30

[51] Vien N A, Ertel W, Dang V H and Chung T 2013 Monte-Carlo tree search for Bayesian reinforcement learning *Appl. Intell.* **39** 345–53

[52] Jang B, Kim M, Harerimana G and Kim J W 2019 Q-learning algorithms: a comprehensive classification and applications *IEEE Access* **7** 133653–67

[53] Bommasani R *et al* 2021 On the opportunities and risks of foundation models arXiv: 2108.07258v3

[54] Radford A and Narasimhan K 2018 Improving language understanding by generative pre-training *Open AI Blog* https://cdn.openai.com/research-covers/language-unsupervised/language_understanding_paper.pdf

[55] Devlin J, Chang M W, Lee K and Toutanova K 2019 BERT: pre-training of deep bidirectional transformers for language understanding *Proc. Conf. of the North American Chapter of the Association for Computational Linguistics: Human Language Technologies* vol 1 pp 4171–86

[56] Gu Y *et al* 2020 Domain-specific language model pretraining for biomedical natural language processing *ACM Trans. Comput. Healthc.* **3** 24

[57] Bolton E *et al* 2024 BioMedLM: a 2.7B parameter language model trained on biomedical text arXiv: 2403.18421v1

[58] Huang K, Altosaar J and Ranganath R 2019 ClinicalBERT: modeling clinical notes and predicting hospital readmission arXiv: 1904.05342v3

[59] Caron M *et al* 2021 Emerging properties in self-supervised vision transformers *Proc. of the IEEE Int. Conf. on Computer Vision* (Piscataway, NJ: IEEE) pp 9630–40

[60] He K, Chen X, Xie S, Li Y, Dollar P and Girshick R 2022 Masked autoencoders are scalable vision learners *Proc. of the IEEE Computer Society Conf. on Computer Vision and Pattern Recognition (2022-June)* pp 15979–88

[61] Radford A *et al* 2021 Learning transferable visual models from natural language super-vision *Proc. Mach. Learn. Res* **139** 8748–63

[62] Liu H, Li C, Wu Q and Lee Y J 2023 Visual instruction tuning arXiv: 2304.08485v2

[63] Cai L, Gao J and Zhao D 2020 A review of the application of deep learning in medical image classification and segmentation *Ann. Transl. Med.* **8** 713

[64] Zhu W *et al* 2019 AnatomyNet: deep learning for fast and fully automated whole-volume segmentation of head and neck anatomy *Med. Phys.* **46** 576–89

[65] Isensee F, Jaeger P F, Kohl S A A, Petersen J and Maier-Hein K H 2021 nnU-Net: a self-configuring method for deep learning-based biomedical image segmentation *Nat. Methods* **18** 203–11

[66] Chen X *et al* 2021 A deep learning-based auto-segmentation system for organs-at-risk on whole-body computed tomography images for radiation therapy *Radiother. Oncol.* **160** 175–84

[67] Wong J *et al* 2021 Implementation of deep learning-based auto-segmentation for radiotherapy planning structures: a workflow study at two cancer centers *Radiat. Oncol.* **16** 101

[68] Urago Y *et al* 2021 Evaluation of auto-segmentation accuracy of cloud-based artificial intelligence and atlas-based models *Radiat. Oncol.* **16** 175

[69] Korte J C, Hardcastle N, Ng S P, Clark B, Kron T and Jackson P 2021 Cascaded deep learning-based auto-segmentation for head and neck cancer patients: organs at risk on T2-weighted magnetic resonance imaging *Med. Phys.* **48** 7757–72

[70] Lei Y *et al* 2021 Male pelvic multi-organ segmentation on transrectal ultrasound using anchor-free mask CNN *Med. Phys.* **48** 3055–64

[71] Podobnik G, Strojan P, Peterlin P, Ibragimov B and Vrtovec T 2023 HaN-seg: the head and neck organ-at-risk CT and MR segmentation dataset *Med. Phys.* **50** 1917–27

[72] Valindria V V *et al* 2018 Multi-modal learning from unpaired images: application to multi-organ segmentation in CT and MRI *Proc. IEEE Winter Conf. on Applications of Computer Vision(January)* (Piscataway, NJ: IEEE) pp 547–56

[73] Cardenas C E *et al* 2021 Generating high-quality lymph node clinical target volumes for head and neck cancer radiation therapy using a fully automated deep learning-based approach *Int. J. Radiat. Oncol. Biol. Phys.* **109** 801–12

[74] Qi X, Hu J, Zhang L, Bai S and Yi Z 2022 Automated segmentation of the clinical target volume in the planning CT for breast cancer using deep neural networks *IEEE Trans. Cybern.* **52** 3446–56

[75] Liu Z *et al* 2020 Development and validation of a deep learning algorithm for auto-delineation of clinical target volume and organs at risk in cervical cancer radiotherapy *Radiother. Oncol.* **153** 172–9

[76] Fu J, Singhrao K, Qi X S, Yang Y, Ruan D and Lewis J H 2021 Three-dimensional multipath DenseNet for improving automatic segmentation of glioblastoma on pre-operative multimodal MR images *Med. Phys.* **48** 2859–66

[77] Hu S Y *et al* 2019 Multimodal volume-aware detection and segmentation for brain metastases radiosurgery *Artificial Intelligence in Radiation Therapy* Lecture Notes in Computer Science vol 11850 (Cham: Springer) pp 61–9

[78] Wang J Y *et al* 2023 Stratified assessment of an FDA-cleared deep learning algorithm for automated detection and contouring of metastatic brain tumors in stereotactic radiosurgery *Radiat. Oncol.* **18** 61

[79] Groendahl A R *et al* 2021 A comparison of methods for fully automatic segmentation of tumors and involved nodes in PET/CT of head and neck cancers *Phys. Med. Biol.* **66** 065012

[80] Xiang D, Zhang B, Lu Y and Deng S 2023 Modality-specific segmentation network for lung tumor segmentation in PET-CT Images *IEEE J. Biomed. Health Inform.* **27** 1237–48

[81] Ma J, He Y, Li F, Han L, You C and Wang B 2024 Segment anything in medical images *Nat. Commun.* **15** 654

[82] Gibson E 2018 Multi-organ abdominal CT reference standard segmentations *Data Set* Zendono

[83] Lambert Z, Petitjean C, Dubray B and Kuan S 2020 SegTHOR: segmentation of thoracic organs at risk in CT images *2020 10th Int. Conf. on Image Processing Theory, Tools and Applications, IPTA 2020*

[84] Antonelli M *et al* 2022 The medical segmentation decathlon *Nat. Commun.* **13** 4128

[85] Kazerooni A F *et al* 2023 The Brain Tumor Segmentation (BraTS) Challenge 2023: focus on pediatrics (CBTN-CONNECT-DIPGR-ASNR-MICCAI BraTS-PEDs) arXiv: 2305.17033v7

[86] Bilic P *et al* 2023 The liver tumor segmentation benchmark (LiTS) *Med. Image Anal.* **84** 102680

[87] Yan K, Wang X, Lu L and Summers R M 2018 DeepLesion: automated mining of large-scale lesion annotations and universal lesion detection with deep learning *J. Med. Imag.* **5** 036501

[88] Prior F *et al* 2017 The public cancer radiology imaging collections of the cancer imaging archive *Sci. Data* **4** 170124

[89] Weinstein J N *et al* 2013 The Cancer Genome Atlas Pan-Cancer analysis project *Nat. Genet.* **45** 1113

[90] Gronberg M P, Gay S S, Netherton T J, Rhee D J, Court L E and Cardenas C E 2021 Technical note: Dose prediction for head and neck radiotherapy using a three-dimensional dense dilated U-net architecture *Med. Phys.* **48** 5567–73

[91] Ahn S H *et al* 2021 Deep learning method for prediction of patient-specific dose distribution in breast cancer *Radiat. Oncol.* **16** 154

[92] Nguyen D *et al* 2019 A feasibility study for predicting optimal radiation therapy dose distributions of prostate cancer patients from patient anatomy using deep learning *Sci. Rep.* **9** 1076

[93] Bohara G, Sadeghnejad Barkousaraie A, Jiang S and Nguyen D 2020 Using deep learning to predict beam-tunable pareto optimal dose distribution for intensity modulated radiation therapy *Med. Phys.* **47** 3898

[94] Ma J *et al* 2021 A feasibility study on deep learning-based individualized 3D dose distribution prediction *Med. Phys.* **48** 4438–47

[95] Wang W *et al* 2021 Deep learning-based fluence map prediction for pancreas stereotactic body radiation therapy with simultaneous integrated boost *Adv. Radiat. Oncol.* **6** 100672

[96] Li X *et al* 2020 Automatic IMRT planning via static field fluence prediction (AIP-SFFP): a deep learning algorithm for real-time prostate treatment planning *Phys. Med. Biol.* **65** 175014

[97] Li Y *et al* 2023 Simultaneous dose distribution and fluence prediction for nasopharyngeal carcinoma IMRT *Radiat. Oncol.* **18** 110

[98] Shen C *et al* 2020 Operating a treatment planning system using a deep-reinforcement learning-based virtual treatment planner for prostate cancer intensity-modulated radiation therapy treatment planning *Med. Phys.* **47** 2329–36

[99] Zhang J, Späth S S, Marjani S L, Zhang W and Pan X 2018 Characterization of cancer genomic heterogeneity by next-generation sequencing advances precision medicine in cancer treatment *Precis. Clin. Med.* **1** 29–48

[100] Cui Y, Li B, Pollom E L, Horst K C and Li R 2018 Integrating radiosensitivity and immune gene signatures for predicting benefit of radiotherapy in breast cancer *Clin. Cancer Res.* **24** 4754–62

[101] Speers C *et al* 2020 A signature that may be predictive of early versus late recurrence after radiation treatment for breast cancer that may inform the biology of early, aggressive recurrences *Int. J. Radiat. Oncol. Biol. Phys.* **108** 686–96

[102] Liveringhouse C L *et al* 2021 Genomically guided breast radiation therapy: a review of the current data and future directions *Adv. Radiat. Oncol.* **6** 100731

[103] Abdollahi H *et al* 2022 Radiomics-guided radiation therapy: opportunities and challenges *Phys. Med. Biol.* **67** 12TR02

[104] Cui S, Ten Haken R K and El Naqa I 2021 Integrating multiomics information in deep learning architectures for joint actuarial outcome prediction in non-small cell lung cancer patients after radiation therapy *Int. J. Radiat. Oncol. Biol. Phys.* **110** 893–904

[105] Salome P *et al* 2022 Multi-omics classifier of tumor recurrence vs radiation-induced lung fibrosis in NSCLC patients treated with SBRT *Int. J. Radiat. Oncol. Biol. Phys.* **114** e388–9

[106] Wei L *et al* 2023 Artificial intelligence (AI) and machine learning (ML) in precision oncology: a review on enhancing discoverability through multiomics integration *Br. J. Radiol.* **96** 20230211

[107] Ford E C and Evans S B 2018 Incident learning in radiation oncology: a review *Med. Phys.* **45** e100–19

[108] Luk S M H, Ford E C, Phillips M H and Kalet A M 2022 Improving the quality of care in radiation oncology using artificial intelligence *Clin. Oncol. (R. Coll. Radiol.)* **34** 89–98

[109] Han C *et al* 2023 Integrating plan complexity and dosiomics features with deep learning in patient-specific quality assurance for volumetric modulated arc therapy *Radiat. Oncol.* **18** 116

[110] Kalendralis P *et al* 2023 Automatic quality assurance of radiotherapy treatment plans using Bayesian networks: a multi-institutional study *Front. Oncol.* **13** 1099994

[111] Ford E C, Fong De Los Santos L, Pawlicki T, Sutlief S and Dunscombe P 2013 The structure of incident learning systems for radiation oncology *Int. J. Radiat. Oncol. Biol. Phys.* **86** 11–2

[112] Nelson C, Roy L A and Wallace H J 2019 Radiation oncology incident learning system (RO-ILS): increasing stakeholder participation for safety and quality improvement *J. Clin. Oncol.* **37** 232–2

[113] Luximon D C *et al* 2024 Results of an artificial intelligence-based image review system to detect patient misalignment errors in a multi-institutional database of cone beam computed tomography-guided radiation therapy *Int. J. Radiat. Oncol. Biol. Phys.* **120** 243–52

[114] Moor M *et al* 2023 Foundation models for generalist medical artificial intelligence *Nature* **616** 259–65

[115] Azad B *et al* 2023 Foundational models in medical imaging: a comprehensive survey and future vision arXiv: 2310.18689v1

[116] Li Q *et al* 2024 Progress and opportunities of foundation models in bioinformatics *Brief. Bioinform.* **25** bbae548

[117] Moon S, Pakhomov S, Liu N, Ryan J O and Melton G B 2014 A sense inventory for clinical abbreviations and acronyms created using clinical notes and medical dictionary resources *J. Am. Med. Inform. Assoc.* **21** 299–307

[118] Johnson A E W *et al* 2016 MIMIC-III, a freely accessible critical care database *Sci. Data* **3** 160035

[119] Pollard T J, Johnson A E W, Raffa J D, Celi L A, Mark R G and Badawi O 2018 The eICU Collaborative Research Database, a freely available multi-center database for critical care research *Sci. Data* **5** 180178

[120] Pandy A, Harangi B and Hajdu A 2023 Extracting drug names from medical reports *Int. Scientific and Technical Conf. on Computer Sciences and Information Technologies* (Piscataway, NJ: IEEE)

[121] Ayers J W *et al* 2023 Comparing physician and artificial intelligence chatbot responses to patient questions posted to a public social media forum *JAMA Intern. Med.* **183** 589–96

[122] Van Veen D *et al* 2024 Adapted large language models can outperform medical experts in clinical text summarization *Nat. Med.* **30** 1134–42

[123] Agaronnik N D, Lindvall C, El-Jawahri A, He W and Iezzoni L I 2020 Challenges of developing a natural language processing method with electronic health records to identify persons with chronic mobility disability *Arch. Phys. Med. Rehabil.* **101** 1739–46

[124] Li T *et al* 2024 CancerGPT for few shot drug pair synergy prediction using large pretrained language models *npj Digit. Med.* **7** 40

[125] Yousefzadeh M *et al* 2021 AI-corona: radiologist-assistant deep learning framework for COVID-19 diagnosis in chest CT scans *PLoS One* **16** e0250952

[126] Kim C *et al* 2024 Transparent medical image AI via an image–text foundation model grounded in medical literature *Nat. Med.* **30** 1154–65

[127] Betker J *et al* 2023 Improving image generation with better captions *Open AI Blog* https://cdn.openai.com/papers/dall-e-3.pdf

[128] Adams L C, Busch F, Truhn D, Makowski M R, Aerts H J W L and Bressem K K 2023 What does DALL-E 2 know about radiology? *J. Med. Internet Res.* **25** e43110

[129] Barrett T *et al* 2013 NCBI GEO: archive for functional genomics data sets—update *Nucleic Acids Res.* **41** D991–5

[130] Berman H M *et al* 2000 The protein data bank *Nucleic Acids Res.* **28** 235–42

[131] Song B, Li Z, Lin X, Wang J, Wang T and Fu X 2021 Pretraining model for biological sequence data *Brief. Funct. Genom.* **20** 181–95

[132] Cui H *et al* 2024 scGPT: toward building a foundation model for single-cell multi-omics using generative AI *Nat. Methods* **2024** 1470–80

[133] Chen J *et al* 2022 Interpretable RNA foundation model from unannotated data for highly accurate RNA structure and function predictions arXiv: 2204.00300v5

[134] Benegas G, Albors C, Aw A J, Ye C and Song Y S 2023 GPN-MSA: an alignment-based DNA language model for genome-wide variant effect prediction *BioRxiv* **202** 561776

[135] Benary M *et al* 2023 Leveraging large language models for decision support in personalized oncology *JAMA Netw. Open* **6** e2343689–e29

[136] Zhuang F *et al* 2021 A comprehensive survey on transfer learning *Proc. IEEE* **109** 43–76

[137] Saraswat D *et al* 2022 Explainable AI for healthcare 5.0: opportunities and challenges *IEEE Access* **10** 84486–517

[138] Seoni S, Jahmunah V, Salvi M, Barua P D, Molinari F and Acharya U R 2023 Application of uncertainty quantification to artificial intelligence in healthcare: a review of last decade (2013–2023) *Comput. Biol. Med.* **165** 107441

IOP Publishing

Artificial Intelligence in Adaptive Radiation Therapy

Yi Wang and X. Sharon Qi

Chapter 6

Introduction to adaptive radiotherapy

Jack Neylon, Michael Vincent Lauria and Yi Lao

Adaptive radiotherapy (ART) encompasses all practices of modifying a patient's treatment plan in response to anatomical or physiological changes during their treatment course. The frequency and timeline of this can vary widely, from a single adaptation implemented over several days, to daily adaptation performed in the minutes between imaging and treatment. In this chapter, the clinical motivations and technological advancements driving the evolution of radiotherapy techniques will be summarized, followed by an in-depth review of the adaptive workflow and the challenges of clinical implementation.

6.1 The road to ART

The goal of radiotherapy with curative intent is to maximize tumor control probability (TCP) while simultaneously minimizing normal tissue complication probability (NTCP). The ratio of these two values, TCP/NTCP, defines the therapeutic ratio [1].

Ideally, maximal dose to the target increases the TCP, while minimal dose to the normal tissues suppresses the NTCP. But in reality, limitations in technology and technique have dictated how well the treated volume can be conformed to the target anatomy, forcing compromises between these objectives, narrowing the gap between TCP and NTCP, and worsening the therapeutic ratio.

In addition, patient anatomy is constantly changing due to physiological movements, daily anatomical deformations, and treatment-related changes such as tumor shrinkage and weight loss. Yet, until very recently, radiotherapy treatments have been predominantly planned and delivered under the assumption of a static snapshot of the anatomy acquired at the time of simulation. Thus, to avoid compromising the efficacy of treatment in the presence of these many uncertainties, expanded margins around the target volume have been required to ensure coverage with sufficient confidence. These aspects again contribute to diminish the therapeutic ratio.

doi:10.1088/978-0-7503-6119-4ch6

To overcome these challenges, radiotherapy remains one of the fastest evolving medical disciplines. As imaging technologies advance, layers of uncertainty are peeled back, allowing the observation and quantifiable measurement of changes in weight, tumor regression/progression, and physiological motion. However, as each layer of uncertainty is removed, it exposes another underlying assumption and further pushes the field to innovate and adapt to account for this new information.

In the following subsections, we provide brief summaries of the transitions into the eras of 3D conformal radiotherapy (3DCRT), intensity-modulated radiotherapy (IMRT), and image-guided radiotherapy (IGRT). The summaries focus on how technological evolutions affected the source and scale of uncertainties in radiotherapy, providing a path to push the therapeutic ratio. We also remember the major efforts to revise and refine our understanding of normal tissue tolerances in response to these new capabilities.

6.1.1 3D conformal radiotherapy (3DCRT)

Early conventional techniques relied on single-slice geometries, often without a defined target volume, daily set-ups based on external markers only, and required large fields without customized margins. With the advent of computed tomography (CT), several changes were introduced to clinical workflows [2]. Targets could be identified and contoured three dimensionally, along with nearby organs at risk (OARs). Custom margins could then be expanded from the targets. Custom blocks could be molded to the shape of the target from the beam's eye view. Dose could be calculated on the computer in 3D and produce dose–volume histograms. Digitally reconstructed radiographs facilitated set-up adjustments based on x-ray imaging of anatomical structures.

Soon, several studies explored the benefit of utilizing this 3D information in radiotherapy and estimated the required precision for radiotherapy treatments [3–8]. These culminated in a report by the American Association of Physicists in Medicine (AAPM), 'Physical aspects of quality assurance in radiation therapy' [4]. Within this report, they estimated the spatial uncertainties, from all sources, should be within one centimeter, while dosimetric uncertainty should aim to be within 5%.

The prevalence of CT imaging and 3D treatment planning continued to rise. With improved target localization and more conformal treatment plans, the volume of normal tissues being irradiated was reduced. This led to a proliferation of studies examining dose escalation. Higher doses meant better TCP, but to assess if this actually improved the therapeutic ratio, new toxicity endpoints and dose constraints needed to be discerned.

This led to Emami's seminal paper, published in the *Red Journal* in 1991, as the culmination of a monumental effort to interpret previously published dose–response data, and translate these into normal tissue tolerances [9]. The motivation for this work and its relation to 3DCRT is summarized thusly: 'During preliminary experimentation with three-dimensional treatment planning, it became apparent that there is a critical need for more accurate information about the tolerance of normal tissue to radiation.' This work undoubtedly improved radiotherapy treatments over the next two decades, but still had severe limitations, the largest of which being the source data. The lack of volumetric information for the delivered doses forced the authors to arbitrarily proportion organs volumes into thirds. As Emami himself commented in a 2013 article revisiting his prior work: 'It completely pre-dated the 3DCRT/IMRT-IGRT era. Even at that time dose–volume histograms were not in routine clinical use.' [10]

6.1.2 Intensity modulated radiotherapy (IMRT)

As 3D dosimetric data accumulated, new studies attempted to quantify the impact of geometrical uncertainties on radiotherapy treatment. Soon, investigators derived margin equations to account for random uncertainties during treatment planning [11–14]. The widespread incorporation of multi-leaf collimators (MLCs) paved the way for inversely optimized treatment plans, and intensity modulation, able to conform the high-dose region even more compactly around the target volume.

In 1994, AAPM Task Group 40 published their report 'Comprehensive QA for radiation oncology' [15], with recommendations for QA tests, frequencies, and tolerances aimed to maintain an overall dosimetric uncertainty within 5%, and spatial uncertainty within 5 mm.

In 2011, standing on two decades of 3D treatment planning data and outcomes reporting, and amid the transition to widespread intensity-modulated radiotherapy (IMRT), an effort was coordinated to update normal tissue tolerances with the 'Quantitative analyses of normal tissue effects in the clinic (QUANTEC)' papers [16]. One of the driving motivations of this effort was due to the ability of recent technology advances to produce near uniform dose distributions in the target, while only producing partial non-uniform doses to the surrounding normal tissues.

Still, as described by Marcel van Herk in his 2004 overview on the interplay of errors and margins in radiotherapy, the main source of uncertainty remained tumor delineation and set-up variations [17]. Much effort had been made in recent years to reduce geometrical errors. In 1999, Jaffray et al published a review article of advances in uncertainty reduction, stating, 'The geometric precision of radiotherapy treatments must increase if the objectives of dose escalation and increased disease control are to be achieved.' [18] In this article, they expound on the need for improved immobilization and both offline and online correction strategies to improve precision, including more frequent imaging.

6.1.3 Image-guided radiotherapy (IGRT)

Returning to van Herk, he states in a 2007 publication, 'margins overlap organs at risk, thereby limiting dose escalation. The aim of IGRT is to improve the accuracy by imaging tumors and critical structures on the machine just before irradiation.' [19] While this could not reduce random anatomic or physiologic uncertainties, it reduces localization errors, allowing tighter margins during planning.

In another 2007 publication, Dawson and Jaffray discuss advances in IGRT, stating that 'geometric advantages increase the chance of tumor control, reduce the risk of toxicity after radiotherapy, and facilitate the development of shorter radiotherapy schedules.' [20] However, they also describe how 'IGRT increases our awareness of geometric change occurring during radiation therapy'.

The benefits of image guidance and reduced margins were evidenced repeatedly over the years in different treatment settings. For example, Srivastava *et al* found on-board imaging could achieve set-up uncertainties within 5 mm for the head and neck (HN) [21], and emphasized, 'even a small margin increase (e.g. 1 mm) may result in increase of more than 20% in relative extra volume and 15% in NTCP value of organs at risk (OARs).' Similarly, Burnet *et al* considered IMRT and IGRT in neuro-oncology, and concluded, 'Image guidance adds precision and the possibility of careful reduction in planning target volume margins.' [22] Additionally, Grills *et al* demonstrated the benefit of daily cone-beam CT (CBCT) for aggressive margin reduction in lung radiotherapy [23].

IGRT also elucidated how much improved set-up precision had become. Guckenberger *et al* quantified translational and rotational patient set-up errors using CBCT and found 'that the accuracy of the CBCT-guided evaluation of set-up errors is in the region of a voxel size of 1 mm.' [24]

In following with the efforts of Emami in 1991, and QUANTEC in 2011, the next iteration was published in 2021 as 'High dose per fraction, hypofractionated treatment effects in the clinic (HyTEC)' [25]. HyTEC aimed to address the surge in hypofractionated regimens and higher dose-per-fraction stereotactic body radiotherapy (SBRT) in recent years, which followed from the increasingly precise localization capabilities of IGRT in the past decade. In their editorial, Grimm *et al* state, 'Clinical adoption of SBRT has outpaced outcomes analyses, especially considering the strong impact of fraction size on late effects.' [26]

6.1.4 Adaptive radiotherapy (ART)

As described above, the field of radiotherapy adopts and adapts to advances in imaging. Adaptive radiotherapy is the next in a long line of innovative techniques that increase the precision and conformality of radiation delivery. ART will allow the field to push further, reducing the uncertainty of interfractional anatomic changes, and further increasing the therapeutic ratio.

6.2 ART workflow and implementation

In this section, we will introduce the general adaptive workflow. We will discuss what it takes to make ART work, current practices, and what could be preventing the transition from offline ART to online ART (OnART) as common practice.

6.2.1 ART workflow

The ART workflow can be categorized into two major categories: offline and online. In offline ART, the adaptive process takes place outside of the treatment room between fractions. In online ART (OnART), the adaptive process happens while the patient is on the table during a treatment fraction, demanding higher levels of technology, time efficiency, and daily image quality. Figure 6.1 from Lim-Reinders *et al* showcases the different steps in offline versus OnART in a flowchart [27].

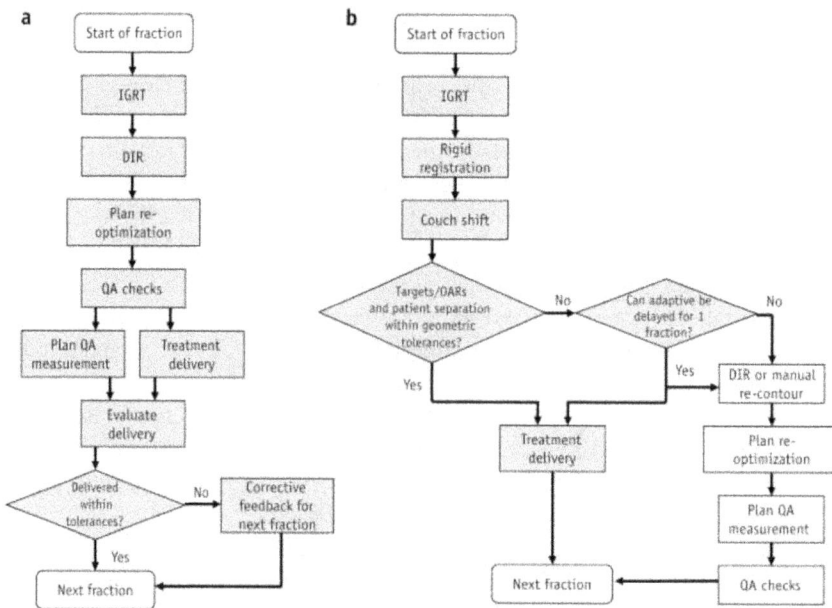

Figure 6.1. Comparison of ART workflows between (a) online ART and (b) offline ART. Abbreviations: DIR = deformable image registration; IGRT = image-guided radiation therapy; OARs = organs at risk; QA = quality assurance. (Reproduced with permission from [27]. Copyright 2017 Elsevier.)

As can be seen from the flowchart in figure 6.1, ART is a technique that not only impacts several stages of the radiotherapy workflow, but also introduces new steps that bring their own demands for technology, required expertise, and clinical considerations. The general approach to ART can be summarized into six key stages: imaging, image registration, re-contouring, re-optimization, dose calculation, and safety/QA.

6.2.1.1 Imaging

There are two imaging requirements for ART: an image for initial planning, and an image at the treatment couch to capture the daily anatomy. The first image follows the traditional radiotherapy workflow. This is commonly a helical CT image. The second image brings more consideration depending on the ART approach.

In offline ART, the daily imaging is straightforward. The same imaging technique used to simulate the patient for initial planning can be used once again to ensure sufficient image quality. This has traditionally been CT but could also be MRI, which we may see increasingly in the future. The key point is that the patient is re-simulated to create a new plan based on the changes in anatomy from the initial simulation, such as weight loss or tumor shrinkage.

Advances in on-board imaging have opened the door to OnART. Primarily, this has resulted from the advent of on-board MRI, which offers real-time, high-quality imaging of soft tissues. Recently, some systems have offered OnART capabilities using on-board MRI. Additionally, with improvements in CBCT, including reduction of artifacts, motion management, and improvements in detector design and image reconstruction, there are now commercially available systems that offer CBCT-based ART capabilities [28]. Perhaps the most recent advancement in on-board imaging for OnART has been the use of PET to guide biologically adaptive radiotherapy, targeting areas of high uptake imaged during the treatment. The choice of imaging may depend on finances, anatomical areas to be treated, and expertise of the clinic.

6.2.1.2 Image registration

To translate the initial plan to the daily anatomy, there needs to be a mapping of the initial image to the new image, whether offline or online. In OnART, the registration is also used to propagate the contours from the initial plan to the new daily image to save considerable time in re-planning. There are two primary choices for mapping these images: rigid registration and deformable image registration (DIR).

Rigid registration is driven by a global translation that matches the image. There are six degrees of freedom (translations in all three directions and rotations on all three axes). Rigid registration allows the clinician to see vast changes in anatomy, target size, or positional accuracy. It also allows a straightforward mapping of the initial plan to the new geometry to review the impacts of those changes on plan quality and help decide if adaptation is needed, or to assess the cumulative dose administered from both the initial and adapted plans.

Unlike rigid registration, DIR allows voxels to expand and contract, and includes individual mapping for each voxel. It therefore has as three degrees of freedom for every voxel. Accurate DIR offers a more sophisticated mapping of voxels, which can lead to more accurate dose accumulation in offline ART, or more accurate contour propagation in OnART. However, DIR can be challenging, particularly in CBCT-based platforms since it relies on high contrast to map anatomical landmarks in the images. The type of image, time constraint, and acceptability of current techniques should all be considered when deciding which registration to use, and the chosen image registration should be heavily tested [27].

A study performed by Hussein *et al* in 2021 surveyed 71 radiotherapy centers in the UK. They received 51 responses with 39% having already implemented DIR and 43% planning to implement DIR clinically [29]. Reported uses of DIR included multi-modality image registration, registration of planning CTs to daily images, dose propagation, and above all, propagation of contours. The survey results also included suggestions to allow more widespread adoption of DIR. The most frequent responses included clear guidelines for different applications, better commissioning tools, and better tools for QA of registration results. These are excellent problems to be addressed by AI tools for DIR commissioning and registration evaluation.

6.2.1.3 Re-contouring

Often, the anatomical changes between the planning image and the daily image include deformation, tumor shrinkage, changes in gas, changes in weight, or other large or unpredictable changes. If rigid registration is used, these will not be captured, so tumors or OARs will need to be re-contoured. If DIR is used, the contours can be propagated to the new image. Even then, these may not deform properly as vast changes can be difficult to describe by the registration's optimization problem, and results should be reviewed closely.

For offline ART, contouring may follow the same procedure as in the initial planning stage with close attention to the anatomical changes. In OnART, there are different approaches to ensure contouring is completed within the adaptive timeframe. For example, one may prescribe a region of interest such as a large ring around the target to focus contouring in the most relevant areas. With DIR, the contours outside of this high-dose region may be accurate enough for plan assessment with relatively limited impact on re-planning.

Re-contouring is an excellent target for automation through AI. For example, the Varian Ethos has an auto-contouring solution that uses a modified convolutional neural network to automatically contour organs from CBCTs. The quality of auto-contours and subsequent treatment plans generated from those contours has been shown to be effective in sites such as pelvic or lung cases [30, 31]. An automatic solution for contouring not only saves time, but also reduces inter-observer variability. However, challenges remain in areas with lack of training, so efforts to improve these solutions will continue to improve their robustness.

At this point in the workflow, we can evaluate the original plan as it applies to the current anatomy. Updated dosimetry can reveal which planning goals are still met, and which planning goals fail with the new anatomy. If there are goals that fail, the next stage is to re-optimize the plan to improve overall plan quality and meet those goals.

6.2.1.4 Re-optimization

Re-optimization is the crux of ART. Without this stage, up to this point in the workflow, we would simply be monitoring accumulated dose (which still has its own value). Re-optimizing is the stage at which the plan is altered to adapt to the changes identified during re-contouring. With an image of the patient's current anatomy, updated contours, and a mapping of our initial plan to the new anatomy, we can re-optimize the plan to meet our planning goals.

A major consideration in re-optimization during OnART is the limited time to try different planning techniques. In offline ART, we can adjust the optimization constraints, field arrangement, or other parameters of the treatment plan to maximize plan quality. There is more time to explore different planning techniques. However, during OnART we do not have that time luxury, and re-optimization must be performed efficiently. This likely means using the same beam arrangement as the initial plan, but re-optimizing the MLC leaf sequences to change the targeting and modulation of the dose.

6.2.1.5 Dose calculation

In offline ART, dose calculation should follow the same approach as the initial planning. With time to re-plan offline, sufficient dose calculation accuracy should be prioritized, and all guidelines of routine planning should be implemented.

Dose calculation during OnART must be both fast and accurate. With recent technological strides in dose calculation, highly accurate models, such as Monte Carlo or Boltzmann transport solvers, have been implemented in common adaptive platforms. The dose grid resolution is another key factor for speed [32–34]. While it is typical to use a 2 mm grid for high doses, a 3 mm grid may be used for large targets, such as a prostate treatment including the lymph nodes, to reduce calculation time.

6.2.1.6 Safety/QA

The ART workflow introduces its own quality assurance (QA) requirements to ensure the quality and integrity of the new plan within the timeframe of the adaptive environment. Figure 6.2 from Cai *et al* neatly summarizes the key workflow steps in OnART with MR-guidance and proposed QA procedures [35]. Many of the processes such as fusion and contour inspection, planning goals comparison, and plan quality check are conventional QA procedures re-established for the adaptive plan.

One key consideration for QA in the OnART workflow is the plan integrity check. Most clinics today use phantoms or on-board detectors to perform IMRT QA, verifying consistency between the planned and delivered dose and demonstrating the deliverability of the plan [36]. However, during adaptive re-planning, there is no time to perform such a test. Therefore, the plan integrity check is often performed as an independent dose calculation and monitor units (MUs) check.

As time is a key concern with the plan integrity check in OnART, it is consistently a concern through the entire QA process. Therefore, automation is a necessary aspect of successfully and efficiently performing QA. In figure 6.2, the processes in green text indicate opportunities for automation, including plan goal comparison, plan integrity checks, independent dose calculation, and post-delivery QA.

Offline ART avoids many of the time-specific concerns in ART QA, but there are still unique safety and accuracy considerations involved. These have been nicely summarized by Yan *et al*. In the offline setting, DIR is used between an initial

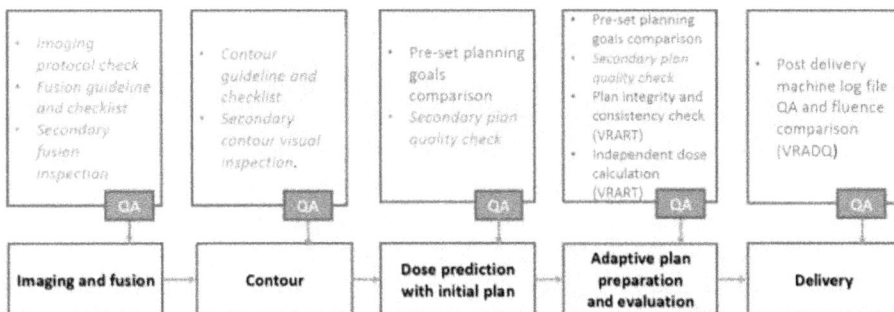

Figure 6.2. QA in the online ART workflow. The lower level shows the ART workflow steps and the upper level shows the related QA procedures. Orange, italic text denotes manual processes while green text denotes automated processes. (Reproduced with permission from [35]. Copyright 2018 Elsevier.)

planning image and multiple daily images, often of a different modality (CT versus CBCT, for example) [37]. As a major component of offline ART QA, the accuracy of this registration needs to be checked thoroughly. Other offline ART considerations highlighted by Yan *et al* include uncertainties in couch or MLC-based aperture corrections, systematic and random errors in treatment positions, uncertainties in dose tracking, and uncertainties in offline adaptive planning modifications. Regular checks for patient positioning accuracy can address many of these concerns, which may already be part of the clinical workflow. However, dose monitoring daily for hypofractionated plans and weekly for fractionated plans as well as checks for unexpected anatomical changes, target changes, and DVH parameter verification are examples of offline ART-specific QA procedures.

Following successful QA checks, the adapted plan can be safely delivered. In OnART, treatment is delivered immediately. In offline ART, the patient returns for their next fraction, and the new plan is delivered in place of the old plan.

6.2.2 Current practice

In current clinical practice, ART is primarily performed offline. One major signal that offline ART may be necessary is weight loss, especially in HN radiotherapy patients. This weight loss can arise from either the tumor itself or treatment-related toxicities [38]. Weight loss impacts planning by shrinking the patient anatomy. The initial plan thus overestimates the distances between OARs and the target, which could lead to overdosing those organs. Furthermore, these treatments are often hyperfractionated and can last more than a month, offering enough time to invite large anatomical changes, and also sufficient time to re-simulate and adapt the treatment plan.

Another common cause for offline ART is tumor regression, which could happen in many sites. For fractionated treatments, the tumor may respond during the course of treatment. In this case, the tumor may shrink, and the original treatment plan may consequently deliver the prescription dose to nearby healthy tissue and OARs. It is thus worthwhile to adapt the plan for a smaller target offline. Tumor regression is a significant indication for adaptation in gynecologic tumors, and can also call for adaptation in rectal cases [39, 40].

Though tumor regression is an important indication for offline ART, organ motion is much more common. In a review of offline and OnART in clinical workflows by Thörnqvist *et al* in 2016, 98% of the reviewed adaptations were due to target motion, as opposed to only 2% due to tumor regression [40]. For the prostate, this often presented as prostate motion relative to the bony anatomy. For the bladder, plans were often adapted for changes in bladder shape and position. The key to offline ART is exploiting geometric differences, whether from changes in the patient, their normal organs, or the tumors themselves.

OnART is a much newer concept than offline ART, but it is becoming increasingly common thanks to the introduction of real-time MRI image guidance, high-quality CBCTs, faster dose calculation, and the growing experience of clinicians. OnART is best suited to address smaller intrafraction changes, such as positional changes of abdominal organs such as bowels, baseline variation of the lungs, and tumor response [41].

Early experience implementing OnART has been reported by Lamb *et al* from UCLA, summarizing their workflow, communication scheme, time considerations, strategies, and QA approach [42]. They estimated a median total workflow time of 54 min (9 min for imaging, 7 min for physician approval of the set-up, 10 min for adaptive re-contouring, and 14 min for planning and QA), so it is critical that we continue to introduce automation to reduce the time spent on each step.

6.2.3 Clinical impact

ART can offer great improvements to plan dosimetry, and ultimately, patient outcomes. Clinical trials have shown the potential for ART to improve plan dosimetry, and more trials are underway to study its impact on patient outcomes [43–45]. However, it also bears great impact on the clinical workflow. This impact extends to all members of the radiation oncology team, including therapists, dosimetrists, physicians, and physicists. Figure 6.3 from Liu *et al* nicely summarizes some of the roles and responsibilities of these groups in the ART workflow [46].

6.2.3.1 Therapists
Therapists, as in traditional radiotherapy, drive the treatment in the ART workflow. They set up the patient in the treatment room and interface with the patient to keep them informed and comfortable during treatment. The increased treatment time leads to more involvement of the therapists in coaching patients. They also acquire the daily images that are used for adaptive re-planning. After adaptation, therapists need to pay careful mind to delivering the correct plan, and thus need to be well-trained on the ART system and interface and need to have a strong understanding of the workflow.

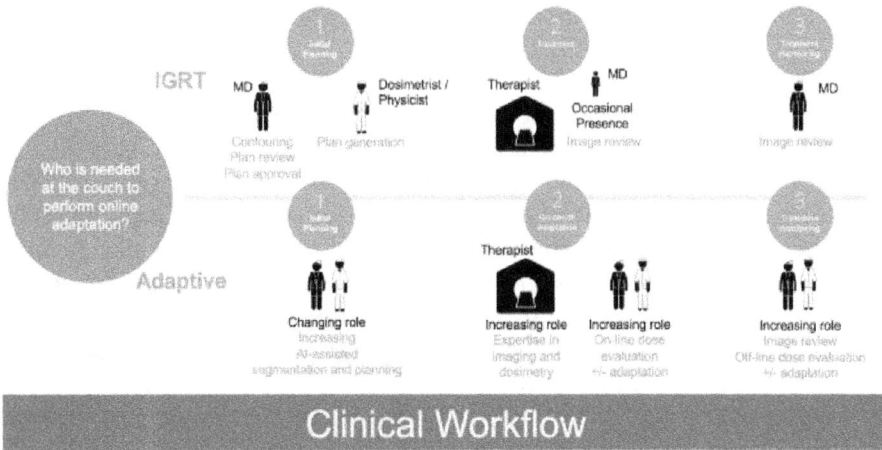

Figure 6.3. Clinical workflow. (Reproduced from [46]. CC BY 4.0.)

6.2.3.2 Dosimetrists

Dosimetrists play a large role in both online and offline ART. In offline ART, their role may be more straightforward—optimizing the new adapted plan using the image from re-simulation following the same approach as the initial plan. However, they need to have an intimate understanding of the planning strategies and concerns in the adaptive approach. Their role in OnART can be much more involved. There is less time to digest the case, and even less time to re-contour and re-optimize the plan. This demands thorough training and experience from dosimetrists so that they are comfortable in the adaptive environment.

6.2.3.3 Physicians

Physicians play an instrumental role in the ART workflow, primarily in deciding when to adapt, and after re-optimizing, whether to accept the new plan or choose to deliver the original plan. They may plan to adapt ahead of time or know when to trigger adaptation based on the circumstances during treatment, such as the changed positions of internal organs or changes in the tumor size and shape. In some cases, they may drive the decision to escalate dose based on what they see during treatment [47]. This demands new expertise from physicians, including new trials to investigate new approaches and the impact of ART. Physicians also play important roles in reviewing and approving imaging, contours, and plans. The fast-paced OnART environment thus demands an increased presence and engagement at the treatment machine.

6.2.3.4 Physicists

Along with sharing the roles of the dosimetrists, physicists provide the technical expertise to commission and implement the ART workflow in their clinics. They must understand the details of the imaging, registration, contouring, optimization, dose calculation, and QA to safely bring each stage to operation. They should also ensure continuous safe operation of all procedures by working with therapists, dosimetrists, and physicians. Physicists are also responsible for establishing QA procedures and educating the rest of the team on executing those procedures [37].

6.2.3.5 Collaboration

Although each member of the radiotherapy team bears many unique responsibilities in the adaptive workflow, it is ultimately a highly collaborative environment. Physician input on imaging and re-planning are crucial to aid the therapists and dosimetrists in their roles. Physics input for safe and effective treatment delivery help inform the physicians. The room is often full of different team members working closely together. Furthermore, a strong collaborative effort is necessary to continue pushing the field of ART forward. Kristy Brock discussed this importance in her 2019 article, calling for collaboration between physicians, physicists, and industry partners to further improve the clinical workflow, increase technical accuracy, and enable the best decision-making ability in ART [28]. AI provides a promising avenue to push the boundaries of every aspect of ART, and it will require a strong effort from all parties to develop and implement this technology safely and accurately.

6.3 Considerations for implementing online ART

6.3.1 Time as a limiting factor

The effective administration of ART, which responds promptly to changes in tumor and surrounding tissue conditions, requires reliable and efficient clinical execution. With advancements in rapid imaging acquisition and computational resources, OnART has emerged to address inter-fraction variations based on pre-treatment in-room imaging. While offline ART primarily targets systematic errors manifested between treatments, OnART can accommodate both random and systematic errors in daily anatomy and set-up changes, thereby maximizing dosimetric benefits [48–50]. However, the successful implementation of OnART imposes unique requirements on time and resource allocation.

Currently, only a limited number of OnART systems are available for clinical use, which can be categorized into CT-based OnART, represented by Varian Ethos, and MR-based OnART, exemplified by ViewRay MRIdian and Elekta Unity.

In an initial investigation into clinical OnART efficiency, a single institutional study examined the treatment logs of 450 CT-based OnART fractions for various sites, including the prostate, GYN, breast, lung, HN, as well as abdomen. They reported an average duration of 37 ± 16 min for daily adaptive treatments, from patient simulation to delivery completion. Specifically, the additional steps for generating online adaptive plans took an average of 20 min [51]. Similarly, another institution implementing CT-based ART reported on over 1000 fractions, indicating an average time of 34.52 ± 11.42 min from start to finish, with physicist/physician-involved steps totaling around 20 min [52].

In MR-based OnART, the current workflow entails slightly prolonged treatment sessions attributable to extended acquisition times and additional steps in treatment planning. An institutional inquiry into 80 adapted pelvic and abdominal SBRT fractions, conducted with the 0.35 T MR-based ViewRay MRIdian system, unveiled an average overall session duration of 54 min, with the adaptive steps pertaining to planning and evaluation consuming 31 min [42]. Similarly, another institution employing a 1.5 T MR-based Elekta platform for 65 liver and pancreas SBRT cases reported an average session duration just below 70 min (ranging from 50 to 90 min) [53].

The extended on-couch time during OnART imposes considerable pressure on patient immobilization, as any movement by the patient during re-planning can compromise the effectiveness of plan adaptation itself. This underscores the critical need for fast and reliable solutions in re-planning, encompassing contouring, registration, re-optimization, plan evaluation, and QA. On the other hand, the increased workload associated with plan regeneration for each treatment fraction stresses departmental resources. Consequently, there is a pressing need for enhanced workflow efficiency and the adoption of automated processes. Considerations for rapid plan generation and workflow automation will be discussed in detail in the following sections.

6.3.2 Implications for fast and reliable re-planning

6.3.2.1 OAR contouring

Based on current institutional reports, the additional time allocated for OnART re-planning varies depending on the imaging modality: approximately 20 min for CT-based systems and 30 min for MR-based systems [42, 49, 53]. The bottleneck in this process remains the contouring of OARs, which consumes over 10 min in both CT- and MR-based OnART sessions, with some complicated treatment sites requiring up to 24 min [54]. While deformable registration-based propagation has been widely adopted in clinical practice to expedite these steps, it still involves significant manual editing and evaluation.

Recently, there has been a surge in the development of deep learning (DL) based auto-contouring algorithms. These algorithms have demonstrated comparable quality to manual delineation on both daily KVCT or MR images and have significantly accelerated contouring procedures to within seconds. Specifically, several DL-based auto-segmentation networks have exhibited high accuracy in OAR delineation and are readily available for clinical integration in prostate, cervical, and HN cancers [55, 56]. Some studies have even achieved one-shot auto-contouring on KVCT for up to 117 OARs throughout the body [57–59]. These developments lay a robust foundation for minimal manual edits in current radiotherapy workflows for a broader range of RT applications, including total marrow irradiation and cranial-spinal irradiation.

Moreover, attempts have been made to integrate labor-free auto-contouring into OnART workflows for pelvic cancer treatments [60, 61]. While these attempts have demonstrated satisfactory quality without manual edits for most patients, there are still instances where manual intervention is required. Hence, continuous scrutiny of daily auto-segmentation is necessary for its full integration into clinical OnART. Additionally, the majority of these DL-based studies are primarily tailored for the pelvic or HN regions [59], which are anatomically more rigid and therefore exhibit fewer interfractional alterations. However, there remains a shortage of auto-contouring methods for the thoracic and abdominal regions, where more interfractional anatomical changes are anticipated. Despite the challenges of auto-contouring in the thoracic and abdominal regions, it is anticipated that OnART will offer greater dosimetric benefits in these areas. Hence, there is an urgent need for further research in this domain.

6.3.2.2 Deformable imaging registration (DIR)

DIR plays a fundamental role in the OnART workflow, encompassing tasks such as aligning planning CT scans with daily imaging, propagating target volumes, and accumulating doses. With the accessibility of parallel computing within modern OnART platforms, DIR operations themselves are not inherently time intensive. However, the inherent uncertainties associated with DIR methodologies pose challenges to downstream processes, necessitating meticulous manual scrutiny and consequently elongating the duration of the OnART workflow.

The primary uncertainties associated with DIR stem from the underlying assumption of homogeneous deformation properties within the image domain [62]. Most current DIR algorithms essentially seek mathematical or numerical solutions for the best match in the image space. Without prior knowledge of differential tissue properties and a physical basis for expansion, contraction, and pose changes, DIR algorithms struggle to effectively distinguish highly elastic structures undergoing substantial morphological transformations, such as the bladder in different fillings, from rigid structures undergoing positional adjustments, such as pelvic bones in different positions. This often leads to implausible movements.

Various algorithms have been proposed to address the heterogeneous biomechanical properties of tissues by introducing non-uniform constraints, including contour-guided registration [63], shape-based regularization [64], or local rigidity penalties [62]. To further leverage biomechanical properties, continuum mechanics have been incorporated into the design of regularizers, enforcing smoothed and diffeomorphic transformations for more physically realistic movement [65, 66]. However, the complexity of domain discretization and resolution schemes limits their clinical integration, particularly in OnART settings.

In addition to the inherent plausibility challenges within current DIR algorithms, complex medical scenarios, such as surgical resections, nasal and pulmonary congestions, and tissue inflammations, can lead to missing correspondences between moving and target images, further augmenting uncertainty [67, 68]. Consequently, to better align with the requirements of the radiotherapy field, there is a need for site-specific fine-tunings that incorporate both physical and medical contexts.

With the adoption of encoder–decoder architectures and spatial transformer networks, deep learning-based DIR, such as Quicksilver [69] and Voxelmorph [70], demonstrate potential in accommodating the heightened computational needs for biomechanically realistic solutions. Coupled with various weakly supervised training strategies adapting to specific medical conditions in radiation oncology, AI-based DIR shows promise in providing solutions to increasingly complex radiotherapy needs within acceptable timeframes in clinical OnART [71].

6.3.2.3 Plan generation

Upon determination of OAR and target volumes, and registration of planning to treatment imaging, subsequent adjustments to plan parameters are necessary. Re-planning procedures can be categorized into two main types: adapt to position (ATP) and adapt to shape (ATS). ATP involves translating the original plan to the new isocenter and optimizing the weights and shapes of MLC segments, while ATS essentially regenerates a new plan. Although ATS affords higher degrees of MLC optimization to adapt to the new anatomy, it is more time-consuming [72]. The time required for plan regeneration can vary from seconds to minutes, depending on the adaptation mode and plan complexity.

ATP has been demonstrated to be cost-effective for adapting daily treatments with minor anatomy variations. For instance, a prospective analysis of HN cancer OnART in ten patients using a 1.5 T MR-linac revealed that the ATP workflow resulted in only a 2% dose difference in target coverage and a high gamma passing rate. Although dose differences in OARs were higher, the delivered dose on the summation plan remained statistically comparable to the reference plan, even with one or more constraint violations in at least two fractions [73]. However, it should be noted that when patient offsets exceed 2 mm, the ATP workflow fails to reproduce clinically acceptable dose distributions [74].

To maximize the dosimetric benefits of OnART, ATS with a higher degree of optimization capability is preferred, if resources allow. Winkel *et al* investigated OnART for five cases with various inter-fraction anatomical changes: single lymph node, prostate, rectum, esophagus, and multiple lymph nodes [72]. In both re-planning modes, various optimization methods with increased degrees of freedom were explored, including adapting segments only, optimizing weights from segments, optimizing weights and shapes from segments, as well as two options available only to ATS: optimizing weights from fluence and optimizing weights and shapes from fluence. As expected, treatments with higher anatomical complexity and inter-fraction changes require optimization methods with greater degrees of freedom to achieve clinically acceptable plans. For instance, while the ATP work-flow with optimization of weights only from segments sufficed for a single lymph node case, ATS workflow with optimization of weights from fluence was necessary for rectum and esophagus cases to meet the same outcome. In the more complex multiple lymph node case, full online ATS optimization had to be used to meet all constraints [72].

To expedite the optimization process, prevalent commercial OnART workflows frequently utilize atlas and protocol-based algorithms [75]. Atlas-based algorithms draw upon a repository of approved contours and plans to establish associations between geometry and DVH, enabling the prediction of achievable DVH for new patients with similar contours and treatment objectives. Conversely, protocol-based algorithms begin with user-defined templates containing clinical goals and priorities, iteratively adjusting the DVH until an optimal plan is achieved. These algorithms can be augmented by DL models [76], which advance DVH prediction to 2D and 3D dose predictions [77]. Moreover, leveraging historical patient plans, additional re-planning steps, such as beam orientation selection, fluence map generation, and delivery parameter generation, can be seamlessly integrated into a single DL task, further enhancing automation [78]. However, despite the demonstrated enhancement in plan efficiency shown by DL-based algorithms in preclinical validation, comprehensive QA procedures are indispensable for their clinical integration into OnART.

Currently, there exists a trade-off between the time and resources allocated for plan regeneration and the dosimetric benefits attained. Future research on sophis-ticated optimization algorithms and large-scale toxicity analysis are imperative to substantiate the appropriate balance between planning time and dosimetric gain.

6.3.2.4 Quality assurance (QA)

Following treatment plan generation, QA becomes imperative prior to treatment delivery. Since on-table patient-specific QA is unfeasible, leading commercially available OnART platforms, including Varian Ethos, Viewray MRIdian, and Elekta Unity, employ a rapid secondary dose calculation (SDC) method [42, 79, 80].

Although vendor-supplied QA tools have demonstrated good agreement with post-treatment QA measurements in small-scale studies [81], failure mode and effects analysis (FMEA) has revealed a 38% increase in the risk priority number for ART, with significant risks associated with segmentation and treatment planning processes [82]. Complementary to vendor-provided SDC, Rippke and colleagues have developed a QA analysis that re-examines additional factors, including absolute volume changes and gaps in structures, electron density maps, and fluence modulation complexity [83]. Their study revealed that errors, particularly those related to contours, which may occur during OnART, can be identified through supplementary QA measures, underscoring the importance of adopting additional QA steps to ensure the safe delivery of OnART.

Moreover, beyond the errors inherent in conventional treatment planning and delivery, OnART introduces distinctive procedures that may contribute to additional uncertainties. Kluter *et al* confirmed the additional risks posed by OnART, with approximately one-third of the risks being specific to MR-linac systems [84]. Additionally, the daily imaging utilized in OnART typically exhibits lower quality compared to planning imaging. This not only affects the delineation of OARs and targets but also influences downstream procedures, such as daily imaging-based dose calculation and accumulation [49]. Consequently, frequent end-to-end verification of the adaptive workflow is recommended [52, 83].

6.3.3 Implications for automated workflow

ART programs are more demanding on clinical staffing levels than SRS/SBRT programs [51, 85]. Despite the widely accepted benefits of reduced toxicity and improved target coverage, the increased logistical and resource burden of OnART limits its widespread implementation. Current clinical decisions within OnART are primarily based on physicians' or physicists' experiences. In the absence of a standardized framework, the implementation of OnART varies with limited consensus on patient selection, time to adapt, and algorithms to choose. Therefore, paramount to the urgent need for fast and accurate re-planning tools, the establishment of a roadmap for automated workflows necessitates a standardized and quantitative framework to support clinical decisions. This framework should not only define action thresholds to initiate an OnART but also guide clinical decisions to progress through each step of the OnART process.

6.3.3.1 Action levels to initiate OnART
To establish a standardized decision-making framework, the first step involves quantifying anatomical deviations, which greatly influence the decision to proceed with OnART. Anatomical deviation primarily arises from inter-fraction motion, which varies in magnitude across treatment sites. For instance, it can be on the scale of millimeters in the prostate, whereas in the liver and pancreas, it can extend to centimeters [86]. However, inter-subject variations exist, as deviations exceeding 1 cm in the prostate are detected occasionally [86]. Adopting the concept of 4D planning, which integrates pre-treatment 4D imaging that is predictive of potential

movement and incorporates adjusted intra-fraction margins into re-planning, has the potential to greatly improve automated workflows and guide session scheduling.

Heterogeneous treatment responses also contribute to anatomical changes, notably through within-course tumor shrinkage, which are commonly reported in lung [87–89] and HN radiotherapy [90]. This shrinkage can vary significantly, ranging from 1.2% per day in lung treatments to as high as 70% in HN treatments [90, 91]. Such changes are often accompanied by secondary shifts in the surrounding OARs. For instance, a reduction in volume of up to 30% in the parotid glands has been observed during HN radiotherapy, along with a tendency to shift towards higher dose regions [92]. Therefore, a quantitative metric comprehensively evaluating the overall anatomical deviation is in demand.

Furthermore, relying solely on univariate distance and volume as the primary descriptors for quantifying anatomical changes may not adequately capture critical changes with the most significant dosimetric impact. In the case of hollow structures such as the bladder, rectum, esophagus, and ventricles, morphological alterations often stem from variations in internal fillings, which may not substantially affect dosimetry. Consequently, parameters developed over tissue wall thickness or surfaces become more relevant for assessing dosimetric changes [93, 94]. Specifically, surface modeling of bladder inter-fraction motion changes has revealed that while significant motion may occur, it predominantly affects the superior–anterior bladder surface, with no discernible dosimetric impact on high-dose regions proximal to the planning target volume (PTV) [95]. Further research is needed to establish a quantitative relationship between anatomical changes and resultant dosimetric consequences to facilitate OnART decision making.

6.3.3.2 Automated plan evaluation

As previously discussed in section 6.3.2, current auto-contouring methods often require manual review. Given the absence of ground-truth contours on daily imaging, expediting the review process necessitates offline selection and tuning of auto-contouring algorithms. Quantitative measurements of contour accuracy commonly fall into two categories: overlapping-based metrics, such as the Dice similarity coefficient (DSC) and Jaccard index [96], and distance-based metrics, such as the Hausdorff distance (HD) [97]. Recently, a surface-based refinement of overlapping metrics, known as surface DSC, has shown higher clinical acceptability compared to traditional metrics [98, 99]. While there is no gold standard available during OnART, evaluating the dosimetric consequences is more relevant for assessing the clinical acceptability of auto-contours in scenarios with limited time and resources.

Several studies have investigated the dosimetric impact of auto-segmented contours on downstream processes and have revealed minimal differences compared to manual contours. For instance, in a study involving 20 lung SBRT patients, Vaassen *et al* compared DVH parameters among plans optimized using five contour sets: fully manual, atlas-based, atlas-based with manual adjustment, deep learning-based, and deep learning-based with manual adjustment [100]. They found that the dose variations resulting from automatic contour variations were comparable to or lower than the intra-observer contour variability. However, manual editing was necessary for OARs with maximum dose constraints, such as the heart [100]. Similarly, in a study with 15 prostate cancer patients, Zabel *et al* found no significant differences in clinically relevant dose–volume metrics between auto-segmented bladder and rectum contours [101]. In a larger study involving 247 cervical cancer patients, Rigaud *et al* reported differences in DVH metrics between auto-segmented and manual contours to be within 1% and 1 Gy [102]. Nonetheless, not all investigated auto-contouring workflows present negligible OAR dosimetric impacts [100, 103]. Additional comparative analyses focused on site-specific dosimetric goals are crucial for determining which OARs require increased scrutiny during online review. This refined approach empowers clinicians to make nuanced decisions aligned with individual patient needs and treatment objectives.

Treatment planning evaluation relies on dosimetric endpoints for both target volumes and OARs. These endpoints are commonly expressed through DVHs, including parameters such as maximum and minimum dose (D_{max} and D_{min}), the dose received by at least n% of the structure's volume ($D_{n\%}$), and the volume of structure receiving at least n Gy (V_{nGy}). Additionally, metrics such as conformity index, homogeneity index, and gradient index provide further insights into dose distribution beyond 1D DVHs. To expedite online plan evaluation, structured checklists of these metrics are generated to assess plan adherence to constraints [104]. The use of auto generated checklists was found to increase the error detection by 20% [105]. However, given that not all constraints can always be met, there is often a trade-off between target coverage and OAR sparing, particularly in cases with close proximity to OARs and limited planning time. In such scenarios, physician input is necessary to prioritize objectives. To integrate both objective and subjective preferences and enable ranked acceptability, Ventura *et al* proposed weighted scoring of dose constraints according to physician preferences, presented in a graphical radar plot [106]. To yield more insights on plan quality other than the commonly used DVH metrics, Ceballos *et al* further extracted 60 non-conventional parameters that specifically probe for hot and cold spots, and 320 radiomic features from the 3D dose distribution to train a random forest regressor for prostate cancer RT plan quality evaluation. The resulting machine learning model using a combination of DVH and dose radiomic features achieved high grading accuracy compared to the physician's evaluation [107].

In addition to determining whether a plan meets certain constraints, an alternative approach to defining plan acceptability involves assessing whether the current plan achieves the best possible dosimetric endpoints. This entails comparing the current DVH or dose distribution with predicted values [108, 109]. By integrating this evaluation criterion with the plan generation process using the predicted DVH or dose to guide plan generation, the resulting plan is deemed 'optimal' without the need for further evaluation. Indeed, several assessments of non-manually intervened auto-planning have demonstrated that such plans are non-inferior to human-generated plans in multiple sites, including prostate, endometrial, lung, and head and neck [110, 111]. Auto-planning even exhibits greater OAR sparing [110], increased dose conformity, and reduction of integral dose [111].

Coupled with the auto-segmentation process, a fully automated contouring and planning workflow tested in nine prostate cancer IMRT patients achieved acceptable target coverage and reduced mean dose to the bladder and rectum [112]. Although still in its nascent stage, with advancements in auto-contouring and auto-planning algorithms, the plan generation process itself shows promise for self-approval in the future.

6.3.4 Clinical considerations

As AI technology continues to advance, it holds the promise of overcoming current technical limitations. With ongoing progress in AI, the generation of treatment plans can become increasingly efficient, with DL algorithms capable of producing plans in as little as 20 s, while knowledge-based planning may take up to 15 min [113, 114]. This reduction in planning time has the potential to significantly decrease the cost of ART, thereby increasing its accessibility and benefits for a larger patient population. Simultaneously, alongside the broader adoption of OnART facilitated by these technical advancements, the concept of 'adaptive' therapy undergoes an expansion. At its fundamental level, adaptive therapy involves modifying existing plans to accommodate known anatomical changes, while at its more sophisticated stage, it encompasses dynamically adjusting clinical objectives in response to tumor behavior and prognosis. However, uncertainties on treatment response, lack of knowledge of toxicity, and inter-patient heterogeneity challenge the clinical decision making.

The integration of functional imaging into ART represents a dynamic area of ongoing research, as functional responses often precede anatomical changes. Advanced imaging modalities, particularly MRI and PET, offer insights into tumor function, enabling early assessment of tumor response and resistance and thereby supporting prescription adjustments [115]. Recent studies have highlighted the predictive and prognostic value of diffusion-weighted imaging (DWI) across various cancers, including rectum, cervix, prostate, HN and brain [116, 117]. Perfusion-weighted MRI, notably dynamic susceptibility contrast (DSC)-MRI, provides additional physiological information and demonstrates correlations with brain glioma progression and treatment response in normal brain tissue [118, 119]. While DWI or DSC imaging modalities have an implicit correlation with the underlying biology and physiology of tumor response [116], PET imaging is more closely related to cellularity and proliferative activity, which are two major indicators of tumor aggressiveness. Furthermore, PET has demonstrated the capability to differentiate necrosis, fibrosis, or radiation therapy-induced inflammation, as well as hypoxic tumor cells, which are a hallmark of radioresistance [120].

With the increasing utilization of MR-linac and the emergence of PET-linac, biologically adaptive OnART becomes feasible. However, the reproducibility of quantitative functional biomarkers depends heavily on imaging devices and protocols, as significant inter-system and inter-sequence variability have been observed [121, 122]. Consequently, quantitative functional measurements developed on diagnostic imaging systems or sequences may not translate reproducibly to hybrid MRI- or PET-linac scanners. Moreover, imaging processing methods introduce additional uncertainties to the development of quantitative biomarkers. For example, the selection of diffusion resultant decay models and the fit quality influence the accuracy of DWI-derived parameters [116]. RT-induced perfusion changes in normal tissue may bias the DSC metrics if selected as a reference region, potentially overestimating tumor physiological response [118]. Additionally, various correction factors can be applied to calculate the standardized uptake value (SUV) in PET, albeit contradictory results have been reported regarding which SUV calculation method best correlates with the glucose metabolic rate [122].

To develop optimal strategies for integrating functional imaging into RT, larger clinical trials with standardized imaging protocols across multiple institutions are imperative. The rising application of DL-based imaging reconstruction and post-processing allows for fast in-room scans with quality comparable to or exceeding state-of-the-art diagnostic standards [123–125]. Complementing the technical advancements in imaging acquisition is the increasing integration of quantitative imaging and machine learning applications into the radiation oncology workflow, notably through radiomics analyses. These developments offer an unprecedented opportunity to refine the assessment of early treatment response, OAR toxicity, and long-term clinical outcomes at an individual level [126, 127]. Such endeavors would enable more robust and reliable outcome prediction, ultimately enhancing clinical decision making.

6.4 Summary

In this chapter, we discussed the evolution of radiotherapy, which has seen significant improvements to conformality and precision over the past few decades. Each technological leap has highlighted the remaining assumptions in our processes and pushed our field further forward. The rise in prevalence of image guidance emphasized how we still plan on a static snapshot of the patient's anatomy. Adaptive radiotherapy evolved to address the day-to-day variations and systematic changes in anatomy. In the early stages, technological limitations relegated adaptation to offline re-simulation and re-planning. Recent years have seen a widespread push toward OnART, but the current solutions remain bottlenecks to clinical throughput. Several tasks in the adaptive workflow have high potential for acceleration through AI automation, and these applications will be discussed in detail in subsequent chapters.

References

[1] Benson R and Mallick S 2020 Therapeutic index and its clinical significance *Practical Radiation Oncology* (Singapore: Springer) pp 191–2

[2] IAEA 2008 Transition from 2-D radiotherapy to 3-D conformal and intensity modulated radiotherapy *Technical Report* IAEA-TECDOC-1588 International Atomic Energy Agency, Vienna

[3] Svensson G K 1984 Quality assurance in radiation therapy: physics efforts *Int. J. Radiat. Oncol. Biol. Phys.* **10** 23–9

[4] Svensson G K *et al* 1984 Physical aspects of quality assurance in radiation therapy *Report* #13 American Association of Physicists in Medicine, New York pp 5–8

[5] Brahme A 1984 Dosimetric precision requirements in radiation therapy *Acta Radiol. Oncol.* **23** 379–91

[6] Dutreix A 1984 When and how can we improve precision in radiotherapy? *Radioth. Oncol.* **2** 275–92

[7] Goitein M 1985 Calculation of the uncertainty in the dose delivered during radiation therapy *Med. Phys.* **12** 608–12

[8] Cunningham J 1984 Quality assurance in radiation therapy: clinical and physical aspects. Quality assurance in dosimetry and treatment planning *Int. J. Radiat. Oncol. Biol. Phys.* **10** 105–9

[9] Emami B *et al* 1991 Tolerance of normal tissue to therapeutic irradiation *Int. J. Radiat. Oncol. Biol. Phys.* **21** 109–22

[10] Emami B 2013 Tolerance of normal tissue to therapeutic radiation *Rep. Radiother. Oncol.* **1** 123–7

[11] Bel A, van Herk M and Lebesque J V 1996 Target margins for random geometrical treatment uncertainties in conformal radiotherapy *Med. Phys.* **23** 1537–45

[12] Van Herk M, Remeijer P and Lebesque J V 2002 Inclusion of geometric uncertainties in treatment plan evaluation *Int. J. Radiat. Oncol. Biol. Phys.* **52** 1407–22

[13] Stroom J C and Heijmen B J 2002 Geometrical uncertainties, radiotherapy planning margins, and the ICRU-62 report *Radiother. Oncol.* **64** 75–83

[14] McKenzie A, Van Herk M and Mijnheer B 2002 Margins for geometric uncertainty around organs at risk in radiotherapy *Radiother. Oncol.* **62** 299–307

[15] Kutcher G J *et al* 1994 Comprehensive QA for radiation oncology: report of AAPM radiation therapy committee task group 40 *Med. Phys.* **21** 581

[16] Bentzen S M *et al* 2010 Quantitative analyses of normal tissue effects in the clinic (QUANTEC): an introduction to the scientific issues *Int. J. Radiat. Oncol. Biol. Phys.* **76** S3–9

[17] van Herk M 2004 Errors and margins in radiotherapy *Semin. Radiat. Oncol.* **14** 52–64

[18] Jaffray D, Yan D and Wong J 1999 Managing geometric uncertainty in conformal intensity-modulated radation therapy *Semin. Radiat. Oncol.* **9** 4–19

[19] van Herk M 2007 Different styles of image-guided radiotherapy *Semin. Radiat. Oncol.* **17** 258–67

[20] Dawson L A and Jaffray D A 2007 Advances in image-guided radiation therapy *J. Clin. Oncol* **25** 938–46

[21] Srivastava S P, Cheng C-W and Das I J 2016 Image guidance-based target volume margin expansion in IMRT of head and neck cancer *Technol. Cancer Res. Treat.* **15** 107–13

[22] Burnet N *et al* 2014 Clinical and practical considerations for the use of intensity-modulated radiotherapy and image guidance in neuro-oncology *Clin. Oncol.* **26** 395–406

[23] Grills I S *et al* 2008 Image-guided radiotherapy via daily online cone-beam CT substantially reduces margin requirements for stereotactic lung radiotherapy *Int. J. Radiat. Oncol. Biol. Phys.* **70** 1045–56

[24] Guckenberger M, Meyer J, Vordermark D, Baier K, Wilbert J and Flentje M 2006 Magnitude and clinical relevance of translational and rotational patient setup errors: a cone-beam CT study *Int. J. Radiat. Oncol. Biol. Phys.* **65** 934–42

[25] Grimm J, Marks L B, Jackson A, Kavanagh B D, Xue J and Yorke E 2021 High dose per fraction, hypofractionated treatment effects in the clinic (HyTEC): an overview *Int. J. Radiat. Oncol. Biol. Phys.* **110** 1–10

[26] Grimm J, Jackson A, Kavanagh B D, Marks L B, Yorke E and Xue J 2021 The HyTEC Project *Med. Phys.* **48** 2699–700

[27] Lim-Reinders S, Keller B M, Al-Ward S, Sahgal A and Kim A 2017 Online adaptive radiation therapy *Int. J. Radiat. Oncol. Biol. Phys.* **99** 994–1003

[28] Brock K K 2019 Adaptive radiotherapy: moving into the future *Semin. Radiat. Oncol.* **29** 181–4

[29] Hussein M, Akintonde A, McClelland J, Speight R and Clark C H 2021 Clinical use, challenges, and barriers to implementation of deformable image registration in radiotherapy—the need for guidance and QA tools *Br. J. Radiol.* **94** 20210001

[30] Sibolt P *et al* 2021 Clinical implementation of artificial intelligence-driven cone-beam computed tomography-guided online adaptive radiotherapy in the pelvic region *Phys. Imaging Radiat. Oncol.* **17** 1–7

[31] Mao W *et al* 2022 Evaluation of auto-contouring and dose distributions for online adaptive radiation therapy of patients with locally advanced lung cancers *Pract. Radiat. Oncol.* **12** e329–e38

[32] Saenz D L, Paliwal B R and Bayouth J E 2014 A dose homogeneity and conformity evaluation between ViewRay and pinnacle-based linear accelerator IMRT treatment plans *J. Med. Phys.* **39** 64–70

[33] Snyder J E *et al* 2020 Commissioning of a 1.5 T Elekta Unity MR-linac: a single institution experience *J. Appl. Clin. Med. Phys.* **21** 160–72

[34] Hu Y, Byrne M, Archibald-Heeren B, Collett N, Liu G and Aland T 2020 Validation of the preconfigured Varian Ethos Acuros XB beam model for treatment planning dose calculations: a dosimetric study *J. Appl. Clin. Med. Phys.* **21** 27–42

[35] Cai B, Green O L, Kashani R, Rodriguez V L, Mutic S and Yang D 2018 A practical implementation of physics quality assurance for photon adaptive radiotherapy *Z. Med. Phys.* **28** 211–23

[36] Miften M *et al* 2018 Tolerance limits and methodologies for IMRT measurement-based verification QA: recommendations of AAPM Task Group No. 218 *Med. Phys.* **45** e53–83

[37] Yan D 2008 Developing quality assurance processes for image-guided adaptive radiation therapy *Int. J. Radiat. Oncol. Biol. Phys.* **71** S28–32

[38] Ottosson S, Zackrisson B, Kjellén E, Nilsson P and Laurell G 2013 Weight loss in patients with head and neck cancer during and after conventional and accelerated radiotherapy *Acta Oncol.* **52** 711–8

[39] Yen A, Shen C and Albuquerque K 2023 The new kid on the block: online adaptive radiotherapy in the treatment of gynecologic cancers *Curr. Oncol.* **30** 865–74

[40] Thörnqvist S *et al* 2016 Adaptive radiotherapy strategies for pelvic tumors—a systematic review of clinical implementations *Acta Oncol.* **55** 943–58

[41] Green O L, Henke L E and Hugo G D 2019 Practical clinical workflows for online and offline adaptive radiation therapy *Semin. Radiat. Oncol.* **29** 219–27

[42] Lamb J *et al* 2017 Online adaptive radiation therapy: implementation of a new process of care *Cureus* **9** e1618

[43] Schwartz D L *et al* 2013 Adaptive radiotherapy for head and neck cancer—dosimetric results from a prospective clinical trial *Radiother. Oncol.* **106** 80–4

[44] Sher D *et al* 2023 Acute toxicity and efficiency outcomes in the DARTBOARD randomized trial of daily adaptive radiotherapy for head and neck squamous cell carcinoma *Int. J. Radiat. Oncol. Biol. Phys.* **117** e6

[45] Chuong M D *et al* 2024 Stereotactic MR-guided on-table adaptive radiation therapy (SMART) for borderline resectable and locally advanced pancreatic cancer: a multi-center, open-label phase 2 study *Radiother. Oncol.* **191** 110064

[46] Liu H *et al* 2023 Review of cone beam computed tomography based online adaptive radiotherapy: current trend and future direction *Radiat. Oncol.* **18** 144

[47] Brabbins D *et al* 2005 A dose-escalation trial with the adaptive radiotherapy process as a delivery system in localized prostate cancer: analysis of chronic toxicity *Int. J. Radiat. Oncol. Biol. Phys.* **61** 400–8

[48] Li X *et al* 2012 Combined online and offline adaptive radiation therapy *Int. J. Radiat. Oncol. Biol. Phys.* **84** S29–30

[49] Lavrova E *et al* 2023 Adaptive radiation therapy: a review of CT-based techniques *Radiol. Imaging Cancer* **5** e230011

[50] Nierer L *et al* 2022 Dosimetric benefit of MR-guided online adaptive radiotherapy in different tumor entities: liver, lung, abdominal lymph nodes, pancreas and prostate *Radiat. Oncol.* **17** 53

[51] Cardenas C, Stanley D, Belliveau J and Popple R 2022 Retrospective analysis to define appropriate physics FTE support for online adaptive radiotherapy programs *Int. J. Radiat. Oncol. Biol. Phys.* **114** e588–e9

[52] Stanley D N *et al* 2023 A roadmap for implementation of kV-CBCT online adaptive radiation therapy and initial first year experiences *J. App. Clin. Med. Phys.* **24** e13961

[53] Stanescu T *et al* 2022 MRI-guided online adaptive stereotactic body radiation therapy of liver and pancreas tumors on an MR-linac system *Cancers* **14** 716

[54] Henke L *et al* 2018 Phase I trial of stereotactic MR-guided online adaptive radiation therapy (SMART) for the treatment of oligometastatic or unresectable primary malignancies of the abdomen *Radiother. Oncol.* **126** 519–26

[55] Astaraki M, Bendazzoli S and Toma-Dasu I 2023 Fully automatic segmentation of gross target volume and organs-at-risk for radiotherapy planning of nasopharyngeal carcinoma arXiv: 2310.02972v1

[56] Savenije M H *et al* 2020 Clinical implementation of MRI-based organs-at-risk auto-segmentation with convolutional networks for prostate radiotherapy *Radiat. Oncol.* **15** 104

[57] Chen X *et al* 2021 A deep learning-based auto-segmentation system for organs-at-risk on whole-body computed tomography images for radiation therapy *Radiother. Oncol.* **160** 175–84

[58] Shi F *et al* 2022 Deep learning empowered volume delineation of whole-body organs-at-risk for accelerated radiotherapy *Nat. Commun.* **13** 6566

[59] Wasserthal J *et al* 2023 TotalSegmentator: robust segmentation of 104 anatomic structures in CT images *Radiol. Artif. Intell.* **5** e230024

[60] Moazzezi M, Rose B, Kisling K, Moore K L and Ray X 2021 Prospects for daily online adaptive radiotherapy via ethos for prostate cancer patients without nodal involvement using unedited CBCT auto-segmentation *J. Appl. Clin. Med. Phys.* **22** 82–93

[61] Breto A L *et al* 2022 Deep learning for per-fraction automatic segmentation of gross tumor volume (GTV) and organs at risk (OARs) in adaptive radiotherapy of cervical cancer *Front. Oncol.* **12** 854349

[62] König L, Derksen A, Papenberg N and Haas B 2016 Deformable image registration for adaptive radiotherapy with guaranteed local rigidity constraints *Radiat. Oncol.* **11** 122

[63] Gu X *et al* 2013 A contour-guided deformable image registration algorithm for adaptive radiotherapy *Phys. Med. Biol.* **58** 1889

[64] Weistrand O and Svensson S 2015 The ANACONDA algorithm for deformable image registration in radiotherapy *Med. Phys.* **42** 40–53

[65] Burger M, Modersitzki J and Ruthotto L 2013 A hyperelastic regularization energy for image registration *SIAM J. Sci. Comput.* **35** B132–B48

[66] Genet M, Stoeck C T, Von Deuster C, Lee L C and Kozerke S 2018 Equilibrated warping: finite element image registration with finite strain equilibrium gap regularization *Med. Image Anal.* **50** 1–22

[67] Lao Y, Yu V, Chang E, Yang W and Sheng K 2020 Deformable alignment of longitudinal postoperative brain GBM scans using deep learning *Proc. SPIE* **11313** 1131300

[68] McKenzie E M, Tong N, Ruan D, Cao M, Chin R K and Sheng K 2021 Using neural networks to extend cropped medical images for deformable registration among images with differing scan extents *Med. Phys.* **48** 4459–71

[69] Yang X, Kwitt R, Styner M and Niethammer M 2017 Quicksilver: fast predictive image registration—a deep learning approach *NeuroImage* **158** 378–96

[70] Balakrishnan G, Zhao A, Sabuncu M R, Guttag J and Dalca A V 2019 VoxelMorph: a learning framework for deformable medical image registration *IEEE Trans. Med. Imaging* **38** 1788–800

[71] Alvarez P and Cotin S (ed) 2024 Deformable image registration with stochastically regularized biomechanical equilibrium *2024 IEEE International Symposium on Biomedical Imaging (ISBI)* (Piscataway, NJ: IEEE)

[72] Winkel D *et al* 2019 Adaptive radiotherapy: the Elekta Unity MR-linac concept *Clin. Transl. Radiat. Oncol.* **18** 54–9

[73] McDonald B A *et al* 2021 Initial feasibility and clinical implementation of daily MR-guided adaptive head and neck cancer radiation therapy on a 1.5 T MR-linac system: prospective R-IDEAL 2a/2b systematic clinical evaluation of technical innovation *Int. J. Radiat. Oncol. Biol. Phys.* **109** 1606–18

[74] Gupta A *et al* 2022 Online adaptive radiotherapy for head and neck cancers on the MR linear accelerator: introducing a novel modified Adapt-to-Shape approach *Clin. Transl. Radiat. Oncol.* **32** 48–51

[75] Hussein M, Heijmen B J, Verellen D and Nisbet A 2018 Automation in intensity modulated radiotherapy treatment planning—a review of recent innovations *Br. J. Radiol.* **91** 20180270

[76] Bohoudi O *et al* 2017 Fast and robust online adaptive planning in stereotactic MR-guided adaptive radiation therapy (SMART) for pancreatic cancer *Radiother. Oncol.* **125** 439–44

[77] Nguyen D *et al* 2019 3D radiotherapy dose prediction on head and neck cancer patients with a hierarchically densely connected U-net deep learning architecture *Phys. Med. Biol.* **64** 065020

[78] Wang M, Zhang Q, Lam S, Cai J and Yang R 2020 A review on application of deep learning algorithms in external beam radiotherapy automated treatment planning *Front. Oncol.* **10** 580919

[79] Nachbar M, Mönnich D, Dohm O, Friedlein M, Zips D and Thorwarth D 2021 Automatic 3D Monte-Carlo-based secondary dose calculation for online verification of 1.5 T magnetic resonance imaging guided radiotherapy *Phys. Imaging Radiat. Oncol.* **19** 6–12

[80] Shen C *et al* 2023 Clinical experience on patient-specific quality assurance for CBCT-based online adaptive treatment plan *J. Appl Clin. Med. Phys.* **24** e13918

[81] Radus R, Epstein D and Levin D 2021 Verifying plan QA for online adaptive treatment in MR linac *Int. J. Radiat. Oncol. Biol. Phys.* **111** e519–e20

[82] Noel C E *et al* 2014 Process-based quality management for clinical implementation of adaptive radiotherapy *Med. Phys.* **41** 081717

[83] Rippke C *et al* 2022 Quality assurance for on-table adaptive magnetic resonance guided radiation therapy: a software tool to complement secondary dose calculation and failure modes discovered in clinical routine *J. Appl. Clin. Med. Phys.* **23** e13523

[84] Klüter S *et al* 2021 A practical implementation of risk management for the clinical introduction of online adaptive magnetic resonance-guided radiotherapy *Phys. Imaging Radiat. Oncol.* **17** 53–7

[85] Chowdhry V K and Simpson N C 2023 Process modeling a radiation oncology clinic workflow from therapeutic simulation to treatment: identifying impending strain and possible treatment delays *Adv. Radiat. Oncol.* **8** 101261

[86] Langen K M and Jones D T 2001 Organ motion and its management *Int. J. Radiat. Oncol. Biol. Phys.* **50** 265–78

[87] Kupelian P A *et al* 2005 Serial megavoltage CT imaging during external beam radiotherapy for non-small-cell lung cancer: observations on tumor regression during treatment *Int. J. Radiat. Oncol. Biol. Phys.* **63** 1024–8

[88] Fox J, Ford E, Redmond K, Zhou J, Wong J and Song D Y 2009 Quantification of tumor volume changes during radiotherapy for non-small-cell lung cancer *Int. J. Radiat. Oncol. Biol. Phys.* **74** 341–8

[89] Vu N *et al* 2020 Tumor volume shrinkage during stereotactic body radiotherapy is related to better prognoses in patients with stage I non-small-cell lung cancer *J. Radiat. Res.* **61** 740–6

[90] Barker J L Jr *et al* 2004 Quantification of volumetric and geometric changes occurring during fractionated radiotherapy for head-and-neck cancer using an integrated CT/linear accelerator system *Int. J. Radiat. Oncol. Biol. Phys.* **59** 960–70

[91] Hamming-Vrieze O *et al* 2017 Analysis of GTV reduction during radiotherapy for oropharyngeal cancer: implications for adaptive radiotherapy *Radiother. Oncol.* **122** 224–8

[92] Buciuman N and Marcu L G 2022 Adaptive radiotherapy in head and neck cancer using volumetric modulated arc therapy *J. Pers. Med.* **12** 668

[93] Willigenburg T *et al* 2022 Accumulated bladder wall dose is correlated with patient-reported acute urinary toxicity in prostate cancer patients treated with stereotactic, daily adaptive MR-guided radiotherapy *Radiother. Oncol.* **171** 182–8

[94] Kleijnen J-P J *et al* 2018 Does setup on rectal wall improve rectal cancer boost radiotherapy? *Radiat. Oncol.* **13** 61

[95] Lao Y *et al* 2021 Bladder surface dose modeling in prostate cancer radiotherapy: an analysis of motion-induced variations and the cumulative dose across the treatment *Med. Phys.* **48** 8024–36

[96] Eelbode T *et al* 2020 Optimization for medical image segmentation: theory and practice when evaluating with Dice score or Jaccard index *IEEE Trans. Med. Imaging* **39** 3679–90

[97] Zhao C, Shi W and Deng Y 2005 A new Hausdorff distance for image matching *Pattern Recognit. Lett.* **26** 581–6

[98] Rhee D J et al 2022 Automatic contouring QA method using a deep learning–based autocontouring system J. Appl. Clin. Med. Phys. 23 e13647

[99] Vaassen F et al 2020 Evaluation of measures for assessing time-saving of automatic organ-at-risk segmentation in radiotherapy Phys. Imaging Radiat. Oncol. 13 1–6

[100] Vaassen F, Hazelaar C, Canters R, Peeters S, Petit S and van Elmpt W 2021 The impact of organ-at-risk contour variations on automatically generated treatment plans for NSCLC Radiother. Oncol. 163 136–42

[101] Zabel W J et al 2021 Clinical evaluation of deep learning and Atlas-based auto-contouring of bladder and rectum for prostate radiation therapy Pract. Radiat. Oncol. 11 e80–e9

[102] Rigaud B et al 2021 Automatic segmentation using deep learning to enable online dose optimization during adaptive radiation therapy of cervical cancer Int. J. Radiat. Oncol. Biol. Phys. 109 1096–110

[103] Hwee J et al 2011 Technology assessment of automated atlas based segmentation in prostate bed contouring Radiat. Oncol. 6 110

[104] Covington E L et al 2016 Improving treatment plan evaluation with automation J. Appl. Clin. Med. Phys. 17 16–31

[105] Nealon K A, Court L E, Douglas R J, Zhang L and Han E Y 2022 Development and validation of a checklist for use with automatically generated radiotherapy plans J. Appl. Clin. Med. Phys 23 e13694

[106] Ventura T et al 2020 Clinical validation of a graphical method for radiation therapy plan quality assessment Radiat. Oncol. 15 64

[107] Liu L, Silva E A, Wu C and Wang H 2017 A machine learning-based method for the large-scale evaluation of the qualities of the urban environment Comput. Environ. Urban Syst. 65 113–25

[108] Moore K L 2019 Automated radiotherapy treatment planning Semin. Radiat. Oncol. 29 209–18

[109] Sun Z et al 2022 A hybrid optimization strategy for deliverable intensity-modulated radiotherapy plan generation using deep learning-based dose prediction Med. Phys. 49 1344–56

[110] Cornell M et al 2020 Noninferiority study of automated knowledge-based planning versus human-driven optimization across multiple disease sites Int. J. Radiat. Oncol. Biol. Phys. 106 430–9

[111] Cilla S et al 2020 Template-based automation of treatment planning in advanced radio-therapy: a comprehensive dosimetric and clinical evaluation Sci. Rep. 10 423

[112] Li X et al 2013 A fully automated method for CT-on-rails-guided online adaptive planning for prostate cancer intensity modulated radiation therapy Int. J. Radiat. Oncol. Biol. Phys. 86 835–41

[113] Craft D L, Hong T S, Shih H A and Bortfeld T R 2012 Improved planning time and plan quality through multicriteria optimization for intensity-modulated radiotherapy Int. J. Radiat. Oncol. Biol. Phys. 82 e83–90

[114] Foy J J et al 2017 An analysis of knowledge-based planning for stereotactic body radiation therapy of the spine Pract. Radiat. Oncol. 7 e355–e60

[115] Zhou Q, Xue C, Ke X and Zhou J 2022 Treatment response and prognosis evaluation in high-grade glioma: an imaging review based on MRI J. Magn. Reson. Imaging 56 325–40

[116] Leibfarth S, Winter R M, Lyng H, Zips D and Thorwarth D 2018 Potentials and challenges of diffusion-weighted magnetic resonance imaging in radiotherapy *Clin. Transl. Radiat. Oncol.* **13** 29–37

[117] Jones K M, Michel K A, Bankson J A, Fuller C D, Klopp A H and Venkatesan A M 2018 Emerging magnetic resonance imaging technologies for radiation therapy planning and response assessment *Int. J. Radiat. Oncol. Biol. Phys.* **101** 1046–56

[118] Fahlström M, Blomquist E, Nyholm T and Larsson E-M 2018 Perfusion magnetic resonance imaging changes in normal appearing brain tissue after radiotherapy in glioblastoma patients may confound longitudinal evaluation of treatment response *Radiol. Oncol.* **52** 143–51

[119] Wang L *et al* 2020 Evaluation of perfusion MRI value for tumor progression assessment after glioma radiotherapy: a systematic review and meta-analysis *Medicine* **99** e23766

[120] Shen L-F, Zhou S-H and Yu Q 2020 Predicting response to radiotherapy in tumors with PET/CT: when and how? *Transl. Cancer Res.* **9** 2972

[121] Kolff-Gart A *et al* 2015 Diffusion-weighted imaging of the head and neck in healthy subjects: reproducibility of ADC values in different MRI systems and repeat sessions *Am. J. Neuroradiol.* **36** 384–90

[122] Adams M C, Turkington T G, Wilson J M and Wong T Z 2010 A systematic review of the factors affecting accuracy of SUV measurements *Am. J. Roentgenol.* **195** 310–20

[123] Ueda T *et al* 2022 Deep learning reconstruction of diffusion-weighted MRI improves image quality for prostatic imaging *Radiology* **303** 373–81

[124] Ichikawa Y *et al* 2021 Deep learning image reconstruction for improvement of image quality of abdominal computed tomography: comparison with hybrid iterative reconstruction *Jpn. J. Radiol.* **39** 598–604

[125] Yang C *et al* 2023 Deep learning image reconstruction algorithms in low-dose radiation abdominal computed tomography: assessment of image quality and lesion diagnostic confidence *Quant. Imag. Med. Surg.* **13** 3161

[126] Desideri I, Loi M, Francolini G, Becherini C, Livi L and Bonomo P 2020 Application of radiomics for the prediction of radiation-induced toxicity in the IMRT era: current state-of-the-art *Front. Oncol.* **10** 1708

[127] Shi L *et al* 2018 Radiomics for response and outcome assessment for non-small cell lung cancer *Technol. Cancer Res. Treat.* **17**

Chapter 7

Overview of artificial-intelligence driven adaptive therapy workflow

Chenyang Shen, Justin Visak, Andrew Godley and Mu-Han Lin

In the landscape of adaptive therapy, which includes offline, online, and real-time approaches, two clinically relevant workflows for adaptive radiation therapy (ART) are distinguished: offline and online [1]. Offline ART is the less time constrained of the pair and typically aims to address anatomical changes throughout the treatment course via offline re-planning with or without patient re-simulation. While artificial intelligence (AI) holds the potential to enhance both online and offline adaptive therapy workflows, we will specifically concentrate on its application in online adaptive therapy in this chapter, given its seamless translation to offline scenarios. Online ART addresses inter-fraction changes by creating a new treatment plan while the patient remains on the treatment unit. This departs from traditional image guided RT (IGRT) where typically the same reference plan is delivered repeatedly throughout the treatment course. Online ART plans can be delivered using x-ray [2] or MRI guidance, both available commercially [3, 4]. Regardless of the imaging guidance, the online ART components can be generalized into simulation, pre-planning, daily imaging/re-planning, and quality assurance, all of which can be enhanced with AI-driven workflows. Delivering a robust and successful online ART treatment demands a specialized treatment team and workflow compared to conventional delivery methods. The intricacies of online ART often necessitate heightened clinical resources. However, the integration of AI in online ART streamlines workflows, enhancing efficiency and facilitating a more coordinated approach. Automating optimization tasks with advanced algorithms lowers the entry barriers for general clinics, widening the spectrum of clinical adoption. This chapter explores the integration of AI into ART workflows, emphasizing its transformative potential in enhancing efficiency, precision, and accessibility. ART, encompassing offline, online, and real-time approaches, adapts treatment to anatomical and functional changes, necessitating specialized workflows and clinical resources. The chapter delineates the components of ART—simulation, pre-planning, daily imaging and re-planning, and quality

doi:10.1088/978-0-7503-6119-4ch7

assurance—highlighting AI's role in automating processes such as segmentation, dose prediction, and treatment optimization. AI-driven advancements in synthetic CT generation, auto-contouring, and real-time plan adaptation streamline ART workflows, enabling widespread clinical adoption. The discussion extends to future directions, envisioning AI-enabled real-time ART and functional adaptation, which incorporate physiological responses to personalize treatments further. This integration of AI into ART paves the way for more dynamic, precise, and patient-specific radiation therapy, setting the stage for its evolution into a standard of care.

7.1 Components of ART workflow

7.1.1 Simulation

One fundamental difference between an image guided RT (IGRT) and online adaptive radiation therapy (ART) workflow is the expected patient time on table. The objective of a successful online ART program is to expedite the typical 5–7 days simulation-to-treatment workflow to a more rapid timeframe, aiming for completion within 1 hour. Early publications indicate this is now clinically feasible for select sites due to recent emergence of commercial technology [5]. Whether x-ray or MR-guided online ART is utilized, it is reasonable and practical to expect a patient's time on the table will be increased for treatment [6]. Therefore, one important component of the online ART workflow is simulation to ensure the patient is comfortable and in a reproducible position. Once images are acquired, and the plan adaptation begins, it is imperative to minimize patient movement. Striking a balance between effective immobilization and patient comfort is essential. For instance, consider the use of compression in treating mobile tumors—while maximum compression may be dosimetrically advantageous, patients may find it challenging to endure the extended periods of online ART under full compression. Therefore, adopting a more moderate level of compression that aligns with patient comfort becomes a pragmatic approach, ensuring both effective treatment and patient tolerance in the dynamic landscape of online adaptive therapy.

The simulation process of adaptive therapy closely resembles conventional radiotherapy, with the key distinction lying in the evaluation of whether a patient is a suitable candidate who would significantly benefit from adaptive therapy. This consideration plays a crucial role in guiding clinical resource allocation. Minimally, a 3D computed tomography CT simulation should be acquired with reproducible patient marking. For patients with intra-fractional motion, a ten-phase 4DCT can also be acquired to encompass the motion of the gross tumor volume referred to as the internal target volume (ITV). For MR-guided workflows, an MR simulation may also be completed in addition or in place of the CT simulation to improve target delineation and assess MR image quality at the time of simulation. These reference images will be brought into an offline treatment planning system for delineation and planning. For MR-guided workflows, the MR images may be used as the primary planning images for the patient's treatment. AI can further enhance this decision-making process by predicting patient candidacy based on various factors, such as optimizing the choice of imaging modalities for simulation and treatment or estimating the expected time a patient might spend on adaptive therapy. This predictive capability contributes to efficient resource management, enabling the optimization of clinical slot times and ensuring a streamlined and personalized approach to adaptive therapy. Additionally, MR-only simulation workflows are becoming of increasing interest [7, 8], where AI is a critical component in synthetic CT image generation.

7.1.2 Pre-planning

After simulation, all the images, including requested diagnostic images, will be imported into the offline planning system and a reference plan will be generated. The first step of preparing a treatment plan is identifying organs-at-risk (OARs) and target delineation on the reference images. It is well understood that AI will enhance this process through various means of automating segmentation [9–11].

In order to facilitate an efficient online re-planning workflow, meticulous attention must be given to the pre-plan process. Unlike a conventional workflow where all relevant OARs and targets are delineated on the reference image, the practicality of considering all OARs during online ART may be limited. Therefore, a strategic focus should be placed on the most proximal OARs to the intended target, such as those within 3 cm of the planning target volume, streamlining the planning process. To enhance the precision and efficiency of online contouring and re-planning, it is crucial to prioritize and define the high-dose impact OARs during pre-planning. Rather than including all OARs and requesting physicians to re-contour each during online ART, the identification of key OARs allows for a more targeted and streamlined approach to strike on the key elements of generating high-quality plans during online ART. Similarly, any tuning structures essential for the adaptive process should be designed in a manner that enables automatic replication and dynamic adjustment based on the new anatomy of the day. This strategic approach optimizes the adaptation workflow, ensuring not only precision but also efficiency in the creation of adaptive plans during online ART.

Current ART workflows for x-ray and MR-guided treatments require inverse planning techniques where the planner upfront defines patient-specific or population-based dose–volume histogram (DVH) objectives [12]. These objectives are transferred to an optimization problem where a computer algorithm attempts to find the most optimal solution. Similar to conventional treatments, inverse planning for online ART is as much of an art as a science and is highly dependent on a planner's skill and experience [13]. It is well-documented that any institution is subject to this 'inter-planner variability' and therefore this carves an important aspect in the online ART process for AI to enhance the reference planning process. Over the past decade, it has been of global interest to the radiation therapy community to deploy AI during the optimization process. Some examples are direct DVH prediction, 2D/3D dose prediction, beam angle geometry, and attempts at mimicking a human-like planning process [14–17]. Notably, the integration of AI in pre-plan holds the promise of bridging the gap in planner experience levels. More details on this topic will be covered later in the chapter.

In many clinics, once an inverse plan is generated, patient-specific quality assurance (PSQA) is typically conducted through either measurement-based or calculation-based methods, a practice also observed in pre-plans. Measurement-based QA involves transferring and recalculating the plan on a QA phantom (film/chamber, 2D array, 3D array) and performing a gamma analysis between the measured and expected dose distribution [18]. Although measurement-based QA is a common and reliable practice, efficiently identifying catastrophic delivery errors, it has limitations. Critics argue that in most instances, IMRT QA passes, and it is inefficient in detecting subtle plan delivery errors [19]. As covered later, it is also impractical to remove the patient during online adaptive to QA the plan. However, this approach faces practical challenges. Performing measurement-based QA during online adaptive therapy, where the goal is to shorten treatment duration, is impractical. This limitation will be further detailed in section 7.1.4, where alternatives for online adaptive therapy QA will be explored.

7.1.3 Online imaging and daily re-planning

During online ART it is crucial to acquire daily images suitable for contouring and planning. For x-ray guided ART, cone-beam CT (CBCT) or fan beam CT images are typically acquired while in MR-guided ART. In the case of MR-guided ART, a daily MRI is acquired, offering additional flexibility. Different weighted MR images can be acquired, providing users with enhanced contrast to various OARs or targets. For both workflows, following the daily image acquisition, contouring of anatomy occurs.

One common challenge in most online ART workflows, excluding fan beam CT, is the inability to directly employ daily images for dose calculation. Currently, this issue is addressed by generating a synthetic CT or utilizing density overrides for dose calculation. In x-ray guided ART, the reference planning CT undergoes automatic deformation using the daily CBCT. In MR-guided ART workflows, the system extracts the mean electron density of each delineated organ from CT and applies a bulk density override based on the daily MR contours. One system offers two solutions: direct dose calculation on CT through rigid/deformable registration with the daily MR or utilizing bulk density overrides. Another system has the capability to directly calculate the dose on a higher quality CBCT.

For online contour delineation, several AI-based approaches have been developed that will be covered in more detail in later sections of the chapter [20]. Various delineation capabilities are also at the disposal to enhance workflow efficiency. Many systems can propagate contours onto the daily image through either rigid or deformable registration, offering a head start in the contouring process. As a common practice, targets are often rigidly propagated, while OARs undergo deformable propagation. Furthermore, AI-based methods can be employed for initial contouring of targets and OARs on the daily image, providing an additional layer for review and editing. Before progressing to the planning phase, contours, especially those of targets, typically undergo approval by the physician.

Various advanced systems strive to enhance optimization efficiency using distinct approaches in their online planning methodologies. One such system employs an intelligent optimization engine (IOE) to facilitate online re-optimization, acting as a mediator between the human planner and the optimization algorithm. This system utilizes a predefined set of clinical goals and priorities, creating a structured online re-optimization process in line with the reference strategy.

Another system offers two types of online adaptation: adapt-to-position (ATP) and adapt-to-shape (ATS). The system maintains a fixed isocenter and couch position, restricting user adjustments during the online process. ATP compensates for this constraint through a segment aperture morphing (SAM) algorithm, adapting the multi-leaf collimator (MLC) based on the beams' eye view of the old and new target projections. In this workflow, the user can only register reference contours to the daily image without alterations [21]. Conversely, the ATS workflow allows changes to the target and OAR, followed by warm-start optimization based on the pre-planning strategy. Unlike the IOE system, users can modify the optimization strategy on-the-fly.

Lastly, another system provides several online optimization strategies, including BOT Optimize and Optimize Dose or Add Segments. BOT Optimize involves basic segment weight optimization, while Optimize Dose utilizes the reference strategy, initiating a new optimization or continuing from a previous starting point. This system employs an ultra-fast Monte Carlo and optimizer, enabling multiple iterations over the expected timeframe of online ART to achieve the optimal plan for the day's anatomy. The specific AI-related capabilities of these systems are not disclosed.

7.1.4 Quality assurance

As previously mentioned, it is impractical to remove the patient from the table to perform a measurement-based QA. The emergence of calculation-based PSQA utilizing independent dose calculation engines and treatment unit log file analysis is very timely and well suited to QA of online adapted plans [22–26]. For calculation-based QA, in lieu of a physical measurement the planner can export the plan to an independent second check (often Monte Carlo based) where gamma analysis can be performed between the treatment planning system calculated dose and the recalculated dose. For log-based PSQA, the treatment machine log files that record the location of multi-leaf collimators, gantry and collimator locations and can be used to compare between expected and actual positions of the plan [27]. It is then possible to reconstruct a 3D dose following treatment delivery and compare the delivered dose distributions [28, 29]

Prior work has been completed that compares measurement-based and calculation-based PSQA methods. Commercially available platforms utilize an independent convolution–superposition dose calculation algorithm to verify the TPS. An alternative option is utilizing Monte Carlo based methods [30–32]. After plan review and QA, typically a physicist and physician will sign off on the treatment plan and QA.

One area where AI can be utilized is in the decision-making process to decide whether to adapt or not.

7.2 AI-driven ART

Technically speaking, artificial intelligence (AI) broadly refers to any intelligence achieved by computer systems in contrast to human intelligence. Deep learning (DL), as a subtype of techniques within the scope of AI, has achieved tremendous success in a wide spectrum of different areas including medicine. With recent increasing interest, AI and DL have been used interchangeably in many scenarios. This practice is followed in the rest of this chapter unless mentioned otherwise.

Following the order of the major steps in the ART workflow as listed previously, we will introduce the detailed applications of AI techniques in each step, and how these AI techniques could improve the current ART workflow.

7.2.1 Simulation

As the crucial initial step of the ART workflow, simulation can benefit from the emerging AI techniques in many different aspects. One of the most popular applications of AI algorithms in simulation is CT image synthesis. A number of studies have been carried out recently to convert images acquired from other modalities, e.g. magnetic resonance images (MRI) [33–37], or on-board CBCT [7, 38–41], to synthetic CT (sCT) images which can be employed to generate the initial plan for ART. Specifically, AI-based sCT generation algorithms based on MRI have the potential to enable the MR-only simulation workflow [42, 43] for RT treatment planning, eliminating the necessity of CT simulation. On top of the obvious benefit of simplified workflow and reduced imaging dose, AI-based sCT images also share the identical anatomy with the MR images. The treatment target and OARs delineated from MR images can be directly utilized in sCT, removing the uncertainty introduced by anatomical discrepancy between simulation MR and CT images. CBCT-based sCT generation permits both online and offline re-planning directly based off the most recent patient anatomy from CBCT without requiring re-simulation. Given that CBCT is the most widely available on-board imaging guidance, AI-based sCT generation holds great potential of realizing ART on a wide range of conventional treatment platforms, particularly current c-arm linacs.

Generating sCT directly based on diagnostic scans can completely eliminate the currently required extra step of simulation, introducing a brand new concept of AI-driven virtual simulation. A pioneering study [44] has been conducted to develop and implement virtual simulation for hippocampus sparing whole brain treatment on the x-ray guided ART system. This virtual simulation workflow not only saves the overall cost and time from the patient side, but also helps clinics to release the heavy scheduling and scanning burden on their CT simulators. It opens up the possibility to substantially reduce the waiting time from diagnosis to radiation treatment leading to further benefit in treatment quality and outcome [45].

7.2.2 Pre-planning

Planning in ART commonly consists of two stages, i.e. the initial, reference or pre-planning stage, and the re-planning stage, either online or offline. The pre-planning process of ART is similar to that in the conventional workflow, but with some key difference covered previously. Re-planning, on the other hand, has a more stringent constraint on planning efficiency as it is highly desired to complete re-planning and deliver treatment prior to further anatomical changes or patient movement. AI-based algorithms developed for conventional treatment planning are applicable to improve the planning quality and efficiency of ART pre- and adaptive planning while specifically designed approaches may provide better performance.

AI-based auto-segmentation. Both the pre- and adaptive planning process of ART starts with defining contours of the treatment target and OARs in planning images, which typically takes extensive manual work from both physicians and planners. AI-based automatic segmentation algorithms have been designed and are now implemented frequently in clinical practice to reduce the manual contouring time. Substantial research efforts have initially been devoted to automate the OAR segmentation process since it is tedious, time-consuming, and relatively more straightforward compared to target delineation, which is often performed by physicians only, with the target appearing markedly different from patient to patient. Numerous AI segmentation tools have been developed to perform automatic OAR segmentation for different body regions or disease sites. Head and neck (HN) cancer [46–49] is commonly considered as a challenging site to contour since it involves more than 20 OARs of significantly distinct shapes and volumes. These studies demonstrated equivalent human-level accuracy of the developed AI-based methods in defining most of the OARs for HN cancer. Similar performance was also observed for other sites. Comprehensive clinical evaluations have shown that AI-generated OAR contours with minor manual edits were able to greatly reduce the time and inter-observer variations in OAR contouring [50, 51]. Further improvement in performance is warranted for some challenging OARs with complex topologies, e.g. the sigmoid colon [52–54].

Novel AI-based tools [55–61] have been developed for automatic target delineation. Despite their encouraging performance, treatment targets in RT are still primarily contoured by physicians. One reason is that treatment target definition frequently needs to account for information from multiple resources including diagnostic images, planning images, as well as the patient specific clinical characteristics extracted from radiology and pathology reports, which is beyond the capability of the most current AI models. Further development on novel multi-modal algorithms incorporating state-of-the-art segmentation models jointly with the emerging large language models (LLMs) [62, 63] are highly desired.

AI-based automatic segmentation algorithms [64–68] have also been designed specifically to serve the purpose of online ART re-planning. These methods often take advantage of the readily available contours from the initial planning stage as well as the previous ART sessions to enhance the segmentation performance for successful adaptive planning. This is a relatively new topic and continued research efforts are required to fully utilize the rich patient-specific information embedded in the contours and images available.

AI-based dose prediction. Predicting dose for high-quality treatment plans provides explicit objectives for both pre- and adaptive planning of ART, and hence can substantially reduce the time and efforts spent in the planning process. Since its feasibility has been demonstrated in several pioneering studies [69–73], accurate prediction of three-dimensional (3D) dose distribution uniquely enabled by AI techniques have become an active research area [15, 74–81]. Several recent studies have been conducted to further tailor the algorithms to fit the novel treatment paradigm of ART specifically. For example, an intentional over-fit algorithm was developed to adapt a population-based dose prediction model to a specific patient for enhanced ART dose prediction performance [82]. This method was then further extended to use training data from the initial plan and the first ART plan of only a single patient to predict the patient-specific dose for subsequent ART sessions [83].

Motivated by the success of AI-based dose prediction, preliminary studies have been performed to further model physician preference in treatment planning [84, 85] using AI. Using prostate cancer stereotactic body RT as a test bed, this study [84] illustrated the feasibility of training an AI-model to predict the probability for a given plan being approved by physicians along with suggestions in plan improvement. These models representing physician treatment intent can be used to guide the treatment planning process and pre-check the generated plan, improving the overall efficiency, consistency, and quality of treatment planning.

AI-based auto-planning. Treatment planning, aimed at designing personalized high-quality plans, is typically accomplished jointly by human planners and physicians in a time-consuming and labor-extensive trial-and-error manner. Given the time constraints in clinical practice, suboptimal treatment plans can often be accepted [86–88], deteriorating treatment quality [89]. It is highly desired to fully automate and accelerate the planning process, particularly for the ART workflow, which has far more stringent requirement on planning efficiency.

The goal of treatment planning is fundamentally different from dose prediction and the reason is two-fold: first, treatment planning directly tackles the machine parameters required to deliver the designed high-quality plan, while dose prediction models only estimate a dose distribution. Realizing the predicted dose on a treatment machine still needs to go through the planning process. Second, it is possible that the predicted dose is not feasible to achieve on a treatment machine, while treatment planning guarantees the feasibility by taking realistic machine specifications and constraints into account in the planning process.

Extensive research efforts have been devoted to develop AI algorithms for direct treatment planning. A typical approach is to incorporate AI models to predict the fluence map based on the planning images as well as the treatment targets and OAR contoured for the patient [90–96]. Post-processing is further required to determine the machine parameters from the predicted fluence map in order to make it deliverable. Note that a discrepancy often exists between the predicted and the final fluence map calculated based on machine parameters as the machine constraints and limitations are not explicitly modeled. Another group of methods incorporate reinforcement learning [97–99] (RL) techniques to establish AI planning agents [100–108] for automatic planning. The training process of RL-based AI agents is very similar to the trail-and-error strategy of humans. The established AI agents can automatically operate the TPS to generate high-quality treatment plans, in lieu of human planners. These plans are likely deliverable plans since they are directly optimized and calculated using the TPS, identical to the way of generating clinical treatment plans.

7.2.3 AI for delivery

Patient-specific quality assurance for online adapted plans has traditionally relied heavily on calculation-based methods. While some studies have supported the clinical feasibility of such approaches, there remains a gap in understanding the correlation between the complexity of adapted plans and the quality of their delivery. The advent of AI models presents a promising avenue for more efficient real-time predictions without the need for extensive measurements and resources. Initial efforts in patient-specific quality assurance focused on conventional IMRT or VMAT, leveraging treatment plan complexity and linear accelerator performance metrics to directly predict the gamma passing rate [109–114]. Building upon this foundation, Hirashima *et al* took a pioneering step by incorporating radiomics features extracted from dose distribution. This addition helped quantify plan complexity, and machine learning techniques were employed to further enhance prediction accuracy [115]. These advanced methods, initially applied to conventional therapies, hold great potential for adaptation to the dynamic landscape of online adaptive therapy. By integrating radiomics and machine learning, these models offer a more comprehensive approach to predict the deliverability of adaptive plans, representing a notable advancement in the field of patient-specific quality assurance for adaptive therapy.

7.3 Outlook and future directions

ART is currently in its nascent stage, with its application primarily confined to specific clinical scenarios or patients with the most pressing needs. Its full potential is yet to be realized, and the trajectory of its advancement is poised for a significant leap with the integration of AI. Throughout this chapter, we have delved into the ways in which AI can markedly enhance the efficiency and precision of ART—two critical domains that must undergo substantial improvements to elevate ART to the status of standard care for all patients.

Now, let us explore the frontier of possibilities where AI could usher in the ultimate evolution in both efficiency and precision—real-time ART. The concept of real-time ART envisions a dynamic and adaptive treatment approach that seamlessly adjusts to the immediate physiological state of the patient during each session. AI is anticipated to play a pivotal role in orchestrating this real-time adaptation, ensuring that treatment strategies are continually refined based on the most up-to-date information.

Beyond real-time adaptation, another frontier emerges in the potential to tailor patient treatments based on both the physics of radiation delivery and the functional response of individual patients. This concept envisions a level of personalization that extends beyond anatomical considerations to account for the unique physiological responses of each patient. AI is poised to become a cornerstone in this paradigm, contributing to the dynamic adaptation of treatment plans based on the interplay between the physical attributes of radiation and the specific functional responses exhibited by individual patients.

In essence, as AI continues to advance, its integration into the realm of ART holds the promise of not only enhancing the efficiency and precision of existing practices but also catalyzing the evolution of real-time adaptive therapies and personalized treatments. The journey towards realizing the full potential of ART is intricately entwined with the advancements AI brings to the field, marking a paradigm shift towards a future where adaptive radiation therapy becomes a standard and tailored approach for all patients

7.3.1 Real-time ART with AI

Having observed the current applications of AI in ART, it is worth considering how AI could enable real-time ART. In this dynamic approach, there is no single adaptive plan; instead, the system continuously adapts during the course of treatment, accounting for any changes in anatomy as treatment is delivered.

Prior to the commencement of real-time ART, a pivotal phase involves a substantial refinement of the pre-treatment workflow, benefitting both the patient and the physician. This transformative process initiates with the assistance of AI, which collaborates with the physician in reviewing an exhaustive set of available data, encompassing imaging, pathology, and patient history. The objective is to recommend a comprehensive course of treatment, delineating the optimal modality, radiation dose, and fractionation schedule.

In the subsequent steps, AI takes on the responsibility of contouring the target and pertinent OARs by leveraging the highest quality image available for each organ. These contours are amalgamated onto a synthetic CT, meticulously generated to replicate the treatment position. Following this, a collaborative review involving both the physician and physicist ensures the accuracy and suitability of the scan and contours.

Moving forward, AI takes a proactive role in generating a pre-plan designed for deliverability, accompanied by specific optimization goals tailored for real-time adaptive planning. To fortify the robustness of the pre-plan, AI continuously refines its optimization goals through the generation of a range of daily images. These images serve as testing grounds for the optimization goals, allowing AI to adapt and update them based on the evolving nuances in the patient's anatomy.

In essence, the integration of AI into the pre-treatment workflow not only streamlines decision-making processes for the physician but also forms the foundation for subsequent real-time adaptive planning. Once AI generates a deliverable pre-plan along with specific optimization goals, it employs its acquired knowledge from the pre-plan phase and continually adapts to changes observed in daily images. This iterative process ensures that AI refines and updates its optimization goals dynamically, fostering robustness in the adaptive planning phase.

At treatment, 4D imaging would occur on which AI would predict the dose that will be delivered today for review. This prediction would be based on the daily anatomy imaged, and both the observed motion in the 4D image, and an AI expanded range of motion to provide a given certainty of coverage. Once the expected dose distribution is approved, treatment would start.

Real-time ART could take many forms, one of which is imagined here. From a 2D image, AI would predict the full 3D image, contour target and OARs within the field of view and re-optimize the plan, accounting for the dose already delivered, knowing which beam angles were still available, and which of those could provide better chances to deliver dose to the target and avoid OARs. After completion of one arc, AI would determine if a second arc is needed to paint in any remaining areas of coverage, using information from the first arc delivery to find the optimal gantry angle and motion phase to deliver this dose.

Real-time adaptation represents the pinnacle of dose delivery, potentially eliminating the requirement for patient immobilization. Given its dynamic nature, the implementation of advanced AI algorithms becomes imperative for seamless delivery. Upon completion of treatment, AI assumes the role of furnishing a comprehensive summary of the delivered dose, encompassing both the current session and the cumulative dose to date, coupled with an analysis of anatomical changes.

7.3.2 Dose escalation and functional adaption with AI

The decision-making process for dose escalation will then rest in the capable hands of both AI and the physician, strategically determining when such escalation is justified. This pivotal decision will draw insights from the unique combination of disease type and patient history, accentuated by the specific response of the individual to the treatment. Here, AI emerges as a valuable ally, contributing nuanced insights into both the physical and functional changes indicative of treatment response, with a distinct emphasis on the significance of functional alterations—an aspect that holds paramount importance in the pursuit of optimal treatment outcomes.

Tools are already available to highlight changes in physical characteristics of tumors between images [116]. AI will be able to review and collate the data to identify relevant changes, requiring an increased target dose, or allowing treatment to be shortened. Incorporated into this decision will be information about adjuvant treatment the patient is receiving, particularly immunotherapy. AI may be able to differentiate the response of the tumor to the different modalities and help the physician decide how to proceed. In addition, AI will predict the best time to deliver the therapies, where gaps in treatment may be beneficial to allow the tumor to respond to treatment, in a manner described by PULSAR [88].

Functional imaging, encompassing both positron emission tomography (PET) and quantitative magnetic resonance imaging (MRI), has already made substantial contributions to the pre-planning stage in radiation therapy. Furthermore, its utility has extended to dynamic use during treatment adjustments, as evidenced in trials such as the PET Lung trial [117]. The natural progression in this trajectory is functional adaptation, heralding a transformative phase in cancer treatment. This could be based on daily PET, by quantitative MR sequences on MR-guided adaptive machines, or by importing separate PET and MR images into x-ray guided systems to help with the adaption. A key realization is that a tumor's reduction in size may not necessarily correlate with a decrease in its core functionality. In instances where the core remains highly functional, it could signify the need for an increase in dose rather than a reduction due to conventional measures such as tumor shrinkage. This nuanced understanding of both physical and functional tumor characteristics necessitates the intervention of AI to determine the optimal course of action.

The envisaged coupling of real-time adaptive therapy with AI-generated treatment predictions based on functional imaging marks a monumental leap forward in patient care. This integration holds the promise of revolutionizing cancer treatment by harnessing the dynamic capabilities of AI to navigate and adapt to the ever-evolving physical and functional aspects of tumors. The anticipation and development of sophisticated AI tools to actualize this vision underscore a progressive and promising frontier in the realm of adaptive radiation therapy.

7.4 Summary

In summary, artificial intelligence (AI) serves as a catalyst for advancing adaptive radiation therapy (ART) into mainstream clinical practice. By addressing key challenges such as workflow efficiency, planning accuracy, and resource optimization, AI empowers clinicians to deliver more personalized and effective treatments. The integration of AI into ART workflows not only reduces the complexity of real-time adaptation but also enhances decision-making through predictive modeling and functional imaging insights. The chapter underscores the potential of AI-driven ART to achieve superior treatment outcomes, paving the way for innovative, patient-centered care in radiation oncology.

References

[1] Green O L, Henke L E and Hugo G D 2019 Practical clinical workflows for online and offline adaptive radiation therapy *Semin. Radiat. Oncol.* **29** 219–27

[2] Archambault Y *et al* 2020 Making on-line adaptive radiotherapy possible using artificial intelligence and machine learning for efficient daily re-planning *Med. Phys. Intl. J.* **8** 77–86

[3] Raaymakers B W *et al* 2017 First patients treated with a 1.5 T MRI-linac: clinical proof of concept of a high-precision, high-field MRI guided radiotherapy treatment *Phys. Med. Biol.* **62** L41–50

[4] Mutic S and Dempsey J F 2014 The ViewRay system: magnetic resonance-guided and controlled radiotherapy *Semin. Radiat. Oncol.* **24** 196–9

[5] Byrne M *et al* 2022 Varian ethos online adaptive radiotherapy for prostate cancer: early results of contouring accuracy, treatment plan quality, and treatment time *J. Appl. Clin. Med. Phys.* **23** e13479

[6] Corradini S *et al* 2019 MR-guidance in clinical reality: current treatment challenges and future perspectives *Radiat. Oncol.* **14** 92

[7] Chen L, Liang X, Shen C, Jiang S and Wang J 2020 Synthetic CT generation from CBCT images via deep learning *Med. Phys.* **47** 1115–25

[8] Han X 2017 MR-based synthetic CT generation using a deep convolutional neural network method *Med. Phys.* **44** 1408–19

[9] Elmahdy M S *et al* 2021 Joint registration and segmentation via multi-task learning for adaptive radiotherapy of prostate cancer *IEEE Access* **9** 95551–68

[10] Fu Y *et al* 2018 A novel MRI segmentation method using CNN-based correction network for MRI-guided adaptive radiotherapy *Med. Phys.* **45** 5129–37

[11] Rigaud B *et al* 2021 Automatic segmentation using deep learning to enable online dose optimization during adaptive radiation therapy of cervical cancer *Int. J. Radiat. Oncol. Biol. Phys.* **109** 1096–110

[12] Visak J *et al* 2023 Evaluating machine learning enhanced intelligent-optimization-engine (IOE) performance for ethos head-and-neck (HN) plan generation *J. Appl. Clin. Med. Phys.* **24** e13950

[13] Good D, Lo J, Lee W R, Wu Q J, Yin F F and Das S K 2013 A knowledge-based approach to improving and homogenizing intensity modulated radiation therapy planning quality among treatment centers: an example application to prostate cancer planning *Int. J. Radiat. Oncol. Biol. Phys.* **87** 176–81

[14] Fogliata A *et al* 2014 On the pre-clinical validation of a commercial model-based optimisation engine: application to volumetric modulated arc therapy for patients with lung or prostate cancer *Radiother. Oncol.* **113** 385–91

[15] Nguyen D *et al* 2019 3D radiotherapy dose prediction on head and neck cancer patients with a hierarchically densely connected U-net deep learning architecture *Phys. Med. Biol.* **64** 065020

[16] Barragan-Montero A M *et al* 2019 Three-dimensional dose prediction for lung IMRT patients with deep neural networks: robust learning from heterogeneous beam configurations *Med. Phys.* **46** 3679–91

[17] Francolini G *et al* 2020 Artificial intelligence in radiotherapy: state of the art and future directions *Med. Oncol.* **37** 50

[18] Miften M *et al* 2018 Tolerance limits and methodologies for IMRT measurement-based verification QA: recommendations of AAPM Task Group No. 218 *Med. Phys.* **45** e53–83

[19] Stojadinovic S, Ouyang L, Gu X, Pompoš A, Bao Q and Solberg T D 2015 Breaking bad IMRT QA practice *J. Appl. Clin. Med. Phys.* **16** 5242

[20] Nachbar M *et al* 2023 Automatic AI-based contouring of prostate MRI for online adaptive radiotherapy *Z. Med. Phys.* **34** 197–207

[21] Qiu Z, Olberg S, den Hertog D, Ajdari A, Bortfeld T and Pursley J 2023 Online adaptive planning methods for intensity-modulated radiotherapy *Phys. Med. Biol.* **68** 10TR01

[22] Yang B *et al* 2021 Initial clinical experience of patient-specific QA of treatment delivery in online adaptive radiotherapy using a 1.5 T MR-linac *Biomed. Phys. Eng. Express* **7** 035022

[23] Shen C *et al* 2023 Clinical experience on patient-specific quality assurance for CBCT-based online adaptive treatment plan *J. Appl. Clin. Med. Phys.* **24** e13918

[24] Zhao X, Stanley D N, Cardenas C E, Harms J and Popple R A 2023 Do we need patient-specific QA for adaptively generated plans? Retrospective evaluation of delivered online adaptive treatment plans on Varian Ethos *J. Appl. Clin. Med. Phys.* **24** e13876

[25] Xu Y, Xia W, Ren W, Ma M, Men K and Dai J 2024 Is it necessary to perform measurement-based patient-specific quality assurance for online adaptive radiotherapy with Elekta Unity MR-linac? *J. Appl. Clin. Med. Phys.* **25** e14175

[26] Cai B, Green O L, Kashani R, Rodriguez V L, Mutic S and Yang D S 2018 A practical implementation of physics quality assurance for photon adaptive radiotherapy *Z. Med. Phys.* **28** 211–23

[27] Rangaraj D *et al* 2013 Catching errors with patient-specific pretreatment machine log file analysis *Pract. Radiat. Oncol.* **3** 80–90

[28] Qian J *et al* 2010 Dose reconstruction for volumetric modulated arc therapy (VMAT) using cone-beam CT and dynamic log files *Phys. Med. Biol.* **55** 3597–610

[29] Teke T, Bergman A M, Kwa W, Gill B, Duzenli C and Popescu I A 2010 Monte Carlo based, patient-specific RapidArc QA using linac log files *Med. Phys.* **37** 116–23

[30] Cheng B *et al* 2023 Development and clinical application of a GPU-based Monte Carlo dose verification module and software for 1.5 T MR-linac *Med. Phys.* **50** 3172–83

[31] Lin J *et al* 2024 ART2Dose: a comprehensive dose verification platform for online adaptive radiotherapy *Med. Phys.* **51** 18–30

[32] Wang Y, Mazur T, Park J, Yang D, Mutic S and Li H 2017 Development of a fast Monte Carlo dose calculation system for online adaptive radiation therapy quality assurance *Med. Phys.* **44** 3130–1

[33] Bahrami A, Karimian A and Arabi H 2021 Comparison of different deep learning architectures for synthetic CT generation from MR images *Phys. Med.* **90** 99–107

[34] Han X 2017 MR-based synthetic CT generation using a deep convolutional neural network method *Med. Phys.* **44** 1408–19

[35] Hsu S-H, Cao Y, Huang K, Feng M and Balter J M 2013 Investigation of a method for generating synthetic CT models from MRI scans of the head and neck for radiation therapy *Phys. Med. Biol.* **58** 8419

[36] Lei Y *et al* 2019 MRI-only based synthetic CT generation using dense cycle consistent generative adversarial networks *Med. Phys.* **46** 3565–81

[37] Liang X *et al* 2023 Bony structure enhanced synthetic CT generation using Dixon sequences for pelvis MR-only radiotherapy *Med. Phys.* **50** 7368–82

[38] Chen L, Liang X, Shen C, Nguyen D, Jiang S and Wang J 2021 Synthetic CT generation from CBCT images via unsupervised deep learning *Phys. Med. Biol.* **66** 115019

[39] Gao L *et al* 2021 Generating synthetic CT from low-dose cone-beam CT by using generative adversarial networks for adaptive radiotherapy *Radiat. Oncol.* **16** 202

[40] Liu Y *et al* 2020 CBCT-based synthetic CT generation using deep-attention cycleGAN for pancreatic adaptive radiotherapy *Med. Phys.* **47** 2472–83

[41] Liang X *et al* 2019 Generating synthesized computed tomography (CT) from cone-beam computed tomography (CBCT) using CycleGAN for adaptive radiation therapy *Phys. Med. Biol.* **64** 125002

[42] Jonsson J, Nyholm T and Söderkvist K 2019 The rationale for MR-only treatment planning for external radiotherapy *Clin. Transla. Radiat. Oncol.* **18** 60–5

[43] Bird D, Henry A M, Sebag-Montefiore D, Buckley D L, Al-Qaisieh B and Speight R 2019 A systematic review of the clinical implementation of pelvic magnetic resonance imaging-only planning for external beam radiation therapy *Int. J. Radiat. Oncolo. Biol. Phys.* **105** 479–92

[44] Chen L *et al* 2023 AI empowered diagnostic MRI based simulation-omitted hippocampal-sparing whole brain radiation therapy on Ethos *Annual Meeting of the American Association of Physicists in. Medicine (Houston, TX, 23–27 July)*

[45] Chen Z, King W, Pearcey R, Kerba M and Mackillop W J 2008 The relationship between waiting time for radiotherapy and clinical outcomes: a systematic review of the literature *Radiother. Oncol.* **87** 3–16

[46] Nikolov S *et al* 2018 Deep learning to achieve clinically applicable segmentation of head and neck anatomy for radiotherapy arXiv:1809.04430

[47] Nikolov S *et al* 2021 Clinically applicable segmentation of head and neck anatomy for radiotherapy: deep learning algorithm development and validation study *J. Med. Internet Res.* **23** e26151

[48] Tong N, Gou S, Yang S, Ruan D and Sheng K 2018 Fully automatic multi-organ segmentation for head and neck cancer radiotherapy using shape representation model constrained fully convolutional neural networks *Med. Phys.* **45** 4558–67

[49] Vrtovec T, Močnik D, Strojan P, Pernuš F and Ibragimov B 2020 Auto-segmentation of organs at risk for head and neck radiotherapy planning: from atlas-based to deep learning methods *Med. Phys.* **47** e929–50

[50] Cardenas C E, Yang J, Anderson B M, Court L E and Brock K B 2019 Advances in auto-segmentation *Semin. Radiat. Oncol.* **29** 185–97

[51] van der Veen J, Gulyban A, Willems S, Maes F and Nuyts S 2021 Interobserver variability in organ at risk delineation in head and neck cancer *Radiat. Oncol.* **16** 120

[52] Gonzalez Y, Shen C, Jung H and Jia X 2019 A human behavior-driven deep-learning approach for automatic sigmoid segmentation *Int. J. Radiat. Oncol. Biol. Phys.* **105** S93–4

[53] Gonzalez Y *et al* 2021 Semi-automatic sigmoid colon segmentation in CT for radiation therapy treatment planning via an iterative 2.5-D deep learning approach *Med. Image Anal.* **68** 101896

[54] Ibrahim S S and Ravi G 2023 Deep learning based brain tumour classification based on recursive sigmoid neural network based on multi-scale neural segmentation *Int. J. Recent Innov. Trends Comput. Commun.* **11** 77–86

[55] Balagopal A *et al* 2021 A deep learning-based framework for segmenting invisible clinical target volumes with estimated uncertainties for post-operative prostate cancer radiotherapy *Med. Image Anal.* **72** 102101

[56] Bi N *et al* 2019 Deep learning improved clinical target volume contouring quality and efficiency for postoperative radiation therapy in non-small cell lung cancer *Front. Oncol.* **9** 1192

[57] Elguindi S *et al* 2019 Deep learning-based auto-segmentation of targets and organs-at-risk for magnetic resonance imaging only planning of prostate radiotherapy *Phys. Imaging Radiat. Oncol.* **12** 80–6

[58] Jin D *et al* 2021 DeepTarget: gross tumor and clinical target volume segmentation in esophageal cancer radiotherapy *Med. Image Anal.* **68** 101909

[59] Liu Z *et al* 2020 Development and validation of a deep learning algorithm for auto-delineation of clinical target volume and organs at risk in cervical cancer radiotherapy *Radiother. Oncol.* **153** 172–9

[60] Ma C Y *et al* 2022 Deep learning-based auto-segmentation of clinical target volumes for radiotherapy treatment of cervical cancer *J. Appl. Clin. Med. Phys.* **23** e13470

[61] Men K *et al* 2018 Fully automatic and robust segmentation of the clinical target volume for radiotherapy of breast cancer using big data and deep learning *Phys. Med.* **50** 13–9

[62] Nori H, King N, McKinney S M, Carignan D and Horvitz E 2023 Capabilities of GPT-4 on medical challenge problems arXiv: 2303.13375

[63] Thirunavukarasu A J, Ting D S J, Elangovan K, Gutierrez L, Tan T F and Ting D S W 2023 Large language models in medicine *Nat. Med.* **29** 1930–40

[64] Li Z *et al* 2022 Patient-specific daily updated deep learning auto-segmentation for MRI-guided adaptive radiotherapy *Radiother. Oncol.* **177** 222–30

[65] Elmahdy M S, Ahuja T, Heide U A V D and Staring M 2020 Patient-specific finetuning of deep learning models for adaptive radiotherapy in prostate CT *2020 IEEE 17th Int. Symp. on Biomedical Imaging (ISBI) (3–7 April 2020)* pp 577–80

[66] Ding J, Zhang Y, Amjad A, Xu J, Thill D and Li X A 2022 Automatic contour refinement for deep learning auto-segmentation of complex organs in MRI-guided adaptive radiation therapy *Adv. Radiat. Oncol.* **7** 100968

[67] Kim N, Chun J, Chang J S, Lee C G, Keum K C and Kim J S 2021 Feasibility of continual deep learning-based segmentation for personalized adaptive radiation therapy in head and neck area *Cancers* **13** 702

[68] Ma L *et al* 2022 Registration-guided deep learning image segmentation for cone beam CT-based online adaptive radiotherapy *Med. Phys.* **49** 5304–16

[69] Chen X, Men K, Li Y, Yi J and Dai J 2019 A feasibility study on an automated method to generate patient-specific dose distributions for radiotherapy using deep learning *Med. Phys.* **46** 56–64

[70] Nguyen D *et al* 2019 A feasibility study for predicting optimal radiation therapy dose distributions of prostate cancer patients from patient anatomy using deep learning *Sci. Rep.* **9** 1076

[71] Fan J, Wang J, Chen Z, Hu C, Zhang Z and Hu W 2019 Automatic treatment planning based on three-dimensional dose distribution predicted from deep learning technique *Med. Phys.* **46** 370–81

[72] Liu Z *et al* 2019 A deep learning method for prediction of three-dimensional dose distribution of helical tomotherapy *Med. Phys.* **46** 1972–83

[73] Kearney V, Chan J W, Haaf S, Descovich M and Solberg T D 2018 DoseNet: a volumetric dose prediction algorithm using 3D fully-convolutional neural networks *Phys. Med. Biol.* **63** 235022

[74] Götz T I, Schmidkonz C, Chen S, Al-Baddai S, Kuwert T and Lang E W 2020 A deep learning approach to radiation dose estimation *Phys. Med. Biol.* **65** 035007

[75] Bakx N, Bluemink H, Hagelaar E, van der Sangen M, Theuws J and Hurkmans C 2021 Development and evaluation of radiotherapy deep learning dose prediction models for breast cancer *Phys. Imaging Radiat. Oncol.* **17** 65–70

[76] Kandalan R N *et al* 2020 Dose prediction with deep learning for prostate cancer radiation therapy: model adaptation to different treatment planning practices *Radiother. Oncol.* **153** 228–35

[77] Ma J *et al* 2021 A feasibility study on deep learning-based individualized 3D dose distribution prediction *Med. Phys.* **48** 4438–47

[78] Barragán-Montero A M *et al* 2021 Deep learning dose prediction for IMRT of esophageal cancer: the effect of data quality and quantity on model performance *Phys. Med.* **83** 52–63

[79] Chen X *et al* 2021 DVHnet: a deep learning-based prediction of patient-specific dose volume histograms for radiotherapy planning *Med. Phys.* **48** 2705–13

[80] Nguyen D *et al* 2018 Three-dimensional radiotherapy dose prediction on head and neck cancer patients with a hierarchically densely connected U-Net deep learning architecture arXiv: 1805.10397

[81] Barragán-Montero A M *et al* 2019 Three-dimensional dose prediction for lung IMRT patients with deep neural networks: robust learning from heterogeneous beam configurations *Med. Phys.* **46** 3679–91

[82] Maniscalco A, Liang X, Lin M-H, Jiang S and Nguyen D 2023 Intentional deep overfit learning for patient-specific dose predictions in adaptive radiotherapy *Med. Phys.* **50** 5354–63

[83] Maniscalco A, Liang X, Lin M-H, Jiang S and Nguyen D 2023 Single patient learning for adaptive radiotherapy dose prediction *Med. Phys.* **50** 7324–37

[84] Gao Y, Shen C, Gonzalez Y and Jia X 2022 Modeling physician's preference in treatment plan approval of stereotactic body radiation therapy of prostate cancer *Phys. Med. Biol.* **67** 115012

[85] Gonzalez Y, Shen C, Albuquerque K and Jia X 2020 Deep-learning based prediction of physicians intention for high-dose-rate brachytherapy with tandem-and-ovoids applicator *Med. Phys.* **47** E454–4

[86] Das I J, Cheng C-W, Chopra K L, Mitra R K, Srivastava S P and Glatstein E 2008 Intensity-modulated radiation therapy dose prescription, recording, and delivery: patterns of variability among institutions and treatment planning systems *J. Natl Cancer Inst.* **100** 300–7

[87] Nelms B E *et al* 2012 Variation in external beam treatment plan quality: an inter-institutional study of planners and planning systems *Pract. Radiat. Oncol.* **2** 296–305

[88] Moore K L, Brame R S, Low D A and Mutic S 2011 Experience-based quality control of clinical intensity-modulated radiotherapy planning *Int. J. Radiat. Oncol. Biol. Phys.* **81** 545–51

[89] Ohri N, Shen X, Dicker A P, Doyle L A, Harrison A S and Showalter T N 2013 Radiotherapy protocol deviations and clinical outcomes: a meta-analysis of cooperative group clinical trials *JNCI: J. Natl Cancer Inst.* **105** 387–93

[90] Li X *et al* 2020 Automatic IMRT planning via static field fluence prediction (AIP-SFFP): a deep learning algorithm for real-time prostate treatment planning *Phys. Med. Biol.* **65** 175014

[91] Lee H *et al* 2019 Fluence-map generation for prostate intensity-modulated radiotherapy planning using a deep-neural-network *Sci. Rep.* **9** 15671

[92] Ma L, Chen M, Gu X and Lu W 2020 Deep learning-based inverse mapping for fluence map prediction *Phys. Med. Biol.* **65** 235035

[93] Vandewinckele L, Willems S, Lambrecht M, Berkovic P, Maes F and Crijns W 2022 Treatment plan prediction for lung IMRT using deep learning based fluence map generation *Physica Med.* **99** 44–54

[94] Wang W *et al* 2021 Deep learning-based fluence map prediction for pancreas stereotactic body radiation therapy with simultaneous integrated boost *Adv. Radiat. Oncol.* **6** 100672

[95] Wang W *et al* 2020 Fluence map prediction using deep learning models—direct plan generation for pancreas stereotactic body radiation therapy *Front. Artif. Intell.* **3** 68

[96] Yuan Z *et al* 2022 Accelerate treatment planning process using deep learning generated fluence maps for cervical cancer radiation therapy *Med. Phys.* **49** 2631–41

[97] Mnih V *et al* 2015 Human-level control through deep reinforcement learning *Nature* **518** 529

[98] Silver D *et al* 2017 Mastering the game of Go without human knowledge *Nature* **550** 354

[99] Silver D *et al* 2016 Mastering the game of Go with deep neural networks and tree search *Nature* **529** 484

[100] Hrinivich W T and Lee J 2020 Artificial intelligence-based radiotherapy machine parameter optimization using reinforcement learning *Med. Phys.* **47** 6140–50

[101] Liu Y *et al* 2022 Automatic inverse treatment planning of Gamma Knife radiosurgery via deep reinforcement learning *Med. Phys.* **49** 2877–89

[102] Shen C, Chen L, Gonzalez Y and Jia X 2021 Improving efficiency of training a virtual treatment planner network via knowledge-guided deep reinforcement learning for intelligent automatic treatment planning of radiotherapy *Med. Phys.* **48** 1909–20

[103] Shen C, Chen L and Jia X 2021 A hierarchical deep reinforcement learning framework for intelligent automatic treatment planning of prostate cancer intensity modulated radiation therapy *Phys. Med. Biol.* **66** 134002

[104] Shen C *et al* 2019 Intelligent inverse treatment planning via deep reinforcement learning, a proof-of-principle study in high dose-rate brachytherapy for cervical cancer *Phys. Med. Biol.* **64** 115013

[105] Shen C *et al* 2020 Operating a treatment planning system using a deep-reinforcement learning-based virtual treatment planner for prostate cancer intensity-modulated radiation therapy treatment planning *Med. Phys.* **47** 2329–36

[106] Sprouts D, Gao Y, Wang C, Jia X, Shen C and Chi Y 2022 The development of a deep reinforcement learning network for dose–volume-constrained treatment planning in prostate cancer intensity modulated radiotherapy *Biomed. Phys. Eng. Express* **8** 045008

[107] Zhang J *et al* 2021 An interpretable planning bot for pancreas stereotactic body radiation therapy *Int. J. Radiat. Oncol. Biol. Phys.* **109** 1076–85

[108] Gao Y, Shen C, Jia X and Park Y K 2023 Implementation and evaluation of an intelligent automatic treatment planning robot for prostate cancer stereotactic body radiation therapy *Radiother. Oncol.* **184** 109685

[109] Valdes G, Scheuermann R, Hung C Y, Olszanski A, Bellerive M and Solberg T D 2016 A mathematical framework for virtual IMRT QA using machine learning *Med. Phys.* **43** 4323

[110] Valdes G, Chan M F, Lim S B, Scheuermann R, Deasy J O and Solberg T D 2017 IMRT QA using machine learning: a multi-institutional validation *J. Appl. Clin. Med. Phys.* **18** 279–84

[111] Li J *et al* 2019 Machine learning for patient-specific quality assurance of VMAT: prediction and classification accuracy *Int. J. Radiat. Oncol. Biol. Phys.* **105** 893–902

[112] Tomori S *et al* 2018 A deep learning-based prediction model for gamma evaluation in patient-specific quality assurance *Med. Phys.* **45** 4055–65

[113] Tomori S *et al* 2021 Systematic method for a deep learning-based prediction model for gamma evaluation in patient-specific quality assurance of volumetric modulated arc therapy *Med. Phys.* **48** 1003–18

[114] Du W, Cho S H, Zhang X, Hoffman K E and Kudchadker R J 2014 Quantification of beam complexity in intensity-modulated radiation therapy treatment plans *Med. Phys.* **41** 021716

[115] Hirashima H *et al* 2020 Improvement of prediction and classification performance for gamma passing rate by using plan complexity and dosiomics features *Radiother. Oncol.* **153** 250–7

[116] Lee C C *et al* 2021 Applying artificial intelligence to longitudinal imaging analysis of vestibular schwannoma following radiosurgery *Sci Rep.* **11** 3106

[117] Kong F M *et al* 2017 Effect of midtreatment PET/CT-adapted radiation therapy with concurrent chemotherapy in patients with locally advanced non-small-cell lung cancer: a phase 2 clinical trial *JAMA Oncol.* **3** 1358–65

Chapter 8

Imaging, imaging processing, and synthetic computed tomography

Tonghe Wang and Xiaofeng Yang

Computed tomography (CT) image synthesis from cone-beam computer tomography (CBCT) and magnetic resonance imaging (MRI) has been explored for various applications within the adaptive radiation therapy workflow. Synthesized CT images have demonstrated feasibility for quantitative tasks such as dose calculation, image segmentation, registration, and PET attenuation correction. These images offer improved quality over CBCT images and provide complementary information to MR images. Deep learning techniques, ranging from convolutional networks to generative models, have been extensively applied in these studies, offering significant advantages in performance compared to traditional image processing methods. This chapter reviews the deep learning methods employed in CT synthesis and examines their potential applications in adaptive radiation therapy.

This chapter is adapted from 'A review on medical imaging synthesis using deep learning and its clinical applications' by Wang *et al* [1], used under a CC BY 4.0 license.

8.1 Introduction

Synthesizing CT images from alternative imaging modalities constitutes a pioneering avenue in medical image synthesis, representing a focal point of extensive research efforts within the field. Building upon its initial success, numerous applications dedicated to the synthesis between diverse imaging modalities have garnered active attention. The primary clinical motivation behind CT synthesis lies in mitigating the exposure of patients to ionizing radiation, a factor associated with potential side effects [2]. Additionally, the synthesis of CT images holds promise for various clinic-oriented advantages, including cost reduction in hardware and maintenance, as well as enhanced patient throughput.

This chapter concentrates on the synthesis of CT images, acknowledging that current studies reveal synthetic CT results that still exhibit noticeable disparities from authentic CT scans. This disparity presently precludes direct diagnostic

doi:10.1088/978-0-7503-6119-4ch8

application. Nevertheless, a wealth of research underscores the feasibility of synthetic CT for non- or indirect-diagnostic purposes, such as its utility in treatment planning for radiation therapy and PET attenuation correction.

8.2 Synthetic CT: deep learning methods

8.2.1 Conventional methods

The absence of a direct correspondence between magnetic resonance (MR) voxel intensity and CT Hounsfield unit (HU) values gives rise to significant disparities in image appearance and contrast, rendering intensity-based calibration methods impractical. Notably, CT depicts air as dark and bone as bright, while MR portrays both as dark. As a result, conventional calibration methods face challenges in aligning these distinct characteristics. Existing approaches in the literature either segment MR images into material-specific groups and assign corresponding CT HU numbers, [3–8] or register MR images with an atlas possessing known CT HU values [9–11].

The technique of CT number bulk-assignment can be traced back to Lee *et al* in 2003 [3]. They manually delineated the entire bone in the pelvic region on MR images and assigned a bone value, designating the remaining region as water. Building upon this, Jonsson *et al* extended a similar methodology to other anatomical sites [4]. Keereman *et al* introduced the use of ultrashort echo time (UTE) sequences as a replacement for conventional magnetic resonance imaging (MRI) sequences [12]. The UTE sequence allows the derivation of an R2 map, which represents bone with high values and soft tissue with low values. Subsequently, a straightforward thresholding method is applied to the R2 map to assign piece-wise constant attenuation coefficient values for air, soft tissue, and bone. In a similar vein, Catana *et al* proposed a dual-echo UTE approach and devised associated image processing procedures to generate a map suitable for thresholding [13]. With UTE, Johansson *et al* developed a Gaussian mixture regression model to link the intensities in MRs (two dual-echo UTE with different flip angles and one T2w image) to CT images [7]. These advancements highlight the efforts to refine and enhance the bulk-assignment of CT numbers, particularly in the context of utilizing alternative imaging sequences and methodologies for improved accuracy and efficiency.

On the other hand, atlas-based registration methods have been introduced as an alternative approach. For instance, Kops and Herzog devised a method where a common attenuation template was created from ten normal volunteers and spatially normalized to the SPM2 standard brain shape [14]. Individual MR images were subsequently registered with this template to obtain an attenuation map. It is important to note that this method was originally developed for brain imaging and necessitates a reliable and locally precise inter-subject registration, as mentioned by the authors. Addressing the challenges posed by whole-body images characterized by high inter-subject variability, Hofmann *et al* proposed a novel approach that combines pattern recognition and atlas registration [15]. This hybrid method effectively captures the global variation in anatomy, making it more suitable for the complexities associated with whole-body imaging applications.

These methodologies rely heavily on the efficacy of segmentation and registration techniques, which proves to be particularly challenging due to the ambiguous air/bone boundary and substantial inter-patient variation. The complexities involved in distinguishing these elements hinder the reliability and accuracy of these calibration methods, emphasizing the need for innovative solutions in addressing the inherent differences between MR and CT imaging modalities.

8.2.2 U-Net

In one of the pioneering studies utilizing deep learning for CT synthesis, Han employed an autoencoder to synthesize CT images from MR images, adopting and modifying a U-Net architecture [16]. The U-Net model in Han's study comprised an encoding and a decoding part. The encoder extracted hierarchical features from an MR image input using convolutional, batch normalization, rectified linear unit (ReLU), and pooling layers. Meanwhile, the mirrored decoder replaced pooling layers with deconvolution layers, transforming the features and reconstructing the predicted CT images from low to high-resolution levels. Short-cut connections were introduced between the two parts on multiple layers. These short-cuts facilitated the concatenation of early layers with late layers, allowing late layers to learn simple features captured in early layers. In Han's study, these short-cuts enabled high-resolution features from the encoding part to be used as extra inputs in the decoding part. Moreover, the original autoencoder design included fully connected 'hidden layers', which connect every neuron in the previous layer to every neuron in the next. However, these fully connected layers, crucial for image classification tasks, were found to be less relevant for dense pixel-wise prediction. Therefore, Han's model eliminated fully connected layers, significantly reducing the number of parameters. The study trained the model using pairs of MR and CT 2D slices, with a training process minimizing a mean absolute error (MAE) loss function between the predictions and ground truth. The use of an L1-norm loss function such as MAE contributes to improved robustness to noise, artifacts, and misalignment among the training images. Han's work represents a significant advancement in the application of deep learning to CT synthesis.

Most studies employing the U-Net architecture have generally adhered to the outlined structure, yet there have been numerous proposed variants and improvements. For instance, in comparison to Han's model, Jang *et al* and Liu *et al* applied a similar encoder and decoder model without the inclusion of skip connections [17, 18]. Instead of utilizing CT images directly as ground truth in their MR-based CT synthesis studies, they employed discretized maps from CTs, categorizing three materials and framing CT synthesis as a segmentation problem. The final layer of the decoder incorporated a multi-class softmax classifier, assigning probabilities to each material class within each voxel (e.g. 0.5 for bone, 0.3 for air, and 0.1 for soft tissue).

An additional noteworthy feature introduced by Jang *et al* is the inclusion of a fully connected conditional random field, considering neighboring voxels during label predictions [18]. This provided complementary information to the base classifier, which focused on single voxels. In this application, the conditional random field supplied 3D context to 2D image slices, establishing pairwise potentials between all pairs of voxels by utilizing the model's output and the original 3D volume when predicting voxel labels.

A landmark advancement in U-Net architecture occurred when Dong *et al* identified that the information carried in the long skip connection from the encoding path often contained high-frequency and irrelevant components from noisy input images [19]. To address this, they introduced a self-attention strategy that utilized feature maps extracted from the coarse-scale early in the encoder module to identify the most relevant emerging features. These features were assigned attention scores, enabling the elimination of noise before concatenation. Alternatively, Hwang *et al* adopted a strategy that employed skip connections only in deeper layers, offering an alternative approach to handling noise and enhancing the efficiency of information flow within the network [20].

The selection of building blocks within the encoding and decoding modules has been a subject of exploration. Fu *et al* made several enhancements based on Han's architecture [21]. Notably, they replaced batch normalization layers, where normalization is applied across image subsets of the original sample to expedite convergence, with instance normalization layers. The latter performs normalization at the level of image channels, contributing to further performance improvements, particularly when training with a small batch size. Additionally, in the decoder, the unpooling layers, responsible for up-sampling and reversing the pooling layers in the encoder, were substituted with deconvolutional layers. These deconvolutional layers produce dense feature maps, and the skip connections were replaced with residual short-cuts inspired by ResNet. This alteration aims to conserve computational memory more efficiently. Neppl *et al* opted to replace the ReLU layer with a generalized parametric ReLU (PReLU) to adaptively adjust the activation function [22]. In a similar vein, Torrado-Carvajal *et al* introduced a dropout layer before the first transposed convolution in the decoder to mitigate overfitting concerns [23].

Various loss functions have been explored in the studies reviewed. In addition to the commonly used L1-norm and L2-norms, which enforce voxel-wise similarity, the total loss function often incorporates other functions describing different image properties. For instance, Leynes *et al* employed a total loss function that was a combination of MAE loss, gradient difference loss, and Laplacian difference loss [24]. The latter two components aimed to enhance image sharpness. Similarly, Chen *et al* combined MAE loss with structure dissimilarity loss to promote whole-structure-wise similarity [25]. To prevent overfitting, L2-regularization has been integrated into the loss function in some studies [26, 27]. Kazemifar *et al* introduced mutual information, widely employed in loss functions for image registration, into their loss function. They demonstrated its advantages over MAE loss in better compensating for misalignment between CT and MR images. Another innovative addition is the perceptual loss introduced by Largent *et al*. This loss function, which mimics human visual perception by considering similar features rather than solely intensities, was implemented in three different versions of increasing complexity: on a single convolutional layer, on multiple layers with uniform weights, and on multiple layers with different weights assigning greater importance to layers yielding lower MAE [28].

8.2.3 Generative adversarial networks

A generative adversarial network (GAN) comprises a generative network and a discriminative network that undergo simultaneous training. The generative network is tasked with producing synthetic images, while the discriminative network learns to distinguish between real and synthetic images. The overarching training objective of a GAN is to enable the generative network to generate synthetic images of utmost realism, deceiving the discriminator. In tandem, the discriminative network strives to accurately classify images as either real or synthetic. The training process involves adversarial competition between these networks until equilibrium is achieved. In a production setting, the trained generative network is applied to generate synthetic images for new inputs.

Similar to autoencoders, GANs have found application in early publications on medical image synthesis using deep learning. In a study by Nie *et al* a fully convolutional autoencoder, devoid of fully connected layers, served as the generative network, while a standard AE was employed for the discriminative network [29]. Both networks utilized a binary cross-entropy loss function. Notably, the discriminative network's loss aimed to minimize the difference between assigned labels and ground truth conventionally. In contrast, the generative network's loss was formulated to maximize the error of the discriminative network by minimizing the disparity between the labels assigned by the discriminative network and an incorrect label. Given that the study employed a patch-to-patch training approach, limiting the contextual information available in training samples, an auto-context model was introduced. This model integrates low-level and contextual information derived from low-level appearance features to refine the synthesis results.

Various iterations of GANs have been explored, each tailored to specific tasks. Emami *et al* introduced the conditional GAN (cGAN) in their work on CT synthesis from MR [30]. In contrast to the traditional unconditional GAN, both the generative and discriminative networks of the cGAN are exposed to input images, such as MR images in CT synthesis from MR. This design involves conditioning the loss function of the discriminator on the input images, proving to be particularly effective for image-to-image translation tasks [31].

Liang *et al* incorporated CycleGAN into their study on synthetic CT generation based on cone beam computed tomography (CBCT) [32]. The CycleGAN features two generators: a CBCT/CT generator and a CT/CBCT generator, alongside two discriminators: a real CT/synthetic CT discriminator and a real CBCT/synthetic CBCT discriminator. The first cycle involves transforming the input CBCT into a synthesized CT using the CBCT/CT generator, and then regenerating a cycle CBCT from the synthetic CT using the CT/CBCT generator. This cycle CBCT is compared to the original input CBCT, generating CBCT cycle consistency loss. Simultaneously, a real CT-synthetic CT discriminator distinguishes between the real and synthetic CT to produce CT adversarial loss, akin to a standard GAN. To enforce a one-to-one mapping between CT and CBCT, a second cycle transformation from CT to CBCT is performed, mirroring the first cycle but swapping the roles of CBCT and CT. CycleGAN introduces an innovative approach by including an inverse mapping network through cycle consistency loss. This addition enhances network performance, in particular in scenarios where exact matching image pairs in training sets are unavailable. CycleGAN exhibits a robust tolerance for misalignment in paired training datasets, a critical advantage in inter-modality synthesis where acquiring precisely matched image pairs is challenging. Many studies employ registration to pair training images, preserving quantitative pixel values and minimizing baseline geometric discrepancies [33]. This approach enables the network to concentrate on mapping details and accelerates training while addressing the inherent difficulties associated with achieving exact image pair matches.

Diverse architectures of feature extraction blocks have demonstrated efficacy across various applications. Several studies have highlighted the effectiveness of autoencoders with residual blocks, particularly in tasks involving image transformation where source and target images exhibit significant similarity, such as the transition between CT and CBCT. Given the visual resemblance but quantitative differences between these image pairs, residual blocks, comprising a residual connection coupled with multiple hidden layers, have been incorporated into the network to discern and learn the distinctions within these pairs. In this configuration, an input traverses these hidden layers via the residual connection. Consequently, the hidden layers work to minimize a residual image between the source and the ground truth target images, aiming to reduce noise and artifacts. This approach stands in contrast to standard autoencoder blocks where a feed-forward summation is used. The residual connection in the blocks effectively enforces the minimization of differences, contributing to the refinement of image synthesis [33–37].

On the other hand, dense blocks adopt a different strategy by concatenating outputs from preceding layers rather than utilizing feed-forward summation. This design choice enables the capture of multi-frequency information, encompassing both high and low-frequency details. Dense blocks prove particularly advantageous in scenarios of inter-modality image synthesis, such as MR-to-CT and PET-to-CT [19, 38–42]. By capturing a broader spectrum of information, dense blocks enhance the representation of the mapping from the source image modality to the target image modality, resulting in more comprehensive and accurate synthesis outcomes.

In the realm of GANs, autoencoders and their variants are frequently employed for both generative and discriminative networks. Notably, Emami et al opted for a ResNet architecture in their generative network [30]. They modified the architecture by eliminating fully connected layers and introducing two transposed convolutional layers following residual blocks, effectively leveraging deconvolution. Meanwhile, Kim et al innovatively combined the U-Net architecture with a residual training scheme in their generative network [43]. Olberg et al proposed a deep spatial pyramid convolutional framework, incorporating an atrous spatial pyramid pooling (ASPP) module within a U-Net architecture [44]. This module performs atrous convolution at multiple rates concurrently, allowing for the exploitation of multi-scale features to characterize a single pixel. The encoder in this framework captures rich multi-scale contextual information, enhancing its ability for image translation. In contrast to the complexity often found in the generator, the discriminator is commonly implemented in a more straightforward fashion. Liu *et al* introduced a common example comprising a few down-sampling convolutional layers, followed by a sigmoid activation layer to binarize the output [41].

GANs and their variants incorporate adversarial loss functions alongside image quality and accuracy loss functions embedded within architectures such as U-Net. The adversarial term, distinct from the reconstruction term that ensures image intensity accuracy, gauges the correctness of the discriminator's decision regarding real or synthetic images. Commonly used loss functions include binary cross-entropy or similar sigmoid cross-entropy, as well as negative log-likelihood functions outlined in the original GAN publication within computer vision. However, training challenges may arise, including divergence due to vanishing gradients and mode collapse when the discriminator is optimized for a fixed generator [45]. To mitigate these issues, Emami *et al* introduced the use of least-square loss, which has demonstrated greater stability during training and yields higher quality results [30]. Another alternative is the Wasserstein distance loss function, known for its smoother gradient flow and faster convergence. In GANs, providing true or false labels from the discriminator to the generator may not be sufficient for improvement and can lead to numerical instability due to vanishing or exploding gradients. To address this, Ouyang *et al* employed a feature-matching technique. This involves specifying a new objective function where the generator aims to synthesize images that match the expected values of features on intermediate layers of the discriminator, rather than directly maximizing the final output of the discriminator [46].

8.2.4 Denoising diffusion probabilistic model

The denoising diffusion probabilistic model (DDPM) is emerging as one of the most promising deep generative models, showcasing impressive capabilities in various tasks such as image generation, superresolution, and image inpainting. This model operates in two stages: a forward stage that progressively introduces noise, and a reverse stage aimed at denoising and reconstructing the original sample incrementally. The forward stage comprises multiple small steps, where the image undergoes slight corruption by Gaussian noise. In the reverse stage, a trained neural network is employed to estimate the noise at each reverse diffusion step.

In contrast to GANs, DDPM exhibits greater stability during training, displaying reduced susceptibility to mode collapse and diminished sensitivity to hyperparameters [47]. However, given the relative novelty of DDPM, as of the writing of this chapter, no publications in peer-reviewed journals have been identified. The current insights are drawn from pioneering studies available as preprints, providing a preliminary glimpse into the capabilities and characteristics of DDPM in comparison to other generative models.

Lyu *et al* proposed diffusion and score-matching models for conversion between MRI and CT images.[48] In their study, they explored four distinct sampling strategies, one of which involved the use of the DDPM. The authors demonstrated that the CT images generated through their proposed method exhibited favorable results when compared to those produced by conventional convolutional neural network and GAN models.

Pan *et al* introduced an innovative approach in the form of an MRI-to-CT transformer-based DDPM (MC-DDPM) [49]. This model utilizes diffusion processes in conjunction with a shifted-window transformer network to generate synthetic CT images from MRI data. Specifically, a shifted-window transformer V-Net (Swin-V-Net) is employed in the reverse process to denoise noisy CT images conditioned on MRI input, resulting in the generation of high-quality, noise-free CT images. The proposed MC-DDPM demonstrated statistically significant improvements across various metrics for both brain and prostate sites when compared to competing GAN-based networks. However, it is worth noting that the MC-DDPM is not without limitations. One notable drawback is its heavy computational burden, leading to longer inference times in comparison to GAN-based methods. Despite this drawback, the model's superior performance in terms of image quality metrics underscores its potential in addressing the MRI-to-CT synthesis task, offering a valuable alternative to existing approaches. Additionally, the feasibility of conditional DDPM in generating synthetic CT from CBCT has also been demonstrated by Peng *et al* and Fu *et al*, further expanding the applicability of this innovative approach [50, 51].

8.3 Synthetic CT from CBCT

CBCT and CT image reconstruction share fundamental physics principles related to x-ray attenuation and back projection. However, their practical implementation in terms of acquisition and reconstruction, as well as their clinical applications, varies significantly. Consequently, in the context of this review, they are treated as two distinct imaging modalities.

CBCT has found extensive application in image-guided radiation therapy (IGRT), primarily for assessing patient set-up errors and inter-fractional motion. This is achieved by comparing the displacement of anatomical landmarks relative to the treatment planning CT images. As adaptive radiation therapy techniques gain prevalence, more sophisticated applications of CBCT are being explored. These include challenging tasks such as daily dose estimation and automated contouring, facilitated by deformable image registration (DIR) with CT imaging acquired during the simulation process. The evolving role of CBCT in these advanced applications reflects its increasing significance in improving the precision and adaptability of radiation therapy procedures.

In contrast to CT scanners that employ fan-shaped x-ray beams with multi slice detectors, CBCT utilizes a cone-shaped x-ray beam directed onto a flat panel detector. While the flat panel detector provides high spatial resolution and extensive coverage along the *z*-axis, it is susceptible to increased scatter signal due to x-ray scatter generated throughout the entire body volume reaching the detector. The presence of scatter signals gives rise to pronounced streaking and cupping artifacts in CBCT images, contributing to substantial quantitative CT errors. These errors pose challenges in the calibration of the CBCT Hounsfield unit (HU) to electron density, particularly when utilizing CBCT images for dose calculation. Furthermore, the compromised image contrast and bone suppression can introduce significant errors in DIR for the propagation of contours from planning CT to CBCT. The diminished image quality of CBCT thus limits its utility in advanced quantitative applications within the realm of radiation therapy.

8.3.1 Noise and artifact reduction

Deep learning-based methods, as listed in table 8.1, have been proposed to address and enhance CBCT HU values in comparison to CT, leveraging the advantages offered by image translation techniques. CBCT images are reconstructed from numerous 2D projections captured from various angles. In certain studies, neural

Table 8.1. Summary of studies on CBCT-based synthetic CT for image quality improvement. (Adapted from [1]. CC BY 4.0.)

Network	Projection or image domain	Site, and # of patients in training/testing	Key findings in synthetic CBCT quality	Author, year
U-Net	Image	Pelvis: 20, 5-fold cross validation	PSNR (dB): 50.9	Kida *et al* [52]
AE	Image	Lung: 15 training/5 testing	PSNR (dB):8.823	Xie *et al* [53]
U-Net	Image	Head and neck: 30 training/ 7 validation/7 testing Pelvis: 6 training/5 testing	MAE (HU): 18.98 (head and neck) 42.40 (pelvis)	Chen *et al* [25]
CycleGAN	Image	Brain: 24, leave-one-out Pelvis: 20, leave-one-out	MAE (HU): 13.0 ± 2.2 (brain) 16.1 ± 4.5 (pelvis)	Harms *et al* [33]
U-Net	Projection	1800 projections in training (simulation)/200 validation (simulation)/ 360 testing (phantom)	MAE (HU): 17.9 ± 5.7	Nomura *et al* [54]
U-Net	Image	Head and neck: 40 training/ 15 testing	MAE (HU): 49.28	Yuan *et al* [55]
CycleGAN	Image	Pelvis: 16 training/4 testing	Mean error (HU): (2, 14)	Kida *et al* [56]

networks have been applied in the projection domain, focusing on the enhancement of 2D projection images to improve the overall quality before volume reconstruction. The refined projection images are then employed in the reconstruction process to generate CBCT image volumes with improved quality. Alternatively, some methods operate in the image domain, directly taking the reconstructed CBCT image volumes as input and producing synthetic CT images with enhanced quality as output.

Projection-domain methods offer advantages when dealing with a larger number of training 2D projection images (typically >300) compared to image-domain methods, where the number of training image slices is generally fewer (<100) for each scan. Moreover, projection-domain methods can be more effective in addressing the unpredictable cupping and streaking artifacts caused by scatter in CBCT images, as these artifacts are less predictable than those in projection images. Neural networks find it easier to learn from projection images due to the reduced variability in per-patient artifactual features compared to the image domain. In the image domain, where the variability in artifactual features is greater, models are typically not trained on non-anthropomorphic phantoms because the learned features may not be applicable across different patient image sets.

Nomura *et al* demonstrated that features characterizing scatter distribution in anthropomorphic phantom projections can be successfully learned from non-anthropomorphic phantom projections in the projection domain [54]. This success is attributed to the neural network effectively capturing the inherent relationship between scatter distribution and objective thickness in the projection domain. In contrast, the relationship between scatter artifact and objective appearance is more intricate in the image domain, making it challenging for neural networks to learn and generalize easily.

8.3.2 Online dose calculation

Synthetic CTs have shown substantial improvements over original CBCTs in terms of dosimetric accuracy, bringing them closer to planning CT for photon dose calculations. Some reviewed literature is summarized in table 8.2. The feasibility of synthetic CTs in volumetric modulated arc therapy (VMAT) planning has been investigated across various body sites, assessing select dose–volume histogram (DVH) metrics, dose, and/or gamma differences. As shown in figure 8.1, it is demonstrated that significant local dosimetric errors occur in regions with severe artifacts in original CBCTs. Synthetic CTs effectively mitigate these artifacts and the associated dosimetric errors [37].

However, it is worth noting that achieving acceptable dosimetric accuracy with synthetic CT in proton planning is more challenging compared to photon planning. This is primarily due to the presence of range shifts, which can be as substantial as 5 mm. Managing these range shifts poses a significant challenge in proton planning with synthetic CTs, highlighting the importance of carefully addressing such complexities for accurate dose calculations in proton therapy [57–59].

Table 8.2. Summary of studies on CBCT-based synthetic CT for dose calculation in radiation therapy. (Adapted from [1]. CC BY 4.0.)

Network	Projection or image domain	Site, and # of patients in training/testing	Key findings in dosimetry	Author, year
U-Net	Projection	Pelvis: 15 training/7 testing/ 8 evaluation	Passing rate for 2% dose difference: 100% for photon plan, 15%–81% for proton plan	Hansen *et al* [58]
CycleGAN	Image	Pelvis: 18 training/7 validation/8 testing	Passing rate for 2% dose difference: 100% for photon plan, 71%–86% for proton plan	Kurz *et al* [57]
U-Net	Image	Pelvis: 27 training/7 validation/8 testing	Passing rate for 2% dose difference: > 99.5% for photon plan, > 80% for proton plan	Landry *et al* [59]
U-Net	Image	Head and neck: 50 training/ 10 validation/10 testing	Average DVH metrics difference: 0.2% ± 0.6%	Li *et al* [60]
CycleGAN	Image	Head and neck: 81 training/ 9 validation/20 testing	Gamma passing rate at (1%, 1 mm): 96.26 ± 3.59%	Liang *et al* [32]
U-Net	Image	Head and neck: 33, 3-fold cross validation	Gamma passing rate at (2%, 2 mm): 93.75%–99.75% (proton)	Adrian *et al* [61]
CycleGAN	Image	Pancreas: 30. leave-one-out	DVH metrics difference < 1 Gy	Liu *et al* [37]

8.3.3 Online image segmentation

The segmentation of targets and organs at risk (OARs) on daily imaging is a crucial yet time-consuming step in the adaptive re-planning process. Manual delineation can significantly prolong the entire process, making it imperative to explore more efficient methods. CBCT-based auto organ delineation has been investigated, involving contour propagation through rigid or deformable registration between daily CBCT and planning CT. However, the accuracy of contour propagation is highly dependent on the quality of registration, often requiring manual editing and verification. While semi-automated methods have been explored to speed up OAR contouring, their improvement is limited, prompting the need for faster organ delineation methods for CBCT-based plan adaptation.

Deep learning-based segmentation algorithms have shown promising performance in CT contouring for various anatomical sites. Nevertheless, the inferior image quality of CBCT compared to CT poses challenges in directly applying existing convolutional neural network-based algorithms on CBCT images. Dai *et al* proposed a two-in-one deep learning model that first utilizes a cycleGAN network to

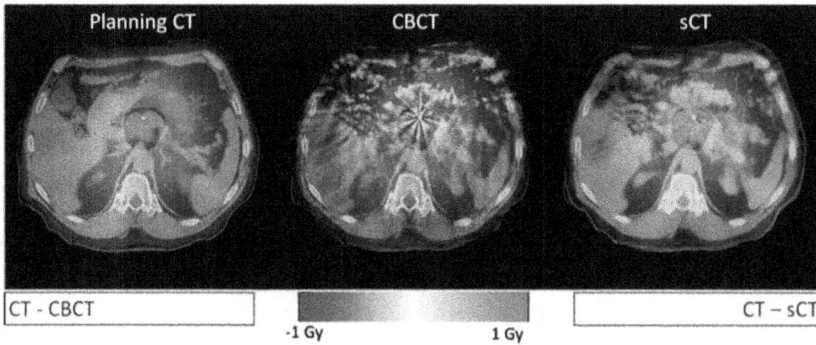

Figure 8.1. Dose comparison between CT- and CBCT-, as well as between CT- and sCT-based plans. CBCT = cone-beam CT; sCT = synthetic CT. (Reproduced from [37] with permission from John Wiley & Sons. Copyright 2020 American Association of Physicists in Medicine.)

convert CBCT to synthetic CT [62]. Subsequently, a mask scoring regional convolutional neural network is applied to the synthetic CT to obtain organ contours. The enhanced image quality of synthetic CT from CBCT is expected to facilitate the image segmentation task. Evaluated on pancreas cancer patients, the proposed method has demonstrated significant improvements across all metrics for the majority of selected organs compared to direct segmentation on CBCT.

8.4 Synthetic CT from MRI

The current standard for radiation therapy planning involves the sequential use of both MRI and CT imaging modalities on patients. This approach is driven by the complementary strengths of each modality, with MR images offering superior soft-tissue contrast crucial for delineating tumors and OARs [63], while CT images provide electron density maps essential for accurate dose calculations and serve as reference images for pre-treatment positioning. The delineation of tumor and OAR contours typically begins with MR images and is then transferred to CT images through image registration, facilitating treatment planning and dose assessment.

However, the dual-modality approach incurs additional costs and time for patients and introduces systematic positioning errors of up to 2 mm during the CT-MRI image registration process [64–66]. Furthermore, the CT scan contributes a non-negligible ionization dose to patients, particularly those necessitating re-simulation [67]. Consequently, there is a compelling need to explore alternatives, such as a treatment planning workflow solely reliant on MRI, to address these challenges. The advent of MR-linac technology further encourages the exclusive use of MRI in radiotherapy [68, 69]. Despite the potential advantages, it is important to note that MR cannot directly substitute CT in current radiotherapy workflows. This limitation arises from the fact that MR images derive signal from hydrogen nuclei, precluding the direct provision of material attenuation coefficients necessary for electron density calibration and subsequent dose calculations.

The preference for replacing CT with MR is extending into current PET imaging practices. Traditionally, CT is frequently combined with PET, allowing both imaging examinations to be conducted sequentially on the same table. CT images play a crucial role in this set-up, as they are utilized to generate a 511 keV linear attenuation coefficient map. This map, derived through a piece-wise linear scaling algorithm [70, 71], is then employed to correct PET images for attenuated annihilation photons within the patient's body, ensuring a satisfactory level of image quality. The integration of MR with PET has emerged as a promising alternative to the established PET/CT systems. MR offers notable advantages as mentioned above. However, akin to the challenges faced in radiation therapy, MR images cannot directly provide the 511 keV attenuation coefficients required for the attenuation correction process in PET imaging. Consequently, the solution lies in the incorporation of MR-to-CT image synthesis within PET/MR systems to enable accurate photon attenuation correction. This innovative approach capitalizes on the strengths of MR imaging while addressing the specific needs of PET imaging for enhanced diagnostic capabilities.

8.4.1 Synthetic image accuracy

An overview of studies focused on synthesizing CT from MR images for radiation therapy and PET attenuation correction is listed in tables 8.3 and 8.4, respectively. In the context of CT synthesis applications for radiation therapy, the mean absolute error (MAE) emerges as the predominant and well-defined metric used to assess image quality. Nearly every study in this domain reported the image quality of its synthetic CT using MAE as a key evaluation criterion. On the other hand, when it comes to synthetic CT in PET attenuation correction, the assessment of synthetic CT quality is more commonly conducted indirectly. Instead of directly evaluating the synthetic CT itself, studies tend to assess the quality of PET attenuation correction. This suggests that, in this application, the focus is often on the impact of synthetic CT on PET image quality and attenuation correction accuracy. In instances where studies present multiple variants of methods, it is noted that the selected method for inclusion in the tables is based on achieving the best MAE for radiation therapy or the best PET quality for PET attenuation correction. This approach allows for a concise representation of the most effective variants in terms of image quality metrics for each respective application.

Table 8.3. Summary of studies on MR-based synthetic CT for radiation therapy. (Adapted from [1]. CC BY 4.0.)

Author, year	Network	MR parameters	Site, and # of patients in training/testing	Key findings in image quality	Key findings in dosimetry
Han [16] Nie et al [29]	U-Net GAN	1.5 T T1w without contrast N/A	Brain: 18, 6-fold cross validation Brain: 16 Pelvis: 22	MAE (HU): 84.8 ± 17.3 MAE (HU): 92.5 ± 13.9	N/A* N/A
Xiang et al [87]	AE	T1w	Brain: 16, leave-one-out Pelvis: 22, leave-one-out	MAE (HU): 85.4 ± 9.24 (brain) 42.4 ± 5.1 (pelvis)	N/A
Dinkla et al [75] Arabi et al [76] Chen et al [73]	AE U-Net U-Net	1.5 T T1w 3 T T2w 3 T T2w	Brain: 52, 2-fold cross validation Pelvis: 39, 4-fold cross validation Pelvis: 36 training/15 testing	MAE (HU): 67 ± 11 MAE (HU): 32.7 ± 7.9 MAE (HU): 29.96 ± 4.87	Dose difference < 1% Dose difference < 1% Dose difference of max dose in PTV < 1.01%
Emami et al [30] Maspero et al [88]	GAN GAN	1 T post-gadolinium T1w Dixon in-phase, fat and water	Brain: 15, 5-fold cross validation Pelvis: 91 (59 prostate + 18 rectal + 14 cervical cancer), 32 (prostate) training/59 (rest) testing	MAE (HU): 89.3 ± 10.3 MAE (HU): 65 ± 10 (prostate) 56 ± 5 (rectum) 59 ± 6 (cervix)	N/A Dose difference < 1.6%
Dinkla et al [72]	U-Net	3 T in-phase Dixon T2w	Head and neck: 22 training/12 testing	MAE (HU): 75 ± 9	Mead dose difference – 0.03% ± 0.05% overall, −0.07% ± 0.22% in > 90% of prescription dose volume
Fu et al [21]	U-Net	1.5 T T1w without contrast	Pelvis: 20, 5-fold cross validation	MAE (HU): 40.5 ± 5.4 (2D) 37.6 ± 5.1 (3D)	N/A

Reference	Method	Field/sequence	Dataset	MAE	Metrics
Gupta et al [74]	U-Net	3 T in-phase Dixon T1w	Brain: 47 training/13 testing	MAE (HU): 17.6 ± 3.4	Mean target dose difference 2.3 ± 0.1%
Kazemifar et al [85]	GAN	1.5 T post-gadolinium T1w	Brain: 77, 70% training/12% validation/18% testing	MAE (HU): 47.2 ± 11.0	Mean DVH metrics difference < 1%
Largent et al [28]	GAN	3 T T2w	Pelvis: 39, training/testing: 25/14, 25/14, 25/11	MAE (HU): 34.1 ± 7.5	PTV V95% difference < 0.6%
Lei et al [39]	CycleGAN	Brain: T1w Pelvis: T2w	Brain: 24, leave-one-out cross validation Pelvis: 20, leave-one-out cross validation	MAE (HU): 55.7 ± 9.4 (brain) 50.8 ± 15.5 (pelvis)	N/A
Liu et al [89]	U-Net	1.5 T T1w	Brain: 30 training/10 testing	MAE (HU): 75 ± 23	PTV V95% difference 0.27% ± 0.79%
Liu et al [40, 42]	CycleGAN	3 T/1.5 T T1w	Liver: 21, leave-one-out cross validation	MAE (HU): 72.87 ± 18.16	Mean DVH metrics difference < 1% for both photon and proton plans
Liu et al [42]	CycleGAN	1.5 T T2w	Pelvis: 17, leave-one-out cross validation	MAE (HU): 51.32 ± 16.91	Mean DVH metrics difference < 1% (proton plan)
Neppl et al [22]	U-Net	1.5 T T1w	Brain: 57 training/28 validation/4 testing	MAE (HU): (82, 147)[+]	Gamma passing rate: > 95% at (1%, 1 mm) for photon plan, > 90% at (2%, 2 mm) for proton plan
Olberg et al [44]	GAN	0.35 T T1w	Breast: 48 training/12 testing	MAE (HU): 16.1 ± 3.5	PTV D95 difference < 1%
Shafai-Erfani et al [90]	CycleGAN	1.5 T T1w	Brain: 50	MAE (HU): 54.55 ± 6.81	PTV D95 difference < 0.5% (proton plan)

(Continued)

Table 8.3. (*Continued*)

Author, year	Network	MR parameters	Site, and # of patients in training/testing	Key findings in image quality	Key findings in dosimetry
Wang et al [91]	U-Net	1.5 T T2w	Head and neck: 23 training/10 testing	MAE (HU): 131 ± 24	N/A
Florkow et al [82]	U-Net	3 T T1w Dixon	Pelvis: 27, 3-fold cross validation	MAE (HU): (33, 40)	N/A
Koike et al [92]	GAN	T1w + T2w + FLAIR	Brain: 15	MAE (HU): 108.1 ± 24.0	DVH metrics difference < 1%
Qi et al [81]	GAN	T1w + T2w + contrast-enhanced T1w + contrast-enhanced T1w Dixon water	Head and neck: 30 training/15 testing	MAE (HU): 69.98 ± 12.02	Mean average dose difference < 1%
Tie et al [83]	GAN	1.5 T pre-contrast T1w + post-contrast T1w + T2w	Head and neck: 32, 8-fold cross validation	MAE (HU): 75.7 ± 14.6	N/A
Brou Boni et al [93]	GAN	1.5 T and 3 T T2w from three scanners	Pelvis: 11 training from two scanner/8 testing from one scanner	MAE (HU): 48.5 ± 6	Maximum dose difference in target = 1.3%

AE: Autoencoder.
* N/A: not available, i.e. not explicitly indicated in the publication.
+ Numbers in parentheses indicate minimum and maximum values.

Table 8.4. Summary of studies on MR-based synthetic CT for PET attenuation correction. (Adapted from [1]. CC BY 4.0.)

Author, year	Network	MR parameters	Site, and # of patients in training/testing	Key findings in PET quality
Gong et al [84]	U-Net	Dixon and ZTE	Brain: 14, leave-two-out	Absolute bias < 3% among 8 VOIs
Jang et al [18]	U-Net	3 T UTE	Brain: 30 pre-training/6 training/8 testing	Bias (%): −0.8 ± 0.8–1.1 ± 1.3 among 23 VOIs
Leynes et al [24]	U-Net	3 T Dixon and ZTE	Pelvis: 26, 10 training/16 testing	RMSE (%): 2.68 among 30 bone lesions, 4.07 among 60 soft-tissue lesions
Liu et al [17]	U-Net	1.5 T T1w	Brain: 30 training/10 testing	Bias (%): −3.2 ± 1.3–0.4 ± 0.8
Spuhler et al [27]	U-Net	1.5 T T1w	Brain: 44 training/11 validation/11 testing	Global bias (%): −0.49 ± 1.7 for 11C-WAY-100 635–1.52 ± 0.73 for 11C-DASB
Torrado-Carvajal et al [23]	U-Net	Dixon-VIBE	Pelvis: 28 pairs from 19 patients, 4-fold cross validation	Bias (%): 0.27 ± 2.59 for fat −0.03 ± 2.98 for soft tissue −0.95 ± 5.09 for bone
Blanc-Durand et al [79]	U-Net	ZTE	Brain: 23 training/47 testing	Bias (%): −1.8 ± 1.9–1.7 ± 2.6 among 70 VOIs
Ladefoged et al [80]	U-Net	UTE	Brain: 79 (pediatric), 4-fold cross validation	Bias (%): −0.2–0.5 in 95% CI
Arabi et al [94]	GAN	3 T T1w	Brain: 40, 2-fold cross validation	Absolute bias < 4% among 63 VOIs

In the majority of the studies, the MAE of the synthetic CT within the patient's body typically falls within the range of 40–70 HU. Some reported results even approach the uncertainties observed in standard CT simulation. Specifically, several studies highlight MAEs for soft tissue that are less than 40 HU [21, 28, 30, 72–75], demonstrating relatively accurate intensity mapping in this region. However, due to the indistinguishable contrast of bone or air on MR images, the MAE for these tissues tends to exceed 100 HU, indicating higher discrepancies. Misalignment between CT and MR images in patient datasets emerges as a common source of error. This misalignment, particularly on bone structures, not only contributes to intensity mapping errors during training but also results in an overestimation of error during evaluation. This is because the error from misalignment registers as synthetic error in the assessment metrics. Notably, two studies reported significantly higher MAE for the rectum (∼70 HU) compared to other soft tissues [28, 76]. This discrepancy may be attributed to mismatches in CT and MR imaging, potentially arising from variable filling of the rectum. Considering that the number of bone pixels is considerably fewer than those of soft tissue, the training process may tend to map pixels to the low HU region during the prediction stage. Potential solutions to address these challenges could include assigning higher loss weights on bone structures or incorporating bone-only images during the training process [21].

In multiple studies, learning-based methods consistently outperform conventional methods, showcasing superior accuracy in generating synthetic CTs [16, 29, 73, 76]. This highlights the advantage of adopting a data-driven approach over traditional model-based methods. For instance, synthetic CTs generated by atlas-based methods were observed to be more susceptible to noise and registration errors, resulting in significantly greater MAE compared to learning-based methods. Despite the advantages of learning-based methods, there are limitations to consider. The performance of these methods can be unpredictable when applied to datasets that significantly differ from the training sets. Such differences may stem from unusual or abnormal anatomy, or images with degraded quality due to severe artifacts and noise. In contrast, atlas-based methods generate a weighted average of templates derived from prior knowledge. This characteristic makes them less prone to failure in handling unexpected or unusual cases, contributing to their robustness in scenarios with significant variations in image quality [76].

The diverse datasets, training approaches, and testing strategies employed across these studies make the direct comparison of results challenging, precluding the determination of a single best methodology for all applications. However, some studies have conducted comparisons with competing methods using the same datasets, shedding light on relative advantages and limitations. For example, in a study involving fifteen brain cancer patients, a GAN-based method demonstrated better preservation of detail and closer similarity to real CT with less noise when compared to an autoencoder-based method [30]. The GAN-based synthetic CT exhibited higher accuracy at the bone–air interface and in determining fine structures, with approximately 10HU less error by MAE. Another study comparing U-Net and GAN with different loss functions on 39 patients with prostate cancer revealed quantitative results indicating that U-Net methods had significantly higher MAE than their GAN counterparts. Interestingly, the perceptual loss in both U-Net and GAN did not contribute to reducing MAE or provide benefits for dose calculation accuracy [28]. A comparison between CycleGAN and GAN-based methods on patients with brain and prostate cancer demonstrated a significant improvement in MAE with CycleGAN. CycleGAN also exhibited better visual results in terms of fine structural detail and contrast. Notably, CycleGAN results were less sensitive to local mismatches in the training CT/MR pairs, resulting in less blurry bone boundaries compared to GAN results [39]. Similar comparison results were reported in a study comparing CycleGAN and GAN on liver stereotactic body radiation therapy (SBRT) cases. While dosimetry comparison showed minimal difference, attributed to the insensitivity of volumetric modulated arc therapy (VMAT) plans to HU inaccuracy, CycleGAN exhibited improved MAE and visual results over GAN [40].

Among the reviewed studies, various MR sequences have been employed for synthetic CT generation, with the choice often dictated by their availability.

The optimal sequence yielding the best performance has not been conclusively determined. T1-weighted and T2-weighted sequences, being two of the most common general diagnostic MR sequences, are widely used due to their availability. These sequences enable models to be trained on relatively large datasets containing co-registered CT and T1- or T2-weighted MR images. T2-weighted images may be preferable to T1-weighted ones due to their intrinsically superior geometric accuracy within regions of significant anatomic variability, such as the nasal cavity, and reduced chemical shift artifacts at fat and tissue boundaries. However, both T1- and T2-weighted MR images lack contrast for air and bone, which can impede the extraction of features corresponding to these structures in learning-based methods.

The two-point Dixon sequence, capable of separating water and fat, has been utilized in commercial PET/MR applications for segmentation [77, 78]. However, its limitation lies in poor bone contrast, resulting in the misclassification of bone as fat. To enhance bone contrast and facilitate feature extraction in learning-based methods, ultrashort echo time (UTE) and/or zero echo time (ZTE) MR sequences have been employed recently to generate positive image contrast from bone [17]. While studies by Ladefoged et al and Blanc-Durand et al demonstrated the feasibility of UTE and ZTE MR sequences using U-Net in PET/MR attenuation correction, respectively [79, 80], a direct comparison with conventional MR sequences under the same deep learning network is lacking. Therefore, the advantage of these specialized sequences has not been conclusively validated. Moreover, compared with conventional T1- or T2-weighted MR images, UTE/ ZTE MR images may have limited diagnostic value for soft tissue and longer acquisition times. This may potentially reduce their clinical utility, particularly in poorly tolerated, long-duration exams such as whole-body PET/MR.

Several studies have explored the use of multiple MR images with varying contrasts as training inputs to enhance the overall predictive power and accuracy of synthetic CT generation. Qi et al proposed a four-channel input comprising T1, T2, contrast-enhanced T1, and contrast-enhanced T1 Dixon water images. The results from the four-channel input demonstrated lower mean absolute error (MAE) compared to results from fewer channels, highlighting the potential benefits of incorporating diverse contrast information [81]. Florkow et al investigated single- and multi-channel inputs using magnitude MR images and Dixon-reconstructed water and fat images obtained from a single T1 multi-echo gradient-echo acquisition [82]. Their findings indicated that multi-channel input can improve synthetic CT generation over single-channel input, with the Dixon sequence input outperforming other configurations. Tie et al employed T2 and pre- and post-contrast T1 MR images in a multi-channel, multi-path architecture, demonstrating additional improvement over multi-channel single-path and single-channel results [83]. Combining UTE or ZTE sequences with Dixon sequences, which provide contrast for bone against air and fat against soft tissue, respectively, has been considered an attractive combination [24, 84]. Leynes et al showed that synthetic CT using both ZTE and Dixon MR sequences has less error than using Dixon alone, showcasing the potential benefits of combining these contrast sources [24]. While the resulting improvement in image quality has been validated, the necessity of performing additional MR sequences for synthetic CT generation requires further study in specific applications to justify the associated costs and acquisition time.

In the reviewed studies, CT and MR images in the training datasets were acquired separately on different machines, necessitating image registration between the CT and MR images to create CT-MR pairs for training. The registration error is generally minimal at the level of the brain but may be more significant within the pelvis, owing to variable bladder and rectum filling, and in the abdomen, due to variations introduced by respiratory motion and peristalsis. Methods such as U-Net and GAN-based approaches can be susceptible to registration errors, particularly when utilizing a pixel-to-pixel loss function. These errors can be exacerbated by physiological motion, making accurate registration challenging. To address this issue, Kazemifar *et al* proposed a potential solution using mutual information as the loss function in the GAN generator. This approach aims to bypass the registration step during training, potentially mitigating the impact of registration errors on the performance of the model [85]. CycleGAN-based methods, developed for unpaired image-to-image translation, exhibit greater robustness to registration errors. This is attributed to the role of the cycle consistency loss, which enforces structural consistency between the original and cycle-generated images. For instance, in the context of synthetic CT generation from MR images, the cycle consistency loss ensures that a cycle MRI generated from synthetic CT remains similar to the original MRI. This characteristic makes CycleGAN-based methods more resilient to registration errors, contributing to their effectiveness in scenarios where accurate image registration is challenging [19, 33, 35, 86].

8.4.2 Dose calculation in MR-only radiation therapy

In studies with applications in radiation therapy, many have evaluated the dosimetric accuracy of synthetic CT by calculating the radiation treatment dose from the original treatment plan and comparing it against ground truth CT simulation imaging. It has been observed that the dose difference is approximately 1%, which is relatively small compared to typical total dose delivery uncertainties over an entire treatment course (5%). For reference, in the bulk-density assignment method, Lee *et al* observed that the differences between the dose of CRT plans on bulk-density, when compared to CT, were less than 2% [3]. Similarly, Jonsson *et al* reported a comparable result, noting that the maximum difference in monitor units (MU) required to reach the prescribed dose was 1.6% [4]. The improvement in dosimetric accuracy provided by deep learning-based methods in radiation therapy, when compared to image accuracy, is relatively small and may lack clinical relevance [73, 76]. One potential reason for this phenomenon is that dose calculation on photon plans tends to be forgiving to image inaccuracy, particularly within homogeneous regions such as the brain. In VMAT, the contribution to dosimetric error from random image inaccuracy also tends to cancel out within an arc. However, the small dosimetric improvement observed may be of significance in scenarios such as stereotactic radiosurgery (SRS) and stereotactic body radiation therapy (SBRT), where small volumes are treated to very high doses. In such cases, significant dosimetric errors may arise from otherwise negligible errors in CT synthesis, particularly in the region surrounding the target volume [95]. These findings underscore the importance of considering the clinical context and the specific treatment scenario when assessing the impact of synthetic CT accuracy on dosimetry in radiation therapy applications.

Studies have also assessed the use of synthetic CT in the context of proton therapy for various cancers, including prostate, liver, and brain cancer [41, 42, 90]. Proton beams, unlike photon beams, exhibit a sharp dose gradient (Bragg peak) at the distal end of the beam, allowing for highly conformal dose delivery to the target by superimposing proton beams from several angles. Any inaccuracies in HU along the beam path on the planning CT can lead to a shift in the highly conformal high-dose area. This shift may result in the tumor being substantially under-dosed or the organs at risk being over-dosed [96]. In studies such as the one by Liu *et al* most of the dose differences resulting from the use of synthetic CT were observed at the distal end of the proton beam [42]. Liu *et al* reported that the largest and mean absolute range differences were 0.56 and 0.19 cm among their 21 liver cancer patients, and 0.75 and 0.23 cm among 17 prostate cancer patients, respectively [41, 42]. These findings emphasize the critical importance of accurate synthetic CT generation in proton therapy, where precision in dose delivery is crucial due to the unique characteristics of proton beams.

In addition to dosimetric accuracy for treatment planning, the evaluation of synthetic CT imaging must also consider geometric fidelity for treatment set-up. However, studies specifically focusing on synthetic CT positioning accuracy are limited. Fu *et al* conducted patient alignment testing by rigidly aligning synthetic CT and real CT to the CBCT acquired during the delivery of the first fraction of a fractionated radiotherapy treatment course [21]. The average translation vector distance and absolute Euler angle difference between the two alignments were found to be less than 0.6 mm and 0.5°, respectively. Gupta *et al* performed a similar study and reported that the translation difference was less than 0.7 mm in one direction [74]. Although studies have addressed alignment with CBCT, the alignment between the digitally reconstructed radiograph (DRR) derived from the synthetic CT and on-board kilovolt (kV) imaging of the patient is also clinically important. However, no studies on DRR alignment accuracy were found in the reviewed literature. It is worth noting that the geometric accuracy of synthetic CT is influenced not only by the synthetic methods employed but also by the geometric distortion on MR images caused by magnetic field inhomogeneity, as well as subject-induced susceptibility and chemical shift. Therefore, methods to mitigate MR distortion are crucial for improving synthetic CT accuracy in patient positioning, contributing to the overall success of radiotherapy treatment set-up.

8.4.3 PET attenuation correction

In studies focused on PET attenuation correction, the evaluation has primarily centered around the bias introduced in PET quantification due to synthetic CT errors. While it is challenging to define a specific error tolerance that significantly impacts clinical decision-making, a general consensus is that quantitative errors of 10% or less typically do not have a substantial impact on decisions in diagnostic imaging [15]. A thresholding on MR images of UTE sequences resulted into an average error of 5% in brain PET images [12]. Kops and Herzog demonstrated that the segmentation-based and the registration-based methods proposed by them have similar performance in PET image reconstruction [14]. A thresholding on MR images of UTE sequences resulted in an average error of 5% in brain PET images [12]. Kops and Herzog demonstrated that the segmentation-based and the registration-based methods proposed by them have similar performance in PET image reconstruction [14]. Most of the proposed deep learning methods in the reviewed studies met this criterion based on the average relative bias reported. However, it is essential to note that due to variation among study subjects, the bias in some volumes-of-interest (VOIs) may exceed 10% for certain patients [24, 79]. This emphasizes the importance of considering both the mean and standard deviation of the bias when interpreting results, as proposed methods may exhibit poor local performance affecting specific patients. Reporting alternative results that list or plot all data points, or at least their range, could provide a more comprehensive understanding of the proposed methods' performance.

Bone accuracy on synthetic CT is crucial for PET attenuation correction since bone has the highest capacity for attenuation due to its high density and atomic number. Unlike applications in radiation therapy, the bias and geometric accuracy of bone on synthetic CT are more frequently evaluated for PET attenuation correction. Several studies have demonstrated that improved accuracy of bone representation in CT synthesis leads to more globally accurate PET [23, 79, 84, 94]. In the reviewed studies, PET attenuation correction by conventional CT synthesis methods exhibited an average bias of about 5% among selected VOIs. In contrast, learning-based methods reduced the bias to around 2%, highlighting the significant improvements achieved in PET accuracy with more accurate synthetic CT images generated by these methods [17, 18, 23, 24, 84].

8.4.4 Image registration

In addition to its applications in radiation treatment planning and PET attenuation correction, MR-based CT synthesis has demonstrated promise in facilitating inter-modality image registration. Direct registration between CT and MR images is challenging due to disparate image contrast, and this challenge is further amplified in deformable registration, where significant geometric distortion is allowed. McKenzie *et al* proposed a CycleGAN-based method to synthesize CT images, utilizing the synthetic CT to replace MR imaging in MR-CT registration in the head and neck [97]. By doing so, they transformed an inter-modality registration problem into an intra-modality one. As summarized in table 8.5, their findings revealed that, using the same deformable registration algorithm, the average landmark error decreased from 9.8 ± 3.1 mm in direct MR-CT registration to 6.0 ± 2.1 mm when using synthetic CT as a bridge. Similar positive results were reported in the inverse CT-MR registration task.

Table 8.5. Summary of study on MR-based synthetic CT for registration. (Adapted from [1]. CC BY 4.0.)

Author, year	Network	MR parameters	Site, and # of patients in training/testing	Key findings in registration accuracy
McKenzie *et al* [97]	CycleGAN	0.35 T	Head and neck: 25, 5-fold cross validation	Landmark error (mm): 6.0 ± 2.1 (MR-to-CT) 6.6 ± 2.0 (CT-to-MR)

8.5 Discussion and outlook

Recent years have seen a surge in the utilization of deep learning within the realm of medical imaging. Cutting-edge networks and techniques borrowed from computer vision have been adapted to cater to specific clinical tasks in radiology and radiation oncology. This chapter reviews the emerging and active field of CT synthesis, with most of the studies covered being published within the last three years. With ongoing advancements in both artificial intelligence and computing hardware, it is anticipated that more advanced learning-based methods will further enhance the clinical workflow with novel applications. While the reviewed literature showcases the success of deep learning-based image synthesis in various applications, there are still some open questions that need addressing in future studies.

The incorporation of novel network architectures, including transformers and diffusion models, holds great promise for advancing the field of CT synthesis. The transformer architecture, renowned for its success in natural language processing and image recognition, may offer enhanced capabilities in capturing long-range dependencies and contextual information within medical images. The attention mechanism in transformers enables the model to focus on relevant image regions, potentially improving the synthesis accuracy, particularly in complex anatomical structures. Similarly, the diffusion model, such as the DDPM, has emerged as a powerful tool for deep generative tasks. Its unique two-stage approach involving noise addition and subsequent denoising offers stability during training, making it less susceptible to issues such as mode collapse and hyperparameter sensitivity. As research in this area progresses, the application of diffusion models could contribute to more robust and accurate CT synthesis, addressing challenges faced by current deep learning-based methods.

The selection between 2D and 3D models for CT synthesis is a pivotal decision that hinges on the specific demands and constraints of the application. 2D models exhibit advantages in computational efficiency and training data availability, making them suitable for scenarios with limited resources and large datasets. However, challenges arise in their ability to capture 3D context and potential slice discontinuities. On the other hand, 3D models inherently provide spatial context and more homogeneous synthesis but demand greater computational resources and extensive training data. Fu *et al* compared the performance of 2D and 3D models using the same U-Net implementation, finding that 3D-generated synthetic CT exhibited smaller MAE and more accurate bone regions [21]. Hybrid approaches, combining 3D patches or multiple adjacent slices, offer a compromise [98]. The ongoing development of techniques that optimize both 2D and 3D models may provide a balanced solution, ensuring that the choice aligns with the unique requirements of medical imaging tasks, such as CT synthesis, where understanding volumetric relationships is critical for accurate clinical applications.

The reviewed studies underscore the superiority of learning-based methods over conventional approaches in terms of performance and clinical utility. Learning-based methods consistently surpass conventional ones by producing synthetic images that closely resemble real images and exhibit superior quantitative metrics. While the training process for learning-based methods demands hours to days, the application of a trained model to new patients enables the rapid generation of synthetic images within seconds to minutes. In contrast, conventional methods display a broad spectrum of run times due to diverse methodologies, with iterative approaches such as compressed sensing (CS) proving less favorable due to substantial time and computational resource requirements.

While learning-based methods have demonstrated clear advantages, it is crucial to acknowledge the potential unpredictability of their performance when dealing with input images during production that significantly differ from the training images. Many reviewed studies tend to exclude unusual cases, but the clinical reality may present scenarios that deviate from the norm. Instances such as hip prostheses, causing severe artifacts on both CT and MR images, could impact the application of learning-based methods, and understanding such effects is essential. Unusual cases, ranging from medical implants introducing artifacts to challenges posed by obesity and anatomic deformities, may arise in various imaging modalities, warranting further investigation to ensure the robustness and reliability of learning-based models in diverse clinical scenarios.

Before integrating learning-based models into the clinical workflow, addressing several challenges is paramount. To accommodate potentially unpredictable synthetic images arising from non-compliance with imaging protocols in the training data or unexpected anatomic variations, the implementation of additional quality assurance (QA) steps becomes essential in clinical practice. QA procedures would be designed to routinely assess or verify the consistency of model performance, either through periodic checks or after upgrades, involving re-training the network with additional patient datasets. This approach ensures the reliability of synthetic image quality across a range of cases in diverse clinical scenarios.

8.6 Summary

In recent years, the increasing integration of deep learning into medical imaging has been notable. Borrowing from computer vision, advanced techniques of AI are now being tailored for clinical use in radiology and radiation oncology. Adaptive radiation therapy is an emerging concept that involves complex imaging operations. AI with its superior ability in image style transferring can facilitate the adaptive radiation therapy workflow by synthesizing CT images from CBCT or/and MRI images for dose calculation, image segmentation, registration and PET attenuation correction. While feasibility has been demonstrated in recent studies, addressing challenges remains pivotal prior to clinical implementation.

References

[1] Wang T, Lei Y, Fu Y, Wynne J F, Curran W J, Liu T and Yang X 2020 A review on medical imaging synthesis using deep learning and its clinical applications *J. Appl. Clin. Med. Phys.* **22** 11–36

[2] Yang X, Lei Y, Shu H-K, Rossi P, Mao H, Shim H, Curran W J and Liu T 2017 Pseudo CT estimation from MRI using patch-based random forest *Proc. SPIE* **10133** 101332Q

[3] Lee Y K, Bollet M, Charles-Edwards G, Flower M A, Leach M O, McNair H, Moore E, Rowbottom C and Webb S 2003 Radiotherapy treatment planning of prostate cancer using magnetic resonance imaging alone *Radiother. Oncol.* **66** 203–16

[4] Jonsson J H, Karlsson M G, Karlsson M and Nyholm T 2010 Treatment planning using MRI data: an analysis of the dose calculation accuracy for different treatment regions *Radiat. Oncol.* **5** 62

[5] Lambert J *et al* 2011 MRI-guided prostate radiation therapy planning: Investigation of dosimetric accuracy of MRI-based dose planning *Radiother. Oncol.* **98** 330–4

[6] Kristensen B H, Laursen F J, Løgager V, Geertsen P F and Krarup-Hansen A 2008 Dosimetric and geometric evaluation of an open low-field magnetic resonance simulator for radiotherapy treatment planning of brain tumours *Radiother. Oncol.* **87** 100–9

[7] Johansson A, Karlsson M and Nyholm T 2011 CT substitute derived from MRI sequences with ultrashort echo time *Med. Phys.* **38** 2708–14

[8] Hsu S-H, Cao Y, Huang K, Feng M and Balter J M 2013 Investigation of a method for generating synthetic CT models from MRI scans of the head and neck for radiation therapy *Phys. Med. Biol.* **58** 8419

[9] Dowling J A, Lambert J, Parker J, Salvado O, Fripp J, Capp A, Wratten C, Denham J W and Greer P B 2012 An atlas-based electron density mapping method for magnetic resonance imaging (MRI)-alone treatment planning and adaptive MRI-based prostate radiation therapy *Int. J. Radiat. Oncol. Biol. Phys.* **83** e5–e11

[10] Uh J, Merchant T E, Li Y, Li X and Hua C 2014 MRI-based treatment planning with pseudo CT generated through atlas registration *Med. Phys.* **41** 051711

[11] Sjölund J, Forsberg D, Andersson M and Knutsson H 2015 Generating patient specific pseudo-CT of the head from MR using atlas-based regression *Phys. Med. Biol.* **60** 825

[12] Keereman V, Fierens Y, Broux T, De Deene Y, Lonneux M and Vandenberghe S 2010 MRI-based attenuation correction for PET/MRI using ultrashort echo time sequences *J. Nucl. Med.* **51** 812–8

[13] Catana C, van der Kouwe A, Benner T, Michel C J, Hamm M, Fenchel M, Fischl B, Rosen B, Schmand M and Sorensen A G 2010 Toward implementing an MRI-based PET attenuation-correction method for neurologic studies on the MR-PET brain prototype *J. Nucl. Med.* **51** 1431–8

[14] Kops E R and Herzog H 2007 Alternative methods for attenuation correction for PET images in MR-PET scanners *2007 IEEE Nuclear Science Symp. Conf. Record* (Piscataway, NJ: IEEE) pp 4327–30

[15] Hofmann M, Steinke F, Scheel V, Charpiat G, Farquhar J, Aschoff P, Brady M, Scholkopf B and Pichler B J 2008 MRI-based attenuation correction for PET/MRI: a novel approach combining pattern recognition and atlas registration *J. Nucl. Med.* **49** 1875–83

[16] Han X 2017 MR-based synthetic CT generation using a deep convolutional neural network method *Med. Phys.* **44** 1408–19

[17] Liu F, Jang H, Kijowski R, Bradshaw T and McMillan A B 2018 Deep learning MR imaging-based attenuation correction for PET/MR imaging *Radiology* **286** 676–84

[18] Jang H, Liu F, Zhao G, Bradshaw T and McMillan A B 2018 Technical note: deep learning based MRAC using rapid ultrashort echo time imaging *Med. Phys.* **45** 3697–704

[19] Dong X, Wang T, Lei Y, Higgins K, Liu T, Curran W J, Mao H, Nye J A and Yang X 2019 Synthetic CT generation from non-attenuation corrected PET images for whole-body PET imaging *Phys. Med. Biol.* **64** 215016

[20] Hwang D, Kim K Y, Kang S K, Seo S, Paeng J C, Lee D S and Lee J S 2018 Improving the accuracy of simultaneously reconstructed activity and attenuation maps using deep learning *J. Nucl. Med.* **59** 1624–9

[21] Fu J, Yang Y, Singhrao K, Ruan D, Chu F I, Low D A and Lewis J H 2019 Deep learning approaches using 2D and 3D convolutional neural networks for generating male pelvic synthetic computed tomography from magnetic resonance imaging *Med. Phys.* **46** 3788–98

[22] Neppl S *et al* 2019 Evaluation of proton and photon dose distributions recalculated on 2D and 3D Unet-generated pseudoCTs from T1-weighted MR head scans *Acta Oncol.* **58** 1429–34

[23] Torrado-Carvajal A, Vera-Olmos J, Izquierdo-Garcia D, Catalano O A, Morales M A, Margolin J, Soricelli A, Salvatore M, Malpica N and Catana C 2019 Dixon-VIBE deep learning (DIVIDE) pseudo-CT synthesis for pelvis PET/MR attenuation correction *J. Nucl. Med.* **60** 429–35

[24] Leynes A P, Yang J, Wiesinger F, Kaushik S S, Shanbhag D D, Seo Y, Hope T A and Larson P E Z 2018 Zero-echo-time and Dixon deep pseudo-CT (ZeDD CT): direct generation of pseudo-CT images for pelvic PET/MRI attenuation correction using dep convolutional neural networks with multiparametric MRI *J. Nucl. Med.* **59** 852–8

[25] Chen L, Liang X, Shen C, Jiang S and Wang J 2019 Synthetic CT generation from CBCT images via deep learning *Med. Phys.* **47** 1115–25

[26] Son S J, Park B Y, Byeon K and Park H 2019 Synthesizing diffusion tensor imaging from functional MRI using fully convolutional networks *Comput. Biol. Med.* **115** 103528

[27] Spuhler K D, Gardus J 3rd, Gao Y, DeLorenzo C, Parsey R and Huang C 2019 Synthesis of patient-specific transmission data for PET attenuation correction for PET/MRI neuro-imaging using a convolutional neural network *J. Nucl. Med.* **60** 555–60

[28] Largent A *et al* 2019 Comparison of deep learning-based and patch-based methods for pseudo-CT generation in MRI-based prostate dose planning *Int. J. Radiat. Oncol. Biol. Phys.* **105** 1137–50

[29] Nie D, Trullo R, Lian J, Wang L, Petitjean C, Ruan S, Wang Q and Shen D 2018 Medical image synthesis with deep convolutional adversarial networks *IEEE Trans.Biomed. Eng.* **65** 2720–30

[30] Emami H, Dong M, Nejad-Davarani S P and Glide-Hurst C K 2018 Generating synthetic CTs from magnetic resonance images using generative adversarial networks *Med. Phys.* **47** 3627–36

[31] Isola P, Zhu J-Y, Zhou T and Efros A A 2016 Image-to-image translation with conditional adversarial networks arXiv:1611.07004

[32] Liang X, Chen L, Nguyen D, Zhou Z, Gu X, Yang M, Wang J and Jiang S 2019 Generating synthesized computed tomography (CT) from cone-beam computed tomography (CBCT) using CycleGAN for adaptive radiation therapy *Phys. Med. Biol.* **64** 125002

[33] Harms J, Lei Y, Wang T, Zhang R, Zhou J, Tang X, Curran W J, Liu T and Yang X 2019 Paired cycle-GAN-based image correction for quantitative cone-beam computed tomography *Med. Phys.* **46** 3998–4009

[34] Dong X, Lei Y, Wang T, Higgins K, Liu T, Curran W J, Mao H, Nye J A and Yang X 2019 Deep learning-based attenuation correction in the absence of structural information for whole-body PET imaging *Phys. Med. Biol.* **65** 055011

[35] Lei Y, Dong X, Wang T, Higgins K, Liu T, Curran W J, Mao H, Nye J A and Yang X 2019 Whole-body PET estimation from low count statistics using cycle-consistent generative adversarial networks *Phys. Med. Biol.* **64** 215017

[36] Wang T, Lei Y, Tian Z, Dong X, Liu Y, Jiang X, Curran W J, Liu T, Shu H K and Yang X 2019 Deep learning-based image quality improvement for low-dose computed tomography simulation in radiation therapy *J. Med. Imaging* **6** 043504

[37] Liu Y, Lei Y, Wang T, Fu Y, Tang X, Curran W J, Liu T, Patel P and Yang X 2020 CBCT-based synthetic CT generation using deep-attention cycleGAN for pancreatic adaptive radiotherapy *Med. Phys.* **47** 2472–83

[38] Dong X, Lei Y, Tian S, Wang T, Patel P, Curran W J, Jani A B, Liu T and Yang X 2019 Synthetic MRI-aided multi-organ segmentation on male pelvic CT using cycle consistent deep attention network *Radiother. Oncol.* **141** 192–9

[39] Lei Y, Harms J, Wang T, Liu Y, Shu H K, Jani A B, Curran W J, Mao H, Liu T and Yang X 2019 MRI-only based synthetic CT generation using dense cycle consistent generative adversarial networks *Med. Phys.* **46** 3565–81

[40] Liu Y, Lei Y, Wang T, Kayode O, Tian S, Liu T, Patel P, Curran W J, Ren L and Yang X 2019 MRI-based treatment planning for liver stereotactic body radiotherapy: validation of a deep learning-based synthetic CT generation method *Br. J. Radiol.* **92** 20190067

[41] Liu Y *et al* 2019 Evaluation of a deep learning-based pelvic synthetic CT generation technique for MRI-based prostate proton treatment planning *Phys. Med. Biol.* **64** 205022

[42] Liu Y *et al* 2019 MRI-based treatment planning for proton radiotherapy: dosimetric validation of a deep learning-based liver synthetic CT generation method *Phys. Med. Biol.* **64** 145015

[43] Kim K H, Do W J and Park S H 2018 Improving resolution of MR images with an adversarial network incorporating images with different contrast *Med. Phys.* **45** 3120–31

[44] Olberg S *et al* 2019 Synthetic CT reconstruction using a deep spatial pyramid convolutional framework for MR-only breast radiotherapy *Med. Phys.* **46** 4135–47

[45] Yang Q, Yan P, Zhang Y, Yu H, Shi Y, Mou X, Kalra M K, Zhang Y, Sun L and Wang G 2018 Low-dose CT image denoising using a generative adversarial network with wasserstein distance and perceptual loss *IEEE Trans. Med. Imaging* **37** 1348–57

[46] Ouyang J, Chen K T, Gong E, Pauly J and Zaharchuk G 2019 Ultra-low-dose PET reconstruction using generative adversarial network with feature matching and task-specific perceptual loss *Med. Phys.* **46** 3555–64

[47] Müller-Franzes G *et al* 2023 A multimodal comparison of latent denoising diffusion probabilistic models and generative adversarial networks for medical image synthesis *Sci. Rep.* **13** 12098

[48] Lyu Q and Wang G 2022 Conversion between CT and MRI images using diffusion and score-matching models arXiv:2209.12104

[49] Pan S *et al* 2023 Synthetic CT generation from MRI using 3D transformer-based denoising diffusion model arXiv:2305.19467

[50] Fu L, Li X, Cai X, Miao D, Yao Y and Shen Y 2023 Energy-guided diffusion model for CBCT-to-CT synthesis arXiv:2308.03354

[51] Peng J *et al* 2023 CBCT-based synthetic CT image generation using conditional denoising diffusion probabilistic model arXiv:2303.02649

[52] Kida S, Nakamoto T, Nakano M, Nawa K, Haga A, Kotoku J, Yamashita H and Nakagawa K 2018 Cone beam computed tomography image quality improvement using a deep convolutional neural network *Cureus* **10** e2548

[53] Xie S, Yang C, Zhang Z and Li H 2018 Scatter artifacts removal using learning-based method for CBCT in IGRT system *IEEE Access* **6** 78031–7

[54] Nomura Y, Xu Q, Shirato H, Shimizu S and Xing L 2019 Projection-domain scatter correction for cone beam computed tomography using a residual convolutional neural network *Med. Phys.* **46** 3142–55

[55] Yuan N, Dyer B, Rao S, Chen Q, Benedict S, Shang L, Kang Y, Qi J and Rong Y 2020 Convolutional neural network enhancement of fast-scan low-dose cone-beam CT images for head and neck radiotherapy *Phys. Med. Biol.* **65** 035003

[56] Kida S, Kaji S, Nawa K, Imae T, Nakamoto T, Ozaki S, Ohta T, Nozawa Y and Nakagawa K 2020 Visual enhancement of cone-beam CT by use of CycleGAN *Med. Phys.* **47** 998–1010

[57] Kurz C, Maspero M, Savenije M H F, Landry G, Kamp F, Pinto M, Li M, Parodi K, Belka C and van den Berg C A T 2019 CBCT correction using a cycle-consistent generative adversarial network and unpaired training to enable photon and proton dose calculation *Phys. Med. Biol.* **64** 225004

[58] Hansen D C, Landry G, Kamp F, Li M, Belka C, Parodi K and Kurz C 2018 ScatterNet: a convolutional neural network for cone-beam CT intensity correction *Med. Phys.* **45** 4916–26

[59] Landry G, Hansen D, Kamp F, Li M, Hoyle B, Weller J, Parodi K, Belka C and Kurz C 2019 Comparing Unet training with three different datasets to correct CBCT images for prostate radiotherapy dose calculations *Phys. Med. Biol.* **64** 035011

[60] Li Y, Zhu J, Liu Z, Teng J, Xie Q, Zhang L, Liu X, Shi J and Chen L 2019 A preliminary study of using a deep convolution neural network to generate synthesized CT images based on CBCT for adaptive radiotherapy of nasopharyngeal carcinoma *Phys. Med. Biol.* **64** 145010

[61] Adrian T, Paolo Z, Arturs M, Gabriel G M, Joao S, Roel J H M S, Johannes A L, Stefan B, Maria Francesca S and Antje-Christin K 2020 Comparison of CBCT based synthetic CT methods suitable for proton dose calculations in adaptive proton therapy *Phys. Med. Biol.* **65** 095002

[62] Dai X, Lei Y, Wynne J, Janopaul-Naylor J, Wang T, Roper J, Curran W J, Liu T, Patel P and Yang X 2021 Synthetic CT-aided multiorgan segmentation for CBCT-guided adaptive pancreatic radiotherapy *Med. Phys.* **48** 7063–73

[63] Khoo V S and Joon D L 2006 New developments in MRI for target volume delineation in radiotherapy *Br. J. Radiol.* **79** S2–15

[64] Nyholm T, Nyberg M, Karlsson M G and Karlsson M 2009 Systematisation of spatial uncertainties for comparison between a MR and a CT-based radiotherapy workflow for prostate treatments *Radiat. Oncol.* **4** 54

[65] Ulin K, Urie M M and Cherlow J M 2010 Results of a multi-institutional benchmark test for cranial CT/MR image registration *Int. J. Radiat. Oncol. Biol. Phys.* **77** 1584–9

[66] van der Heide U A, Houweling A C, Groenendaal G, Beets-Tan R G and Lambin P 2012 Functional MRI for radiotherapy dose painting *Magn. Reson. Imaging* **30** 1216–23

[67] Devic S 2012 MRI simulation for radiotherapy treatment planning *Med. Phys.* **39** 6701–11

[68] Lagendijk J J W, Raaymakers B W, Raaijmakers A J E, Overweg J, Brown K J, Kerkhof E M, van der Put R W, Hårdemark B, van Vulpen M and van der Heide U A 2008 MRI/linac integration *Radiother. Oncol.* **86** 25–9

[69] Fallone B G, Murray B, Rathee S, Stanescu T, Steciw S, Vidakovic S, Blosser E and Tymofichuk D 2009 First MR images obtained during megavoltage photon irradiation from a prototype integrated linac-MR system *Med. Phys.* **36** 2084–8

[70] Kinahan P E, Townsend D W, Beyer T and Sashin D 1998 Attenuation correction for a combined 3D PET/CT scanner *Med. Phys.* **25** 2046–53

[71] Burger C, Goerres G, Schoenes S, Buck A, Lonn A H and Von Schulthess G K 2002 PET attenuation coefficients from CT images: experimental evaluation of the transformation of CT into PET 511-keV attenuation coefficients *Eur. J. Nucl. Med. Mol. Imaging* **29** 922–7

[72] Dinkla A M *et al* 2019 Dosimetric evaluation of synthetic CT for head and neck radiotherapy generated by a patch-based three-dimensional convolutional neural network *Med. Phys.* **46** 4095–104

[73] Chen S, Qin A, Zhou D and Yan D 2018 Technical note: U-Net-generated synthetic CT images for magnetic resonance imaging-only prostate intensity-modulated radiation therapy treatment planning *Med. Phys.* **45** 5659–65

[74] Gupta D, Kim M, Vineberg K A and Balter J M 2019 Generation of synthetic CT images from MRI for treatmentplanning and patient positioning using a 3-channel U-Net trained on sagittal images *Front. Oncol.* **9** 964

[75] Dinkla A M, Wolterink J M, Maspero M, Savenije M H F, Verhoeff J J C, Seravalli E, Išgum I, Seevinck P R and van den Berg C A T 2018 MR-only brain radiation therapy: dosimetric evaluation of synthetic CTs generated by a dilated convolutional neural network *Int. J. Radiat. Oncol. Biol. Phys.* **102** 801–12

[76] Arabi H, Dowling J A, Burgos N, Han X, Greer P B, Koutsouvelis N and Zaidi H 2018 Comparative study of algorithms for synthetic CT generation from MRI: consequences for MRI-guided radiation planning in the pelvic region *Med. Phys.* **45** 5218–33

[77] Freitag M T *et al* 2017 Improved clinical workflow for simultaneous whole-body PET/MRI using high-resolution CAIPIRINHA-accelerated MR-based attenuation correction *Eur. Radiol.* **96** 12–20

[78] Izquierdo-Garcia D, Hansen A E, Förster S, Benoit D, Schachoff S, Fürst S, Chen K T, Chonde D B and Catana C 2014 An SPM8-based approach for attenuation correction combining segmentation and nonrigid template formation: application to simultaneous PET/MR brain imaging *J. Nucl. Med.* **55** 1825–30

[79] Blanc-Durand P, Khalife M, Sgard B, Kaushik S, Soret M, Tiss A, El Fakhri G, Habert M-O, Wiesinger F and Kas A 2019 Attenuation correction using 3D deep convolutional neural network for brain 18F-FDG PET/MR: comparison with Atlas, ZTE and CT based attenuation correction *PLoS One* **14** e0223141

[80] Ladefoged C N, Marner L, Hindsholm A, Law I, Hojgaard L and Andersen F L 2018 Deep learning based attenuation correction of PET/MRI in pediatric brain tumor patients: evaluation in a clinical setting *Front. Neurosci.* **12** 1005

[81] Qi M *et al* 2020 Multi-sequence MR image-based synthetic CT generation using a generative adversarial network for head and neck MRI-only radiotherapy *Med. Phys.* **47** 1880–94

[82] Florkow M C *et al* 2020 Deep learning-based MR-to-CT synthesis: The influence of varying gradient echo-based MR images as input channels *Magn. Reson. Med.* **83** 1429–41

[83] Tie X, Lam S K, Zhang Y, Lee K H, Au K H and Cai J 2020 Pseudo-CT generation from multi-parametric MRI using a novel multi-channel multi-path conditional generative adversarial network for nasopharyngeal carcinoma patients *Med. Phys.* **47** 1750–62

[84] Gong K, Yang J, Kim K, El Fakhri G, Seo Y and Li Q 2018 Attenuation correction for brain PET imaging using deep neural network based on Dixon and ZTE MR images *Phys. Med. Biol.* **63** 125011

[85] Kazemifar S, McGuire S, Timmerman R, Wardak Z, Nguyen D, Park Y, Jiang S and Owrangi A 2019 MRI-only brain radiotherapy: assessing the dosimetric accuracy of synthetic CT images generated using a deep learning approach *Radiother. Oncol.* **136** 56–63

[86] Lei Y, Harms J, Wang T, Liu Y, Shu H K, Jani A B, Curran W J, Mao H, Liu T and Yang X 2019 MRI-only based synthetic CT generation using dense cycle consistent generative adversarial networks *Med. Phys.* **46** 3565–81

[87] Xiang L, Wang Q, Nie D, Zhang L, Jin X, Qiao Y and Shen D 2018 Deep embedding convolutional neural network for synthesizing CT image from T1-weighted MR image *Med. Image Anal.* **47** 31–44

[88] Maspero M, Savenije M H F, Dinkla A M, Seevinck P R, Intven M P W, Jurgenliemk-Schulz I M, Kerkmeijer L G W and van den Berg C A T 2018 Dose evaluation of fast synthetic-CT generation using a generative adversarial network for general pelvis MR-only radiotherapy *Phys. Med. Biol.* **63** 185001

[89] Liu F, Yadav P, Baschnagel A M and McMillan A B 2019 MR-based treatment planning in radiation therapy using a deep learning approach *J. Appl. Clin. Med. Phys.* **20** 105–14

[90] Shafai-Erfani G *et al* 2019 MRI-based proton treatment planning for base of skull tumors *Int. J. Part. Ther.* **6** 12–25

[91] Wang Y, Liu C, Zhang X and Deng W 2019 Synthetic CT generation based on T2 weighted MRI of nasopharyngeal carcinoma (NPC) using a deep convolutional neural network (DCNN) *Front. Oncol.* **9** 1333

[92] Koike Y, Akino Y, Sumida I, Shiomi H, Mizuno H, Yagi M, Isohashi F, Seo Y, Suzuki O and Ogawa K 2020 Feasibility of synthetic computed tomography generated with an adversarial network for multi-sequence magnetic resonance-based brain radiotherapy *J. Radiat. Res.* **61** 92–103

[93] Brou Boni K N D, Klein J, Vanquin L, Wagner A, Lacornerie T, Pasquier D and Reynaert N 2020 MR to CT synthesis with multicenter data in the pelvic area using a conditional generative adversarial network *Phys. Med. Biol.* **65** 075002

[94] Arabi H, Zeng G, Zheng G and Zaidi H 2019 Novel adversarial semantic structure deep learning for MRI-guided attenuation correction in brain PET/MRI *Eur. J. Nucl. Med. Mol. Imaging* **46** 2746–59

[95] Wang T, Manohar N, Lei Y, Dhabaan A, Shu H-K, Liu T, Curran W J and Yang X 2019 MRI-based treatment planning for brain stereotactic radiosurgery: dosimetric validation of a learning-based pseudo-CT generation method *Med. Dosim.* **44** 199–204

[96] Li B, Lee H C, Duan X, Shen C, Zhou L, Jia X and Yang M 2017 Comprehensive analysis of proton range uncertainties related to stopping-power-ratio estimation using dual-energy CT imaging *Phys. Med. Biol.* **62** 7056–74

[97] McKenzie E M, Santhanam A, Ruan D, O'Connor D, Cao M and Sheng K 2019 Multimodality image registration in the head-and-neck using a deep learning-derived synthetic CT as a bridge *Med. Phys.* **47** 1094–104

[98] Schilling K G *et al* 2019 Synthesized b0 for diffusion distortion correction (Synb0-DisCo) *Magn. Reson. Imaging* **64** 62–70

Chapter 9

Artificial intelligence-based image registration and segmentation

Brian M Anderson and Kristy K Brock

This chapter delves into the integration of artificial intelligence (AI) into adaptive radiation therapy (ART), emphasizing AI-based image registration and segmentation. It begins by introducing ART's three categories—offline, online, and real-time—and the challenges they pose, such as accurately adapting treatment plans to patient-specific changes. The chapter then explains fundamental AI concepts, including machine learning and deep learning, highlighting components such as convolutional neural networks and activation functions. It explores how these AI techniques enhance image registration and segmentation, which are crucial for precise targeting and dose calculation in ART. By addressing both the potential benefits and challenges of AI in this context, the chapter provides insights into how AI can optimize ART workflows and improve personalized patient care.

9.1 AI-based image registration and segmentation for ART

9.1.1 Adaptive radiation therapy

Historically in radiation therapy, a single radiation treatment plan is generated for an individual patient, which will be used for the duration of care [1]. Adaptive radiation therapy (ART) is a broad umbrella which encompasses any changes from this single radiation treatment plan regiment, based on changes present in the patient. These changes in the patient can be inter-fractional (reduction/increase in tumor burden, inflammation, changes in bowel location/filling, bladder filling, etc) or intra-fractional (respiratory motion, cardiac motion, peristalsis, skeletal motion).

ART can be categorized into three groups: offline ART, online ART, and real-time ART. All these approaches have the potential to dose escalate and/or reduce normal tissue dose [2–4]. However, they also raise a number of challenges and difficulties which might require accurate segmentation of target and tissues at risk (segmentation), recalculation of dose and summation of previously delivered

doi:10.1088/978-0-7503-6119-4ch9

treatments (via deformable registration) re-planning based on patient geometry, and quality assurance ensuring safe adaptation of a plan.

9.1.1.1 Offline ART

Offline ART is commonly performed as part of routine clinical practice in many radiation oncology clinics. This involves the evaluation of imaging (daily or weekly) acquired throughout a patient's treatment for changes in normal tissue and tumor volumes. Patients with bulky disease that is expected to diminish throughout treatment can often be scheduled proactively for mid-treatment simulation scans, e.g. evaluation at fraction 15, or on an ad hoc basis driven by assessments at time of treatment: such as increased difficulty with patient setup. There are several examples of success in dose escalation/normal tissue sparing seen by multiple clinics using offline ART [5–8].

9.1.1.2 Online ART

Online ART is focused on adapting a treatment plan based on inter-fractional changes *while the patient is on the table/in the treatment position*. There are several successful examples with active online ART programs for multiple treatment sites [9–17]. This has the added difficulty of a compressed time frame for many of the steps listed above.

When adapting and recalculating a new treatment plan, a major consideration is the ability to accurately calculate dose on the image acquired in-room during treatment. The Varian Ethos (Varian Medical Systems, Palo Alto, CA) system focuses on CBCT-guided adaptive radiation therapy [18]. The Elekta Unity (Elekta Stockholm, Sweden) 1.5 T MR linac system and the ViewRay MRIdian 0.35 T MR linac system focuses on using an integrated MR linac to visualize changes occurring throughout the treatment process and can be used for both online [19] and real-time ART [20].

9.1.1.3 Real-time ART

Real-time ART aims to account for intra-fractional changes occurring during the patient treatment and enable automatic adjustments to optimize delivery/treat the target. This is not limited to the definition of a complete re-planning for the patient, but can include respiratory gating [21], MLC target tracking via KV monitoring [22] and implanted fiducials [23] (CyberKnife system), MR imaging [24] (with both Elekta Unity and ViewRay MRIdian), and external surface tracking.

9.1.1.4 Challenges

As stated previously, ART requires a concert of moving parts to either acquire a new planning image or adapt the daily image for dose accumulation, segmentation of targets and normal tissues for dose evaluation, accumulation of previously delivered radiation on the new image, perform re-planning, and quality assurance. To expedite these time restricted steps, AI is often leveraged to register, deform, and propagate not only previously defined contours, but also accumulate previously delivered dose. In the following sections we will discuss AI in registration (rigid and deformable), image segmentation, and discuss how these solutions can help alleviate some of these challenges, while creating some new ones as well.

9.2 Artificial intelligence

What defines artificial intelligence (AI)? While the phrase AI can sometimes feel like a creation of the twenty-first century, it is something which has been a part of the user experience with computers for quite some time. AI can be defined as anything which enables computers to mimic human behavior. This behavior can be something as simple as identifying a spam email, or as complex as diagnosing a patient's disease. A more extensive explanation of both machine learning and deep learning is beyond the immediate scope of the information presented later in this chapter. For a mathematical explanation of deep learning, particularly as it applies to deep learning in Python, we highly recommend the books *Deep Learning* by Ian Goodfellow *et al* [25] and *Deep Learning with Python* [26].

9.2.1 What is machine learning?

Within the broad scope of AI there exists a smaller distinction known as machine learning. Machine learning can be defined as an AI model which is generated from a loss-minimization or separation. A model 'loss' function can be imaged as a measure of how incorrect the model is; hence, we often express the desire to 'minimize loss'. For example, imagine a model is created to separate Honeycrisp apples (a reddish-yellow sweet apple) from Granny Smith apples (a green, sour apple). The user could create a variety of features (size, taste, color) that they feel can be quantified between the two apples. A machine learning model would then try to use these features to separate the apples into two groups. A very basic idea of this is shown on the left in figure 9.1, where the features are used directly to make an output prediction.

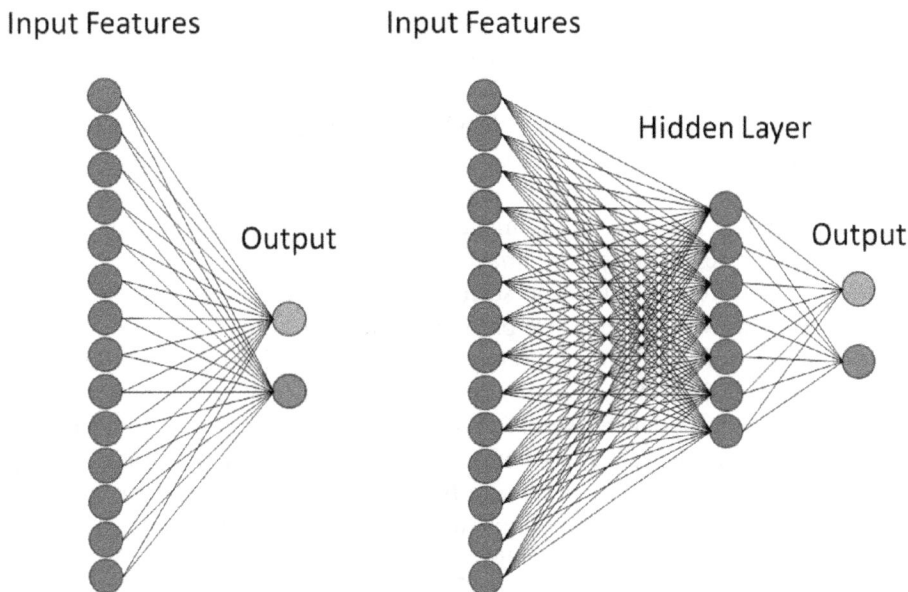

Figure 9.1. (Left) Basic level of a machine learning model: combining input features to an output. (Right) Basic level of a 'shallow' learning model: combining features with some number of hidden layers into an output.

9.2.2 What is deep learning?

Deep learning can be defined as a subset within machine learning. Whereas machine learning combines several features directly into an output, 'deep' learning is often associated as having several intermediary or 'hidden' layers. A single hidden layer, as shown in figure 9.1, would most appropriately be referred to as a 'shallow' network, with 'deep' requiring two or more hidden layers. The benefit of multiple hidden layers is the ability to represent predictions beyond simple linear regression when non-linear activation functions are used (activation functions are spoken of more in the following sections). The downside to the increase in the prediction capabilities of the model is the decrease in interpretability of the model predictions. Deep learning is often cited as being a 'black box', although this does not mean it is impossible to crack open the box and take a peek inside now and again.

9.3 Deep learning: the basic components

While deep learning has evolved considerably over the past decades, most models can be broken down into a combination of several key components. Having a solid understanding of each part will help one understand better how more complex models are generated in the future.

9.3.1 Convolutional neural networks: looking at the picture

Convolutional layers form the bedrock of deep learning image classification, segmentation, and registration models. The basis of these three tasks all relies on the same thing: the computer needs to understand what is occurring within an image. Humans, as well as most animals, have the benefit of eyes which enable us to capture a large amount of information within our field of view. For a computer this can be a relatively daunting task.

The first thing which needs to be defined is the computer's receptive field of view. A convolution is very simply the creation of a new matrix by multiplication and resultant addition of elements on an image. A visual representation of this concept is shown in figure 9.2. Here, the input image is convolved with a simple three-by-three kernel to create a resultant feature image.

If the kernel were a vertical line surrounded by zeros, the output feature map would show where vertical lines are present in the image.

One of the downsides of convolutions is that they are locally dependent. This means that since a kernel size is fixed, images of varying zoom or scale might not properly align with a previously defined kernel. A natural question which arises from this, is why not push towards large kernels which are able to cover large portions of the input image? There are two main concerns with this approach: (i) the larger the kernel, the more computational resources are required to perform the convolution and addition and (ii) larger kernels have more variables present, where an n by m matrix will have $n \times m + 1$ variables. A three-by-three kernel has nine variables (plus a bias to make ten total), while a nine-by-nine kernel has 81 variables (plus a bias to make 82).

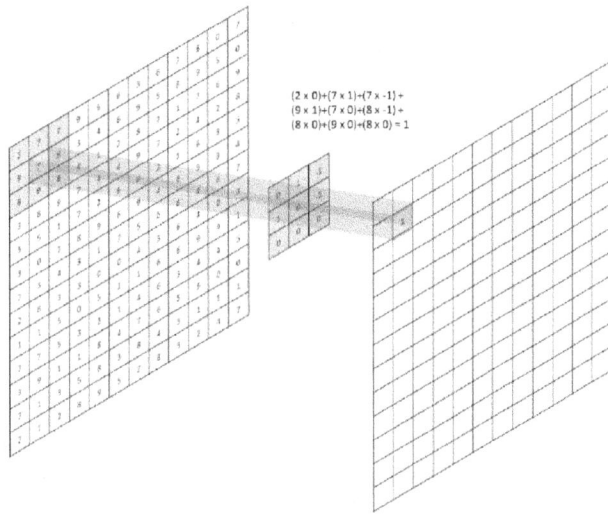

$$(2 \times 0) + (7 \times 1) + (7 \times -1) +$$
$$(9 \times 1) + (7 \times 0) + (8 \times -1) +$$
$$(8 \times 0) + (9 \times 0) + (8 \times 0) = 1$$

Figure 9.2. General representation of a convolution. The input image (left) convolved with the 3×3 kernel (middle) creates a feature map (right).

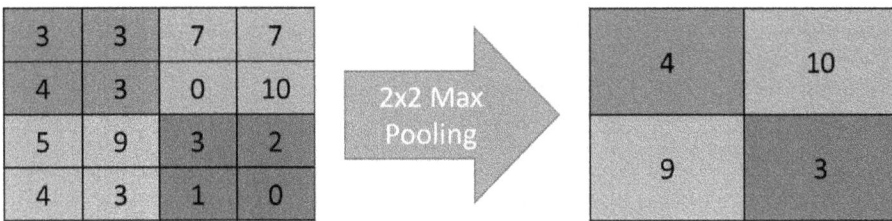

Figure 9.3. Example of a two-by-two max-pooling layer.

This modest increase in kernel size creates significantly more variables to train. A remedy to this local dependency issue comes in the form of pooling layers.

9.3.2 Pooling layers: keeping what matters most

Pooling layers are a way of taking only the most important aspect of a generated feature map. While they come in a variety of forms, a very commonly used pooling layer is max-pooling. Pooling layers are like convolutional layers in that they are a matrix, typically of size two-by-two for two-dimensional images, but rather than multiplying and adding, a max-pooling layer will simply take the maximum value within the defined matrix size, figure 9.3.

One of the most immediate implications of this is that the feature map itself has now decreased in size by a factor of 2 in each direction. This can either be seen as beneficial or detrimental, depending on the desired output. From a positive perspective, max-pooling layers have multiple benefits. The first of these benefits is that the most intense, or important, feature is maintained, while presumably less important features are removed. Second, subsequent convolutions on the post-max-pooled image require significantly less memory—as stated before, the feature map has been reduced in size. A 2 × 2 max-pooled image will be 1/4 the original image size, meaning less memory is required for the convolutional operation. Third, subsequent convolutions now cover a relative area that is larger than the original image size. A three-by-three kernel on an image with resolution of 1 mm × 1 mm per voxel would have a receptive field size of 3 mm by 3 mm. After max-pooling, the resolution of the image is 2 mm × 2 mm per voxel, so a three-by-three kernel has a relative receptive field of view of 6 mm by 6 mm. This is particularly useful in images where the scale/zoom of the image can vary. If the model is designed to identify that a dog is present within an image, it should not matter how large or small the dog presented is.

Despite these benefits for image classification, if the user wishes to identify individual voxels relating to a class (segmentation), the pooling layers can lead to a significant decrease in resolution. A representation of max-pooling followed by bilinear up sampling to the original image size is shown in figure 9.4. Note how the fine resolution text is quickly lost by the fourth pooling, while general features such sa color can be maintained for multiple layers. Maintaining the higher-resolution information for later decision making is a main factor in the popularity of the U-Net style architecture discussed later in this chapter.

One thing we have yet to cover is how these features can lead to a prediction. A model needs a method of combining these features into a final prediction; this combination of features is defined as a fully connected layer.

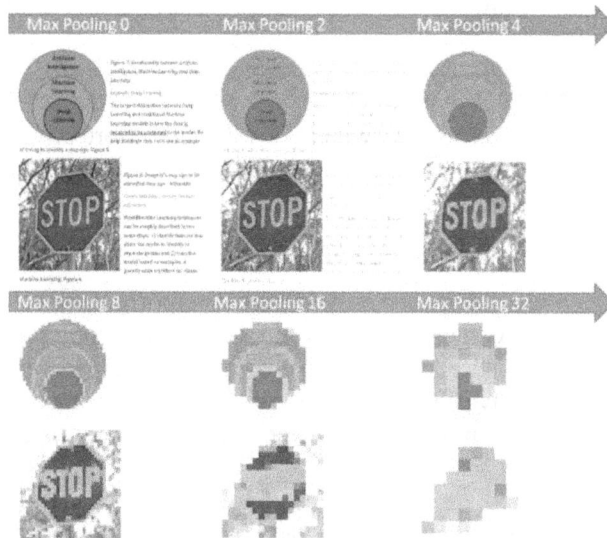

Figure 9.4. Illustration of multiple max-pooling layers and bilinear resampling to illustrate how fine resolution information (text) is quickly lost, while large information (general colors) remains.

9.3.3 Fully connected (dense) layers: bringing it all together

Fully connected, or dense, layers can be imaged as the opposites of convolutional layers. While convolutional layers are locally dependent, the fully connected layer will combine every aspect of the input into an output, figure 9.5. The number of inputs and outputs in a dense layer can vary and are user defined. The mathematical value of each output is $h_i^{\text{out}} = F_i(h_{i-1}^{\text{out}} \times W_i + B_i)$, where F is an activation function, W is the weighting matrix, and B is the bias.

Within convolutional neural networks there can be any number of convolutions and pooling layers. These maps can be represented as several n by m matrices, where n and m are likely smaller than the original image dimensions. In order to feed these features into a dense layer they must first be 'flattened'. This can be imaged as taking the feature image and laying it into a single vector: converting the n-by-m matrix into an $n \times m$ vector. These features can then be used in the final classification. For the example in figure 9.6, we might say that if ears, whiskers, and paws are present, then a dog is present in the image.

The low-level and abstract features of lines, curves, or fuzziness are most likely to appear early in the architecture. Higher level features, such as ears and whiskers, can be imagined arising deeper, as a combination of overlapping low-level features. Finally, all of these features can be combined together after flattening to identify if a dog is present *somewhere* in the image. Note that our output does nothing to identify *where* the dog is present. Furthermore, if the model is truly identifying whether ears, whiskers, and paws are present, it very likely confuses a cat for a dog.

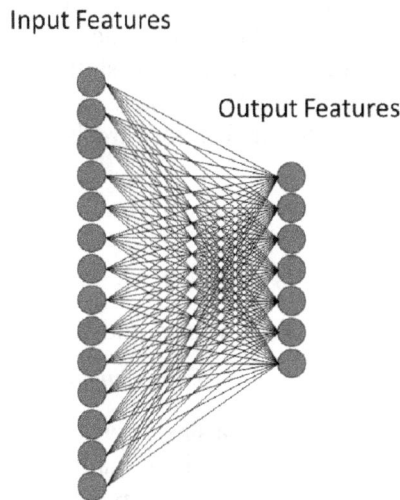

Figure 9.5. A fully connected, or 'dense' layer. Output features are a function of weights from each input feature.

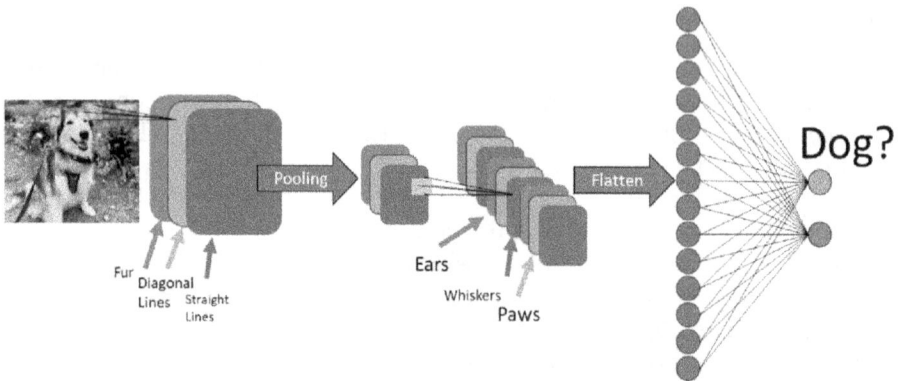

Figure 9.6. Generalized example of a convolutional neural network for the identification of a dog. The first convolutional layers are very low-level; lines, edges, fuzziness. Further down, these features combine to identify ears, paws, or whiskers, before finally feeding into the decision-making process of a fully connected layer.

9.3.4 Activations

Throughout the previous sections we have discussed features, convolutions, and dense layers, but have purposefully been neglecting a very important step in the process. Part of the true power in deep learning comes not only from these critical parts, but also from the final step after each: the activation function.

9.3.4.1 Linear activations

The activation function is a deceivingly simple thing. A simple statement can summarize its purpose: using a defined function, map an input value to an output value. One of the most basic forms of activation is a linear activation: $f(x) = mx + b$, which can have a scaling (m) and bias (b) impact on the outputs. While linear activations can be a useful way of scaling and shifting values, stacking multiple linearly activated layers does not add any new information to the system. To demonstrate this, imagine two linear feed-forward layers, where x is the original values:

$$y_1 = m_1 x + b_1$$

$$y_2 = m_2 y_1 + b_2.$$

The entirety of this network y_2 can be defined and simplified as

$$y_2 = m_2(m_1 x + b_1) + b_2 \rightarrow m_2 m_1 x + m_2 b_1 + b_2 \rightarrow Mx + B,$$

where $m_2 \times b_1 + b_2$ can be combined as a single bias, B, and $m_2 \times m_1$ can be a single scalar, M. This means that regardless of how many linearly activated layers are placed together, they are only capable of expressing linear relationships. For modeling something with non-linear such as gravity, they would inevitably fall short.

9.3.4.2 Non-linear activations

The power of multiple layers becomes more apparent as we transition towards non-linear activation functions. Stacking multiple non-linearly activating layers can add increasing complexity to the model's predictive abilities. For example, if the activation function were $f(x) = mx^2 + gx + c$, two such layers would have the representational ability of several polynomials: x^4, x^3, x^2, x, and bias.

A set of four commonly seen non-linear activation functions is shown in figure 9.7.

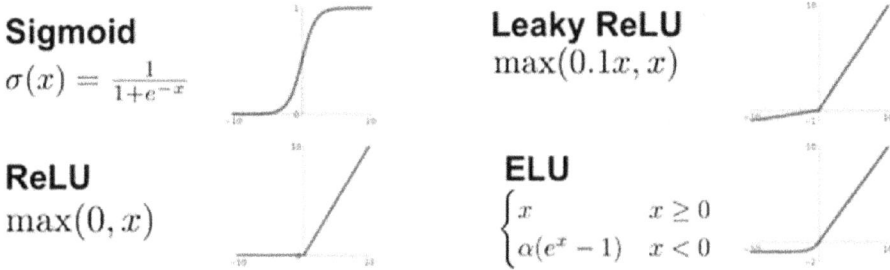

Sigmoid

$\sigma(x) = \frac{1}{1+e^{-x}}$

Leaky ReLU

$\max(0.1x, x)$

ReLU

$\max(0, x)$

ELU

$\begin{cases} x & x \geq 0 \\ \alpha(e^x - 1) & x < 0 \end{cases}$

Figure 9.7. List of common activation functions, sigmoid, rectified linear unit (ReLU), leaky ReLU, and exponential linear unit (ELU).

9.3.4.3 Sigmoid activation

The sigmoid activation function, while not the most commonly seen in the intermediate layers of deep learning architectures, is a common *final* activation function for a binary prediction. This function is commonly expressed as being synonymous with neurons firing within the brain. Given a number of inputs, if the value exceeds some critical threshold the neuron will fire. A sigmoid activation is an appropriate activation for a binary classification system such as our dog model shown in figure 9.6, where '0' would indicate no dog, and '1' would indicate the presence of a dog.

In the case of multiple classification options, the sigmoid activation is often exchanged for the soft-max activation. This provides a probability of a class scaled to the sum of all class's probability:

$$P(y = c|x) = \frac{e^{z_c}}{\sum_{j=1}^{C} e^{z_j}},$$

where c is a particular class and C is the total number of classes.

9.3.4.4 Non-linear activations: rectified linear

The rectified linear unit activation (ReLU) was one of the first and most popular activation functions used in modern deep learning architectures. The function is relatively simple: if x is less than 0, the returned value is 0, otherwise the returned value is x. The 'leaky' ReLU and exponential linear unit (ELU) are both variations on the ReLU, where the differences focus on what occurs when values less than 0 are presented to the function. One of the major issues with ReLU was 'dying' nodes, meaning if a kernel initialized at a value less than 0, all gradient through the node 'died'. The leaky and ELU activation allow at least some gradient.

An important question to raise at this point is 'Why use these non-linear activations?' The answer to this lies in the most interesting part of deep learning: loss and back-propagation.

9.3.5 Loss: driving the model

When making a prediction, we need some method of identifying the 'correctness' of the model prediction. This metric is referred to as the loss. There are several ways of expressing a model loss, although, for mathematical reasons, it is desired that this loss is something that the model is attempting to minimize. An in-depth discussion of back-propagation and gradient descent is beyond the scope of this chapter, please refer to other texts discussed at the beginning of this chapter [25, 26] for a detailed explanation.

9.3.6 Auto-encoders: remove the noise

If one were to be told to draw a bicycle, remove while playing a game of Telestrations, they would likely draw out two simple circles as wheels, a frame connecting them, and a set of handlebars. Perhaps peddles and spokes on the wheels would be included for the more artistically inclined, and yet, this drawing of a bicycle would be relatively far removed from the appearance of an *actual* bicycle. While there are hundreds, if not thousands, of different types of bicycles, most people would be able to review this crude drawing and conclude that the image is supposed to be that of a bicycle. The human brain is amazing in this regard: a bicycle, in all its many shapes and forms, can be condensed down to just a few simple aspects. This 'condensing of important features or removing of unnecessary parts (noise) is the basis of auto-encoders [27].

The goal of an auto-encoder is to simplify, or compress, a set of inputs into its most important aspects, figure 9.8. By reducing the number of features and accurately reproducing the input, the model is able to identify what are the most important aspects of the input. This can similarly be used as a form of principal component analysis (PCA) [28] and is a common building block of both supervised and unsupervised learning models. The so-called 'stacked' auto-encoder is simply a combination of auto-encoders with significantly noted improvement in model predictive capability [29]. The training of these models is often pieced together, with each layer trained separately before being combined and fine-tuned in the final model.

9.3.7 Supervised versus unsupervised learning

Distinctions between supervised and unsupervised learning can be simplified as a statement about data labeling. If the user understands what the desired output should be, e.g. 'is a stop sign present in this image?' and uses those labels to train a

Input Features   Output Features

Compression

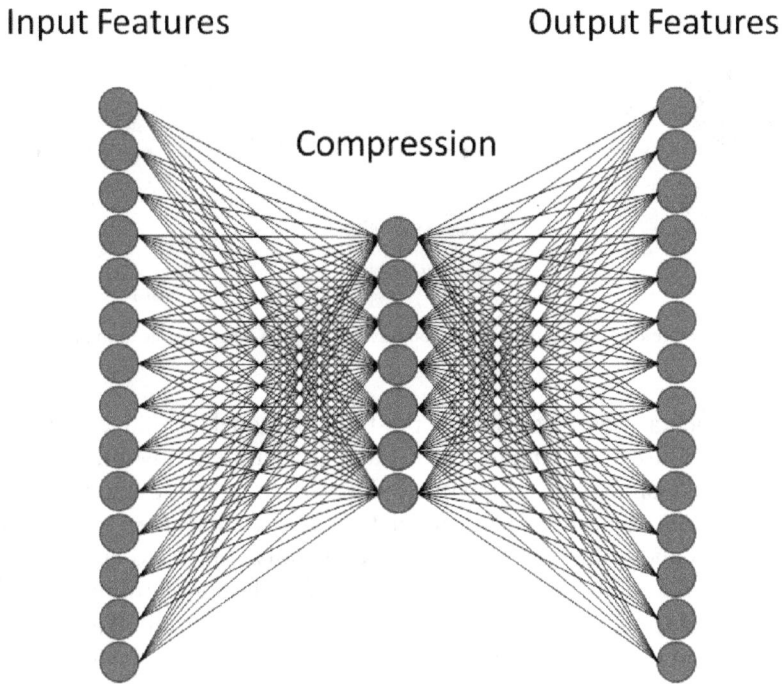

Figure 9.8. Basic example of an auto-encoder.

model, we are operating under 'supervised' learning. However, if we simply had many pictures of stop signs and other signs with no 'ground truth' labeling, we would require an unsupervised learning technique. *This is not to say that unsupervised learning does not require an equal amount of work for training as a supervised learning model.*

9.3.8 Pre-trained convolutional neural networks

Much of the previous discussion revolves around feature extraction (convolutions), refinement (pooling), and combination of those features (dense layers), all with the understanding that relevant features are being identified by the model. However, this is not a guarantee. When first creating a convolutional network, such as one for image classification by the visual geometry group 16 (VGG-16) [30], figure 9.9, every convolutional kernel is going to be a randomly generated distribution of numbers.

Deep learning researchers all suffer from this issue. Updating these random kernels based on correct predictions is a labor intensive and sensitive process that occupies most, if not all, of a researcher's time and effort when beginning a new classification process. The VGG-16 model was trained on the ImageNet challenge, which contains more than 14 million images. This is far above what most medical researchers have available for training their own models. However, this can still be used to our advantage with the concept of using this pre-trained model.

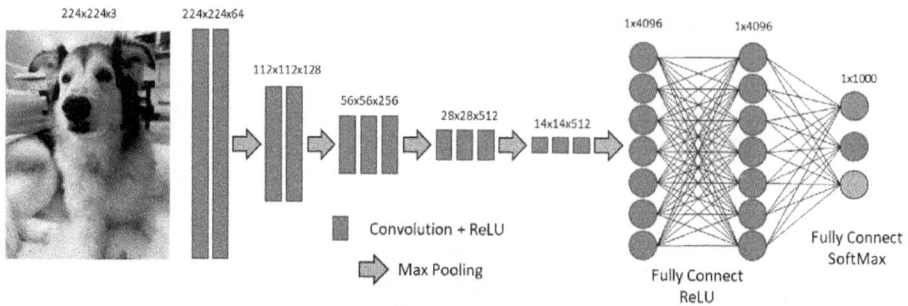

Figure 9.9. Representation of the visual geometry group (VGG-16) classification architecture.

The fundamental basis of using a pre-trained model is that certain low-level features are ubiquitous. As humans, we are able to identify many different objects all of which are built on the same fundamental pieces: lines, curves, edges, etc. We are then able to take this pre-trained model that has been trained on thousands of different images and utilize everything before the fully connected layers as a feature extraction network. This saves potentially countless hours of training; by freezing the convolution layers, we can simply train the end classification. *Note*: Even after a new classification model is trained, it is common to un-freeze the earlier layers in a process of fine tuning.

9.4 Image registration: bringing two images together

Throughout the course of a patient's care there is a potential for multiple forms of medical imaging to be acquired for various purposes, e.g. defining tumor boundaries, identifying surrounding critical normal tissue, and characterizing tumor and normal tissue function. For example, a magnetic resonance image (MRI) can exhibit exquisite contrast of soft tissues in ways that computed tomography (CT) scans cannot, and an FDG positron emission tomography (PET) scan is able to identify regions of metabolic hyperactivity. Currently, standard practice within radiation oncology includes a CT scan enabling the visualization of a desired treatment site and enabling radiation dose calculation, although there is significant research into MRI based generation of electron density.

An ability to refer to multiple imaging modalities to evaluate tumor extent or normal tissues is vital to the decision-making and treatment planning process. Unfortunately, these PET, MRI, and CT scans are rarely acquired at the same time or with exactly consistent positioning of the patient. These changes in time, positioning, and/or anatomy have led to the necessity of tools to align different modalities/images about a region of interest in the anatomy. This aligning of different modalities or images is referred to as image registration.

This is not to say that image registration is only important during the planning process. Accurate alignment of the planning images with treatment imaging (cone-beam CT, fan-beam CT, MRI) is equally vital to a safe and successful treatment.

With ART, it is often vital to understand the distribution of previously delivered radiation for guidance in future planning. This understanding relies on accurate representation and registration of the new imaging with previous plans. It is equally important to understand how a registration is evaluated and functions, the 'registration metric', per AAPM Task Group 132 [31]. After all, when registering two images, how does one know when the registration is 'good'?

There are multiple ways in which a registration can be evaluated. Often, the registration is focused on a particular region of clinical relevance. *Identifying the region of relevance is the first and most important aspect of image registration.*

9.4.1 Registration similarity metrics

There are broadly two ways of evaluating/driving a registration: intensity-based and feature-based.

9.4.1.1 Intensity based registration

Intensity based registration can be defined as a comparison of intensities between the two images, either as a whole, or about a defined sub-region of interest in the image [32–34]. When operating between two images of the same modality, simple comparisons of the intensity values between the two can offer a reasonable evaluation of the registration, possible as the sum of squared differences (SSD) [35, 36]:

$$\text{SSD} = \frac{1}{N}\sum_{i=1}^{N}(I_{X_i} - I_{Y_i})^2,$$

where I is the intensity and subscript X and Y refer to two images across the total number of voxels being evaluated. While this metric can be very useful, it suffers when the voxel intensities throughout the two images vary (a multi-phase contrast enhanced CT). To this end, the normalized cross-correlation (NCC) [36–38] is a wonderful metric, accounting for the differences in intensity between the two images, although assuming that relatively high and low intensities correlate with each other:

$$\text{NCC} = \frac{\sum_{i=1}^{n}(x_i - \bar{x})(y_i - \bar{y})}{\sqrt{\sum_{i=1}^{n}(x_i - \bar{x})^2}\sqrt{\sum_{i=1}^{n}(y_i - \bar{y})^2}}.$$

An important note from both methods is that they require the intensities between the images to be correlated: a bright spot in one image corresponds to a bright spot in the other, etc. For multi-modality images (CT to MR), this is not a guarantee.

A commonly used metric for the registration of images of different modalities is mutual information [39, 40]. This metric is based on the mutual probabilities between the two images and has no reliance on the absolute intensity of the images:

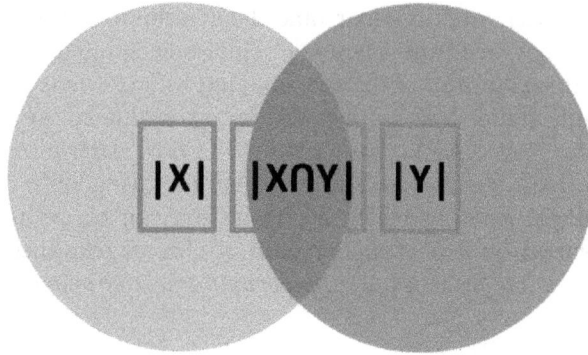

Figure 9.10. Visual representation of the DSC.

$$\text{MI}(I_X, I_Y) = \sum_X \sum_Y P(I_X I_Y) \log_2 \left(\frac{p(I_X, I_Y)}{p(I_X)p(I_Y)} \right),$$

where p is the probability distribution function of the intensities of X and Y, respectively, and $p(I_x, I_y)$ is the joint probability distribution function.

9.4.1.2 Feature-based registration

Feature-based registrations focus not on intensities between the two images, but instead on a defined feature present between the two [41, 42]. These features could be points, lines, or entire structures, such as a contoured brainstem.

Feature-based registrations can broadly be described as minimizing the distance between points or surfaces of interest. When evaluating points, the sum of squared distances between the points appears very similar to the SSD equation shown previously:

$$\text{point difference} = \frac{1}{N}\sum_{i=1}^{N}(P_{X_i} - P_{Y_i})^2.$$

With a surface, this equation changes to evaluate the sum of differences from each point to that of the surface of interest.

A common metric of evaluating the overlap between two surfaces (2D or 3D) is the Dice similarity coefficient (DSC):

$$\text{DSC} = 2\frac{X \cap Y}{Y + X}.$$

When two surfaces/volumes completely overlap, the DSC will be equal to 1, and when there is no overlap present it will be equal to 0, figure 9.10.

9.4.1.3 AI-based feature registration

Both intensity and feature-based registrations as shown above can be roughly called pre-made/hand-crafted features, that have been selected over time because of their success. There are a variety of other options available as well, such as Gabor filters [43] and hand-crafted features that a user identifies to best match their respective images [44–46].

One of the most common uses of convolutional neural networks is in asking the question 'Are these the *best* features to guide our registration?' and 'Can the model figure out what features are most useful?'.

9.4.2 Types of registrations

Image registration algorithms have three main components: similarity index, transformation algorithm, and optimization method. For comprehensive descriptions, the reader is referred to existing chapters and review articles; here we will summarize for the context of AI in adaptive radiotherapy. Transformation algorithms are broadly classified into rigid and deformable.

9.4.2.1 Rigid registration

Rigid registration is characterized by applying a series of translations and rotations to the image. There are three potential translations relating to the left–right, superior–inferior, and posterior–anterior directions of the image, and three potential rotations relating to the pitch, roll, and yaw. These values can be used to directly relate any point in one image to another via the following transformation matrix, where M_1, M_2, and M_3 are the three translations, and T_x, T_y, and T_z are the three rotations, figure 9.11.

A particular thing to note from this transformation is that there is a single, direct relationship between every point in reference B to reference A.

9.4.2.2 Deformable registration

Deformable, or non-rigid registrations, can be broadly categorized as anything that falls outside of the framework of rigid registration. Rather than maintaining a linear and direct relationship from each point in one image space to another, deformable registration enables each voxel to have its own individual transformation. The transformation of a single voxel from one space to the next can be described as the deformation vector field: a matrix of vectors in the x-, y-, and z-plane which describe how an individual voxel from image A transforms into image B. Common deformable registration algorithms used in medical applications include Demons [47] based algorithms, B-spline [48], and the finite element model (FEM) [49, 50].

One of the concerns in deformable registration is this lack of consistent transformation. There is no requirement that every voxel in image A be present in image

$$\begin{bmatrix} ^{A}x \\ ^{A}y \\ ^{A}z \\ 1 \end{bmatrix} = \begin{bmatrix} M_{11} & M_{12} & M_{13} & T_x \\ M_{21} & M_{22} & M_{23} & T_y \\ M_{31} & M_{32} & M_{33} & T_z \\ 0 & 0 & 0 & 1 \end{bmatrix} \begin{bmatrix} ^{B}x \\ ^{B}y \\ ^{B}z \\ 1 \end{bmatrix}$$

Figure 9.11. Transformation matrix describing how a point (x, y, z) transforms from image B to image A.

B, and vice versa. Deformable registrations often have very complex optimization issues, with difficulty interpreting results on a voxel-by-voxel basis. For this reason, there are many considerations regarding the optimization and evaluation of deformable registration models that need to be considered before clinical use.

When interacting with non-rigid registrations it is equally important to understand the implications of the registration results. For example, bone is not an object we would expect to readily deform. *Just because the evaluation metric is optimal does not mean the deformation is realistic or accurate.* The user should not evaluate a registration based solely on the same method used to guide the registration, as there is an implicit bias towards a positive result. For example, if the registration is driven by contour matching, the DSC between the contours is expected to be very high, however, this does not promise accurate or physiologically reasonable registration within the contoured structure.

9.5 AI-based image registration

Within image registration in AI there are multiple groups: supervised learning, unsupervised learning, reinforcement learning, and generative adversarial networks (GANs). For all techniques, the metric and methodologies used to evaluate the final registration is vital as an indication of model efficacy. For all these groups, feature extraction via convolutional neural networks (new or pre-trained) is the common bedrock that connects them all. The features extracted can then be fed into existing models (Demons [47, 51], histogram matching [46], etc) as methods of registration, or used as inputs for new models.

9.5.1 Supervised learning

Within supervised learning, a previously determined registration between two images exists and is defined as the 'correct' answer. This is often the case in image registration, although this now limits the model's ability to learn based on the accuracy of the previous registration and will perpetuate any systematic errors present in the ground truth training data.

9.5.1.1 Convolutional neural network registrations

Convolutional neural networks (CNNs) operate by convolving a number of kernels (typically 3×3 or 5×5 matrix in a 2D image) to identify features present in the images being registered. One of the advantages of CNNs is that these convolutions are not computationally expensive, the same kernel is applied across the space. However, a disadvantage is that the kernel itself has a relatively small receptive field. If we imagine a single convolutional kernel used to identify diagonal lines (an ear), shown in blue in figure 9.12, we can easily see that while the kernel might be able to identify the ear, the receptive field size might not be large enough to see enough of the image to overcome a poor initialization of the two images.

This represents a very important concept in many deep learning image registration programs: both image initialization and the overall receptive field size of the model can have significant impacts on the final accuracy of the prediction. For this

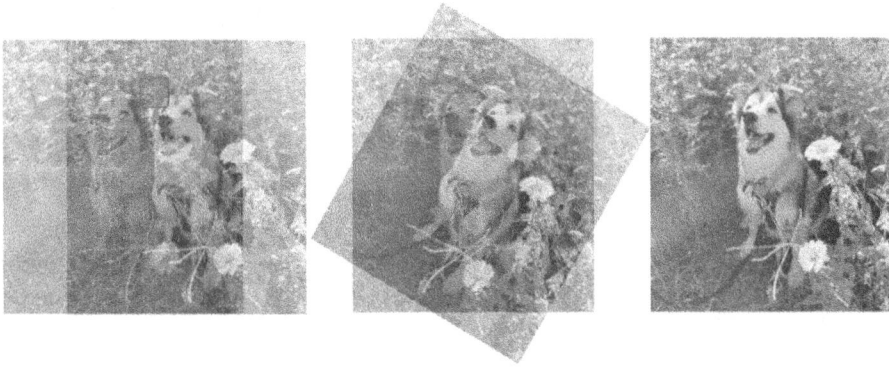

Figure 9.12. (Left) Representation of two images with an applied shift. The blue box represents a kernel for identifying diagonal lines (ear kernel). (Middle) Because of a poor initialization point and a lack of a larger receptive field, the model could incorrectly register the final two images based on this feature as a local minimum, rather than the (right) ideal registration.

reason, networks often include several layers of convolution and pooling, extracting both fine and coarse image information to guide the final registration.

9.5.1.2 Generative adversarial networks

Generative adversarial networks (GANs) exist as a combination of two networks: a decoder which attempts to produce a realistic registration/deformation based on the input and target, and an encoder which attempts to differentiate between 'real' registrations and generated registrations. GANs have shown success in the creation of synthetic modality images (synthetic CT from MRI [62–64], T1-weighted to T2-weighted and vice versa [65]) and applied towards the medical registration task [61].

9.5.2 Unsupervised learning

Rather than be forced to train on explicitly defined answers, unsupervised learning for image registration requires that the image, either in whole or in part, be reducible to some form of feature vector that represents the patch/image. This can take the form of independent component analysis (ICA) [66] or PCA [28]. The model's driving goal then is to reduce a complicated space/patch (2D or 3D MRI of the brain for example) into the principal components/features that represent that space. The model can then try to reduce the separation between these found features.

9.5.2.1 Reinforcement learning

These architectures are often built with some aspect of long-short-term memory (LSTM), the goal of which is to make an informed decision based on previous historical information. In the context of image evaluations, the convolutional LSTM [67] is often seen [55]. This imagines a 3D scan as a series of 2D images, each highly correlated to the image immediately above and below. The largest benefit seen by reinforcement learning, is the 'reward' feedback. Other regression-based methods rely heavily on the image initialization point. Reinforcement learning provides the model an 'action', with a predefined 'reward' acting as a feedback mechanism. Hu *et al* have shown that a simple transformation matrix: rotation, scale, and translation can be used as the driving 'action', with a landmark based error acting as the reward function [55].

9.5.3 Registration in ART

The architectures presented in table 9.1 represent only a small portion of the work performed in AI-based registrations. These rapid registrations can alleviate temporal burden of recontouring targets and organs at risk, which would preclude online or real-time ART. They can further enable plan adaption by calculating a pre-determined plan on daily anatomy, representing 'dose of the day' [68–70]. With propagated contours and dose, the users can create a new plan going forward, or summate the dose on the original plan [71].

9.5.4 Commonalities in architectures

There are several deep learning components that are often seen in both supervised and unsupervised training. Auto-encoders and stacked auto-encoders are often set as the bedrock of deep learning models in image registration. The goal of such components is to remove unnecessary information and identify the principal components of the image.

We have previously identified both feature- and intensity-based metrics that can drive the registration process. Several AI models have instead flipped the question to ask: 'Why not allow the model to figure out what features are important?'

9.5.4.1 Pre-trained convolutional neural networks

A common requirement from these architectures is the ability to identify useful features to guide the registration process. These features/intensities can be local or global and can either be user defined or determined by the model itself.

When using pre-trained models, the user must take extra care to match the new image intensities to that of the images used for original training. Further explanation of utilizing pre-trained networks is elaborated on later in this chapter within section 9.6.

9.6 Image segmentation

9.6.1 Introduction: coloring by the numbers

In the creation of a 3D treatment plan, the voxel-wise identification, or segmentation, of targets and normal tissues/organs-at-risk (OARs) is a vital part of the planning process, with significant downstream repercussions [72–74]. Across a number of treatment sites, there can be a large number of OARs and targets required for the treatment planning process, creating barriers to re-planning, adaptation, and dose accumulation efforts due to the significant time required for manual segmentation. Providing rapid and accurate segmentations is a vital part of the overall workflow in ART, particularly in the online and real-time setting.

Table 9.1. List of various authors and techniques for rigid and deformable image registration. This list is by no means exhaustive but represents a small sampling of the work done by various groups.

Author (year)	Title	Dataset	Technique	Explanation
Wu et al [52]	Unsupervised deep feature learning for deformable registration of MR brain images	Brain MRI	CNN	CNN used for feature extraction, learned features fed into histogram matching algorithm
Yang et al [53]	Fast predictive multimodal image registration	T1/T2 Brain MRI	CNN	Encoder–decoder for deformation prediction
Miao et al [54]	A CNN regression approach for real-time 2D/3D registration	Fluoroscopic video, x-ray and transesophageal echocardiography probe	CNN	Pose estimation via hierarchical learning (PEHL) —> facilitates 2D/3D registration via local feature extraction
Hu et al [55]	End-to-end multimodal image registration via reinforcement learning	Paired CT/MR nasopharyngeal carcinoma patients	Reinforcement learning	LSTM post convolutional layers
Sokooti et al [56]	Non-rigid image registration using multi-scale 3D convolutional neural networks	SPREAD CT [57]	CNN	Pair of 3D patches generates 3D registration vector field
Zhao et al [51]	Deep adaptive log-Demons: diffeomorphic image registration with very large deformations	Brain MRI	CNN	2D affine —> 3D affine with Demons iterative approach
Liu et al [58]	Multimodal medical image registration via common representations learning and differentiable geometric constraints	DR and DRR	CNN	Xception [59] pre-trained network used for feature extraction, warping transform from feature distances

(Continued)

Table 9.1. (*Continued*)

Author (year)	Title	Dataset	Technique	Explanation
Wu et al [60]	Scalable high-performance image registration framework by unsupervised deep feature representation learning	Brain MRI	CNN with stacked auto-encoders	Auto-encoders identify features from 3D patches, decoder network provides larger FOV context
Mahapatra et al [61]	Deformable medical image registration using generative adversarial networks	Retinal, cardiac images	GAN	Deformation fields generated from GAN network, evaluated based on Dice
Simonovsky et al (2016) [112]	A deep metric for multimodal registration	Neonatal brain MRI Adult brain MRI	CNN	CNN estimating dissimilarity of two cubic patches, evaluated based on Dice
Veiga et al [70]	Toward adaptive radiotherapy for head and neck patients: Feasibility study on using CT-to-CBCT deformable registration for 'dose of the day' calculations	CT-CBCT	Not AI, Nifty-Reg	Evaluating dose summation as a 'dose of the day' registration between daily CBCT and planning CT
Konig et al (2016) [113]	Deformable image registration for adaptive radiotherapy with guaranteed local rigidity constraints	CT-CBCT	Not AI, normalized gradient field measure distance and smoothing regularizer	Algorithm comparison of structure propagation in male pelvis from CT to daily CBCT

As discussed previously, rigid, and deformable registration solutions offer opportunities for contour propagation from previous imaging. However, these methodologies all rely on the accuracy of the guiding registration and the accuracy of the previously defined structures. Strategies of identifying a subset of OARs based on disease site proximal to the target has also shown success in online ART [9].

Deep learning, particularly convolutional neural networks, have been shown to be highly successful in the task of OAR segmentation. For OARs, there are multiple vendor solutions available (MIM Contour Protégé [75], Raystation Deep Learning Segmentation [76], Radformation AutoContour [77], and Varian AI-Rad Companion [78]). Likewise, several groups have successfully created models for the segmentation of OARs present in the brain [79], head and neck [80–83], lung [84–86], abdomen [87–90], and pelvis [91–94].

Target delineations offer several new difficulties when creating predictive models: inter- and interobserver variabilities tend to be larger for targets compared to OARs [72–74, 95–98]. Particularly for clinical target volumes (CTVs) 'a volume encompassing visible gross tumor volume and subclinical malignant disease' per ICRU 50 [99], there is often discussion about how generous to make certain contours, which leads to significant challenges in automating this process.

Convolutional networks of CTVs and gross tumor volumes (GTVs) have been successfully implemented in a number of sites for brain tumors [100], rectal cancer [101], nasopharyngeal cancer [102, 103], breast cancer [104], oropharyngeal cancer [105], and arteriovenous malformations [106].

It is important to note that that with supervised machine learning, there is an implicit bias of the created model towards the training data. Models trained on manual contours from institution X could create suboptimal contours for institution Y if there is a systematic difference in practice between institutions. Furthermore, quantitative metrics do not always provide adequate clinical relevance of generated segmentations [94, 107–109]. Including a qualitative assessment of the model's predictions is vital for clinical feasibility.

9.6.2 Segmentation networks

A small sampling of convolutional neural networks tasked with the segmentation of OARs and targets is presented in table 9.2. While these studies all have unique qualities specifically designed to address the task at hand, there are several elements present across a majority of the networks. First is the difficulty of both small field high resolution and large field context. As discussed previously in section 9.3, convolutions suffer from local dependence. Pooling layers can alleviate this dependence by reducing the overall search space for successive convolutions. However, as demonstrated in figure 9.4, recovering to the original image resolution after consecutive pooling layers results in a severe loss of fine resolution information. For this reason, many segmentation architectures incorporate skip connections. The most famous example of this is the fully convolutional neural network called U-Net [110]. Here high-resolution information from each part of the encoding path is directly transferable to the decoding path (figure 9.13).

Table 9.2. List of various authors and techniques for the segmentation of OARs and targets. This list is by no means exhaustive, but represents a small sampling of the work done by various groups.

Author (year)	Title	Dataset	Technique	Goal
Laiton-Bonadiez et al [79]	Deep 3D neural network for brain structures. Segmentation using self-attention modules in MRI images.	Mindboggle-101 Brain MRI	3D U-Net with skip connections multi-head attention	OAR segmentation
Cubero et al [80]	Deep learning-based segmentation of head and neck OARs with clinical partially labeled data.	ARTIX HN CT	3D organ-specific residual U-Net —> nn-U-Net	OAR segmentation
Van Dijk et al [83]	Improving automatic delineation for head and neck organs at risk by deep learning contouring.	HN CT	Mirada medical CNN	OAR segmentation
Morris et al [84]	Cardiac substructure segmentation with deep learning for improved cardiac sparing.	Left-sided whole breast MR/CT	U-Net	OAR segmentation
Dong et al [88]	Automatic multiorgan segmentation in thorax CT images using U-Net-GAN.	2017 AAPM thoracic challenge CT	U-Net-GAN	OAR segmentation
Ranjbarzadeh et al [100]	Brain tumor segmentation based on deep learning and an attention mechanism using MRI multi-modality brain images.	BRATS 2018 Brain MR	Cascaded CNN —> dense connection	Tumor core, enhancing tumor, edema segmentation
Cardenas et al [105]	Deep learning algorithm for auto-delineation of high-risk oropharyngeal clinical target volumes with built-in Dice similarity coefficient parameter optimization function.	CT HN	Stacked auto-encoder	GTV, high-risk CTV segmentation

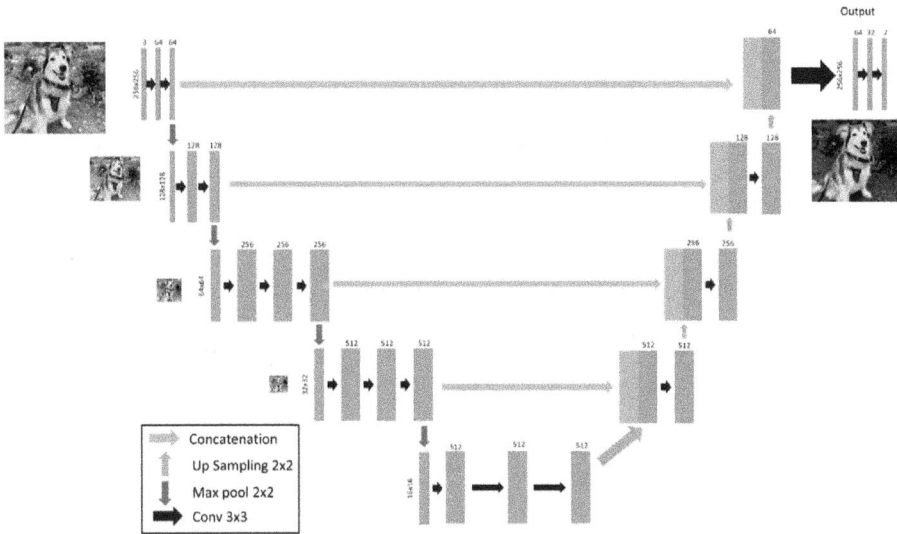

Figure 9.13. Basic representation of the U-Net style architecture, called such because of its 'U' shape. Note that information from the encoding (left) side of the architecture is maintained to the decoding (right) side, facilitating finer resolution segmentation.

Several alternative strategies exist, although at the fundamental level the goal stays the same: enabling fine resolution evaluation for voxel-wise segmentation, while gaining coarse resolution information for guided context.

9.6.2.1 Pre-trained convolutional neural networks

Pre-trained classification networks (VGG-16 [30], Xception [111], InceptionV3) can equally be applied for the task of semantic segmentation. Just as the features which are being extracted can be applied to other tasks in classification, the early convolutional layers can be useful in training a new segmentation model. Users often apply skip connections to the architecture encoder, freezing the previously trained layers and specifically training an entirely new decoder. After an initial learning process, the original encoder layers can be 'unfrozen' for fine tuning, figure 9.14.

9.6.3 Best practices

9.6.3.1 Preprocessing

9.6.3.1.1 Intensity values

A major consideration for any convolutional neural network is data pre-processing. It is always beneficial to normalize input images about the intensity values of interest. For example, if trying to segment the lungs, thresholding the HUs about values present in the lungs can help the model focus on important regions.

This window/leveling and thresholding is especially important when utilizing pre-trained networks. Recall that many pre-trained networks are trained on

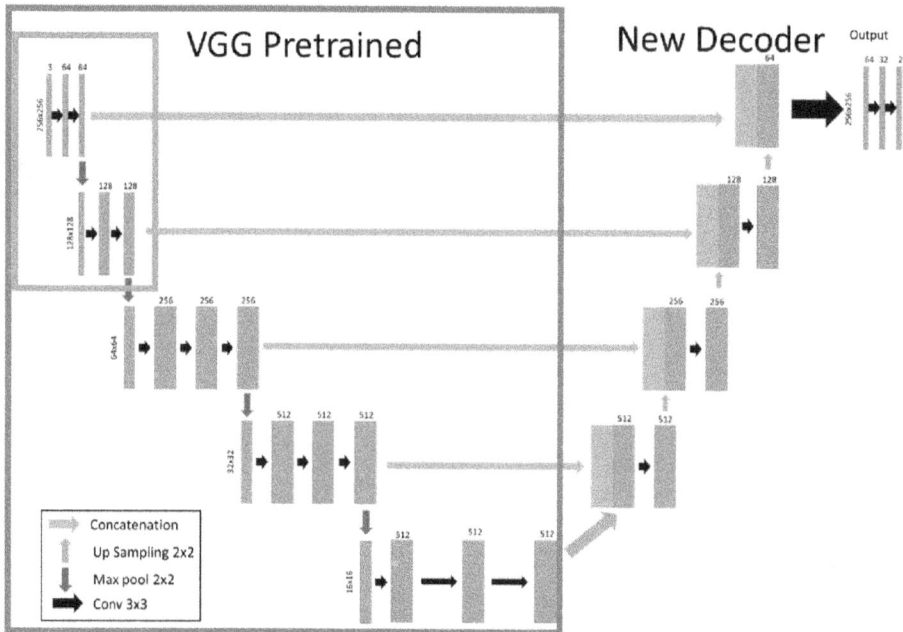

Figure 9.14. A basic representation of utilizing a pre-trained network such as the VGGNet for semantic segmentation. The red box indicates the original classification network, and the green box indicates early layers which are often frozen in the initial training process.

non-medical images (RGB 0–255). Therefore, the kernels which come from this training process are specifically tuned to these values. This does not mean that simply translating the input image to a range of 0–255 is the complete solution! Many models have other pre-processing steps which occur prior to incorporation into the model. Multiple pre-trained architectures in Tensorflow and PyTorch have available pre-processing layers which can convert images from 0 to 255 into the desired range for a pre-trained model during model creation[1].

9.6.3.1.2 Image size

Within medicine we are often interested in not only 2D images, but 3D images as well (CT, MRI, PET). The voxel dimensions of these images can vary greatly depending on the acquisition parameters (field of view, slice thickness, etc). When using convolutional neural networks, the kernels are invariant in size; meaning that if a kernel is trained on a 3D image set with dimensions of $1 \times 1 \times 1$ mm, that same kernel will not likely have the same output if the input is scaled to $3 \times 3 \times 3$ mm.

Proper understanding and accountability of the voxel size for training/validation/ test can be vital to an accurate knowledge of a model's potential weaknesses and biases. It is highly recommended that images be sampled to a uniform resolution, or

---

[1] https://www.tensorflow.org/api_docs/python/tf/keras/applications/xception/preprocess_input

that the model be presented with an equal sampling of the resolution images that it will later be expected to predict.

9.6.3.2 Deep learning

Deep learning is often criticized (fairly) as being a black box. While an explicit explanation of everything which is occurring within a trained model can be difficult to obtain, there are still several strategies which can be beneficial. First, an evaluation of the kernels generated by a model can offer insight into the model's decision-making process. Second, when making a hand-crafted model, properly visualizing the connections between each layer is an efficient method of trouble-shooting errors. Both Tensorflow[2] and PyTorch[3] offer solutions for visualizing a model which can help identify incorrect connections.

9.7 Summary

As we navigate the ever-expanding horizons of AI, the intersection of excitement and caution becomes increasingly vital. Our discussions on AI registration and segmentation underscore the transformative potential it has within ART. However, while AI promises remarkable advancements, its implementation must be grounded by the awareness of limitations and biases in every AI model. AI and adaptive radiation therapy heralds a new era in personalized medicine, where each patient's treatment is guided by cutting-edge technology and personalized care.

We cannot wait to see what the future holds.

'Do the best you can until you know better. Then when you know better, do better.'—Maya Angelou

References

[1] Lim-Reinders S, Keller B M, Al-Ward S, Sahgal A and Kim A 2017 Online adaptive radiation therapy *Int. J. Radiat. Oncol. Biol. Phys.* **99** 994–1003

[2] Vargas C *et al* 2005 Phase II dose escalation study of image-guided adaptive radio-therapy for prostate cancer: use of dose–volume constraints to achieve rectal isotoxicity *Int. J. Radiat. Oncol. Biol. Phys.* **63** 141–9

[3] Dawson L A, Eccles C and Craig T 2006 Individualized image guided iso-NTCP based liver cancer SBRT *Acta Oncol.* **45** 856–64

[4] Liu M *et al* 2017 Individual isotoxic radiation dose escalation based on V20 and advanced technologies benefits unresectable stage III non-small cell lung cancer patients treated with concurrent chemoradiotherapy: long term follow-up *Oncotarget* **8** 51848

[5] Kong F M *et al* 2017 Effect of midtreatment PET/CT-adapted radiation therapy with concurrent chemotherapy in patients with locally advanced non-small-cell lung cancer: a phase 2 clinical trial *JAMA Oncol.* **3** 1358

[6] Nigay E, Bonsall H, Meyer B, Hunzeker A and Lenards N 2019 Offline adaptive radiation therapy in the treatment of prostate cancer: a case study *Med. Dosim.* **44** 1–6

---

[2] https://www.tensorflow.org/tensorboard/graphs
[3] https://pytorch.org/tutorials/intermediate/tensorboard_tutorial.html

[7] Bhandari V, Patel P, Gurjar O P and Gupta K L 2014 Impact of repeat computerized tomography replans in the radiation therapy of head and neck cancers *J. Med. Phys. Assoc. Med. Phys. India* **39** 164

[8] Feng M *et al* 2018 Individualized adaptive stereotactic body radiotherapy for liver tumors in patients at high risk for liver damage: a phase 2 clinical trial *JAMA Oncol.* **4** 40

[9] Henke L *et al* 2018 Phase I trial of stereotactic MR-guided online adaptive radiation therapy (SMART) for the treatment of oligometastatic or unresectable primary malignancies of the abdomen *Radiother. Oncol.* **126** 519–26

[10] Hoffmann L, Alber M, Jensen M F, Holt M I and Møller D S 2017 Adaptation is mandatory for intensity modulated proton therapy of advanced lung cancer to ensure target coverage *Radiother. Oncol.* **122** 400–5

[11] Heijkoop S T *et al* 2014 Clinical implementation of an online adaptive plan-of-the-day protocol for nonrigid motion management in locally advanced cervical cancer IMRT *Int. J. Radiat. Oncol. Biol. Phys.* **90** 673–9

[12] Mohan R *et al* 2005 Use of deformed intensity distributions for on-line modification of image-guided IMRT to account for interfractional anatomic changes *Int. J. Radiat. Oncol. Biol. Phys.* **61** 1258–66

[13] Ahunbay E E *et al* 2010 Online adaptive replanning method for prostate radiotherapy *Int. J. Radiat. Oncol. Biol. Phys.* **77** 1561–72

[14] Court L E *et al* 2005 An automatic CT-guided adaptive radiation therapy technique by online modification of multileaf collimator leaf positions for prostate cancer *Int. J. Radiat. Oncol. Biol. Phys.* **62** 154–63

[15] Li X A *et al* 2011 Development of an online adaptive solution to account for inter- and intra-fractional variations *Radiother. Oncol.* **100** 370–4

[16] El-Bared N *et al* 2019 Dosimetric benefits and practical pitfalls of daily online adaptive MRI-guided stereotactic radiation therapy for pancreatic cancer *Pract Radiat. Oncol.* **9** e46–54

[17] Ahunbay E E, Peng C, Godley A, Schultz C and Li X A 2009 An on-line replanning method for head and neck adaptive radiotherapy *Med. Phys.* **36** 4776–90

[18] Archambault Y *et al* 2020 Making on-line adaptive radiotherapy possible using artificial intelligence and machine learning for efficient daily re-planning *Med. Phys. Int. J.* **8** 77–86

[19] Kontaxis C, Bol G H, Kerkmeijer L G W, Lagendijk J J W and Raaymakers B W 2017 Fast online replanning for interfraction rotation correction in prostate radiotherapy *Med. Phys.* **44** 5034–42

[20] Stemkens B *et al* 2017 Effect of intra-fraction motion on the accumulated dose for free-breathing MR-guided stereotactic body radiation therapy of renal-cell carcinoma *Phys. Med. Biol.* **62** 7407–24

[21] Anastasi G *et al* 2020 Patterns of practice for adaptive and real-time radiation therapy (POP-ART RT) part I: intra-fraction breathing motion management *Radiother. Oncol.* **153** 79

[22] Keall P *et al* 2017 The first clinical implementation of real-time adaptive radiation therapy using a standard linear accelerator *Int. J. Radiat. Oncol. Biol. Phys.* **99** S223–4

[23] Schweikard A, Shiomi H and Adler J 2004 Respiration tracking in radiosurgery *Med. Phys.* **31** 2738–41

[24] Elekta Unity *Elektra* https://elekta.com/products/radiation-therapy/unity/

[25] Goodfellow I, Bengio Y and Courville A 2016 *Deep Learning* (Cambridge, MA: MIT Press)

[26] Chollet F 2017 *Deep Learning with Python* (New York: Manning)

[27] Hinton G E and Salakhutdinov R R 2006 Reducing the dimensionality of data with neural networks *Science* **313** 504–7

[28] Comon P 1994 Independent component analysis, a new concept? *Signal Process.* **36** 287–314

[29] Bengio Y, Courville A and Vincent P 2012 Representation learning: a review and new perspectives *IEEE Trans. Pattern Anal. Mach. Intell.* **35** 1798–828

[30] Simonyan K and Zisserman A 2014 Very deep convolutional networks for large-scale image recognition arXiv: 1409.1556v6

[31] Brock K K, Mutic S, McNutt T R, Li H and Kessler M L 2017 Use of image registration and fusion algorithms and techniques in radiotherapy: report of the AAPM radiation therapy committee task group no. 132 *Med. Phys.* **44** e43–76

[32] Zhang J, Lu Z T, Pigrish V, Feng Q J and Chen W F 2013 Intensity based image registration by minimizing exponential function weighted residual complexity *Comput. Biol. Med.* **43** 1484–96

[33] Lee M E, Kim S H and Seo I H 2009 Intensity-based registration of medical images *Proc. Int. Symp. Test Meas.* **1** 239–42

[34] Xing C and Qiu P 2011 Intensity based image registration by nonparametric local smoothing *IEEE Trans. Pattern Anal. Mach. Intell.* **33** 2081–92

[35] Khosravi J, Shams Esfand Abadi M and Ebrahimpour R 2018 Image registration based on sum of square difference cost function *J. Electr. Comput. Eng. Innov.* **6** 273–81

[36] Hisham M B, Yaakob S N, Raof R A A, Nazren A B A and Embedded N M W 2015 Template matching using sum of squared difference and normalized cross correlation *2015 IEEE Student Conf. on Research and Development* (Piscataway, NJ: IEEE) pp 100–4

[37] Rutesic P and Stosic Z 2018 Image registration based on normalized cross correlation and discrete cosine transform *Int. J. Signal Process.* **3** 16–20

[38] Wang C, Ren Q, Qin X and Yu Y 2018 The same modality medical image registration with large deformation and clinical application based on adaptive diffeomorphic multi-resolution demons *BMC Med. Imaging* **18** 21

[39] Chen H M and Varshney P K 2003 Mutual information-based CT-MR brain image registration using generalized partial volume joint histogram estimation *IEEE Trans. Med. Imaging* **22** 1111–9

[40] Maes F, Loeckx D, Vandermeulen D and Suetens P 2015 Image registration using mutual information *Handbook of Biomedical Imaging: Methodologies and Clinical Research* **vol 295** (Boston, MA: Springer) p 308

[41] Ma J, Jiang X, Fan A, Jiang J and Yan J 2021 Image matching from handcrafted to deep features: a survey *Int. J. Comput. Vis.* **129** 23–79

[42] Canny J 1986 A computational approach to edge detection *IEEE Trans. Pattern. Anal. Mach. Intell.* **PAMI8** 679–98

[43] Gabor D 1946 Theory of communication *J. Inst. Electr. Eng.* **93** 429–41

[44] Wu G, Wang Q, Jia H and Shen D 2012 Feature-based groupwise registration by hierarchical anatomical correspondence detection *Hum. Brain. Mapp.* **33** 253–71

[45] Wang Q, Yap P T, Wu G and Shen D 2009 Attribute vector guided groupwise registration *Med. Image. Comput. Comput. Assist. Interv.* **12** 656–63

[46] Wu G, Kim M, Wang Q and Shen D 2014 S-HAMMER: hierarchical attribute-guided, symmetric diffeomorphic registration for MR brain images *Hum. Brain. Mapp.* **35** 1044–60

[47] Peyrat J M, Delingette H, Sermesant M, Xu C and Ayache N 2010 Registration of 4D cardiac CT sequences under trajectory constraints with multichannel diffeomorphic demons *IEEE Trans. Med. Imaging* **29** 1351–68

[48] Rueckert D 1999 Nonrigid registration using free-form deformations: application to breast MR images *IEEE Trans. Med. Imaging* **18** 712–21

[49] Velec M *et al* 2017 Validation of biomechanical deformable image registration in the abdomen, thorax, and pelvis in a commercial radiotherapy treatment planning system *Med. Phys.* **44** 3407–17

[50] Zhang J, Wang J, Wang X and Feng D 2013 The adaptive FEM elastic model for medical image registration *Phys. Med. Biol.* **59** 97

[51] Zhao L and Jia K 2015 Deep adaptive log-demons: diffeomorphic image registration with very large deformations *Comput. Math. Methods. Med.* **2015** 836202

[52] Wu G *et al* 2013 Unsupervised deep feature learning for deformable registration of MR brain images *Med. Image. Comput. Comput. Assist. Interv.* **16** 649

[53] Yang X, Kwitt R, Styner M and Niethammer M 2017 Fast predictive multimodal image registration *IEEE 14th International Symposium on Biomedical Imaging* (Piscataway, NJ: IEEE) pp 858–62

[54] Miao S, Wang Z J and Liao R 2016 A CNN regression approach for real-time 2D/3D registration *IEEE Trans. Med. Imaging* **35** 1352–63

[55] Hu J *et al* 2021 End-to-end multimodal image registration via reinforcement learning *Med. Image Anal.* **68** 101878

[56] Sokooti H *et al* 2017 Nonrigid image registration using multi-scale 3D convolutional neural networks *Medical Image Computing and Computer Assisted Intervention* Lecture Notes in Computer Science vol 10433 *(Cham: Springer)* pp 232–9

[57] Stolk J *et al* 2007 Progression parameters for emphysema: a clinical investigation *Respir. Med.* **101** 1924–30

[58] Liu C, Ma L, Lu Z, Jin X and Xu J 2019 Multimodal medical image registration via common representations learning and differentiable geometric constraints *Electron. Lett.* **55** 316–8

[59] Chollet F 2017 Xception: deep learning with depthwise separable convolutions arXiv: 1610.02357v3

[60] Wu G, Kim M, Wang Q, Munsell B C and Shen D 2016 Scalable high-performance image registration framework by unsupervised deep feature representations learning *IEEE Trans. Biomed. Eng.* **63** 1505–16

[61] Mahapatra D, Antony B, Sedai S and Garnavi R 2018 Deformable medical image registration using generative adversarial networks *Proc. Int. Symp. Biomed. Imaging* **2018** 1449–53

[62] Hsu S H *et al* 2022 Synthetic CT generation for MRI-guided adaptive radiotherapy in prostate cancer *Front. Oncol.* **12** 969463

[63] Fu J *et al* 2019 Deep learning approaches using 2D and 3D convolutional neural networks for generating male pelvic synthetic computed tomography from magnetic resonance imaging *Med. Phys.* **46** 3788–98

[64] Cusumano D *et al* 2020 A deep learning approach to generate synthetic CT in low field MR-guided adaptive radiotherapy for abdominal and pelvic cases *Radiother. Oncol.* **153** 205–12

[65] Kawahara D and Nagata Y 2021 T1-weighted and T2-weighted MRI image synthesis with convolutional generative adversarial networks *Rep. Pract. Oncol. Radiother.* **26** 35

[66] Hyvärinen A and Hoyer P 2000 Emergence of phase- and shift-invariant features by decomposition of natural images into independent feature subspaces *Neural. Comput.* **12** 1705–20

[67] Shi X *et al* Convolutional LSTM network: a machine learning approach for precipitation nowcasting *NIPS'15: Proc. 29th Int. Conf. on Neural Information Processing Systems* vol 1 (Cambridge, MA: MIT Press) pp 802–10

[68] Chan Y *et al* 2007 Evaluation of on-board kV cone beam CT (CBCT)-based dose calculation *Med. Biol. Phys. Med. Biol.* **52** 685–705

[69] Yang Y, Schreibmann E, Li T, Wang C and Xing L 2007 Evaluation of on-board kV cone beam CT (CBCT)-based dose calculation *Phys. Med. Biol.* **52** 685–705

[70] Veiga C *et al* 2014 Toward adaptive radiotherapy for head and neck patients: feasibility study on using CT-to-CBCT deformable registration for 'dose of the day' calculations *Med. Phys.* **41** 031703

[71] Wu Q *et al* 2009 Adaptive replanning strategies accounting for shrinkage in head and neck IMRT *Int. J. Radiat. Oncol. Biol. Phys.* **75** 924–32

[72] Peters L J *et al* 2010 Critical impact of radiotherapy protocol compliance and quality in the treatment of advanced head and neck cancer: results from TROG 02.02 *J. Clin. Oncol.* **28** 2996–3001

[73] Jameson M G, Kumar S, Vinod S K, Metcalfe P E and Holloway L C 2014 Correlation of contouring variation with modeled outcome for conformal non-small cell lung cancer radiotherapy *Radiother. Oncol.* **112** 332–6

[74] Eminowicz G, Rompokos V, Stacey C and McCormack M 2016 The dosimetric impact of target volume delineation variation for cervical cancer radiotherapy *Radiother. Oncol.* **120** 493–9

[75] Contour ProtégéAI+™ *MIM Software* https://mimsoftware.com/radiation-oncology/contour-protegeai-plus

[76] Machine Learning in RayStation *RaySearch Laboratories* https://raysearchlabs.com/machine-learning-in-raystation/

[77] AutoContour *Radformation* https://radformation.com/autocontour/autocontour

[78] Centerline 2023 AI-driven contouring software integrated with Varian's treatment planning services *Varian Blog* 18 April https://varian.com/resources-support/blogs/ai-driven-contouring-software-integrated-varians-treatment

[79] Laiton-Bonadiez C, Sanchez-Torres G and Branch-Bedoya J 2022 Deep 3D neural network for brain structures segmentation using self-attention modules in MRI images *Sensors* **22** 2559

[80] Cubero L *et al* 2022 Deep learning-based segmentation of head and neck organs-at-risk with clinical partially labeled data *Entropy* **24** 1661

[81] Vrtovec T, Močnik D, Strojan P, Pernuš F and Ibragimov B 2020 Auto-segmentation of organs at risk for head and neck radiotherapy planning: from atlas-based to deep learning methods *Med. Phys.* **47** e929–50

[82] Koo J *et al* 2022 Development of a deep learning-based auto-segmentation of organs at risk for head and neck radiotherapy planning *Int. J. Radiat. Oncol. Biol. Phys.* **112** e8

[83] van Dijk L V *et al* 2020 Improving automatic delineation for head and neck organs at risk by deep learning contouring *Radiother. Oncol.* **142** 115–23

[84] Morris E D *et al* 2020 Cardiac substructure segmentation with deep learning for improved cardiac sparing *Med. Phys.* **47** 576

[85] Hu Q *et al* 2020 An effective approach for CT lung segmentation using mask region-based convolutional neural networks *Artif. Intell. Med.* **103** 101792

[86] Zhang T *et al* 2020 Comparison between atlas and convolutional neural network based automatic segmentation of multiple organs at risk in non-small cell lung cancer *Medicine* **99** e21800

[87] Feng X, Qing K, Tustison N J, Meyer C H and Chen Q 2019 Deep convolutional neural network for segmentation of thoracic organs-at-risk using cropped 3D images *Med. Phys.* **46** 2169–80

[88] Dong X *et al* 2019 Automatic multiorgan segmentation in thorax CT images using U-Net-GAN *Med. Phys.* **46** 2157

[89] Chen S *et al* 2020 Automatic multi-organ segmentation in dual-energy CT (DECT) with dedicated 3D fully convolutional DECT networks *Med. Phys.* **47** 552–62

[90] Zhu J *et al* 2019 Comparison of the automatic segmentation of multiple organs at risk in CT images of lung cancer between deep convolutional neural network-based and atlas-based techniques *Acta. Oncol.* **58** 257–64

[91] Rigaud B *et al* 2021 Automatic segmentation using deep learning to enable online dose optimization during adaptive radiation therapy of cervical cancer *Int. J. Radiat. Oncol. Biol. Phys.* **109** 1096–110

[92] Kawula M *et al* 2022 Dosimetric impact of deep learning-based CT auto-segmentation on radiation therapy treatment planning for prostate cancer *Radiat. Oncol* **17** 21

[93] Nikolov S *et al* 2021 Clinically applicable segmentation of head and neck anatomy for radiotherapy: deep learning algorithm development and validation study *J. Med. Internet. Res.* **23** e26151

[94] Anderson B M *et al* 2020 Automated contouring of contrast and noncontrast computed tomography liver images with fully convolutional networks *Adv. Radiat. Oncol* **6** 100464

[95] Loo S W, Martin W M C, Smith P, Cherian S and Roques T W 2012 Interobserver variation in parotid gland delineation: a study of its impact on intensity-modulated radiotherapy solutions with a systematic review of the literature *Br. J. Radiol.* **85** 1070

[96] Hellebust T P *et al* 2013 Dosimetric impact of interobserver variability in MRI-based delineation for cervical cancer brachytherapy *Radiother. Oncol.* **107** 13–9

[97] Yee Chang A T, Tan L T, Duke S and Ng W T 2017 Challenges for quality assurance of target volume delineation in clinical trials *Front. Oncol.* **7** 221

[98] Moghaddasi L, Bezak E and Marcu L G 2012 Current challenges in clinical target volume definition: tumour margins and microscopic extensions *Acta. Oncol.* **51** 984–95

[99] Jones D 1994 ICRU report 50—Prescribing, recording, and reporting photon beam therapy *Med. Phys.* **21** 833–4

[100] Ranjbarzadeh R *et al* 2021 Brain tumor segmentation based on deep learning and an attention mechanism using MRI multi-modalities brain images *Sci. Rep.* **11** 10930

[101] Men K, Dai J and Li Y 2017 Automatic segmentation of the clinical target volume and organs at risk in the planning CT for rectal cancer using deep dilated convolutional neural networks *Med. Phys.* **44** 6377–89

[102] Men K *et al* 2017 Deep deconvolutional neural network for target segmentation of nasopharyngeal cancer in planning computed tomography images *Front. Oncol.* **7** 315

[103] Lin L *et al* 2019 Deep learning for automated contouring of primary tumor volumes by MRI for nasopharyngeal carcinoma *Radiology* **291** 677–86

[104] Schreier J, Attanasi F and Laaksonen H 2019 A full-image deep segmenter for CT images in breast cancer radiotherapy treatment *Front. Oncol.* **9** 677

[105] Cardenas C E *et al* 2018 Deep learning algorithm for auto-delineation of high-risk oropharyngeal clinical target volumes with built-in dice similarity coefficient parameter optimization function *Int. J. Radiat. Oncol. Biol. Phys.* **101** 468

[106] Wang T *et al* 2019 Learning-based automatic segmentation of arteriovenous malformations on contrast CT images in brain stereotactic radiosurgery *Med. Phys.* **46** 3133

[107] Moeskops P *et al* 2018 Evaluation of a deep learning approach for the segmentation of brain tissues and white matter hyperintensities of presumed vascular origin in MRI *Neuroimage Clin.* **17** 251–62

[108] Bakx N *et al* 2023 Clinical evaluation of a deep learning segmentation model including manual adjustments afterwards for locally advanced breast cancer *Tech. Innov. Patient Support Radiat. Oncol.* **26** 100211

[109] van den Oever L B *et al* 2022 Qualitative evaluation of common quantitative metrics for clinical acceptance of automatic segmentation: a case study on heart contouring from CT images by deep learning algorithms *J. Digit. Imaging.* **35** 240–7

[110] Shelhamer E, Long J and Darrell T 2017 Fully convolutional networks for semantic segmentation *IEEE Trans. Pattern Anal. Mach. Intell.* **39** 640–51

[111] Chollet F 2016 Xception: deep learning with depthwise separable convolutions arXiv: 1610.02357v3

[112] Simonovsky M, Gutiérrez-Becker B, Mateus D, Navab N and Komodakis N 2016 A Deep Metric for Multimodal Registration arXiv: 1609.05396

[113] König L, Derksen A, Papenberg N and Haas B 2016 Deformable image registration for adaptive radiotherapy with guaranteed local rigidity constraints *Rad. Oncol.* **11** 122

IOP Publishing

Artificial Intelligence in Adaptive Radiation Therapy

Yi Wang and X. Sharon Qi

Chapter 10

Artificial intelligence-assisted dose prediction and re-planning

Ivan Vazquez, Laurence E Court and Ming Yang

Artificial intelligence (AI), particularly deep learning, is revolutionizing adaptive radiation therapy (ART) by enabling rapid dose prediction and treatment re-planning. This chapter examines cutting-edge applications of deep learning for dose prediction and re-planning in ART, highlighting their potential to dramatically reduce planning time while maintaining or improving plan quality. Key topics covered include convolutional neural network architectures for volumetric dose prediction, strategies for training and evaluating dose prediction models, and challenges in clinical implementation. The integration of AI tools into re-planning workflows is discussed, including applications in auto-segmentation, beam orientation selection, and treatment parameter optimization. Emerging techniques such as deep reinforcement learning for mimicking human planners are also discussed. While deep learning approaches show immense promise for enhancing ART efficiency and personalization, important considerations around data quality, model interpretability, and quality assurance must be addressed for safe clinical deployment. Overall, this chapter provides a comprehensive overview of the current state and future directions of AI-assisted dose prediction and re-planning in adaptive radiation therapy.

10.1 Introduction

The integration of artificial intelligence (AI) into adaptive radiation therapy (ART) represents a paradigm shift, with AI-powered tools showing promise in various aspects of the treatment process, such as contouring, dose prediction, treatment planning, and quality assurance. ART, as discussed in previous chapters, is a transformative approach that enables clinicians to modify treatment plans based on anatomical changes and treatment responses throughout the treatment course. However, to make the most of ART's benefits, it is crucial to estimate dose distributions quickly and precisely and re-plan effectively when needed [1–4].

doi:10.1088/978-0-7503-6119-4ch10

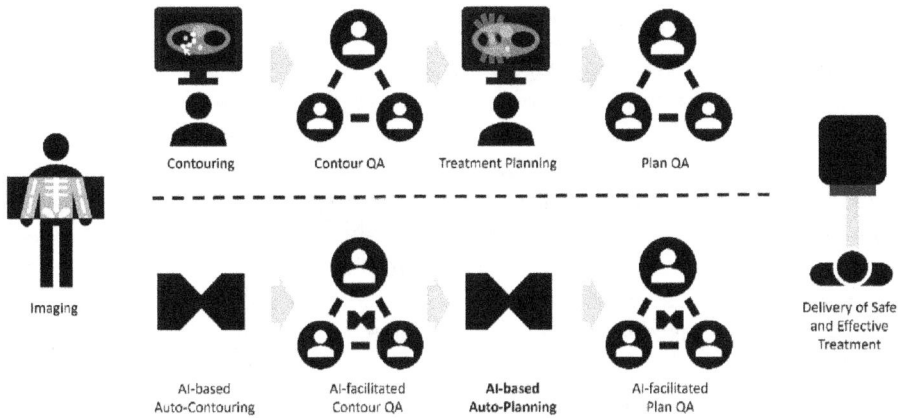

Figure 10.1. Comparison of the traditional manual radiotherapy planning workflow (top) and the AI-assisted workflow (bottom). AI tools can help streamline or fully automate key steps such as contouring, treatment planning, quality assurance (QA), and treatment delivery.

Conventional radiotherapy planning, depicted in the top portion of figure 10.1, usually demands a considerable amount of effort from human experts, and often takes over one day to complete [5]. This complex task involves contouring of tumors and critical structures, followed by iterative optimizations to maximize target coverage while minimizing harm to healthy organs [6, 7]. Patient-specific factors such as tumor size, location, and proximity to organs at risk (OARs) can add complexity while lengthening the planning process, straining resources, and potentially impacting treatment outcomes [8]. Generally, the quality and consistency of plans depend heavily on the expertise of the planning team, introducing variabilities in patient care between and even within institutions [9–11]. The time-consuming and labor-intensive nature of traditional planning methods, coupled with their reliance on expert human involvement, poses significant challenges, especially in regions facing shortages of trained professionals and limited access to radiotherapy equipment.

Over the past decades, efforts have been made to automate key steps in ART, including the estimation of suitable clinical dose distributions and the determination of treatment parameters. Traditional knowledge-based planning (KBP) tools, which rely on hand-engineered inputs and rule-based algorithms, were among the first promising attempts to automate processes in the ART pipeline. More recently, KBP methods have incorporated classical machine learning algorithms such as shallow artificial neural networks (ANNs) to improve their performance [12, 13]. Nevertheless, typical planning times with KBP methods remain in the range of minutes to hours, which might be unacceptable for online or real-time ART [12].

Currently, there is a growing trend towards the use of deep learning techniques for dose prediction and automatic planning, which are expected to overtake traditional KBP methods. This advancement brings previously unseen speeds and automation capabilities to the ART workflows, fueling new promising ideas and redefining the state-of-the-art in the field.

10.1.1 Overview of chapter content

This chapter focuses on cutting-edge applications of deep learning applicable to AI-assisted dose prediction and re-planning in ART. To establish a baseline for understanding the advantages of deep learning methods, we begin with a brief mention of traditional knowledge-based techniques that rely on rule-based algorithms and classical machine learning. Then, we explore the landscape of deep learning-based dose prediction, including convolutional neural networks (CNNs) that have shown remarkable promise in fast volumetric dose prediction.

The discussion will also cover challenges inherent to using modern AI solutions in the prediction of clinically acceptable dose volumes, including the need for standardized datasets and evaluation metrics, the impact of data quality, model interpretability, and the potential gaps between the predicted dose distributions and a truly optimal and personalized result for a patient.

Following the sections centered on dose prediction, we will discuss exciting possibilities for integrating AI in the re-planning stage of ART workflows, emphasizing the role of AI in enhancing planning efficiency. The chapter will conclude with a forward-looking perspective on the next steps in AI-assisted dose prediction and re-planning, highlighting potential avenues for innovation in this rapidly evolving field.

10.2 The landscape of AI-assisted dose prediction

AI-assisted dose prediction holds immense potential for streamlining radiotherapy treatment planning by shortening the time needed for a planner and a physician to iteratively arrive at a high-quality plan. Indeed, the aim of dose prediction is to generate a dose estimation that closely mimics the desired plan dose, i.e. what a skilled planning team would produce manually. As shown in figure 10.2, the

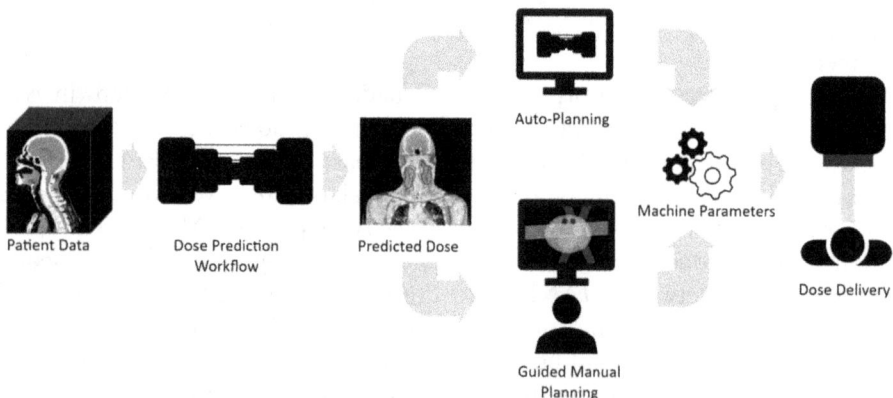

Figure 10.2. Hypothetical workflow showing two pathways for using AI-assisted dose prediction to generate the machine parameters (or instructions) needed to deliver the intended dose. After dose prediction, the resulting dose information can help guide planners in their search for a high-quality treatment or serve as inputs to an automatic-planning platform, where, for instance, it can help define optimization objectives.

predicted dose can then serve as a valuable tool for guiding both physician directives and plan generation, ultimately reducing the time required for subsequent steps in the planning workflow.

In recent years, the landscape of dose prediction research has undergone a significant shift from traditional knowledge-based approaches, including those using classical machine learning, to deep learning methods [3, 12, 14–16]. This section navigates this shift by first giving a brief overview of traditional dose prediction techniques followed by a look at deep learning methods, focusing on characteristics of this technology relevant to dose prediction for ART.

10.2.1 Traditional machine learning for dose prediction

Before the widespread use of traditional machine learning techniques, atlas-based methods and statistical models represented the most common knowledge-based strategies for developing high-quality radiation treatment plans with optimal dose distributions [12, 14, 17]. These rule-based approaches leveraged existing high-quality clinical data to correlate characteristics—such as CT-derived geometric features—of new and previously treated patients. From the correlations, the systems could then recommend possible dosimetric outcomes for a new patient such as dose–volume metrics and dose–volume histogram (DVH) curves.

Early efforts using machine learning often followed a similar philosophy, relying on hand-engineered features as inputs. Nevertheless, these knowledge-based tools leveraged the advantages of machine learning methods, such as the ability to readily model complex non-linear relationships, to achieve superior performance. Today, some commercial tools such as RapidPlan (Varian Medical Systems, Palo Alto, CA, USA), continue to rely on classical machine learning techniques such as support vector machines, random forests, and shallow artificial neural networks trained to predict achievable DVH curves or voxel-wise dose values for new patients [12, 13, 18]. In the case of RapidPlan, the resulting DVH curves can help define optimization objectives that guide the properties of the resulting treatment plan.

Knowledge-based methods, both rule-based or those using classical machine learning, have served to demonstrate the potential of dose prediction and automatic planning in radiotherapy, with some groups integrating them in end-to-end planning pipelines [19]. Commonly reported benefits from the adoption of knowledge-based methods include enhancements in plan quality, improved planning consistency, and reductions in planning times, sometimes exceeding 50% [12, 20–22].

Despite their well-documented advantages, these traditional methods have some limitations. For instance, they rely on a limited set of predefined hand-engineered features, which may fail to capture enough complexity in the data to ensure accuracy, in particular for patients with atypical geometries. Furthermore, many of these methods estimate DVH curves, which lack spatial information and suffer from non-uniqueness, as different volumetric dose distributions can produce identical DVH curves for an organ. Finally, the reported planning times with these tools might exceed what is demanded by online and real-time ART.

10.2.2 Deep learning-based dose prediction

Deep learning methods have emerged as powerful tools for predicting volumetric dose distributions in radiation therapy planning [2, 12, 14, 17]. The core strength of deep learning lies in its ability to automatically discover intricate mappings between input data (e.g. patient anatomy) and the intended output (e.g. dose distributions) [23]. This ability is particularly important when working with complex datasets such as those used in radiation therapy. Moreover, deep learning benefits from the highly optimized and freely available frameworks used for the creation and deployment of models [24, 25]. In combination with powerful graphical processing units (GPUs), models built with these tools can output predictions for entire 3D dose volumes in seconds [2], a speed beneficial to online and real-time ART.

In the last four years, the research momentum behind dose prediction has proved both steady and strong, with about 20–30 scholarly articles published annually including 19 on deep learning-based methods in 2020 alone. While the majority of published works have focused on the prostate [26–34], a common site for proof-of-concept studies, and the head and neck [35–48], considered a highly challenging site to convincingly demonstrate a model's capability, researchers have also investigated other sites, including the lungs [49, 50] cervix [38, 51, 52], and breast [53–55], showcasing the versatility of deep learning methods.

Given the breadth of the research in AI-assisted dose prediction, it is challenging—and outside of our scope—to fully capture the diversity of the existing ideas and implementations. Some of this diversity was captured by a single initiative for the advancement of dose prediction techniques, the OpenKBP Grand Challenge hosted by the American Association of Physicists in Medicine (AAPM) [56]. This competition, the first of its kind, not only saw a strong international involvement, including 195 participants from 28 countries, but also resulted in head-to-head comparisons of 28 unique prediction methods all working with the same data and evaluated equally. The top-performing models, all based on deep learning, highlighted the potential for deep learning to revolutionize dose prediction. The challenge also underscored the importance of model comparison using standardized datasets and evaluation metrics, which enables researchers to objectively evaluate the performance of different dose prediction methods and identify areas for improvement. This collaborative approach to model development and validation is crucial for advancing the field of AI-assisted dose prediction and ultimately improving patient care in radiation therapy.

The versatility of deep learning for dose prediction is demonstrated in figure 10.3, which shows results for example test patients (i.e. left out of the training data), including a head and neck patient treated with volumetric modulated arc therapy (VMAT), a breast cancer patient treated with VMAT, a cervix case treated with VMAT, a head and neck patient treated with scanning proton beams, and a prostate case treated with scanning proton beams. In all cases, predictions were made with models trained using the architecture described in Gronberg *et al*, a variation of the U-Net architecture [57] that ranked second in the OpenKBP Grand Challenge competition [56, 58]. Thus, this figure highlights how a single robust architecture can accurately handle multiple sites and modalities.

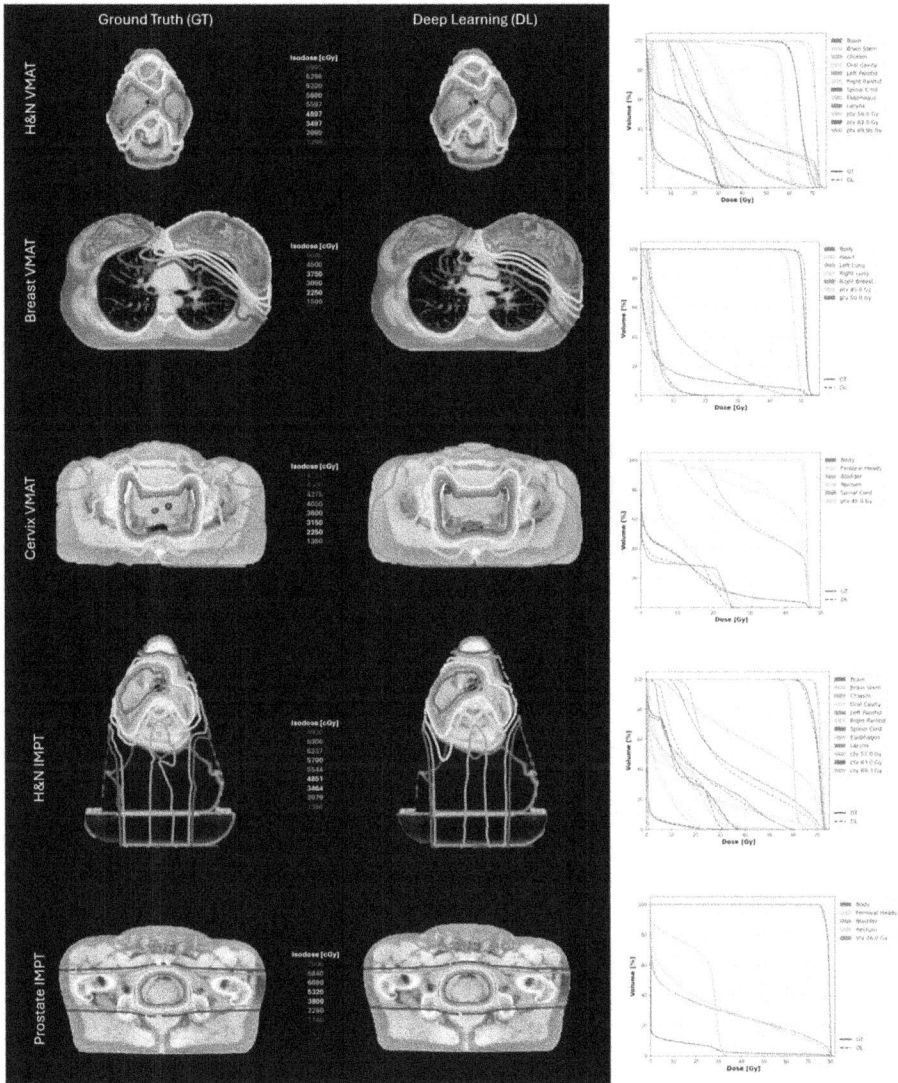

Figure 10.3. The left panel shows axial slices comparing the ground truth (GT) dose to that predicted by a deep learning model (DL) for volumetric modulated arc therapy (VMAT) and intensity-modulated proton therapy (IMPT) cases. The same architecture was used for all cases shown. The right column displays the corresponding dose–volume histograms of each patient comparing the dose predicted (dashed) and ground truth (solid) curves. STV = scanning target volume; PTV = planning target volume; CTV = clinical target volume.

While many of the successful deep learning-based dose prediction methods could benefit ART pipelines, for instance, by being used in the fashion illustrated by figure 10.2, only a couple have explicitly targeted ART. Recently, a method called intentional deep overfit learning (IDOL) was proposed for deep learning strategies targeting ART [42, 59, 60]. For dose prediction, the use of IDOL to generate patient-specific models resulted in significant improvements compared to results from training the same architectures in a more conventional, population-based style [42, 60]. The work of these researchers marks an attempt to predict a truly personalized dose distribution. This is a promising direction, since leveraging the speed of deep learning with methods that enhance the personalization of the predictions can unlock the true potential of AI-assisted dose prediction for ART.

10.2.2.1 Deep learning architectures used in dose prediction

U-Net [57, 61] has emerged as the most widely adopted deep learning architecture for dose prediction tasks. Nguyen et al [62] and Kearney et al [27] were among the pioneering researchers to demonstrate the effectiveness of U-Nets in this domain. Since then, numerous variations of U-Net have been explored for dose prediction across various anatomical sites, each offering unique advantages and trade-offs.

Figure 10.4 illustrates a generalized U-Net model, similar to those employed in dose prediction. The architecture consists of four resolution levels, represented by three sets of gray blocks with varying sizes—linked by 'skip connections'—and a central gray block representing the 'bottleneck' or lowest resolution level. These blocks, referred to here as convolutional blocks, typically apply a sequence of operations involving convolutions, normalization, and activation functions.

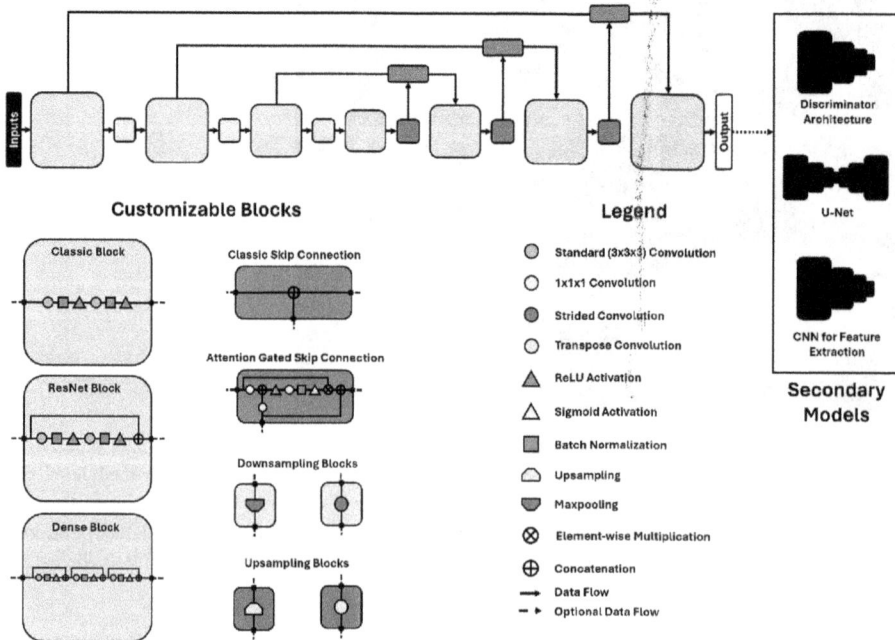

Figure 10.4. Schematic representation of U-Net architecture variations, composed of modular elements such as 'convolutional' blocks that operate on data by applying convolution, activation, and normalization operations. Downsampling, up-sampling, and skip connections, both classic and attention gated, are also illustrated as additional modules. Arrows indicate the direction of data flow, with dashed lines indicating an optional path used when a secondary deep learning architecture is available.

The model's encoder path (left side) progressively reduces the spatial resolution of the feature maps through downsampling operations, such as max pooling or strided convolutions. Conversely, the decoder path (right side) gradually recovers the spatial resolution using up-sampling techniques, such as nearest-neighbor interpolation or transpose convolutions.

Skip connections play a crucial role in U-Net architectures, allowing information to flow directly from the encoder to the decoder at corresponding resolution levels. These connections can be implemented through simple concatenation operations or, for example, using a more sophisticated attention-gated mechanisms [63–65]. Attention-gated skip connections enable the model to selectively focus on relevant features from the encoder, with the intention of enhancing the accuracy of the predicted outputs.

The components of convolutional blocks can significantly impact the model's performance and computational efficiency. Sources of variation in block types and operations used in dose prediction models include:

1. *ResNet-like blocks* [27, 66]: These blocks incorporate skip connections, as proposed in the ResNet architecture [67], allowing for deeper networks and improved gradient flow.

2. *Dense blocks* [45]: Inspired by the DenseNet architecture [68], these blocks utilize a dense set of concatenation operations to propagate the outputs of convolutional layers, effectively reusing features and increasing the cumulative number of forward-propagated features without increasing the number of trainable parameters.

3. *Dilated convolutions* [58, 69]: These convolutions expand the receptive field of the model without sacrificing resolution in the feature maps, enabling the capture of broader contextual information [70, 71].

4. *Activation and normalization functions*: Researchers have experimented with various activation functions, such as replacing the commonly used rectified linear unit (ReLU) [72] with Mish [73], and normalization techniques, such as substituting batch normalization [74] with group normalization [75], to enhance model performance and stability [47].

In some implementations, the outputs of U-Net serve as inputs to a secondary model, as indicated in figure 10.4. When the secondary model acts as a discriminator, the resulting architecture becomes trainable with an adversarial scheme. For example, the discriminator can learn to identify outputs deviating from the distribution of high-quality clinical dose volumes, providing an additional quality check akin to human oversight. For this reason, such architectures, which fall in the category of generative adversarial networks (or GANs), have been proposed to improve the accuracy and realism of dose predictions [30, 63, 76, 77].

Alternatively, a pre-trained CNN network can help extract features from both the clinical and predicted dose, which can be compared in the loss function to introduce additional penalties [47]. The extracted features are based on the trained—and thus task specific—filters of the pre-trained model, e.g. a ResNet 3D trained for video classification [78], and should produce matching results after operating on the clinical and predicted dose volumes if both were identical.

The third possibility illustrated in figure 10.4 involves using a second U-Net in a cascaded manner to further refine the predictions from the first model [46]. While computationally and resource intensive, the cascaded U-Net approach demonstrated superior performance in the OpenKBP Grand Challenge [56]. This technique has also resulted in superior performance for segmentation tasks [79].

The search for an optimal model design for dose prediction remains an empirical process, requiring extensive experimentation and domain expertise. The field of deep learning is highly dynamic, with new and increasingly capable methods being proposed frequently. This rapid progress is reflected in the diverse and complex landscape of architectural designs for dose prediction, which can prove challenging for new practitioners to navigate. Fortunately, well-designed, robust architectures, such as the top performers from the OpenKBP Grand Challenge, serve as excellent starting points for researchers entering the field. These proven models demonstrate remarkable versatility, accurately predicting dose distributions across different anatomical sites and even treatment modalities with minimal modifications. As exemplified by the results in figure 10.3, these architectures showcase the promise of deep learning in dose prediction and provide a solid foundation for further advancements in the field.

As research in this field continues to advance, we can expect further refinements and innovations in deep learning architectures tailored for dose prediction. These advancements will likely focus on improving prediction accuracy, computational efficiency, and adaptability to various clinical scenarios, ultimately enhancing the quality and efficiency of radiotherapy treatment planning.

10.2.2.2 Training and evaluation strategies

Just as there are numerous variations in architectures, the methodology for training and evaluating dose prediction models often differs between studies. One such difference involves dividing the data into random patches (or subregions) as opposed to using full volumes for the inputs. The patch-based approach can reduce the resource requirements while augmenting the effective number of inputs to the model [45]. On the other hand, using full volumes may better capture global contextual information and help a model uncover the underlying physics governing the dose deposition [66].

Input channels play a crucial role in enabling the model to learn an effective mapping between inputs and outputs. Most studies use a CT scan along with a set of contours marking the position of relevant OARs, thus providing anatomical context to the model. Additionally, an input channel with prescription information is often included, typically constructed using the target volumes to communicate the maximum prescribed dose at each voxel in the final dose distribution.

Researchers have also explored incorporating additional inputs to improve prediction accuracy. Some authors have investigated using distance information, e.g. the distance between OARs and the surface of target volumes, similar to the inputs of some traditional knowledge-based techniques [80, 81]. Furthermore, beam geometry information has been used to enhance the accuracy of model predictions, particularly when the training data reflects the use of heterogeneous beam arrangements [49, 76, 82, 83]. This information can be provided as a contour, such as that of an OAR, with nonzero values assigned to voxels with a high probability of receiving dose due to their proximity to the beam path. Alternatively, a fast dose calculation method can be used to produce an initial guess of an unmodulated dose distribution that communicates the desired beam arrangement [49].

The choice of loss function is critical for the success of a dose prediction model [84]. Most applications of dose prediction employ a mean squared error (MSE) or mean absolute error (MAE). In some cases, these popular choices are combined with terms that apply weighted penalties in the predictions inside regions of interest [58] or regularization techniques. Some researchers have also investigated the benefits of loss functions incorporating terms derived from DVH metrics [52] or using approximations of the DVH curves to impart domain-specific knowledge to the training [30, 66, 85]. Other types of loss functions, such as adversarial loss functions, have also been explored in the literature [30, 38, 63, 84].

An understanding of the generalizability and limitations of dose prediction methods can help us learn how to best translate them into clinical settings. To address this, some authors have explored training techniques that investigate the generalizability of models. For instance, studies have examined how pre-trained models performed with data from different anatomical sites [86] and other institutions [80]. This type of work is important, as the ability to use models across different sites and institutions could facilitate the adoption of dose prediction.

To ensure the reliability and robustness of dose prediction models, thorough evaluation using appropriate metrics and validation strategies is essential. Commonly reported metrics include mean absolute error (or dose score), errors in the mean and maximum dose received in regions of interest, errors in the radiation dose delivered to a specific percentage of the volume of relevant structures, errors in the conformity index, gamma passing rate evaluations, and the Dice similarity coefficient to quantify the overlap between isodose surfaces of the predicted and actual dose. In addition to these, Babier *et al* proposed the DVH score, which quantifies the average error in some relevant DVH metrics for both OARs and target volumes [56]. Although the majority of studies include one or more of these metrics, a standardized strategy to evaluate models has yet to be defined.

10.2.3 Challenges in AI-assisted dose prediction

A potential limitation of AI-assisted dose prediction involves the use of data from past plans to train models expected to perform well in today's clinics. This could present serious issues especially when past plans do not reflect state-of-the-art practices. Thus, as treatment techniques evolve over time, models will likely require periodic revisions to ensure that their performance aligns with the latest standards. Some techniques in AI, including transfer learning and online learning [87, 88], can help alleviate or overcome circumstances when sudden changes in standards makes a model unreliable.

Another challenge lies in clearly evaluating the quality—in a clinical sense—of the predicted dose [89]. Many dose prediction models are trained on diverse datasets produced by several planners and, thus, varying in quality. The output of models trained on such data may produce suboptimal results representing the average quality of the training data. This hypothesis should be tested with clinically relevant methods for quantifying the quality of dose distributions.

Furthermore, directly comparing the outputs from dose prediction models with delivered dose volumes, as it is often done, may not adequately convey the clinical utility of the predicted dose distributions. A more informative approach could be to first use the predicted dose to generate a deliverable dose, e.g. through inverse optimization, and then compare how well each deliverable dose volume—predicted and clinical—satisfy clinical directives [39].

The success of deep learning models for dose prediction in clinical settings remains mostly unexplored, with some studies indicating that tools that perform successfully during initial testing might not achieve the same degree of success when deployed in the clinic [90]. To reduce risks and ensure the safe deployment of AI-assisted tools in the clinic, systems designed to identify potential errors and quantify uncertainty are essential. Nguyen *et al* proposed methods to quantify the uncertainty of predictions, providing a feedback mechanism that can reveal to users when and where a model lacks confidence [43]. Such techniques can enhance the interpretability of results, a known challenge in the adoption of AI tools.

Users of AI-assisted tools also run the risk of becoming over-reliant on deep learning algorithms, which may reduce the amount of quality control checks performed and potentially lower treatment quality. This is an observed consequence of the use of automation called automation bias [91]. The establishment of clear guidelines for integrating AI-assisted dose prediction into clinical workflows could help reduce this risk.

The field of AI-assisted dose prediction can also benefit from the development of several standardized datasets and clearly defined evaluation metrics to quantify model effectiveness. The performance of deep learning models is generally proportional to the amount of training data available. In the context of dose prediction, limited data size and high variability in the training data both negatively impact performance. On the other hand, a lack of variability, even for large data volumes, can lead to biased dose prediction tools that produce errors when applied to patients with properties outside the training data distribution. Collaboration between institutions to share knowledge and data is also essential to mitigate problems such as bias and to leverage the data-driven performance of deep learning. However, such collaborations present significant challenges for the medical community, as they can impose resource and time requirements that are difficult for busy clinics to meet. As new technologies become available, tools to facilitate data sharing and their use in data-driven technologies will likely lead to significant improvements in AI-assisted dose prediction.

10.3 Re-planning workflows powered by AI

In ART, when the evaluation of a scheduled plan indicates suboptimal quality, such as demonstrating a high risk for loss in target coverage or unnecessary dose to OARs, re-planning is triggered. Re-planning aims to generate a new plan that enhances both target coverage and normal tissue sparing compared to the scheduled plan, as illustrated in figure 10.5, for a hypothetical online ART pipeline. However, re-planning comes with an undesirable consequence: the potential to significantly increase the overall complexity of the radiotherapy treatment [1, 3, 4, 92, 93]. This increased complexity poses a particular challenge in online ART, where the time window for re-planning is extremely limited, ideally in the order of a few minutes. Under these stringent time constraints, substantial human involvement in plan generation may be limited or even prohibited. Therefore, rapid re-planning techniques are not merely beneficial; they are a technological necessity for online ART [92, 94]. Notably, the development of such techniques not only addresses the challenges of online ART but also has the potential to benefit other forms of adaptive radiotherapy, such as offline ART, by streamlining the re-planning process and reducing the overall workload in a busy clinic.

AI, particularly deep learning, has the potential to accelerate or automate several steps essential for efficient and effective re-planning, including accurate segmentation, dose prediction, plan optimization, and quality assurance. Thus, integrating deep learning techniques into re-planning pipelines could significantly enhance both online and offline ART workflows. Currently, commercially available tools for ART, such as Varian's Ethos system, are leveraging deep learning and classical machine learning to meet the challenges of re-planning in online ART [94, 95]. These systems are actively contributing to the growing body of evidence supporting the benefits of automation and AI in radiation therapy. In this section, we explore four exciting applications of deep learning in radiation therapy and their potential roles in streamlining the re-planning process for both online and offline ART.

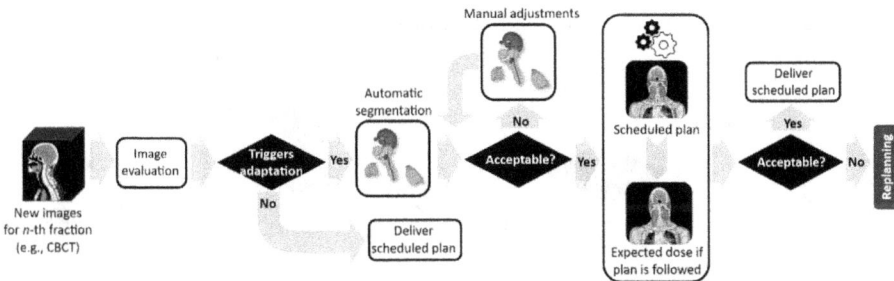

Figure 10.5. Flowchart illustrating the decision-making process in a hypothetical online ART pipeline during an intermediate fraction. When new images (e.g. CBCT) are acquired, the process first determines if adaptation is triggered based on observed anatomical changes. If triggered, a deep learning-based segmentation for the new images begins, and the results are subsequently evaluated. The output of the segmentation step helps in the estimation of the expected dose to the patient if the previous plan was followed. Once the daily dose under the scheduled plan is determined and evaluated, two outcomes become possible: delivering the scheduled plan if it is deemed acceptable or starting re-planning to generate a new plan that satisfies clinical constraints for target coverage and organs-at-risk sparing.

10.3.1 Deep learning for re-planning pipelines

10.3.1.1 Automatic segmentations

Figure 10.5 places auto-segmentation, the topic of chapter 9, near the start of the workflow, illustrating its relevance. This important step currently benefits from deep learning, even in commercial systems. Since segmented structures serve as inputs to subsequent steps in the ART workflow, including re-planning, accurate tools for fast automatic segmentation are essential. In the last decade, medical image segmentation powered by AI has made remarkable progress, significantly outpacing other areas integrating AI, including dose prediction. This advancement is supported by the availability of numerous curated datasets and performance evaluation schemes for both researchers and enthusiasts. While progress will likely continue at an accelerated pace, evidence already exists for cases where auto-segmentation tools matched human performance [96]. Furthermore, these tools have also demonstrated inherent reductions in both interobserver variability and the time needed for this labor-intensive and time-consuming step [96, 97].

10.3.1.2 From dose prediction to deliverable plans

Figure 10.6 illustrates a hypothetical scenario where deep learning is integrated into the re-planning process, with a primary focus on dose prediction. Before predicting the dose, three essential deep learning applications come into play: generating a set of structures (see figure 10.5), estimating the orientation of treatment beams when applicable, and predicting a suitable dose distribution using the outputs of the previous two steps. By integrating these deep learning components together, each with the potential for exceptional performance and a high degree of automation, the pipeline becomes highly autonomous and fast.

Predicting beam orientation, when relevant to the treatment, offers several benefits. For example, it eliminates the need for a planner to search for an optimal beam configuration, saving time. As with dose prediction, automating this step can potentially enhance consistency in plan quality. Using beam geometry information during dose prediction can also lead to gains in prediction accuracy [49, 76, 82].

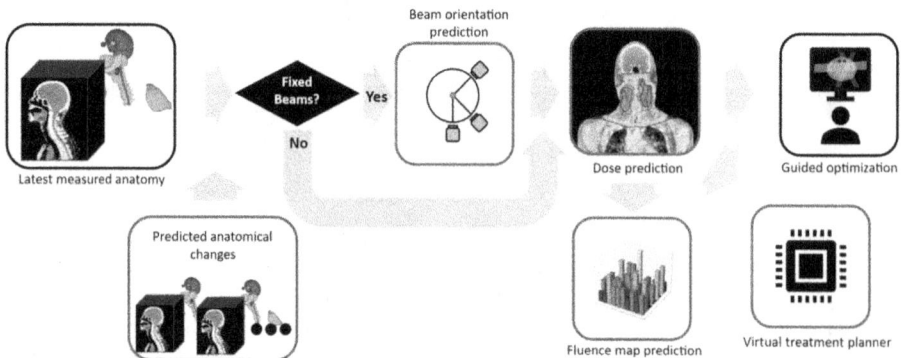

Figure 10.6. Flowchart depicting four potential applications of deep learning (indicated by the red outlines) that could be integrated into re-planning pipelines for online and offline ART.

Researchers have successfully employed deep learning for automatic beam angle selection in applications for intensity-modulated radiation therapy (IMRT) and intensity-modulated proton therapy (IMPT) [98, 99].

Once the dose is predicted based on the desired anatomical information, it serves as a guide for the optimization process, ultimately leading to a deliverable dose that meets the clinical objectives for the treatment. The feasibility of using deep learning-based dose prediction to guide plan optimization has been demonstrated in several studies [39, 48, 77]. Additionally, Mahmood *et al* showed that the deliverable dose obtained from optimizing based on deep learning-predicted doses was better at creating plans that met clinical criteria compared to state-of-the-art knowledge-based planning methods using traditional machine learning and other classical techniques [39].

Another promising application of deep learning is fluence map prediction, which involves generating a fluence map from a dose distribution [29, 100, 101]. The aim of this application is to bypass the need for a separate optimization step. By combining fluence map prediction with dose and angle prediction, a deep learning-based algorithm could generate all the necessary treatment parameters in a single step, potentially resulting in a tremendous reduction in planning time.

Although the approaches mentioned here could plausibly result in highly accelerated re-planning, it is worth noting that they all represent areas of active research. While significant progress has been made in recent years, there are still challenges to overcome before these techniques can be fully and safely integrated into clinical workflows.

10.3.1.3 *Virtualizing the re-planning process with deep reinforcement learning (DRL)*

One of the potential final steps of the flowchart in figure 10.6 shows the use of DRL to automate and expedite re-planning. DRL is a subfield of deep learning, which has been proposed as a tool for mimicking the human decision-making process during treatment planning [102–104]. The resulting networks, known as virtual treatment planner networks (VTPNs), are trained to intelligently tune the treatment planning system by making reasonable parameter adjustments to achieve high-quality plans. In practice, these networks monitor intermediate DVH curves for a developing plan and decide how to improve the plan by adjusting weights and threshold doses in the objective function.

Shen *et al* demonstrated the potential of this approach by training a VTPN on a small dataset of just 10 patients [103]. When applied to a test patient cohort, the trained network led to a substantial increase in plan quality. A subsequent study by Sprouts *et al* further highlighted the ability of VTPNs to improve plan quality and efficiency [104]. On average, the trained VTPN took less than one minute to reach the final treatment plan for each case using their in-house treatment planning system (TPS), while an experienced human planner required about three minutes to finish the same planning steps. These early applications of reinforcement learning suggest that by virtualizing the planning process, the speed and efficiency of deep learning can be leveraged to produce human-like results in a fraction of the time needed by human planners.

10.3.1.4 Anticipating change: deep learning for predicting anatomical variations

In addition to speeding up the planning process, deep learning tools could help in forecasting future anatomical changes for a patient. This possibility is indicated with a process at the start of figure 10.6. The result of such an algorithm, which serves as input to the subsequent steps of the flowchart, represents information that can facilitate the generation of a set of plans with deliverable dose distributions. This approach would resemble the 'plan-of-the-day' scheme used in some offline ART applications [92, 105]. In cases where the anatomical changes are accurately forecasted and a plan is ready, treatment can begin without delay or with minimal initial adjustments. The ability to use deep learning to forecast anatomical changes and potentially create corresponding plans with improved normal tissue sparing showed promise in a recent study [106]. Lee *et al* used a sequence-to-sequence (Seq2Seq) technique based on convolutional long short-term memory (Conv-LSTM) to predict the longitudinal changes of the esophagus and lung tumor.

10.3.1.5 Summary of deep learning for re-planning pipelines

While the scenarios discussed in relation to figure 10.6 are hypothetical, they are grounded in recent research findings. However, it is challenging to predict with certainty which techniques and ideas will drive the ART workflows of the future, particularly in fields well-positioned to benefit from the rapidly advancing domain of deep learning.

In our discussion, we omitted the quality assurance steps. Deep learning has led to impressive outcomes in applications pertinent to quality assurance, e.g. a tool for sub-second Monte Carlo calculations and similarly fast statistical robustness evaluation of IMPT dose distributions [107, 108]. The omission of these steps does not imply the unlikely ideal case of error-free performance by the discussed deep learning implementations. Indeed, if these methods were implemented, several quality control checks would be necessary to assess their performance and alert clinicians when errors or other unwanted circumstances are likely to occur.

10.4 Future directions of AI-assisted dose prediction and re-planning

Deep learning-based dose prediction is a growing field with a lot of untapped potential. The impressive performance of these techniques and their ability to automate tasks create many new possibilities. Figure 10.7 shows one such possibility, displaying two dose prediction outputs for a patient: one for a VMAT photon treatment and one for an IMPT treatment. This kind of volumetric dose information, combined with DVH metrics, could help clinicians compare different treatment modalities before starting formal treatment planning process. This can also benefit in situations when treatment machines become unavailable due to unforeseen circumstances, allowing for quick adaptations and minimizing treatment delays.

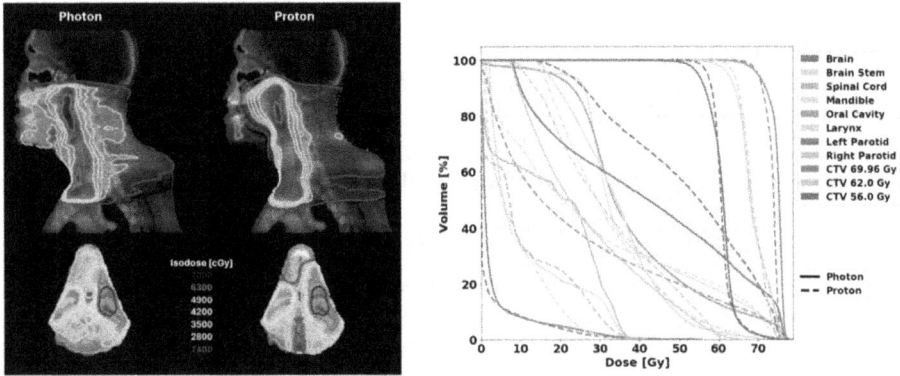

Figure 10.7. Comparison of two treatment modalities for the same patient. The left panel shows dose distributions predicted by a deep learning model for a VMAT plan (left) and IMPT plan (right).

Another example is real-time re-planning, which could be achieved with the help of dose prediction algorithms based on high-speed imaging techniques such as those in MRI-guided radiotherapy. In addition, accurate dose prediction using cone-beam CT could provide a useful quality assurance tool in online ART pipelines.

Dose prediction and deep learning methods for re-planning may also see significant performance improvements, driven by emerging trends such as the use of transformers [109, 110]. Transformer models have achieved remarkable success in natural language processing and computer vision tasks. These architectures excel at handling long-range dependencies and capturing complex spatial relationships, potentially helping achieve new state-of-the-art performance.

Future initiatives to advance collaboration and increase the availability of standardized, high-quality data will be essential in driving the development and validation of AI-assisted dose prediction and re-planning tools. Establishing shared datasets and benchmarks can facilitate the comparison and improvement of different models, while also promoting transparency and reproducibility in research. Collaborative efforts among institutions and researchers can accelerate this progress and ensure that the benefits of these technologies are widely accessible to the radiotherapy community.

Looking ahead, the next steps in AI-powered dose prediction and re-planning will require close collaboration among medical physicists, radiation oncologists, computer scientists, and industry partners. Continued research and development efforts are needed to refine AI models, integrate them into clinical workflows, and evaluate their impact on patient outcomes. By embracing the potential of AI and working towards its responsible and effective implementation, the radiotherapy community can bring about a new era of personalized, adaptive, and precise cancer care.

10.5 Summary

The integration of artificial intelligence, particularly deep learning, into adaptive radiation therapy workflows can have a profound impact on the field of radiation oncology. AI-assisted dose prediction and re-planning techniques offer promising solutions to some of the challenges associated with traditional radiotherapy planning, such as reducing time for otherwise laborious manual processes, increasing consistency in plan quality, and enabling rapid adaptations in response to anatomical changes.

Deep learning-based dose prediction methods have demonstrated remarkable accuracy and speed in estimating volumetric dose distributions across various anatomical sites and treatment modalities. These AI-powered tools can streamline the planning process by providing valuable guidance to clinicians as they aim to create safe and effective treatment plans.

The continued advancement of AI-assisted dose prediction and re-planning hinges on several key areas. The development of standardized datasets and evaluation metrics will be crucial for establishing benchmarks and facilitating meaningful comparisons between different models. Encouraging collaboration among institutions to share knowledge and data will accelerate progress and mitigate potential biases. Additionally, the exploration of innovative deep learning architectures and training strategies holds the promise of unlocking even greater levels of performance and automation. Crucially, addressing the challenges associated with clinical implementation, such as ensuring robust quality control and enhancing the interpretability of AI-generated outcomes, will be necessary to guarantee the safe and effective deployment of these tools in real-world healthcare settings.

The future of AI in adaptive radiation therapy holds immense promise, and much is left to be discovered. To fully harness the potential of AI-assisted dose prediction and re-planning, close collaboration among medical physicists, radiation oncologists, computer scientists, and industry partners is essential. As we look ahead, embracing the transformative power of AI in radiation oncology will be key to improving treatment efficacy, enhancing patient outcomes, and ultimately, advancing the fight against cancer.

References

[1] Yan D, Vicini F, Wong J and Martinez A 1997 Adaptive radiation therapy *Phys. Med. Biol.* **42** 123–32

[2] Nguyen D, Lin M H, Sher D, Lu W, Jia X and Jiang S 2022 Advances in automated treatment planning *Semin. Radiat. Oncol.* **32** 343–50

[3] Paganetti H, Botas P, Sharp G C and Winey B 2021 Adaptive proton therapy *Phys. Med. Biol.* **66** 22TR01

[4] Brock K K 2019 Adaptive radiotherapy: moving into the future *Semin. Radiat. Oncol.* **29** 181–4

[5] Das I J, Moskvin V and Johnstone P A 2009 Analysis of treatment planning time among systems and planners for intensity-modulated radiation therapy *J. Am. Coll. Radiol.* **6** 514–7

[6] Khan F M, Gibbons J P and Sperduto P W 2021 *Khan's Treatment Planning in Radiation Oncology* (Waltham, MA: Wolters Kluwer Health)

[7] Videtic G M, Vassil A D and Woody N M 2020 *Handbook of Treatment Planning in Radiation Oncology* (Berlin: Springer)

[8] Kishan A U, Cui J, Wang P C, Daly M E, Purdy J A and Chen A M 2014 Quantification of gross tumour volume changes between simulation and first day of radiotherapy for patients with locally advanced malignancies of the lung and head/neck *J. Med. Imaging. Radiat. Oncol.* **58** 618–24

[9] Scaggion A, Fusella M, Roggio A, Bacco S, Pivato N, Rossato M A, Peña L M A and Paiusco M 2018 Reducing inter- and intra-planner variability in radiotherapy plan output with a commercial knowledge-based planning solution *Phys. Med.* **53** 86–93

[10] Moore K L *et al* 2015 Quantifying unnecessary normal tissue complication risks due to suboptimal planning: a secondary study of RTOG 0126 *Int. J. Radiat. Oncol. Biol. Phys.* **92** 228–35

[11] Nelms B E, Robinson G, Markham J, Velasco K, Boyd S, Narayan S, Wheeler J and Sobczak M L 2012 Variation in external beam treatment plan quality: an inter-institutional study of planners and planning systems *Pract. Radiat. Oncol.* **2** 296–305

[12] Momin S, Fu Y, Lei Y, Roper J, Bradley J D, Curran W J, Liu T and Yang X 2021 Knowledge-based radiation treatment planning: a data-driven method survey *J. Appl. Clin. Med. Phys.* **22** 16–44

[13] Shiraishi S and Moore K L 2016 Knowledge-based prediction of three-dimensional dose distributions for external beam radiotherapy *Med. Phys.* **43** 378–87

[14] Kui X, Liu F, Yang M, Wang H, Liu C, Huang D, Li Q, Chen L and Zou B 2024 A review of dose prediction methods for tumor radiation therapy *Meta Radiol.* **2** 100057

[15] Glide-Hurst C K *et al* 2021 Adaptive radiation therapy (ART) strategies and technical considerations: a state of the ART review from NRG oncology *Int. J. Radiat. Oncol. Biol. Phys.* **109** 1054–75

[16] Fuglsang Jensen M and Witt Nystrom P 2020 Treatment planning for proton therapy: what is needed in the next 10 years? *Br. J. Radiol.* **93** 20190304

[17] Wang M, Zhang Q, Lam S, Cai J and Yang R 2020 A review on application of deep learning algorithms in external beam radiotherapy automated treatment planning *Front. Oncol.* **10** 580919

[18] Fogliata A, Cozzi L, Reggiori G, Stravato A, Lobefalo F, Franzese C, Franceschini D, Tomatis S and Scorsetti M 2019 RapidPlan knowledge based planning: iterative learning process and model ability to steer planning strategies *Radiat. Oncol.* **14** 187

[19] Huang K *et al* 2024 Automatic end-to-end VMAT treatment planning for rectal cancers *J. Appl. Clin. Med. Phys.* **25** e14259

[20] Creemers I H P, Kusters J M A M, van Kollenburg P G M, Bouwmans L C W, Schinagl D A X and Bussink J 2019 Comparison of dose metrics between automated and manual radiotherapy planning for advanced stage non-small cell lung cancer with volumetric modulated arc therapy *Phys. Imaging. Radiat. Oncol.* **9** 92–6

[21] van Gysen K, O'Toole J, Le A, Wu K, Schuler T, Porter B, Kipritidis J, Atyeo J, Brown C and Eade T 2020 Rolling out RapidPlan: what we've learnt *J. Med. Radiat. Sci.* **67** 310–7

[22] Rhee D J, Jhingran A, Kisling K, Cardenas C, Simonds H and Court L 2020 Automated radiation treatment planning for cervical cancer *Semin. Radiat. Oncol.* **30** 340–7

[23] Lecun Y, Bengio Y and Hinton G 2015 Deep learning *Nature* **521** 436–44

[24] Abadi M *et al* 2016 TensorFlow: large-scale machine learning on heterogeneous distributed systems arXiv: 1603.04467

[25] Paszke A *et al* 2019 PyTorch: an imperative style, high-performance deep learning library arXiv: 1912.01703v1

[26] Kajikawa T, Kadoya N, Ito K, Takayama Y, Chiba T, Tomori S, Nemoto H, Dobashi S, Takeda K and Jingu K 2019 A convolutional neural network approach for IMRT dose distribution prediction in prostate cancer patients *J. Radiat. Res.* **60** 685–93

[27] Kearney V, Chan J W, Haaf S, Descovich M and Solberg T D 2018 DoseNet: a volumetric dose prediction algorithm using 3D fully-convolutional neural networks *Phys. Med. Biol.* **63** 235022

[28] Kontaxis C, Bol G H, Lagendijk J J W and Raaymakers B W 2020 DeepDose: towards a fast dose calculation engine for radiation therapy using deep learning *Phys. Med. Biol.* **65** 075013

[29] Li X, Zhang J, Sheng Y, Chang Y, Yin F F, Ge Y, Wu Q J and Wang C 2020 Automatic IMRT planning via static field fluence prediction (AIP-SFFP): a deep learning algorithm for real-time prostate treatment planning *Phys. Med. Biol.* **65** 175014

[30] Nguyen D, McBeth R, Sadeghnejad Barkousaraie A, Bohara G, Shen C, Jia X and Jiang S 2020 Incorporating human and learned domain knowledge into training deep neural networks: a differentiable dose–volume histogram and adversarial inspired framework for generating Pareto optimal dose distributions in radiation therapy *Med. Phys.* **47** 837–49

[31] Wang W, Chang Y, Liu Y, Liang Z, Liao Y, Qin B, Liu X and Yang Z 2022 Feasibility study of fast intensity-modulated proton therapy dose prediction method using deep neural networks for prostate cancer *Med. Phys.* **49** 5451–63

[32] Wang J, Hu J, Song Y, Wang Q, Zhang X, Bai S and Yi Z 2022 VMAT dose prediction in radiotherapy by using progressive refinement UNet *Neurocomputing* **488** 528–39

[33] Ma J, Nguyen D, Bai T, Folkerts M, Jia X, Lu W, Zhou L and Jiang S 2021 A feasibility study on deep learning-based individualized 3D dose distribution prediction *Med. Phys.* **48** 4438–47

[34] Liu J, Zhang X, Cheng X and Sun L 2024 A deep learning-based dose prediction method for evaluation of radiotherapy treatment planning *J. Radiat. Res. Appl. Sci.* **17** 100757

[35] Chen X, Men K, Li Y, Yi J and Dai J 2019 A feasibility study on an automated method to generate patient-specific dose distributions for radiotherapy using deep learning *Med. Phys.* **46** 56–64

[36] Chen X, Men K, Zhu J, Yang B, Li M, Liu Z, Yan X, Yi J and Dai J 2021 DVHnet: a deep learning-based prediction of patient-specific dose volume histograms for radiotherapy planning *Med. Phys.* **48** 2705–13

[37] Liu Z, Chen X, Men K, Yi J and Dai J 2020 A deep learning model to predict dose–volume histograms of organs at risk in radiotherapy treatment plans *Med. Phys.* **47** 5467–81

[38] Zhang G, Jiang Z, Zhu J and Wang L 2022 Dose prediction for cervical cancer VMAT patients with a full-scale 3D-cGAN-based model and the comparison of different input data on the prediction results *Radiat. Oncol.* **17** 179

[39] Mahmood R, Babier A, McNiven A, Diamant A and Chan T C Y 2018 Automated treatment planning in radiation therapy using generative adversarial networks *Proc. Mach. Learn. Res* **85** 484–99

[40] Mao X, Pineau J, Keyes R and Enger S A 2020 RapidBrachyDL: rapid radiation dose calculations in brachytherapy via deep learning *Int. J. Radiat. Oncol. Biol. Phys.* **108** 802–12

[41] McIntosh C, Welch M, McNiven A, Jaffray D A and Purdie T G 2017 Fully automated treatment planning for head and neck radiotherapy using a voxel-based dose prediction and dose mimicking method *Phys. Med. Biol.* **62** 5926–44

[42] Maniscalco A, Liang X, Lin M H, Jiang S and Nguyen D 2023 Intentional deep overfit learning for patient-specific dose predictions in adaptive radiotherapy *Med. Phys.* **50** 5354–63

[43] Nguyen D, Sadeghnejad Barkousaraie A, Bohara G, Balagopal A, McBeth R, Lin M H and Jiang S 2021 A comparison of Monte Carlo dropout and bootstrap aggregation on the performance and uncertainty estimation in radiation therapy dose prediction with deep learning neural networks *Phys. Med. Biol.* **66** 054002

[44] Osman A F I, Tamam N M and Yousif Y A M 2023 A comparative study of deep learning-based knowledge-based planning methods for 3D dose distribution prediction of head and neck *J. Appl. Clin. Med. Phys.* **24** e14015

[45] Nguyen D, Jia X, Sher D, Lin M H, Iqbal Z, Liu H and Jiang S 2019 3D radiotherapy dose prediction on head and neck cancer patients with a hierarchically densely connected U-Net deep learning architecture *Phys. Med. Biol.* **64** 065020

[46] Liu S, Zhang J, Li T, Yan H and Liu J 2021 Technical note: a cascade 3D U-Net for dose prediction in radiotherapy *Med. Phys.* **48** 5574–82

[47] Zimmermann L, Faustmann E, Ramsl C, Georg D and Heilemann G 2021 Technical note: dose prediction for radiation therapy using feature-based losses and one cycle learning *Med. Phys.* **48** 5562–6

[48] Fan J, Wang J, Chen Z, Hu C, Zhang Z and Hu W 2019 Automatic treatment planning based on three-dimensional dose distribution predicted from deep learning technique *Med. Phys.* **46** 370–81

[49] Barragán-Montero A M, Nguyen D, Lu W, Lin M H, Norouzi-Kandalan R, Geets X, Sterpin E and Jiang S 2019 Three-dimensional dose prediction for lung IMRT patients with deep neural networks: robust learning from heterogeneous beam configurations *Med. Phys.* **46** 3679–91

[50] Shao Y, Zhang X, Wu G, Gu Q, Wang J, Ying Y, Feng A, Xie G, Kong Q and Xu Z 2021 Prediction of three-dimensional radiotherapy optimal dose distributions for lung cancer patients with asymmetric network *IEEE J. Biomed. Health Inform.* **25** 1120–7

[51] Jihong C, Penggang B, Xiuchun Z, Kaiqiang C, Wenjuan C, Yitao D, Jiewei Q, Kerun Q, Jing Z and Tianming W 2020 Automated intensity modulated radiation therapy treatment planning for cervical cancer based on convolution neural network *Technol. Cancer Res. Treat.* **19**

[52] Gronberg M P *et al* 2023 Deep learning-based dose prediction to improve the plan quality of volumetric modulated arc therapy for gynecologic cancers *Med. Phys.* **50** 6639–48

[53] Ahn S H *et al* 2021 Deep learning method for prediction of patient-specific dose distribution in breast cancer *Radiat. Oncol.* **16** 154

[54] Bakx N, Bluemink H, Hagelaar E, van der Sangen M, Theuws J and Hurkmans C 2021 Development and evaluation of radiotherapy deep learning dose prediction models for breast cancer *Phys. Imaging Radiat. Oncol.* **17** 65–70

[55] Lin T C, Lin C Y, Li K C, Ji J H, Liang J A, Shiau A C, Liu L C and Wang T H 2020 Automated hypofractionated IMRT treatment planning for early-stage breast cancer *Radiat. Oncol.* **15** 67

[56] Babier A, Zhang B, Mahmood R, Moore K L, Purdie T G, McNiven A L and Chan T C Y 2021 OpenKBP: the open-access knowledge-based planning grand challenge and dataset *Med. Phys.* **48** 5549–61

[57] Ronneberger O, Fischer P and Brox T 2015 U-Net: convolutional networks for biomedical image segmentation arXiv:1505.04597

[58] Gronberg M P, Gay S S, Netherton T J, Rhee D J, Court L E and Cardenas C E 2021 Technical note: dose prediction for head and neck radiotherapy using a three-dimensional dense dilated U-Net architecture *Med. Phys.* **48** 5567–73

[59] Chun J, Park J C, Olberg S, Zhang Y, Nguyen D, Wang J, Kim J S and Jiang S 2022 Intentional deep overfit learning (IDOL): a novel deep learning strategy for adaptive radiation therapy *Med. Phys.* **49** 488–96

[60] Maniscalco A, Liang X, Lin M H, Jiang S and Nguyen D 2023 Single patient learning for adaptive radiotherapy dose prediction *Med. Phys.* **50** 7324–37

[61] Çiçek Ö, Abdulkadir A, Lienkamp S S, Brox T and Ronneberger O 2016 3D U-Net: learning dense volumetric segmentation from sparse annotation *Medical Image Computing and Computer-Assisted Intervention* Lecture Notes in Computer Science vol 9901 *(Cham: Springer)*

[62] Nguyen D, Long T, Jia X, Lu W, Gu X, Iqbal Z and Jiang S 2019 A feasibility study for predicting optimal radiation therapy dose distributions of prostate cancer patients from patient anatomy using deep learning *Sci. Rep.* **9** 1076

[63] Kearney V, Chan J W, Wang T, Perry A, Descovich M, Morin O, Yom S S and Solberg T D 2020 DoseGAN: a generative adversarial network for synthetic dose prediction using attention-gated discrimination and generation *Sci. Rep.* **10** 11073

[64] Kearney V, Chan J W, Wang T, Perry A, Yom S S and Solberg T D 2019 Attention-enabled 3D boosted convolutional neural networks for semantic CT segmentation using deep supervision *Phys. Med. Biol.* **64** 135001

[65] Oktay O *et al* 2018 Attention U-Net: learning where to look for the pancreas arXiv:1804.03999

[66] Soomro M H, Gabriel V, Alves L, Nourzadeh H and Siebers J V 2021 DeepDoseNet: a deep learning model for 3D dose prediction in radiation therapy arXiv:2111.00077

[67] He K, Zhang X, Ren S and Sun J 2016 Identity mappings in deep residual networks arXiv:1603.05027

[68] Huang G, Liu Z, van der Maaten L and Weinberger K Q 2017 Densely connected convolutional networks *Proc. of the IEEE Conf. on Computer Vision and Pattern Recognition* (Piscataway, NJ: IEEE)

[69] Zhang J, Liu S, Yan H, Li T, Mao R and Liu J 2020 Predicting voxel-level dose distributions for esophageal radiotherapy using densely connected network with dilated convolutions *Phys. Med. Biol.* **65** 205013

[70] Yu F and Koltun V 2015 Multi-scale context aggregation by dilated convolutions arXiv:1511.07122

[71] Yu F, Koltun V and Funkhouser T 2017 Dilated residual networks *2017 IEEE Conf. on Computer Vision and Pattern Recognition* (Piscataway, NJ: IEEE)

[72] Nair V and Hinton G E 2010 Rectified linear units improve restricted Boltzmann machines *Proc. of the 27th Int. Conf. on Machine Learning (ICML-10)* pp 807–14

[73] Misra D 2019 Mish: a self regularized non-monotonic activation function arXiv:1908.08681

[74] Ioffe S and Szegedy C 2015 Batch normalization: sccelerating deep network training by reducing internal covariate shift *Proc. Mach. Learn. Res.* **37** 448–56

[75] Wu Y and He K 2018 Group normalization *Proc. of the European Conf. on Computer Vision (ECCV)* pp 3–19

[76] Gao R, Lou B, Xu Z, Comaniciu D and Kamen A 2023 Flexible-C m GAN: towards precise 3D dose prediction in radiotherapy *Proc. of the IEEE/CVF Conf. on Computer Vision and Pattern Recognition* (Piscataway, NJ: IEEE)

[77] Babier A, Mahmood R, McNiven A L, Diamant A and Chan T C Y 2020 Knowledge-based automated planning with three-dimensional generative adversarial networks *Med. Phys.* **47** 297–306

[78] Tran D, Wang H, Torresani L, Ray J, Lecun Y and Paluri M 2018 A closer look at spatiotemporal convolutions for action recognition *Proc. of the IEEE Computer Society Conf. on Computer Vision and Pattern Recognition* (Los Alamitos, CA: IEEE Computer Society) pp 6450–9

[79] Isensee F *et al* 2018 nnU-Net: self-adapting framework for U-Net-based medical image segmentation *Bildverarbeitung für die Medizin* (Wiesbaden: Springer Vieweg)

[80] Mashayekhi M, Tapia I R, Balagopal A, Zhong X, Barkousaraie A S, McBeth R, Lin M H, Jiang S and Nguyen D 2022 Site-agnostic 3D dose distribution prediction with deep learning neural networks *Med. Phys.* **49** 1391–406

[81] Yue M, Xue X, Wang Z, Lambo R L, Zhao W, Xie Y, Cai J and Qin W 2022 Dose prediction via distance-guided deep learning: initial development for nasopharyngeal carcinoma radiotherapy *Radiother. Oncol.* **170** 198–204

[82] Zhang L *et al* 2023 Beam mask and sliding window-facilitated deep learning-based accurate and efficient dose prediction for pencil beam scanning proton therapy *Med. Phys.* **51** 1484–98

[83] Zhou J, Peng Z, Song Y, Chang Y, Pei X, Sheng L and Xu X G 2020 A method of using deep learning to predict three-dimensional dose distributions for intensity-modulated radiotherapy of rectal cancer *J. Appl. Clin. Med. Phys.* **21** 26–37

[84] Bai X, Zhang J, Wang B, Wang S, Xiang Y and Hou Q 2021 Sharp loss: a new loss function for radiotherapy dose prediction based on fully convolutional networks *Biomed. Eng. Online* **20** 101

[85] Jhanwar G, Dahiya N, Ghahremani P, Zarepisheh M and Nadeem S 2022 Domain knowledge driven 3D dose prediction using moment-based loss function *Phys. Med. Biol.* **67** 185017

[86] Kandalan R N, Nguyen D, Rezaeian N H, Barragán-Montero A M, Breedveld S, Namuduri K, Jiang S and Lin M H 2020 Dose prediction with deep learning for prostate cancer radiation therapy: model adaptation to different treatment planning practices *Radiother. Oncol.* **153** 228–35

[87] Chen T, Goodfellow I and Shlens J 2015 Net2Net: accelerating learning via knowledge transfer arXiv: 1511.05641

[88] Sahoo D, Pham Q, Lu J and Hoi S C H 2017 Online deep learning: learning deep neural networks on the fly arXiv:1 711.03705

[89] Baroudi H *et al* 2023 Automated contouring and planning in radiation therapy: what is 'clinically acceptable'? *Diagnostics* **13** 667

[90] McIntosh C *et al* 2021 Clinical integration of machine learning for curative-intent radiation treatment of patients with prostate cancer *Nat. Med.* **27** 999–1005

[91] Goddard K, Roudsari A and Wyatt J C 2012 Automation bias: a systematic review of frequency, effect mediators, and mitigators *J. Am. Med. Inform. Assoc.* **19** 121–7

[92] Lavrova E, Garrett M D, Wang Y F, Chin C, Elliston C, Savacool M, Price M, Kachnic L A and Horowitz D P 2023 Adaptive radiation therapy: a review of CT-based techniques *Radiol. Imaging. Cancer.* **5** e230011

[93] Qiu Z, Olberg S, den Hertog D, Ajdari A, Bortfeld T and Pursley J 2023 Online adaptive planning methods for intensity-modulated radiotherapy *Phys. Med. Biol.* **68** 10TR01

[94] Pokharel S, Pacheco A and Tanner S 2022 Assessment of efficacy in automated plan generation for Varian Ethos intelligent optimization engine *J. Appl. Clin. Med. Phys.* **23** e13539

[95] Moazzezi M, Rose B, Kisling K, Moore K L and Ray X 2021 Prospects for daily online adaptive radiotherapy via ethos for prostate cancer patients without nodal involvement using unedited CBCT auto-segmentation *J. Appl. Clin. Med. Phys.* **22** 82–93

[96] Nikolov S *et al* 2021 O Clinically applicable segmentation of head and neck anatomy for radiotherapy: deep learning algorithm development and validation study *J. Med. Internet Res.* **23** e26151

[97] Cardenas C E, Yang J, Anderson B M, Court L E and Brock K B 2019 Advances in auto-segmentation *Semin. Radiat. Oncol.* **29** 185–97

[98] Kaderka R *et al* 2022 Toward automatic beam angle selection for pencil-beam scanning proton liver treatments: a deep learning-based approach *Med. Phys.* **49** 4293–304

[99] Sadeghnejad Barkousaraie A, Ogunmolu O, Jiang S and Nguyen D 2020 A fast deep learning approach for beam orientation optimization for prostate cancer treated with intensity-modulated radiation therapy *Med. Phys.* **47** 880–97

[100] Ma L, Chen M, Gu X and Lu W 2020 Deep learning-based inverse mapping for fluence map prediction *Phys. Med. Biol.* **65** 235035

[101] Wang W, Sheng Y, Palta M, Czito B, Willett C, Hito M, Yin F F, Wu Q, Ge Y and Wu Q J 2021 Deep learning-based fluence map prediction for pancreas stereotactic body radiation therapy with simultaneous integrated boost *Adv. Radiat. Oncol.* **6** 100672

[102] Shen C, Chen L and Jia X 2021 A hierarchical deep reinforcement learning framework for intelligent automatic treatment planning of prostate cancer intensity modulated radiation therapy *Phys. Med. Biol.* **66** 134002

[103] Shen C, Chen L, Gonzalez Y and Jia X 2021 Improving efficiency of training a virtual treatment planner network via knowledge-guided deep reinforcement learning for intelligent automatic treatment planning of radiotherapy *Med. Phys.* **48** 1909–20

[104] Sprouts D, Gao Y, Wang C, Jia X, Shen C and Chi Y 2022 The development of a deep reinforcement learning network for dose–volume-constrained treatment planning in prostate cancer intensity modulated radiotherapy *Biomed. Phys. Eng. Express* **8** 045008

[105] Sonke J J, Aznar M and Rasch C 2019 Adaptive radiotherapy for anatomical changes *Semin. Radiat. Oncol.* **29** 245–57

[106] Lee D, Hu Y, Kuo L, Alam S, Yorke E, Li A, Rimner A and Zhang P 2022 Deep learning driven predictive treatment planning for adaptive radiotherapy of lung cancer *Radiother. Oncol.* **169** 57–63

[107] Pastor-Serrano O and Perkó Z 2022 Millisecond speed deep learning based proton dose calculation with Monte Carlo accuracy *Phys. Med. Biol.* **67** 105006

[108] Vazquez I, Gronberg M P, Zhang X, Court L E, Zhu X R, Frank S J and Yang M 2023 A deep learning-based approach for statistical robustness evaluation in proton therapy treatment planning: a feasibility study *Phys. Med. Biol.* **68** 095014

[109] Wen L, Xiao J, Tan S, Wu X, Zhou J, Peng X and Wang Y 2023 A transformer-embedded multi-task model for dose distribution prediction *Int. J. Neural Syst.* **33** 2350043

[110] Jiao Z, Peng X, Wang Y, Xiao J, Nie D, Wu X, Wang X, Zhou J and Shen D 2023 TransDose: transformer-based radiotherapy dose prediction from CT images guided by super-pixel-level GCN classification *Med. Image Anal.* **89** 102902

Chapter 11

Artificial intelligence-based intrafraction motion monitoring for precise adaptive radiation therapy delivery

Lianli Liu and James M Balter

Patient motion during treatment delivery results in discrepancies between the actual dose delivered and the planned dose distribution and is a significant source of radiation treatment uncertainty. Real-time adaptation of treatment delivery parameters based on changing patient anatomy has the potential to reduce dose delivery uncertainty and improve treatment precision. This chapter will review the current status of motion monitoring for real-time adaptive radiation therapy and discuss the challenges and the use of artificial intelligence (AI) in supporting real-time adaptive treatment workflow.

11.1 Introduction

Adaptive radiation therapy (ART) is based on the premise that modifying treatments to changes in patient configuration and/or biology will yield improved tumor control and/or organ-at-risk (OAR) sparing. While there are now a number of systems and workflows in place that enable adaptation as frequently as daily (or even multiple times in a fraction, although this is impractical in most systems at the time of writing due to the complexity of the adaptation workflows currently in place) to such changes, intrafraction patient motion can significantly alter the shape and position of targets, as well as surrounding OARs, thus potentially diminishing the benefit of adaptation. Various physiologic sources contribute to intrafraction motion, with breathing being the most significant for thoracic and abdominal targets, where motions up to 50 mm have been reported [1, 2]. Cardiac motion also contributes to target position uncertainty and has been observed in lung tumors, mediastinal lymph nodes, and liver tumors [3–5]. Peristalsis-induced motions, of a similar magnitude to respiratory motion, have been reported for abdominal cases [6, 7]. Slow internal configuration changes can become significant with elongated treatment times, where position drifts of over 5 mm have been observed within a 20 min time window [8]. Changes in organ filling status, such as the bladder and rectum, also lead to intrafraction motion for both the organs themselves as well as and nearby targeted tissue and OARs, with motion greater than 30 mm being reported [9–11].

The changes of configuration and position of targets and OARs due to intra-fraction motion can result in discrepancies between the actual dose delivered and that planned based on static patient anatomy. Real-time implementation of adaptive radiotherapy ('real-time' ART) aims to adjust treatment delivery parameters based on changing patient anatomy and has the potential to reduce dose delivery uncertainty and improve treatment precision. With the development of both imaging and radiation delivery techniques, the potential for 'real-time' monitoring of, and reaction to, intrafraction motion is emerging. In this chapter, we will first review the current status and challenges of real-time ART for maintaining precise treatment delivery, then describe both practical use and research of AI in supporting real-time ART workflows. Finally, we will discuss potential future areas of development to further support 'real-time' adaptation during treatment delivery.

11.2 Real-time ART during treatment delivery: current status and challenges

To adapt to changes, patient anatomical information needs to be sampled frequently during treatment delivery. Motion information is then estimated based on the sampled data and adjustments to treatment delivery parameters are made accord-ingly. Figure 11.1 outlines the major steps of real-time ART during treatment delivery. Successful implementation of real-time ART therefore requires several technical components including imaging tools that sample patient data at a temporal resolution high enough to capture the motion-induced anatomical changes, data analysis tools that extract motion information from the acquired patient images, and

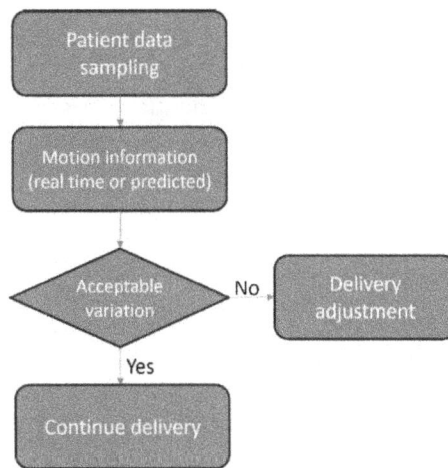

Figure 11.1. Major steps of real-time ART.

treatment delivery tools that adjust treatment parameters quickly based on the motion information.

11.2.1 Imaging-based motion monitoring

Various imaging techniques have been developed to sample patient motion information during treatment delivery. These techniques vary in both imaging frequency and imaging content and are therefore designed to monitor different types of motion. For example, fast breathing motion requires sub-second sampling rates but can be estimated from external patient images. On the other hand, slow prostate motion can be monitored less frequently but requires direct imaging of the internal patient anatomy. The motion information extracted from the images also varies from simple 1D shift information to high-dimensional deformation vector fields. Infrared and optical imaging systems have been developed to image reflective markers or the patient's skin surface [12–15]. External surrogate information, extracted from the marker positions or external body contour, is used to infer changes in internal patient anatomy. External surrogate-based motion imaging is mostly used to monitor respiratory-induced motion or bulk patient movement, given the strong correlation between the surrogate and internal motions. Implanted devices, such as gold fiducials and electromagnetic transponders, serve as internal surrogates and have been combined with x-ray imaging or electromagnetic receivers for motion monitoring, primarily in the prostate [16–19]. During treatment delivery, the positions of the implants are calculated from the acquired images to reflect the position change of the tissue of interest. Hybrid techniques that combine optical imaging of external markers and x-ray imaging of implants or internal anatomy are used in at least one commercial treatment delivery system to take advantage of the high imaging speed of optical imaging and the internal anatomy information from x-ray imaging [20–23]. Internal motion information is inferred from the position changes of external markers and the modeled correlation between internal and external marker motions. Hybrid techniques have been used to monitor respiratory motion in patients with tumors in the lung and liver. Ultrasound and magnetic resonance imaging (MRI) are non-ionizing imaging techniques that provide soft tissue contrast. Ultrasound imaging has been used to monitor prostate motion [24–26], while MRI integrated with a linear accelerator (MR-linac) is in use worldwide for multiple body sites including the abdomen, thorax, and prostate [27–31]. Figure 11.2 shows example elements of surface imaging, marker-based imaging, and anatomical imaging [32] for patient motion monitoring.

11.2.2 Delivery system actions

Based on the motion monitoring results, rapid changes of radiation delivery parameters can be made to account for the changing patient anatomy. The simplest change of delivery parameters is through gating, a binary process where the delivery of radiation is turned on/off when patient motion is inside/outside a treatment gating window that specifies the acceptable range of motion [33–35]. Treatment gating has been implemented on clinical systems in combination with various imaging

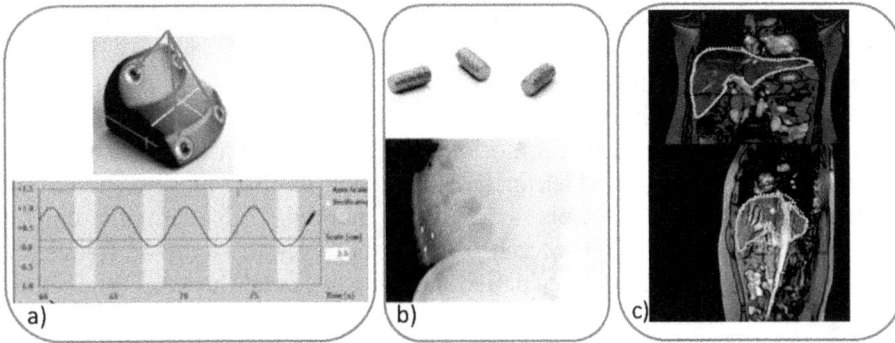

Figure 11.2. Example elements of systems for motion monitoring. (a) Infrared imaging of reflective markers produces 1D breathing motion traces of the patient's surface. (b) X-ray imaging of golden fiducial markers implanted in soft tissue . (c) Anatomical imaging (cine MRI) visualizes tumor location in the sagittal and coronal planes. ((a) and (b) Adapted from [32]. CC BY 3.0. (c) Adapted from [30] with permission from John Wiley & Sons. Copyright 2020 American Association of Physicists in Medicine.)

modalities. Alternatively, treatment tracking keeps the radiation delivery on throughout the treatment. The delivery parameters are adjusted during treatment to adapt the radiation dose distributions to the moving treatment target, so that the tumor is always inside the high-dose region. Treatment tracking has been implemented on the CyberKnife system, where the linac position is adapted to patient motion through a robotic arm [21, 36]. Treatment tracking through beam collimation adaptation has also been implemented on TomoTherapy systems [37, 38] and, more recently, on PET/CT-linac systems [39], where collimator shapes are adjusted to account for patient motion during treatment delivery. Real-time re-planning during treatment delivery has also been investigated to adapt treatment to patient motion, where rapid dose recalculation is performed based on the updated patient anatomy, followed by rapid re-planning to account for the change in dose distributions [40]. While preliminary investigations have suggested the feasibility of such a treatment adaption scheme, it has not been implemented on commercial systems to date.

11.2.3 Challenges for real-time ART implementation

11.2.3.1 Motion monitoring frequency and complexity
To monitor patient motion in real time, a trade-off must be made between motion monitoring frequency and the complexity of the motion information obtained. For example, respiration occurs at a temporal rate of 3–5 s/cycle and the range of motion during a motion cycle can be up to several centimeters. To capture the rapid anatomy changes induced by respiration with sufficient accuracy to limit dose deviations from motion to reasonable levels, patient motion states need to be updated at a sub-second temporal rate through imaging or some other means of motion monitoring. Infrared and optical-based imaging technologies have the advantage of high sampling frequency (>20 Hz) [41, 42]; however, these surface

imaging techniques cannot directly capture internal anatomy changes. Instead, they rely on a correlation model between external and internal motions, potentially degrading the accuracy of obtained motion information. Furthermore, the motion information obtained is limited to low-dimensional signals (1D shift or 3D shift and rotations). These low-dimensional motion signals are simplified representations of complex anatomy changes, which include both rigid motion and non-rigid deformation. X-ray imaging of implanted fiducial markers or patient anatomy can provide direct information on internal motion, however the imaging frequency is usually lower due to concerns over patient imaging dose and the extra time required for image analysis, for example, marker segmentation or image registration, to extract the motion information. An imaging frequency of 9.5 Hz has been reported for prostate motion monitoring [43] and imaging time intervals of 10–50 s has been used when combining x-ray imaging with high frequency optical imaging [44]. The clinically reported imaging interval of CyberKnife orthogonal x-ray projection imaging is sometimes longer than 1 min and is used to monitor erratic movements of patients during craniospinal treatments. The x-ray projection imaging has also been combined with fast surface-based imaging to update a motion model as described in section 11.3.1.1 for breathing motion monitoring.

Cine MRI mode has been used to monitor motion on MR-linac systems for multiple body sites including the thorax, abdomen, pelvis, and prostate. MRI provides superior soft tissue contrast compared to x-ray imaging with no imaging dose. Yet the slower imaging speed and the time required to calculate target deformation based on the acquired image samples limit the imaging frequency of cine MRI to around 4–5 Hz [45, 46]. Cine MRI is also limited to one or a few 2D planes and cannot fully capture the motion in 3D space. Ultrasound is another ionization-free imaging modality with good soft tissue contrast. Currently the only commercial system for ultrasound-based motion tracking is designed for monitoring 3D rigid prostate motion. The system creates a continuously scanned 3D-reconstructed volume with a motor-driven sweeping motion. An image reading frequency of 2 Hz has been used [47]. In-house investigations have also demonstrated the potential of ultrasound in monitoring breathing motion [48], where robotic arms and breathing motion control/compression were used to ensure close contact between the ultrasound probe and the patient surface.

11.2.3.2 System latency

When patient motion occurs, the treatment delivery system processes the motion information and takes action to adapt to the changing anatomy. The processing time results in system latency, which refers to the time delay between the motion occurring and the system acting. Various factors contribute to system latency, including the image acquisition time, the time required to process the images to extract motion information, and the time needed for the system to adjust delivery parameters. The system latency therefore depends on (i) the imaging modality, for example, video camera-based external marker imaging systems generally have a shorter latency than radiographic or tomographic anatomical imaging systems; (ii) the complexity of motion analysis (rigid or deformable); and (iii) the mechanism of system action for motion adaption, for example, the binary action of turning on/off the beam (treatment gating) generally takes less time than treatment tracking or re-planning. A wide range of system latencies have been reported, from below 100 ms for external marker imaging-guided treatment gating/tracking [49, 50], to around 300 ms for MRI-guided treatment gating [51, 52]. The acceptable system latency depends on the velocity of the motion the system is trying to account for. For example, adapting to fast breathing motion will require a system with shorter latency than adapting to slow prostate motion. *In vitro* studies of ultrasound-guided treatment tracking have demonstrated adequate compensation of prostate motion with a total system latency of −1 s [53]. The ability to predict motion trajectories can allow for longer latencies with acceptable residual errors.

11.3 AI in real-time ART workflows

While intrafraction motion-induced anatomy changes are complex, those changes are continuous and correlated both spatially and temporally. Such correlation implies that historic information of patient anatomy and motion might provide valuable knowledge on future anatomical changes of a patient during treatment delivery. Indeed, when medical experts review patient images acquired over time, they can make reasonable conjectures on future patient motion, for example, transition from inhale to exhale, and identify image artifacts that are not caused by patient motion. AI models, by definition, are models that can learn at least somewhat like human beings do [54]. By training AI models from historic patient motion data, prior knowledge embedded in the models can be taken advantage of to support the real-time ART workflow including efficient sampling of patient data during treatment delivery, accurate motion analysis, and fast system reaction based on the motion information. While recently developed AI approaches to address motion are mostly deep learning models, in this chapter we adopt the broad definition of AI and review both clinical and experimental AI models of various architectures for real-time ART workflow.

11.3.1 Improving intrafraction motion monitoring through AI

AI models have been developed to overcome temporal and spatial limitations of different imaging techniques for motion monitoring to produce high-quality motion information at high temporal sampling rates.

11.3.1.1 Correlating external imaging with internal anatomy through AI
External imaging has the advantage of high sampling frequency, yet the motion monitoring accuracy is compromised by monitoring patient surface motion instead of internal anatomy changes. Fiducial and anatomical imaging, on the other hand, can directly monitor internal motion but are limited by lower sampling frequencies. An external–internal correlation model (ECM) has been developed to combine different imaging techniques together for high frequency monitoring of internal motion. As illustrated in figure 11.3, prior knowledge of the correlation between external and internal motion is learnt from a pre-treatment training dataset that

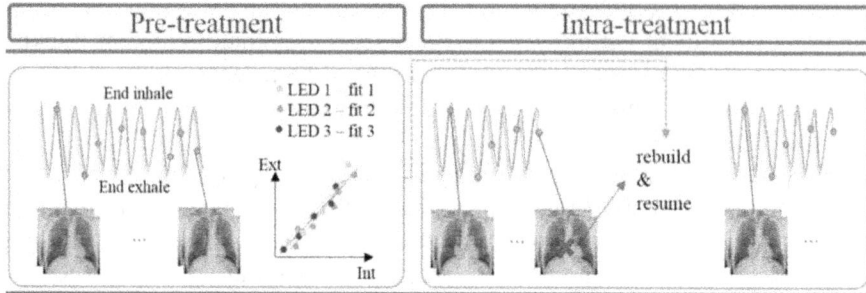

Figure 11.3. Illustration of pre-treatment model training and in-treatment motion monitoring, with the CyberKnife system as an example. (Reproduced from [32]. CC BY 3.0.)

consists of both internal images and external images at different motion states. During treatment delivery, internal motion is predicted by combining the ECM model with external motion information sampled at a high frequency. The ECM model may also be updated online during treatment delivery, when new pairs of internal and external images are acquired.

Different imaging modalities have been investigated for ECM model-based motion monitoring. Bertholet *et al* [55] utilized pre-treatment free-breathing CBCT and infrared images of reflective markers (RPM) to construct the ECM model. The ECM model parameters were optimized to output 3D motion information based on 1D motion traces extracted from an infrared imaging system, which captures the motion of a block placed on the patient's skin surface. Fiducial markers were segmented in CBCT projections, and 3D motion trajectories were estimated through maximum likelihood estimation, assuming a Gaussian spatial distribution of the fiducial markers. The CyberKnife Synchrony system trains the ECM model using orthogonal x-ray images and images of light-emitting diode (LED) markers placed on the patient's surface. During model training, at least eight pairs of x-ray images are acquired at different breathing phases and are used to determine internal target motions. The ECM model is trained to correlate the internal treatment target motion to the external LED marker motion detected by cameras. Chen *et al* [56] investigated the feasibility of estimating internal motion from surface imaging through ECM. 4DCT images of different breathing motion phases and surface images extracted from the 4DCT scan were used for model training. Internal and external motion information was estimated by registering internal organ meshes and external surface meshes, respectively, using a non-rigid point matching algorithm. The ECM model was trained using a composite matrix that consists of both internal and external deformation vector fields, allowing internal motion vectors to be predicted based on external ones.

ECM models are limited to respiratory-induced motions, as other internal anatomy changes, such as prostate motion caused by organ fillings, do not significantly correlate with external surface motion. Various model parameterization strategies have been proposed for ECM. The simplest assumes a linear relationship between the 3D internal motion vectors and the 1D external motion signals.

More complicated quadratic models have also been investigated to better represent the relationship between internal and external motions. Time-delayed samples [57] and the first-order derivative [58] of external motion have been combined with linear or quadratic models to account for breathing hysteresis. Alternatively, the CyberKnife system uses two quadratic models for the inhale phase and exhale phase, respectively. To model higher-dimensional motion signals, such as deformation vector fields, principal component analysis (PCA)-based models have been investigated [56]. Principal motion characteristics are learned from a training dataset that composites external and internal deformation vector fields. By projecting external deformation vector fields onto the subspace spanned by principal components (eigenvectors), the model parameters (eigenvalues) associated with the motion state can be determined and used to calculate the corresponding internal deformation vector fields.

11.3.1.2 Markerless motion monitoring through AI

Implanted markers, such as gold fiducials and electromagnetic transponders, have been used to provide real-time position information of internal targets. However, marker implantation is invasive, adds workflow complexity, and carries the risk of patient bleeding and marker migration. Markerless motion monitoring using x-ray imagers equipped on linacs is desirable. However, the limited soft tissue contrast and tissue overlay in 2D projection images may compromise the accuracy of markerless motion tracking.

AI models have been developed to integrate prior knowledge of high contrast 3D patient images, acquired before treatment, with low contrast 2D images acquired in real time to improve 3D motion monitoring accuracy. Template matching methods have been investigated for lung and spine target tracking, where prior knowledge of patient anatomy was modeled as a template library of digitally reconstructed radiographs (DRRs). During treatment delivery, motion information has been obtained by registering acquired 2D x-ray images to template DRRs. Cai et al generated a template library of both MV and kV DRRs from high-resolution CBCT reconstructions [59]. 3D target shifts were calculated from kV-to-DRR and MV-to-DRR registration results. Motion monitoring using kV images only has also been investigated, where kV DRRs at different gantry angles were created from planning CT images. During treatment, kV projections were acquired at 7 frames per second and matched to the DRR templates to determine 2D target position. 3D motion information was then obtained through triangulation of matched projections.

Deep learning models have also been investigated for markerless motion monitoring, where a neural network was trained to localize tumors from 2D kV x-ray images. During network training, either a 4DCT dataset or a 3D CT dataset undergoing different deformations was used to mimic anatomical changes at the time of treatment delivery. Digitally reconstructed radiographs (DRRs) were generated from the CT datasets to simulate kV images acquired during treatment. The network was optimized to take the simulated DRRs as input and output the corresponding target locations, which are known from the training CT images. Grama et al [60] proposed a Siamese network comprising twin subnetworks to

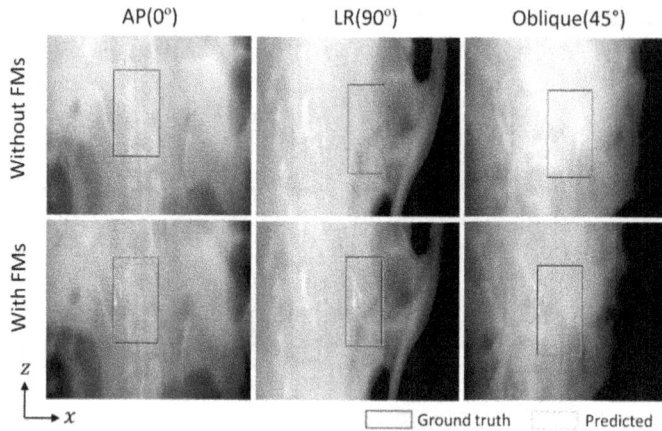

Figure 11.4. Results of pancreatic target localization on x-ray images acquired at various projection angles using a deep learning approach. The deep learning model accurately predicts target location with and without fiducial markers (FMs). (Reproduced with permission from [61]. Copyright 2019 Elsevier.)

process variable-sized input images. Utilizing data-driven features learned by a neural network, deep learning models achieve superior performance in lung tumor motion monitoring compared to template matching-based methods. Deep learning-based methods also show promise in prostate motion monitoring, where the low soft tissue contrast has challenged direct x-ray-based motion monitoring. To improve network localization accuracy, Zhao *et al* [61] proposed concatenating a region proposal network with a target detection network, where the latter network takes the output of the region proposal network as input. As shown in figure 11.4, the network successfully predicted the pancreas target position without fiducial implants, despite the poor soft tissue contrast of the x-ray projection images.

Direct 2D-to-3D registration through AI has also been investigated, where AI models output registration results between the 2D images acquired during treatment delivery and a reference 3D image. The 3D target motion can be inferred from the registration results. Hou *et al* proposed a convolutional neural network to learn a regression function that maps 2D images to their correct position and orientation in 3D space [62]. The network was trained and evaluated for direct registration of digitally reconstructed radiographs (DRR)-to-CT images for thoracic motion monitoring. Foote *et al* combined a patient-specific motion subspace with a convolutional neural network to predict 3D motion from a single x-ray projection [63]. The low-rank motion subspace was constructed through principal component analysis (PCA) of deformation fields between 4DCT scans of different breathing phases and a reference CT image. The network was trained to take DRR projections calculated from deformed reference CT images as inputs, and outputs subspace coordinates that define the deformations associated with the DRR projections. The model is therefore not limited to predicting rigid translation and rotation of the target; instead, voxel-wise deformation over the entire image volume can be obtained.

11.3.1.3 Real-time volumetric imaging through AI

Volumetric imaging provides 3D visualization of patient anatomy and is routinely used for treatment planning and pre-treatment patient set-up. However, the acquisition of volumetric imaging is time-consuming. To reconstruct high-quality CBCT images without artifacts, hundreds of kV projections typically need to be acquired. For MRI imaging, sampling of the Fourier space needs sufficient density to meet the resolution limits set by the Nyquist sampling theorem, which can take up to several minutes depending on scanning volume, contrast and spatial resolution. As a result, despite the advantage of fully characterizing both rigid and non-rigid motions over the entire patient anatomy, volumetric imaging using conventional sampling and reconstruction techniques is not suitable to guide motion monitoring during ART delivery, where changes in patient position and/or configuration need to be determined in real time.

Sparse imaging has been investigated to accelerate volumetric image acquisition, where only a limited set of data samples is acquired for image reconstruction. Direct image reconstruction from the sparse samples will result in subsampling artifacts. Model-based image reconstruction utilizes prior knowledge of the imaging subject to regularize the reconstruction process and remove image artifacts. Manually crafted prior knowledge models, including total variation, low rank, and sparsity in the transform domain, have been investigated. However, the acceleration factors achieved using these methods are still insufficient to support sub-second imaging for motion monitoring. Furthermore, to solve the model-based image reconstruction problem, iterative optimization is needed, which also adds latency to an imaging-guided ART delivery system.

AI models learn prior knowledge in a data-driven manner and have demonstrated advantages over manually crafted models. Zhang *et al* proposed a neural network that combines a DenseNet with a deconvolution-based network [64]. The network takes CT images generated using a sparse set of projections and reconstructed through conventional filtered back projection as inputs and outputs the corresponding fully sampled CT images. Compared to total variation model-based image reconstruction, the network-reconstructed images showed reduced streaking artifacts and increased structural similarity with fully sampled images. The work by Shen *et al* investigated CT imaging with a single x-ray projection, making it possible for real-time CT-based motion monitoring during ART delivery [65]. The network comprises a 2D representation network that learns feature representations from x-ray projections and a 3D generation network that produces volumetric CT images from the learned features. A transformation module was introduced between the 2D and 3D networks to bridge the 2D and 3D feature spaces.

AI models have also been investigated for sparse MRI reconstruction. Zhu *et al* showed that a deep neural network can learn a direct mapping between sensor and image domain MRI data [66]. As shown in figure 11.5, their model (AUTOMAP) is flexible in learning reconstruction transforms for various sparse MRI sampling strategies and demonstrated superior image quality when reconstructing from sparse MRI samples as compared to conventional models. Aggarwal *et al* combined the known signal model of MRI formation with a deep neural network for MRI

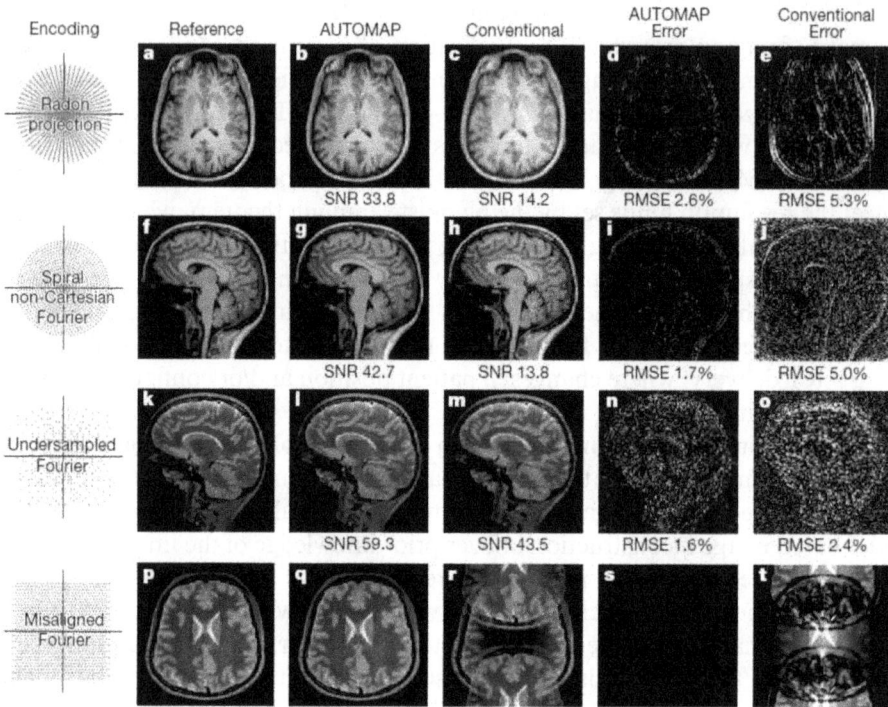

Figure 11.5. MRI acquired with various sparse sampling strategies. AUTOMAP-based reconstruction achieves superior image quality compared to conventional reconstruction. (Reproduced with permission from [66]. Copyright 2018 Springer Nature.)

reconstruction [67]. The deep neural network learns useful features in the image domain and serves as a regularization prior for the model-based image reconstruction process. By incorporating the forward signal model, the authors showed that a smaller network can be trained with fewer training data samples without compromising image reconstruction quality. To achieve real-time volumetric MRI from a single radial projection, Feng *et al* proposed a signature matching-based method [68]. During an initial offline learning stage, a 4D MRI library consisting of different breathing motion states and the corresponding breathing motion signatures was constructed. During the subsequent online matching stage, new motion signatures were acquired in real time and matched to the pre-learnt motion signatures associated with known motion states. The method showed promise in real-time MRI-guided 3D motion monitoring for ART delivery, although handling outlier motion states that were not learned during the offline stage remains a challenging topic. By incorporating prior knowledge of MRI acquisition strategy and the sensor-to-image domain transform into a deep neural network, Liu *et al* demonstrated model robustness to longitudinal patient anatomy changes and eliminated the need for 4D MRI collection before each MRI-guided ART delivery session [69]. The model was trained and tested on MRI datasets acquired months apart and reconstructed high-quality volumetric MRI from sparse samples with sub-second acquisition times.

11.3.2 Mitigating system latency through AI

AI has also begun to show promise to reduce system latency for motion monitoring during ART delivery. AI-based sparsely sampled imaging has reduced not only image acquisition time but also reconstruction time. Compared to conventional methods that take several minutes to iteratively solve the sparse image reconstruction problem [70, 71], a trained AI model can produce images within seconds.

In addition to reducing the imaging time, AI models have also been investigated to support system decision-making during real-time ART. By directly estimating motion information from the acquired image samples, AI models can remove the need of image registration to accelerate system decision-making based on the motion information, thus reducing system latency. The motion monitoring error caused by system latency can also be mitigated through AI-based motion prediction ahead of the acquisition time.

11.3.2.1 Direct motion estimation through AI

Conventionally, motion information is estimated through registration of images acquired during ART delivery with a reference image acquired before treatment. The motion information ranges from low-dimensional vectors describing rigid motion (shift and rotation) up to high-dimensional deformation vector fields (DVFs) with granularity possibly as high as a different transform for each voxel location. Decisions to adapt the treatment are then made based on the motion information. The image registration step adds additional time between motion occurrence and system action to account for the motion. As this time increases, for example for situations where complex registration, such as deformable registration, is needed, the true configuration of the patient has increasing potential to deviate from that measured, leading to reduced effectiveness of motion monitoring which would need to be offset by attempting to add accurate motion predictions to measurements.

To address the temporal efficiency of motion prediction, efforts have been made to directly estimate deformation vector fields (DVFs) from sparse image samples, with the goal of reducing both image acquisition and motion estimation time. Terpstra *et al* proposed a deep learning model to directly estimate 3D DVFs from under-sampled MRI [72]. They collected a population dataset of 4D MRI from 27 patients and calculated ground truth DVFs through deformable registration between fully sampled MRIs at different breathing motion phases. A neural network was trained to take retrospectively under-sampled images as inputs and output the corresponding DVFs (figure 11.6). The authors reported a total time of 200 ms for sparse image acquisition and DVF estimation, with an estimation error of less than 2 mm. Stemkens *et al* introduced a patient-specific subspace model for 3D DVF estimation from 2D MRI [73]. Deformable registration was performed across a patient-specific 4D MRI dataset. The subspace model was constructed by

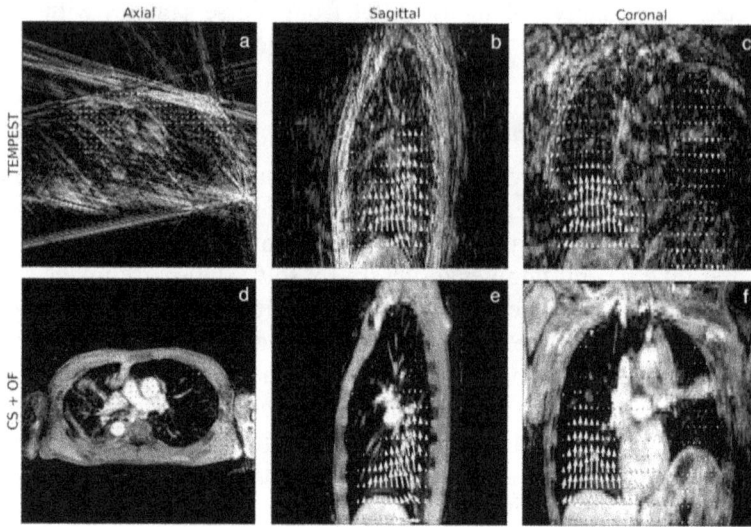

Figure 11.6. (a)–(c) DVFs estimated by a neural network from under-sampled MRI, (d)–(f) compared to DVFs estimated through deformable registration of high-quality images. (Reproduced from [72]. CC BY 4.0.)

performing principal component analysis on the obtained DVFs. The problem of estimating 3D DVF was then reduced to the estimation of principal component coefficients that best match the sparse MRI and the deformed reference MRI at sampled locations. They reported a temporal resolution of less than 500 ms with an average error of 1.45 mm for DVF estimation. Motion estimation from MRI sensor domain samples without image reconstruction has also been explored. Huttinga *et al* incorporated a forward signal model that relates MR sensor domain data to the underlying image subject for motion estimation [74]. A low-rank motion representation was constructed from a pre-treatment 4D dataset to reduce the problem of estimating high-dimensional DVFs to estimating eigenvector coefficients. The method was validated on an MR-linac system, with a reported total latency of 170 ms. Shao *et al* investigated direct motion estimation from sparse sensor domain samples without ground truth DVFs [75]. Instead, the network was trained to output DVFs that optimally wrap a fully sampled prior image to the target sparse samples. The data fidelity loss was calculated in the sensor domain by undersampling the deformed prior image using the same sparse sampling pattern as the target. A regularization loss was also introduced to enforce the smoothness of the DVFs.

Real-time motion estimation from sparse x-ray samples has also been investigated. Li *et al* explored a Bayesian approach to estimate 3D target location from sparse x-ray projections [76]. Probability density functions of tumor locations were estimated from 2D projections acquired with different x-ray imaging directions during patient set-up. During treatment, 2D tumor location information on the imager was used to update the likelihood function and the third dimension of tumor location along the direction of imaging x-ray was estimated by maximizing the posterior probability distribution. Before treatment, the 2D location information was calculated directly from the acquired projections, while the third dimension of motion information was estimated from a probabilistic function that utilizes previously acquired x-ray projections as the prior. Shao *et al* proposed a neural network that estimates deformation vector fields (DVFs) from x-ray projections acquired at arbitrary angles [77]. Similar to motion estimation from sparse MRI samples, a 4DCT dataset was used to train the network with sparse x-ray projections as inputs and ground truth DVFs as outputs. To enforce angle agnosticism, a geometry-informed x-ray feature pooling layer was developed to allow the network to extract angle-dependent image features for motion estimation. The authors reported a liver target localization error of less than 2 mm with the proposed method.

For ultrasound-guided ART delivery, Liu *et al* investigated landmark position tracking using a cascaded Siamese network [78]. Through the cascaded design, the model can increasingly focus on regions with the highest probability of containing the target. The network was trained in an unsupervised manner, where a pseudo tracking target was determined through corner point detection. They reported a tracking error of less than 2.5 mm. Mezheritsky *et al* explored 3D respiratory motion modeling from 2D ultrasound images using convolutional autoencoders [79]. The model comprises a rigid alignment module and a deformable motion module to estimate the 3D DVFs associated with the 2D images. The network was trained using a population database to encode the motion priors into a low-dimensional latent space and decode the corresponding DVFs from the latent codes. They reported a mean tracking error of 3.5 mm.

11.3.2.2 Motion prediction through AI

Utilizing temporal priors of motion patterns, AI models have also been developed to predict motion ahead of time to address issues of latency. For the prediction of low-dimensional motion signals, Teo *et al* implemented a perceptron neural network to predict 1D breathing motion trajectories [80]. The network was trained and tested using breathing motion signals collected from CyberKnife lung patients. It took motion samples acquired over the previous 4 s to predict the future breathing motion signal 650 ms ahead, with submillimeter accuracy. Ruan *et al* proposed a kernel density estimation-based approach to predict 1D breathing motion signals acquired from surface imaging [81]. The joint probability distributions of observed and future motion signals were estimated through Gaussian kernel regression. The authors reported a normalized root mean square error of less than 1 mm under various data sampling strategies and prediction horizons. Ren *et al* developed an autoregressive moving-average model to predict breathing motion in both the superior–inferior and anterior–posterior directions, where motion observations were obtained from marker-based imaging [82]. They also reported that the prediction accuracy depends on the lookahead time and imaging rates, with submillimeter accuracy achieved for a prediction horizon of 200 ms and an imaging rate of 10 Hz.

The prediction of high-dimensional motion information has also been investigated. Ginn *et al* explored an image regression model to predict motion states based on 2D cine MRI acquired on an MR-linac system [83]. Future MR images

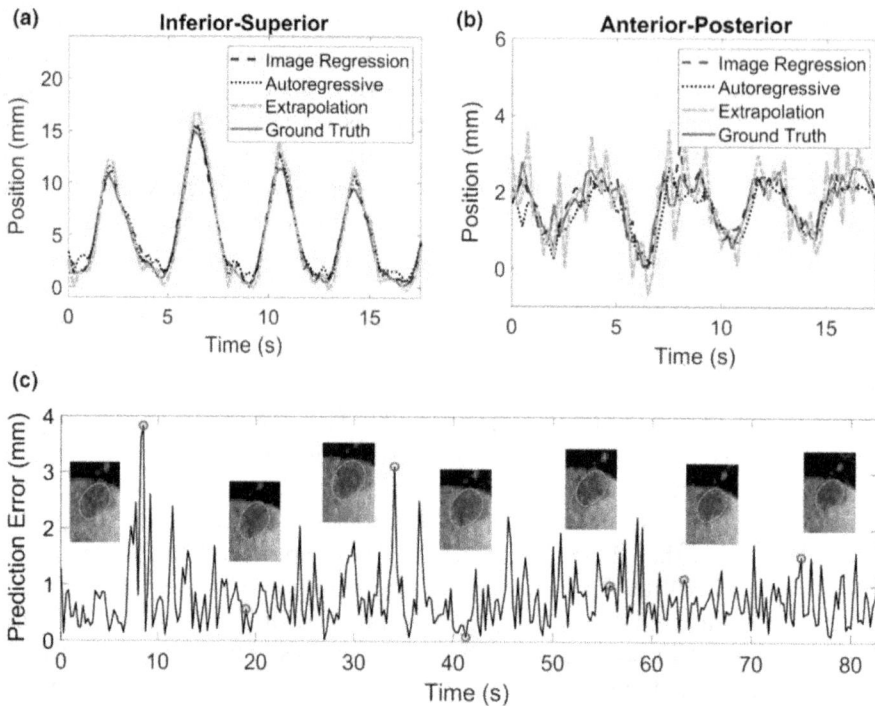

Figure 11.7. Example predicted motion traces and target contours via image regression. (Reproduced from [83] with permission from John Wiley & Sons. Copyright 2019 American Association of Physicists in Medicine.)

with a prediction horizon of 250–330 ms were generated through Gaussian kernel regression over historical image samples acquired at a 4 Hz frame rate. As shown in figure 11.7, future motion information can be calculated from the predicted images to support ART delivery, and the authors reported an averaged gating decision accuracy of 95.8%. Romaguera *et al* predicted in-plane deformation fields via discriminative spatial transformers [84]. The model aimed to learn deformations between consecutive images and extrapolate over time, utilizing image features learned over multiple scales. Submillimeter target position prediction accuracy was achieved when evaluated on MRI, CT, and ultrasound datasets.

While predicting high-dimensional motion information has the advantage of modeling complex motion beyond rigid shifts, it also poses challenges for prediction accuracy. Lombardo *et al* compared three models with similar network structures that predict 2D tumor centroid positions, 2D tumor contours, and DVFs associated with the tumor, respectively, using cine MRI acquired on an MR-linac [85]. Their results suggested that shifting the tumor contour based on the simple 2D centroid position achieved the highest accuracy in predicting tumor boundary, evaluated using Hausdorff distances between the ground truth and predicted tumor contours.

11.4 AI for ART delivery: future directions

11.4.1 Management of non-respiratory motion

While most AI models have focused on managing respiration-induced anatomy changes, recent research has demonstrated that non-respiratory motions, such as peristalsis and slow baseline anatomy drifts also significantly alter patient anatomy and contribute to treatment delivery uncertainty [6–8]. Modeling non-breathing motion to guide ART delivery is challenged by two factors. First, such motion is usually non-cyclic, meaning prior knowledge learnt from historic observations may have limited utility in modeling future motion states. Second, such motion may occur simultaneously with respiration, for example, in the abdomen. The significant magnitudes of respiratory motion can confound the analysis and modeling for non-respiratory motion.

Liu *et al* have investigated simultaneous modeling of breathing motion and slow baseline anatomy drifts for abdomen patients [86]. A multi-temporal resolution image time series was reconstructed from radial MRI samples, where fast breathing motion was extracted from high-temporal-resolution samples and slow drifting motion was extracted from a breathing motion-corrected low-temporal-resolution image time series. A motion prediction scheme was further investigated based on low-rank motion models constructed from principal component analysis of DVFs between different motion states. Model coefficients for future motion states were predicted through Gaussian kernel regression and linear regression, for breathing and slow drifting motions, respectively. Different prediction horizons were also investigated, where breathing motion was predicted 340 ms ahead of time and slow drifting motion was predicted 8.5 s ahead of time (figure 11.8). This longer prediction horizon for slow drifting motion is permitted by the slower motion velocity and is chosen to mitigate the latency resulted from slow drifting motion modeling without compromising the prediction accuracy (submillimeter in centroid position estimation).

Prediction of stomach contractile motion has also been investigated, following a similar approach that separates stomach motion from breathing motion through multi-temporal resolution radial MRI reconstruction [87]. A stomach motion model consisting of ten motion phases was built from a breathing-motion-corrected time

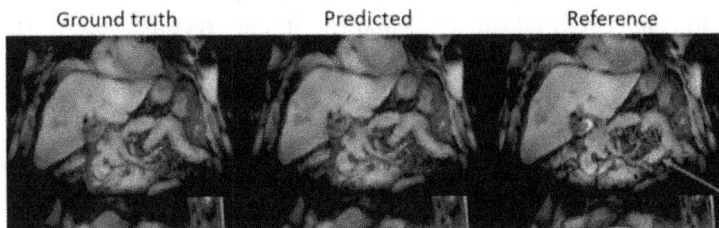

Figure 11.8. Example slow drifting motion prediction results. A DVF was predicted to deform a reference image to reflect motion states 8.5 s ahead of the image acquisition time. (Reproduced with permission from [86]. Copyright 2021 Institute of Physics and Engineering in Medicine.)

series of 2–5 min. Prediction of future stomach motion was achieved through linear extrapolation of motion phases determined using sparse MRI samples. The authors reported submillimeter prediction accuracy using sparse samples of 10 radial MRI spokes with a prediction horizon of 5 s.

While preliminary investigations have demonstrated the feasibility of monitoring non-breathing motion during treatment delivery, how to account for such motion during treatment remains an open question. Zhang *et al* have developed a dose accumulation tool to assess the accumulated dose in gastrointestinal organs [88]. Variations in motion states during treatment delivery were reconstructed retrospectively through multi-temporal resolution reconstruction of radial MRI samples. Delivered dose was calculated for each motion state and accumulated to estimate the total delivered dose. One solution to accounting partially for dose variations due to such motions involves adapting the treatment plan for subsequent treatments based on the accumulated dose from previous fractions. Other motion management schemes, such as MLC tracking or treatment gating, may also help mitigate treatment uncertainty introduced by non-breathing motion. However, accounting for multiple motions simultaneously will complicate the decision-making process for treatment adaptation, add system latency, and elongate treatment time.

11.4.2 Training AI models with small or unpaired datasets

The development of AI models typically requires a training dataset to optimize model parameters. For AI models developed for ART delivery, most training datasets are population-based and consist of motion information (volumetric images or low-dimensional motion signals) collected from a patient population. For the modeling of cyclic motion, such as respiration, patient-specific training datasets have also been used. These patient-specific datasets consist of samples acquired from the same patients but at different motion states. The quality of the training dataset, in terms of both image quality and quantity, directly impacts the model quality. However, due to the variance in data collection protocols and the protected health information associated with medical data, collecting high-quality training data can be time-consuming and may present a bottleneck for clinical implementation.

Shen *et al* investigated a novel machine learning technique, implicit neural representation (INR) learning to develop a patient-specific AI model for sparse imaging [89]. The model required only a single prior image for training and demonstrated the potential of high-quality image reconstruction from sparse samples of 20 CT projections or 40 radial MRI spokes. Liu *et al* leveraged INR to further accelerate volumetric imaging for real-time motion monitoring [90]. The method utilized two volumetric MRIs acquired at different breath-hold states for model training and reconstructed volumetric MRI from sparse samples of two orthogonal cine slices. The method was evaluated for free-breathing abdominal patients and reconstructed high-quality MRI with breathing motion states in between or outside the training images (figure 11.9). As illustrated in figure 11.10, during INR-based sparse image reconstruction, a prior model was trained by optimizing a perceptron network to learn a mapping from prior image coordinates

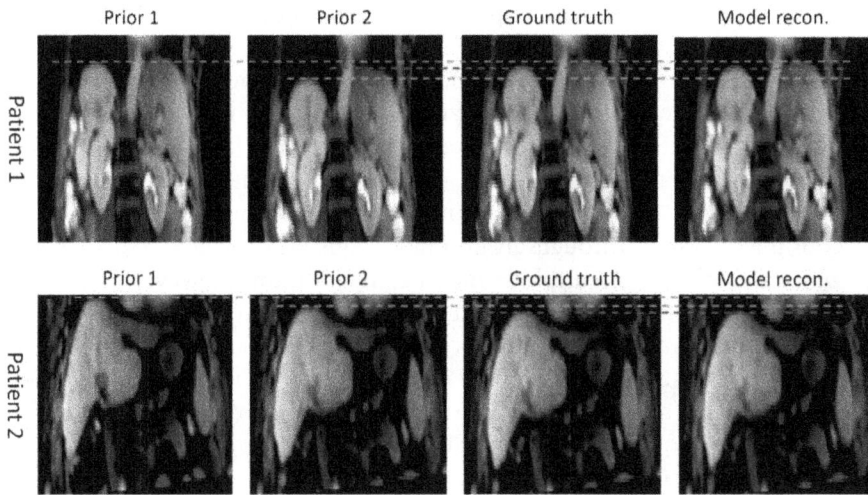

Figure 11.9. INR reconstructs volumetric MRI with motion states in between (patient 1) and outside (patient 2) the 2 prior images. (Reproduced from [90] with permission from John Wiley & Sons. Copyright 2024 American Association of Physicists in Medicine.)

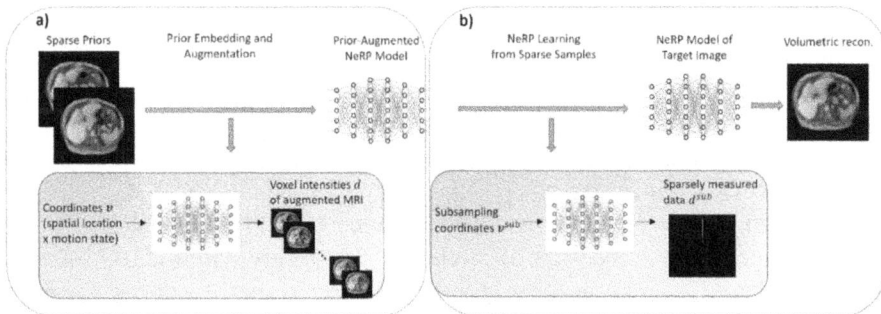

Figure 11.10. Framework of INR learning for real-time volumetric MRI. (Reproduced from [90] with permission from John Wiley & Sons . Copyright 2024 American Association of Physicists in Medicine.)

to prior image voxel values. The optimized network parameterization served as a regularization for the subsequent sparse image reconstruction task, where the network weights were further fine-tuned to fit the sparse samples of the testing images. Volumetric reconstruction was obtained by querying the fine-tuned network at desired 3D image coordinates. By regarding each pair of image coordinate and image voxel value as a training sample, INR requires significantly less training data than conventional machine learning methods.

There is growing interest in population-based learning with unpaired training data samples. Generative models, such as generative adversarial networks and diffusion models, aim to learn a mapping between two probabilistic distributions instead of a mapping between data points. Therefore, the model inputs and ground truth outputs do not have to be perfectly aligned. Generative models have found successful applications in radiotherapy, such as generating 'synthetic CT' from MRI for radiation treatment planning without paired MRI and CT images for model training [91–93]. In computer vision, generative models have demonstrated superior performance in modeling and synthesizing human motions [94, 95]. For motion monitoring during ART delivery, generative models may facilitate the learning of motion priors from population image datasets. To focus on modeling motion-induced anatomical variations, targets and OAR volumes need to be aligned to the same coordinate system through group image registration. The large variances in individual anatomical configurations and imaging positions, however, will challenge the accuracy of group image registration, thus potentially degrading the model quality. Effective learning of motion priors without well-aligned training samples has the potential of simplifying training data collection and preprocessing, improving model accuracy, and guiding ART delivery with high-quality motion information, especially for non-cyclic motions, such as organ fillings, where patient-specific motion modeling may be less effective.

11.4.3 Uncertainty quantification for AI models

While AI models have demonstrated significant potential in supporting ART delivery with improved treatment precision, reliable clinical implementation cannot be achieved without a method to quantify the uncertainty of model outputs. Although ad hoc model validation can be done by comparing model outputs to the ground truth, such ground truth is only available after the delivery of the radiation dose. To ensure patient safety and give clinicians confidence in trusting model outputs, instantaneous feedback on model quality is important for AI models developed for ART delivery.

Confidence intervals have been established for certain statistical machine learning models as a quantitative measure of model output quality. Ginn *et al* investigated confidence interval estimation for a kernel regression model developed for respiratory motion prediction [96]. The estimator consists of three components, including the goodness of model fit, the robustness of prediction quantified through leave-one-out cross-validation, and the velocity of the target. The estimator was evaluated for 20 abdominal subjects imaged with 2D cine MRI for respiratory motion monitoring. An increase of gating accuracy of –2% was reported by overriding the gating decision when the confidence interval estimator suggested a prediction error. Gaussian models have also been utilized to infer target position or motion fields, from surrogate markers or sparse imaging data. The uncertainty was then quantified through the covariance matrix of the linear Gaussian system [97, 98]. As illustrated in figure 11.11, changes of motion patterns can be detected and unreliable motion estimation can be rejected when the associated estimation uncertainty exceeds a certain threshold.

Bayesian networks have been investigated to output both prediction values and prediction uncertainties. Instead of predicting deterministic values, Bayesian networks predict probabilistic distributions based on network weights and inputs, thus

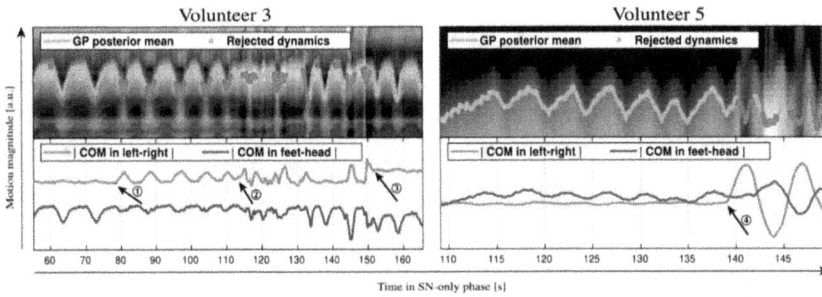

Figure 11.11. Unreliable motion estimations were rejected based on the estimation uncertainty when motion pattern changes, as indicated by the changing patterns in the center of mass-coordinates. (Reproduced from [98]. CC BY 4.0.)

permitting uncertainty quantification based on the probabilistic distribution. Given a set of initial clinical information, the network outputs the probability of obtaining certain radiotherapy parameters. A low probability therefore corresponds to potential errors in the radiotherapy plan. Law *et al* applied a Bayesian network to quantify the uncertainty of synthetic CT generated from MRI for radiation treatment planning [99]. The network outputs were computed using Monte Carlo integration. The synthetic CT values were estimated as the expected values of 100 simulation outputs, and the associated estimation uncertainty was characterized by the Monte Carlo simulation output spread. Uncertainty estimation for image reconstruction has also been investigated using a Markov chain Monte Carlo method, where both the image voxel values, and their associated uncertainties, were calculated from under-sampled MRI data [100]. Future work on uncertainty quantification for motion modeling, in particular for high-dimensional motion modeling such as DVF estimation and prediction, will facilitate clinical translation of AI models to support ART delivery.

11.4.4 Biology-guided ART delivery

Biological imaging modalities such as positron emission tomography (PET) provide tumor functional information that may be used to guide radiotherapy plan and delivery. Several clinical trials are investigating the benefits of biology-guided ART planning, where images providing biological information of the target [101–103] are acquired in the middle of a treatment course for offline plan adaptation. Target motion monitoring using PET has also been investigated through phantom studies [104]. The method combines external surrogate signals with PET signals to reconstruct gated PET images. The target centroid was estimated from the segmented target volume on the gated PET images. The author reported an averaged centroid position estimation error of 1.6 mm for both 1D and 3D motion patterns. The error decreased with time as more coincidence events were accumulated and converged in approximately 90 s.

The advent of PET/CT-linac systems has also permitted PET-guided ART delivery. This technology utilizes CT images for patient set-up and PET detection of outgoing

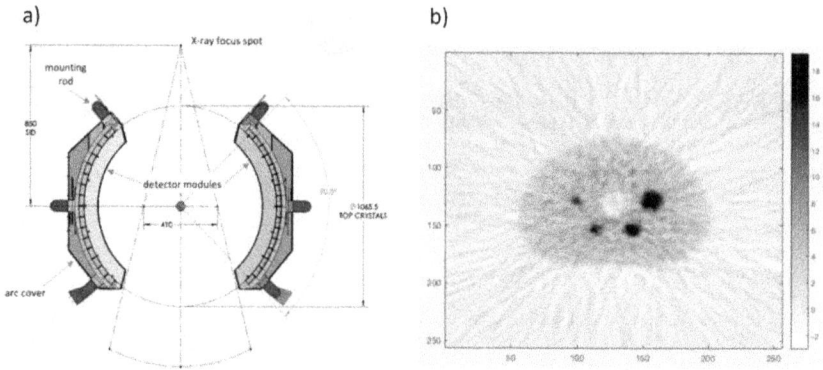

Figure 11.12. (a) Layout of the PET arcs in the gantry. (b) Phantom image acquired using the PET imaging subsystem of the PET-linac system. (Reproduced with permission from [105]. Copyright 2022, 2023 The Authors. Published by the British Institute of Radiology.)

tumor emissions for target motion monitoring during treatment delivery [39]. The motion information is used to guide the system to conform the MV radiation beamlets to the moving target. Preliminary investigations have characterized the imaging quality and tracking accuracy of the PET/CT-linac system [105, 106]. As shown in figure 11.12, a phantom study using the PET imaging subsystem demonstrated comparable spatial resolution and image contrast to diagnostic imaging systems, while the sensitivity and count rate were lower due to the smaller detector area. The tracking accuracy was also characterized through phantom studies with varying levels of PET biodistributions [106]. With good contrast between target and background PET signals (8:1 in PET biodistributions), the tracked dosimetry showed a prescription covering the target of 100%, while for the case with poor contrast (2:1 in PET biodistributions), the prescription covering the target dropped to 88%. In these low contrast cases, the system also flagged warnings based on the low activity concentration within the target.

The accuracy of motion monitoring during PET-guided ART delivery critically depends on PET image quality. To reduce patient motion and imaging dose, it is desirable to lower the injection dose and shorten the PET scan time. However, the low injection dose and the short scan time can lead to image quality degradation, exacerbated by hardware limitations such as smaller detectors that have lower count rates and sensitivity. AI models have demonstrated promising performance in low-dose PET reconstruction. For diagnostic PET reconstruction, generative adversarial networks have been explored to enhance the quality of low-dose PET images [107]. The network was trained using population-based datasets containing both low-dose and high-dose PET images acquired from a patient population. Lim *et al* integrated neural network-learned priors of high-dose PET images with a physical model of the PET imaging system to improve low-dose PET reconstruction [108]. The network served as a data regularization term during the iterative image reconstruction

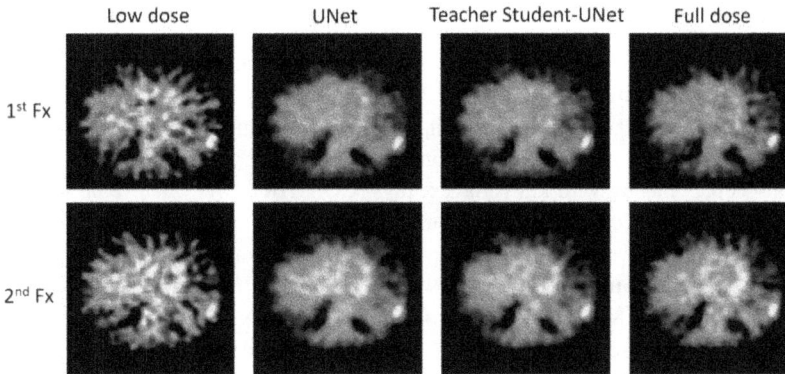

Figure 11.13. Transverse slices from full-dose PET images of different treatment fractions along with the corresponding low-dose images and the images predicted by the U-Net and the teacher–student U-Net for one example patient. (Reproduced from [109]. Courtesy of Cornell University.)

process by penalizing deviations of model estimation from network-learned priors. The method demonstrated good generalizability across different datasets, where the network was trained using PET images of a sphere phantom and tested using PET images of an anthropomorphic torso phantom.

For the image reconstruction of the PET-Linac system, Fu *et al* proposed a patient-specific deep learning model that enhances low-dose PET images using high-dose PET images of the same patient [109]. The model comprises a teacher U-net and a student U-net. The training dataset was created by subsampling coincidence events to generate various low-dose PET images from high-dose acquisitions. The parameters of the student network were optimized to output high-dose PET from low-dose inputs, while the parameters of the teacher network remained constant as the moving-average values of the student network parameters. Consistency loss between the teacher and student network was also incorporated during network training. As shown in figure 11.13, the teacher–student model demonstrated improved image quality compared to a single U-Net model. As more studies are conducted on PET-linac systems, enhancing PET imaging through AI will enable the full exploitation of the advantages of biology-guided ART delivery, with the potential to improve treatment outcomes.

11.5 Summary

While significant advances in adapting treatments have begun to be implemented clinically, they are inherently limited by the motions that occur during treatment. AI has demonstrated the potential to improve treatment monitoring. Simpler AI methods are in clinical use to aid motion tracking, and more advanced methods have shown the potential to dramatically improve the efficiency and accuracy of measuring, predicting, and reacting to changes that occur as treatment is being delivered.

References

[1] Keall P J *et al* 2006 The management of respiratory motion in radiation oncology report of AAPM Task Group 76 a *Med. Phys.* **33** 3874–900

[2] Bertholet J *et al* 2018 Automatic online and real-time tumour motion monitoring during stereotactic liver treatments on a conventional linac by combined optical and sparse monoscopic imaging with kilovoltage x-rays (COSMIK) *Phys. Med. Biol.* **63** 055012

[3] Kitamura K *et al* 2003 Tumor location, cirrhosis, and surgical history contribute to tumor movement in the liver, as measured during stereotactic irradiation using a real-time tumor-tracking radiotherapy system *Int. J. Radiat. Oncol. Biol. Phys.* **56** 221–8

[4] Chen T, Qin S, Xu X, Jabbour S K, Haffty B G and Yue N J 2014 Frequency filtering based analysis on the cardiac induced lung tumor motion and its impact on the radiotherapy management *Radiother. Oncol.* **112** 365–70

[5] Schmidt M L *et al* 2016 Cardiac and respiration induced motion of mediastinal lymph node targets in lung cancer patients throughout the radiotherapy treatment course *Radiother. Oncol.* **121** 52–8

[6] Mostafaei F *et al* 2018 Variations of MRI-assessed peristaltic motions during radiation therapy *PLoS One* **13** e0205917

[7] Johansson A, Balter J M and Cao Y 2021 Gastrointestinal 4D MRI with respiratory motion correction *Med. Phys.* **48** 2521–7

[8] Liu L, Johansson A, Cao Y, Kashani R, Lawrence T S and Balter J M 2021 Modeling intra-fractional abdominal configuration changes using breathing motion-corrected radial MRI *Phys. Med. Biol.* **66** 085002

[9] Fokdal L, Honoré H, Høyer M, Meldgaard P, Fode K and von der Maase H 2004 Impact of changes in bladder and rectal filling volume on organ motion and dose distribution of the bladder in radiotherapy for urinary bladder cancer *Int. J. Radiat. Oncol. Biol. Phys.* **59** 436–44

[10] Chi Y *et al* 2017 A new method to reconstruct intra-fractional prostate motion in volumetric modulated arc therapy *Phys. Med. Biol.* **62** 5509

[11] Stevens M T R, Parsons D D and Robar J L 2016 Continuous monitoring of prostate position using stereoscopic and monoscopic kV image guidance *Med. Phys.* **43** 2558–68

[12] Willoughby T *et al* 2012 Quality assurance for nonradiographic radiotherapy localization and positioning systems: report of Task Group 147 *Med. Phys.* **39** 1728–47

[13] Pan H *et al* 2012 Frameless, real-time, surface imaging-guided radiosurgery: clinical outcomes for brain metastases *Neurosurgery.* **71** 844–52

[14] Rydhög J S *et al* 2017 Target position uncertainty during visually guided deep-inspiration breath-hold radiotherapy in locally advanced lung cancer *Radiother. Oncol.* **123** 78–84

[15] Hoisak J D and Pawlicki T (ed) 2018 The role of optical surface imaging systems in radiation therapy *Seminars in Radiation Oncology* (Amsterdam: Elsevier)

[16] Shirato H, Shimizu S, Kitamura K and Onimaru R 2007 Organ motion in image-guided radiotherapy: lessons from real-time tumor-tracking radiotherapy *Int. J. Clin. Oncol.* **12** 8–16

[17] Prévost J-B G, Nuyttens J J, Hoogeman M S, Pöll J J, Van Dijk L C and Pattynama P M 2008 Endovascular coils as lung tumour markers in real-time tumour tracking stereotactic radiotherapy: preliminary results *Eur. Radiol.* **18** 1569–76

[18] Schmitt D, Nill S, Roeder F, Gompelmann D, Herth F and Oelfke U 2017 Motion monitoring during a course of lung radiotherapy with anchored electromagnetic

transponders: quantification of inter-and intrafraction motion and variability of relative transponder positions *Strahlenther. Onkol.* **193** 840

[19] Shinohara E T *et al* 2012 Feasibility of electromagnetic transponder use to monitor inter- and intrafractional motion in locally advanced pancreatic cancer patients *Int. J. Radiat. Oncol. Biol. Phys.* **83** 566–73

[20] Ozhasoglu C *et al* 2008 Synchrony–cyberknife respiratory compensation technology *Med. Dosim.* **33** 117–23

[21] Hoogeman M, Prévost J-B, Nuyttens J, Pöll J, Levendag P and Heijmen B 2009 Clinical accuracy of the respiratory tumor tracking system of the cyberknife: assessment by analysis of log files *Int. J. Radiat. Oncol. Biol. Phys.* **74** 297–303

[22] Bibault J-E, Prevost B, Dansin E, Mirabel X, Lacornerie T and Lartigau E 2012 Image-guided robotic stereotactic radiation therapy with fiducial-free tumor tracking for lung cancer *Radiat. Oncol.* **7** 1–7

[23] Depuydt T *et al* 2014 Treating patients with real-time tumor tracking using the Vero gimbaled linac system: implementation and first review *Radiother. Oncol.* **112** 343–51

[24] Lachaine M and Falco T 2013 Intrafractional prostate motion management with the Clarity Autoscan system *Med. Phys. Int.* **23** 310–13

[25] Han B *et al* 2018 Evaluation of transperineal ultrasound imaging as a potential solution for target tracking during hypofractionated radiotherapy for prostate cancer *Radiat. Oncol.* **13** 151

[26] Li M *et al* 2017 Prefraction displacement and intrafraction drift of the prostate due to perineal ultrasound probe pressure *Strahlenther. Onkol.* **193** 459

[27] Jassar H *et al* 2023 Real-time motion monitoring using orthogonal cine MRI during MR-guided adaptive radiation therapy for abdominal tumors on 1.5 T MR-linac *Med. Phys.* **50** 3103–16

[28] Menten M J, Fast M F, Nill S, Kamerling C P, McDonald F and Oelfke U 2016 Lung stereotactic body radiotherapy with an MR-linac—quantifying the impact of the magnetic field and real-time tumor tracking *Radiother. Oncol.* **119** 461–6

[29] Paulson E S *et al* 2020 4D-MRI driven MR-guided online adaptive radiotherapy for abdominal stereotactic body radiation therapy on a high field MR-linac: implementation and initial clinical experience *Clin. Transl. Radiat. Oncol.* **23** 72–9

[30] Keiper T D *et al* 2020 Feasibility of real-time motion tracking using cine MRI during MR-guided radiation therapy for abdominal targets *Med. Phys.* **47** 3554–66

[31] Tetar S U, Bruynzeel A M, Lagerwaard F J, Slotman B J, Bohoudi O and Palacios M A 2019 Clinical implementation of magnetic resonance imaging guided adaptive radiotherapy for localized prostate cancer *Phys. Imaging Radiat. Oncol.* **9** 69–76

[32] Bertholet J *et al* 2019 Real-time intrafraction motion monitoring in external beam radiotherapy *Phys. Med. Biol.* **64** 15TR01

[33] Dietrich L, Tücking T, Nill S and Oelfke U 2005 Compensation for respiratory motion by gated radiotherapy: an experimental study *Phys. Med. Biol.* **50** 2405

[34] Vedam S, Keall P, Kini V and Mohan R 2001 Determining parameters for respiration-gated radiotherapy *Med. Phys.* **28** 2139–46

[35] Heerkens H D *et al* 2014 MRI-based tumor motion characterization and gating schemes for radiation therapy of pancreatic cancer *Radiother. Oncol.* **111** 252–7

[36] Antypas C and Pantelis E 2008 Performance evaluation of a CyberKnife® G4 image-guided robotic stereotactic radiosurgery system *Phys. Med. Biol.* **53** 4697

[37] Ferris W A-O, Kissick M W, Bayouth J A-O, Culberson W S and Smilowitz J A-O 2020 Evaluation of Radixact motion synchrony for 3D respiratory motion: modeling accuracy and dosimetric fidelity *J. Appl. Clin. Med. Phys.* **21** 96–106

[38] Chen G-P *et al* 2021 Clinical implementation and initial experience of real-time motion tracking with jaws and multileaf collimator during helical tomotherapy selivery *Pract. Radiat. Oncol.* **11** e486–e95

[39] Oderinde O M, Shirvani S M, Olcott P D, Kuduvalli G, Mazin S and Larkin D 2021 The technical design and concept of a PET/CT linac for biology-guided radiotherapy *Clin. Transl. Radiat. Oncol.* **29** 106–12

[40] Kontaxis C *et al* 2017 Towards fast online intrafraction replanning for free-breathing stereotactic body radiation therapy with the MR-linac *Phys. Med. Biol.* **62** 7233–48

[41] Zhang X, Tang J, Sharp G C, Xiao L, Xu S and Lu H-M 2020 A new respiratory monitor system for four-dimensional computed tomography by measuring the pressure change on the back of body *Br. J. Radiol.* **93** 20190303

[42] Li G 2022 Advances and potential of optical surface imaging in radiotherapy *Phys. Med. Biol.* **67** 16TR02

[43] Hunt M A *et al* 2016 Simultaneous MV–kV imaging for intrafractional motion management during volumetric-modulated arc therapy delivery *J. Appl. Clin. Med. Phys.* **17** 473–86

[44] Pepin E W, Wu H, Fau-Zhang Y, Zhang Y, Fau-Lord B and Lord B 2011 Correlation and prediction uncertainties in the cyberknife synchrony respiratory tracking system *Med. Phys.* **38** 4036–44

[45] Hu P *et al* 2022 Dosimetry impact of gating latency in cine magnetic resonance image guided breath-hold pancreatic cancer radiotherapy *Phys. Med. Biol.* **67** 055008

[46] Hunt B *et al* 2023 Fast deformable image registration for real-time target tracking during radiation therapy using cine MRI and deep learning *Int. J. Radiat. Oncol. Biol. Phys.* **115** 983–93

[47] Sihono D S K *et al* 2018 Determination of intrafraction prostate motion during external beam radiation therapy with a transperineal 4-dimensional ultrasound real-time tracking system *Int. J. Radiat. Oncol. Biol. Phys.* **101** 136–43

[48] Vogel L *et al* 2018 Intra-breath-hold residual motion of image-guided DIBH liver-SBRT: an estimation by ultrasound-based monitoring correlated with diaphragm position in CBCT *Radiother. Oncol.* **129** 441–8

[49] Smith W L and Becker N 2009 Time delays in gated radiotherapy *J. Appl. Clin. Med. Phys.* **10** 140–54

[50] Worm E S, Thomsen J B, Johansen J G and Poulsen P R 2023 A simple method to measure the gating latencies in photon and proton based radiotherapy using a scintillating crystal *Med. Phys.* **50** 3289–98

[51] Liu P Z Y *et al* 2020 First experimental investigation of simultaneously tracking two independently moving targets on an MRI-linac using real-time MRI and MLC tracking *Med. Phys.* **47** 6440–9

[52] Kim T, Lewis B, Lotey R, Barberi E and Green O 2021 Clinical experience of MRI4D QUASAR motion phantom for latency measurements in 0.35T MR-linac *J. Appl. Clin. Med. Phys.* **22** 128–36

[53] Fast M F, O'Shea T P, Nill S, Oelfke U and Harris E J 2016 First evaluation of the feasibility of MLC tracking using ultrasound motion estimation *Med. Phys.* **48** 4628

[54] Manning C 2020 Artificial intelligence definitions *Stanford University Human-Centered Artificial Intelligence* https://hai.stanford.edu/sites/default/files/2020-09/AI-Definitions-HAI.pdf

[55] Bertholet J *et al* 2018 Automatic online and real-time tumour motion monitoring during stereotactic liver treatments on a conventional linac by combined optical and sparse monoscopic imaging with kilovoltage x-rays (COSMIK) *Phys. Med. Biol.* **63** 055012

[56] Chen H *et al* 2018 Internal motion estimation by internal-external motion modeling for lung cancer radiotherapy *Sci. Rep.* **8** 3677

[57] Ruan D *et al* 2008 Inference of hysteretic respiratory tumor motion from external surrogates: a state augmentation approach *Phys. Med. Biol.* **53** 2923–36

[58] Depuydt T *et al* 2013 Initial assessment of tumor tracking with a gimbaled linac system in clinical circumstances: a patient simulation study *Radiother. Oncol.* **106** 236–40

[59] Cai W *et al* 2023 Markerless motion tracking with simultaneous MV and kV imaging in spine SBRT treatment—a feasibility study *Phys. Med. Biol.* **68** 035012

[60] Grama D, Dahele M, van Rooij W, Slotman B, Gupta D K and Verbakel W F 2023 Deep learning-based markerless lung tumor tracking in stereotactic radiotherapy using Siamese networks *Med. Phys.* **50** 6881–93

[61] Zhao W *et al* 2019 Markerless pancreatic tumor target localization enabled by deep learning *Int. J. Radiat. Oncol. Biol. Phys.* **105** 432–9

[62] Hou B *et al* 2017 Predicting slice-to-volume transformation in presence of arbitrary subject motion *Medical Image Computing and Computer-Assisted Intervention—MICCAI 2017* ed M Descoteaux *et al* (Cham: Springer)

[63] Foote M D *et al* 2019 Real-time 2D–3D deformable registration with deep learning and application to lung radiotherapy targeting *Information Processing in Medical Imaging* ed A Chung (Cham: Springer)

[64] Zhang Z, Liang X, Dong X, Xie Y and Cao G 2018 A sparse-view CT reconstruction method based on combination of denseNet and deconvolution *IEEE Trans. Med. Imaging* **37** 1407–17

[65] Shen L, Zhao W and Xing L 2019 Patient-specific reconstruction of volumetric computed tomography images from a single projection view via deep learning *Nat. Biomed. Eng.* **3** 880–8

[66] Zhu B, Liu J Z, Cauley S F, Rosen B R and Rosen M S 2018 Image reconstruction by domain-transform manifold learning *Nature* **555** 487–92

[67] Aggarwal H K, Mani M P and Jacob M 2018 MoDL: model-based deep learning architecture for inverse problems *IEEE Trans. Med. Imaging* **38** 394–405

[68] Feng L A-O, Tyagi N and Otazo R 2020 MRSIGMA: magnetic resonance signature matching for real-time volumetric imaging *Magn. Reson. Med.* **48** 1280–92

[69] Liu L *et al* 2022 Real time volumetric MRI for 3D motion tracking via geometry-informed deep learning *Med. Phys.* **49** 6110–9

[70] Ramani S and Fessler J A 2012 A splitting-based iterative algorithm for accelerated statistical x-ray CT reconstruction *IEEE Trans. Med. Imaging* **31** 677–88

[71] Weller D S, Ramani S and Fessler J A 2014 Augmented Lagrangian with variable splitting for faster non-Cartesian L_1-SPIRiT MR image reconstruction *IEEE Trans. Med. Imaging* **33** 351–61

[72] Terpstra M L, Maspero M, Bruijnen T, Verhoeff J J C, Lagendijk J J W and van den Berg C A T 2021 Real-time 3D motion estimation from undersampled MRI using multi-resolution neural networks *Med. Phys.* **48** 6597–613

[73] Stemkens B, Tijssen R H N, de Senneville B D, Lagendijk J J W and van den Berg C A T 2016 Image-driven, model-based 3D abdominal motion estimation for MR-guided radiotherapy *Phys. Med. Biol.* **61** 5335

[74] Huttinga N R, Bruijnen T, van den Berg C A and Sbrizzi A 2021 Nonrigid 3D motion estimation at high temporal resolution from prospectively undersampled k-space data using low-rank MR-MOTUS *Magn. Reson. Med.* **85** 2309–26

[75] Shao H-C *et al* 2022 Real-time MRI motion estimation through an unsupervised k-space-driven deformable registration network (KS-RegNet) *Phys. Med. Biol.* **67** 135012

[76] Li R, Fahimian B F, Xing L and Xing L 2011 A Bayesian approach to real-time 3D tumor localization via monoscopic x-ray imaging during treatment delivery *Med. Phys.* **38** 4205–14

[77] Shao H-C, Li Y, Wang J, Jiang S and Zhang Y 2023 Real-time liver motion estimation via deep learning-based angle-agnostic x-ray imaging *Med. Phys.* **50** 6649–62

[78] Liu F, Liu D, Tian J, Xie X, Yang X and Wang K 2020 Cascaded one-shot deformable convolutional neural networks: developing a deep learning model for respiratory motion estimation in ultrasound sequences *Med. Image Anal.* **65** 101793

[79] Mezheritsky T, Romaguera L V, Le W and Kadoury S 2022 Population-based 3D respiratory motion modelling from convolutional autoencoders for 2D ultrasound-guided radiotherapy *Med. Image Anal.* **75** 102260

[80] Teo T P *et al* 2018 Feasibility of predicting tumor motion using online data acquired during treatment and a generalized neural network optimized with offline patient tumor trajectories *Med. Phys.* **45** 830–45

[81] Ruan D 2010 Kernel density estimation-based real-time prediction for respiratory motion *Phys. Med. Biol.* **55** 1311

[82] Ren Q, Nishioka S, Shirato H and Berbeco R I 2007 Adaptive prediction of respiratory motion for motion compensation radiotherapy *Phys. Med. Biol.* **52** 6651

[83] Ginn J S, Ruan D, Low D A and Lamb J M 2020 An image regression motion prediction technique for MRI-guided radiotherapy evaluated in single-plane cine imaging *Med. Phys.* **47** 404–13

[84] Romaguera L V, Plantefève R, Romero F P, Hébert F, Carrier J-F and Kadoury S 2020 Prediction of in-plane organ deformation during free-breathing radiotherapy via discriminative spatial transformer networks *Med. Image. Anal.* **64** 101754

[85] Lombardo E *et al* 2023 Evaluation of real-time tumor contour prediction using LSTM networks for MR-guided radiotherapy *Radiother. Oncol.* **182** 109555

[86] Liu L, Johansson A, Cao Y, Lawrence T S and Balter J M 2021 Volumetric prediction of breathing and slow drifting motion in the abdomen using radial MRI and multi-temporal resolution modeling *Phys. Med. Biol.* **66** 175028

[87] Zhang Y, Cao Y, Kashani R, Lawrence T S and Balter J M 2023 Real-time prediction of stomach motions based upon gastric contraction and breathing models *Phys. Med. Biol.* **68** 015001

[88] Zhang Y, Balter J, Dow J, Cao Y, Lawrence T S and Kashani R 2023 Development of an abdominal dose accumulation tool and assessments of accumulated dose in gastrointestinal organs *Phys. Med. Biol.* **68** 075004

[89] Shen L, Pauly J and Xing L 2022 NeRP: implicit neural representation learning with prior embedding for sparsely sampled image reconstruction *IEEE Trans. Neural Netw. Learn. Syst.* **35** 770–82

[90] Liu L *et al* 2024 Volumetric MRI with sparse sampling for MR-guided 3D motion tracking via sparse prior-augmented implicit neural representation learning *Med. Phys.* **51** 2526–37

[91] Lei Y *et al* 2019 MRI-only based synthetic CT generation using dense cycle consistent generative adversarial networks *Med. Phys.* **46** 3565–81

[92] Liu Y *et al* 2021 CT synthesis from MRI using multi-cycle GAN for head-and-neck radiation therapy *Comput. Med. Imaging Graph.* **91** 101953

[93] Liu Y *et al* 2019 Evaluation of a deep learning-based pelvic synthetic CT generation technique for MRI-based prostate proton treatment planning *Phys. Med. Biol.* **64** 205022

[94] Yuan Y, Song J, Iqbal U, Vahdat A and Kautz J 2023 PhysDiff: physics-guided human motion diffusion model *IEEE/CVF Int. Conf. on Computer Vision (ICCV)* (Piscataway, NJ: IEEE)

[95] Dabral R, Mughal M H, Golyanik V and Theobalt C 2023 Mofusion: a framework for denoising-diffusion-based motion synthesis *IEEE/CVF Conf. on Computer Vision and Pattern Recognition (CVPR)* (Piscataway, NJ: IEEE)

[96] Ginn J S, Low D A, Lamb J M and Ruan D 2020 A motion prediction confidence estimation framework for prediction-based radiotherapy gating *Med. Phys.* **47** 3297–304

[97] Remy C, Ahumada D, Labine A, Côté J-C, Lachaine M and Bouchard H 2021 Potential of a probabilistic framework for target prediction from surrogate respiratory motion during lung radiotherapy *Phys. Med. Biol.* **66** 105002

[98] Huttinga N R F, Bruijnen T, van den Berg C A T and Sbrizzi A 2023 Gaussian processes for real-time 3D motion and uncertainty estimation during MR-guided radiotherapy *Med. Image Anal.* **88** 102843

[99] Law M W-K *et al* 2024 A study of Bayesian deep network uncertainty and its application to synthetic CT generation for MR-only radiotherapy treatment planning *Med. Phys.* **51** 1244–62

[100] Luo G, Blumenthal M, Heide M and Uecker M 2023 Bayesian MRI reconstruction with joint uncertainty estimation using diffusion models *Magn. Reson. Med.* **90** 295–311

[101] Guricová K M *et al* 2025 Focal boost to the intraprostatic tumor in external beam radiotherapy for patients with localized prostate cancer: results from the FLAME randomized phase III trial *J. Clin. Oncol.* **0** JCO–25–00274

[102] Kim M M *et al* 2021 A phase 2 study of dose-intensified chemoradiation using biologically based target volume definition in patients with newly diagnosed glioblastoma *Int. J. Radiat. Oncol. Biol. Phys.* **110** 792–803

[103] Fu S *et al* 2022 Diffusion-weighted magnetic resonance imaging-guided dose painting in patients with locoregionally advanced nasopharyngeal carcinoma treated with induction chemotherapy plus concurrent chemoradiotherapy: a randomized, controlled clinical trial *Int. J. Radiat. Oncol. Biol. Phys.* **113** 101–13

[104] Yang J, Yamamoto T, Mazin S R, Graves E E and Keall P J 2014 The potential of positron emission tomography for intratreatment dynamic lung tumor tracking: a phantom study *Med. Phys.* **41** 021718

[105] Hu Z *et al* 2022 Image-mode performance characterisation of a positron emission tomography subsystem designed for biology-guided radiotherapy (BgRT) *Br. J. Radiol.* **96** 20220387

[106] Han B *et al* 2023 Characterization of biology-guided radiotherapy accuracy as a function of PET tracer uptake *Int. J. Radiat. Oncol. Biol. Phys.* **117** e668–e9

[107] Ouyang J, Chen K T, Gong E, Pauly J and Zaharchuk G 2019 Ultra-low-dose PET reconstruction using generative adversarial network with feature matching and task-specific perceptual loss *Med. Phys.* **46** 3555–64

[108] Lim H, Chun I Y, Dewaraja Y K and Fessler J A 2019 Improved low-count quantitative PET reconstruction with an iterative neural network *Med. Phys.* **46** 3512–22

[109] Fu J *et al* 2022 Patient-specific mean teacher UNet for enhancing PET image and low-dose PET reconstruction on RefleXion X1 biology-guided radiotherapy system arXiv:2209.05665

IOP Publishing

Artificial Intelligence in Adaptive Radiation Therapy

Yi Wang and X. Sharon Qi

Chapter 12

Artificial intelligence for quality assurance in adaptive radiation therapy

Sang Kyu Lee and Maria Chan

Quality assurance (QA) within the realm of radiation oncology physics plays a crucial role in ensuring that all patient care processes adhere to predefined quality standards [1]. This comprehensive approach encompasses various policies and procedures designed to establish these standards and outline the methods for monitoring. While artificial intelligence (AI) has the capability to enhance this process by analysing complex data and interpreting system outputs in a comprehensible manner, it is important to recognize that AI serves as a support tool rather than a replacement for QA. The role of AI is to assist in the interpretation and processing of intricate information, thereby facilitating the QA process but not supplanting the foundational principles and practices of QA.

12.1 Introduction

In this chapter, we categorize quality assurance (QA) within the field of radiation therapy into two main divisions—radiotherapy plan QA and machine/instrumentation QA. We delve deeper into radiotherapy plan QA by mapping it across the care chain of a patient, identifying several key processes where medical physicists contribute significantly (figure 12.1). Following this, we explore various scholarly works on the application of artificial intelligence (AI) that can support and enhance QA practices across each sub-category. This review work aims to highlight the potential of AI as a tool to assist in the precision and efficiency of QA processes in radiation therapy.

12.2 Patient QA

12.2.1 Pre-planning QA

12.2.1.1 Contouring QA

Several early investigations used the distribution of the morphological [2–4] or texture [5] features of the contours to detect a contouring error by finding significant

doi:10.1088/978-0-7503-6119-4ch12

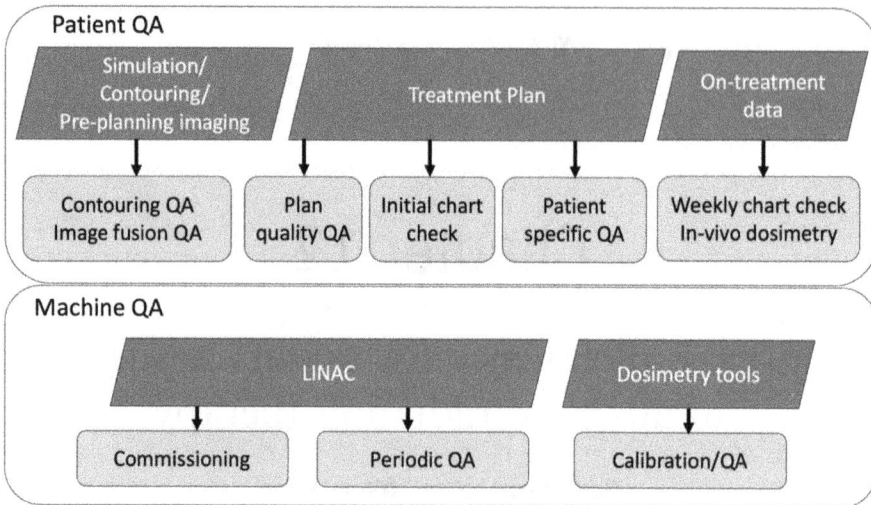

Figure 12.1. Simplified QA workflow in radiation oncology physics. Targets of the QA and QA elements are represented in parallelograms and round-edged rectangles, respectively.

deviation from the ground truth distribution derived from verified contours. Predefined thresholding on the deviation from the mean was applied by Chen *et al* [3] to detect anomalies. Alternatively, a supervised machine-learning approach, such as conditional random forest [2] can be used. A deep-learning-based approach, which had been introduced as an auto-contouring tool [6], can also be used for contouring QA: for example, a convolutional neural network (CNN) was used for verifying atlas-based auto-contours [7].

Care must be taken when adopting the AI contouring QA tools. Many published algorithms are trained to maximize quantitative accuracy metrics such as the Dice similarity coefficient (DSC) or Hausdorff distance (HD). However, these metrics do not always agree with each other [8] or may not be sensitive enough to detect localized errors that could be clinically relevant [7]. Although a correlation between clinical acceptability and surface DSC has been demonstrated [9], other complementary evaluation methods, such as Likert scales [10] or the Turing test [11] could be considered. Moreover, it is important to consider potential mistakes and interoperator variability in manual contours that served as training data—the use of a high-quality contour dataset, such as the manually curated multi-institutional dataset [12] should be considered. Alternatively, tools are available to generate consensus contours from multiple sets of human-generated contours [13]. As such, evaluation of AI contours should be conducted in multiple domains, rather than relying on a single metric [14] (figure 12.2).

12.2.1.2 Image fusion (registration)

Importance of image fusion (registration) QA is growing, particularly in adaptive radiotherapy where registration error between simulation and daily CT propagates

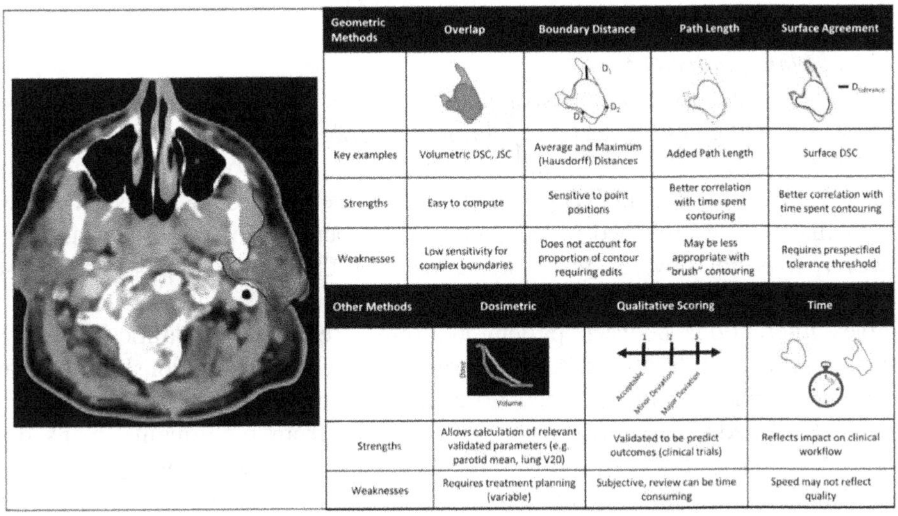

Figure 12.2. Different methods of evaluation of AI-generated contours. (Reproduced with permission from [14]. Copyright 2021 Elsevier.)

to contouring and dose accumulation accuracy and thus negatively impacts plan quality. Image registration QA is conducted mainly at two levels: (i) at the commissioning stage for the registration system and (ii) at a patient-specific level as part of radiotherapy workflow, when image fusion is required for target delineation or plan adaptation. Patient-specific evaluation of image registration is challenging due to a lack of ground truth [17], sources of uncertainties such as anatomical changes or image quality [18], and a lack of consensus on evaluation methods [19]. Consequently, QA practices vary between institutions [19, 20], many of which use qualitative visual inspection in a clinical setting [20]. Although visual inspection is an important element of the patient-specific registration QA, as recommended by TG-132 [15], it is not standardized and relies on the expertise level of a user [16]. Quantitative assessment can be done by identifying and calculating the displacement between homologous anatomical landmarks or contours, or examination of a deformation vector field (DVF) [16]. AI can help in the extraction of homologous structures, which would have been a labor-intensive process if done manually. For this purpose, in addition to the existing image transformation methods [21, 22], the use of machine learning such as the decision tree [23] or deep learning [24] has been investigated. AI can also play an important role in QA of deformable registration and can augment the DVF-based metrics that were already proposed as quantitative QA [25–27]. For example, Neylon *et al* [28] trained a supervised neural network model to calculate the registration error in the physical distance from the registered image and a biomechanical model. Similarly, CNN-based supervised models were used to predict registration accuracy from patches of images [29, 30]. Smolders *et al* [31] trained a deep-learning-based DVF uncertainty prediction model, which can be used for comparing different registration algorithms or estimating uncertainty in accumulated dose.

12.2.2 Pre-treatment plan QA

12.2.2.1 Plan quality QA

One of the most important QAs of plan quality is the planned dose distribution meeting clinical goals in terms of target coverage and organs-at-risk (OARs) sparing. Reviewers often use a table of scoresheets that compares the calculated dose–volume histogram (DVH) parameters for targets and OARs versus the preset criteria that were established based on clinical experience or published guidelines. However, it is not obvious from the scoresheets that the best possible trade-off between target coverage and OAR sparing is achieved, which is determined by complex interactions between patient anatomy, treatment modalities, and other patient-specific considerations. AI can unravel these complex relationships to inform the reviewers whether the planned dose distribution is optimal given these constraints. Knowledge-based planning (KBP) learns from high-quality plans using various AI approaches to estimate a range of achievable dose. A thorough review of KBP is outside the scope of this chapter and can be found in Ge *et al* [32]. The concept of KBP can be used not only for assisting IMRT optimization, but also for automated QA of the completed plans. Tol *et al* [33], and subsequently Cao *et al* [34], used a commercial KBP tool RapidPlan (Varian Medical Systems, Palo Alto, CA) to predict a range of DVH parameters for OARs and showed that the plans for which OAR doses exceeded the predicted range can be improved by further optimization. Stanhope *et al* [35] used their DVH prediction model to identify the clinically unacceptable patient-specific QA (PSQA) results that translate into the DVH falling outside the predicted DVH range. A deep-learning-based approach [36–38] aims at directly predicting 3D dose distribution from simulation CT (figure 12.3); DVH parameters can then be derived from the predicted 3D distribution and used for flagging suboptimal plans [38]

Use of dose prediction models for automatic plan quality QA comes with caveats: in order to achieve precise and accurate prediction and identify more suboptimal plans, it is important to train a model from the carefully selected high-quality plans with consistent OARs sparing [34]. Also, as pointed out in [34, 38], automatic QA does not always align with physicians' judgment, due to the subjective nature of plan quality review where physicians have diverse preferences over target coverage and OAR sparing.

12.2.2.2 Pre-treatment chart review

Pre-treatment chart review is a comprehensive review of a radiotherapy plan by a qualified medical physicist before the treatment begins. Physics chart review comprises various aspects of a plan, including (i) data transfer integrity, (ii) dose calculation accuracy, (iii) plan quality, (iv) consistency of prescription including image guidance requests, and (v) other special considerations [39]. It was shown to be the most effective safety barrier to prevent radiotherapy incidents [40]. However, studies show that a sizable portion of errors pass through the physics chart review [40–42]. Automation and standardization are listed as two major paths to enhance the effectiveness of physics chart review [39, 41]. To this end, software solutions have

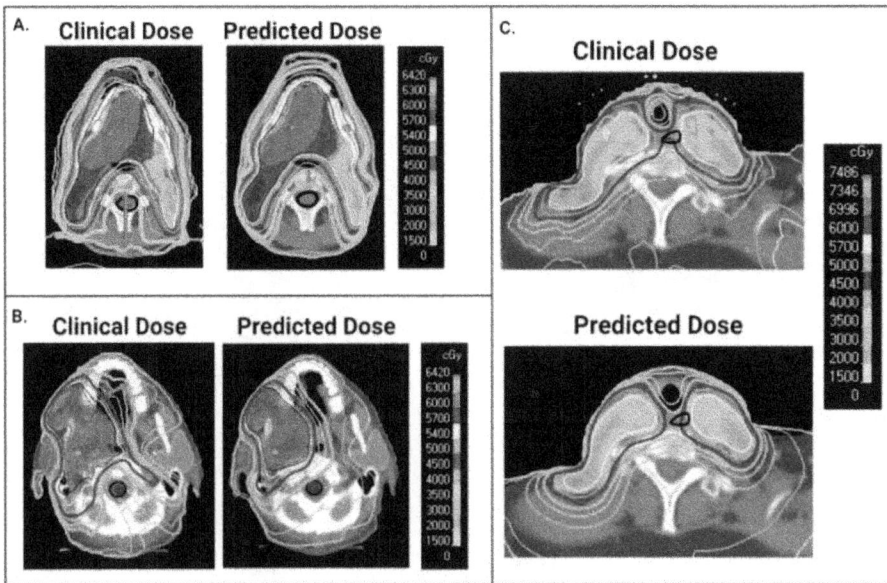

Figure 12.3. Examples of head-and-neck plans flagged by a deep-learning-based 3D dose prediction model by Gronberg *et al* for suboptimal dose to (A) a spinal cord and (B) oral cavity. For (C), the model was not able to predict suboptimal dose to the esophagus. (Reproduced with permission from [38]. Copyright 2023 Elsevier.)

been developed to assist the manual plan checking process [43–46]. These software tools typically apply a set of predefined rules for a given treatment type. As previously mentioned, however, there are many circumstances that these predefined rules cannot apply, and it becomes intractable to set separate rules for every permutation of different scenarios. AI is beneficial in that it can evaluate the plan in the context that it learns from data.

Error detection in chart review can be seen as anomaly detection—identification of the samples that deviate from the rest of the data. A qualitative approach applies data exploration techniques, such as clustering and principal component analysis (PCA), to visually identify outliers. An example is the study by Azmandian *et al* [47] who used the data exploration techniques to detect a gross error in the beam parameters for prostate four-field box treatments (figure 12.4).

One possible quantitative approach is to learn a joint probability distribution of the parameters characterizing a radiotherapy plan (e.g. anatomical sites, fractionation, treatment modality). If the probability model returns a small probability value for a test plan having a certain parameter set, the plan can be flagged for possible presence of errors. A Bayesian network (BN) can calculate joint probability using: (i) a directed acyclic graph (DAG) representing dependent or independent relationships between variables and (ii) conditional probability values that can be learned from training data. BNs have been used for error detection in radiotherapy plans [48–51]. Obtaining network topology for a BN model such as figure 12.5 remains a challenge, often requiring a group of experts to manually define the dependency relationships.

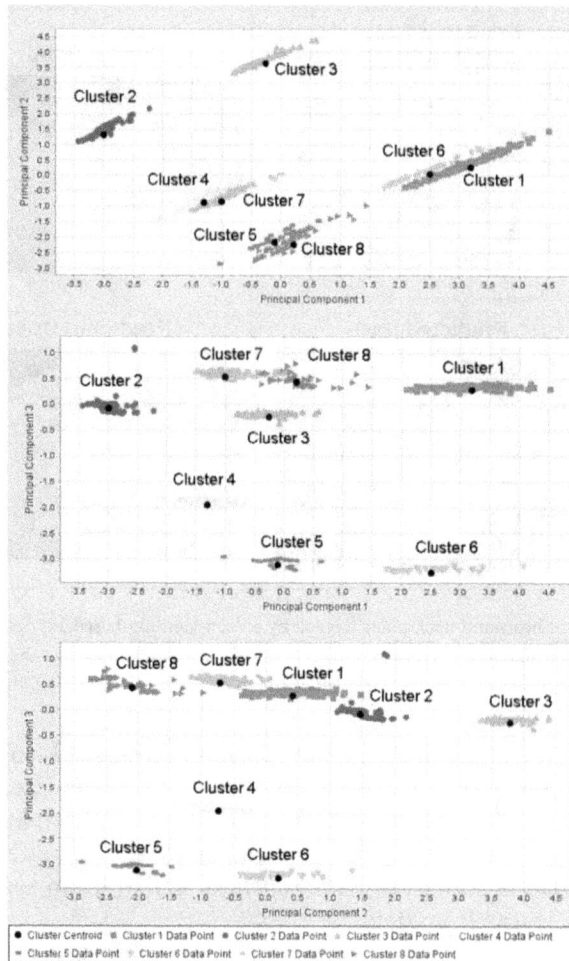

Figure 12.4. Four-field box prostate plans grouped into clusters based on their energy and monitor units. The plans are projected to a two-dimensional plane defined by the first two principal components and clustered using k-means clustering. (Reproduced with permission from [47]. Copyright 2007 IOP Publishing Ltd.)

Kalet *et al* [49] proposed the use of heuristics derived from radiation oncology ontology data to reduce the manual work in learning the network. A combination of data-driven and heuristic approaches can also be used for learning BN DAG [52]. In addition to BN, other machine-learning methods have been applied to detecting outlier radiotherapy plans. The forest-based method, used by Liu *et al* [53], makes it attractive for plan QA in that it can handle categorical variables and is robust to high-dimensional data [54].

When implementing these error detection models in clinic, a 'data drift', a change in data distribution over time, has to be considered. Data drift is prevalent in the medical field [55], including radiation oncology, where treatment practices, such as fractionation schemes, constantly change over time [56]. Thus, these decision

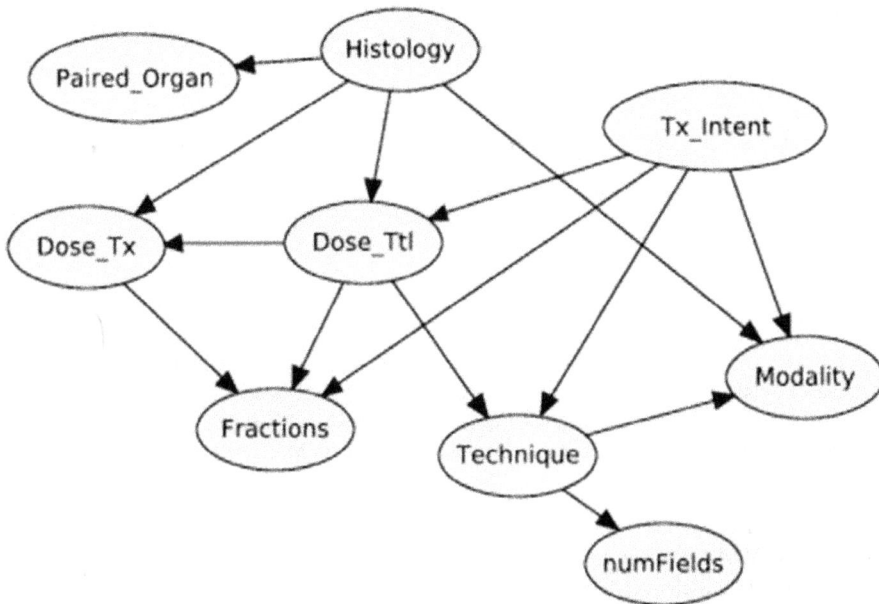

Figure 12.5. A Bayesian network topology by representing the dependency relationships (represented by arrows) between the variables that characterize a treatment plan (represented by nodes). (Reproduced with permission from [48]. Copyright 2015 Institute of Physics and Engineering in Medicine.)

support tools need be regularly monitored and re-calibrated to update the criteria discriminating erroneous plans, in a similar fashion to a study by Ruan *et al* [57]

12.2.2.3 Patient-specific QA

Pre-treatment PSQA was introduced to ensure that IMRT plans involving complex movements of multi-leaf collimators (MLC) are properly calculated, transferred to a machine, and accurately delivered [58]. PSQA is carried out by delivering a plan to a detector and evaluating the agreement between calculation and measurement. The agreement is typically computed using two-dimensional gamma analysis [59] to accommodate two-dimensional detectors. A plan is regarded satisfactory if the gamma passing rate (GPR) is above the fixed threshold: TG-218 [60] recommends a passing rate of 95% under 3%/2 mm criteria. The power of AI can be harnessed to predict GPR from IMRT QA even before delivering the QA plan, based on plan, machine, and measurement device characteristics. Such a prediction system has three potential clinical benefits, as follows. (i) Plan-specific issues, such as the over-optimization use of TPS beyond its capability, can be identified and mitigated ahead of time, thereby minimizing interruption in patient care. (ii) AI can be used to establish a GPR threshold specific to a certain type of plan, enhancing the sensitivity and specificity of the PSQA. (iii) The prediction model can illuminate systematic factors in TPS or delivery systems that can lead to dose discrepancy between calculation and measurement.

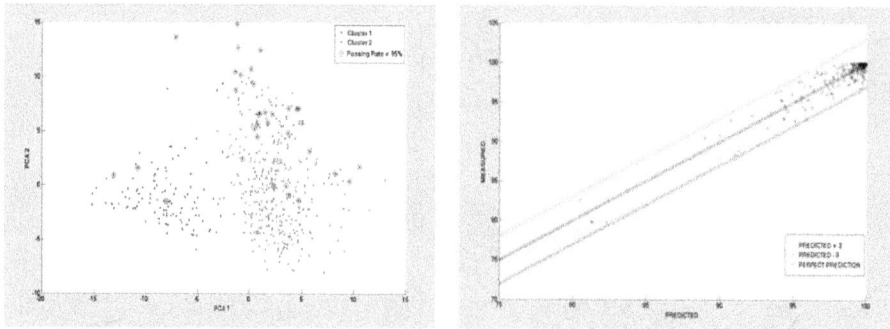

Figure 12.6. Left: Clustering of the examined plans using PCA to demonstrate the plans with low passing rate (circled) can be isolated by a combination of plan characteristics. Right: Agreement between the actual gamma passing rate and prediction by the virtual IMRT QA model. (Reproduced from [70] with permission from John Wiley & Sons. Copyright 2016 American Association of Physicists in Medicine.)

Several plan characteristics have been proposed as predictors of PSQA. First of all, IMRT or VMAT plan complexity metrics that quantify the irregularities in field apertures, MLC motion [61–63], or a fluence map [64], were shown to be correlated with robust deliverability [65] and PSQA GPR [66], and thus have been used for many IMRT QA prediction models. In addition, dosiomics analysis—texture analysis of dose distribution [67]—was proposed as another indicator of plan complexity that can contribute to dose delivery inaccuracies [68], and was shown to have benefits in predicting IMRT QA results [69]. Many machine-learning methods were used for putting together these predictive features into a PSQA prediction model. A seminal work by Valdes *et al* [70], coined as 'virtual IMRT QA' built a Poisson regression-based prediction model that predicts PSQA GPR from 78 plan complexity metrics (figure 12.6). This model was validated in multiple external datasets [71]. Since their work, different machine-learning methods were investigated to enhance GPR prediction, such as CNN [72–74], support vector machine [75], boosted trees [76], and random forest [69, 77].

Several studies highlight the limitation of PSQA, especially in its reliance on GPR, due to lack of sensitivity [78, 79], correlation with dose to targets and OARs [80, 81], or independent audits [82]. One of the criticisms is the use of a fixed GPR threshold for pass/fail, based on empirical evidence that the GPR from PSQA does not follow the Gaussian distribution [70, 83] as assumed for the TG-119 recommendation [58]. AI can be used to overcome the traditional one-size-fits-all approach to better 'explain' the 2D gamma distribution or GPR, by unraveling complex relationships between PSQA results and various sources of uncertainties, such as calculation engines, delivery systems, and detectors. For example, CNN has been used to predict MLC errors from features derived from EPID images [84] or a 3D detector array [85]. Another limitation of GPR is the loss of spatial information. This neural network-based method was extended to detect other types of errors, such as phantom set-up errors [86], monitoring unit scaling errors [87], or MLC modeling in TPS [88].

Some investigators attempted to directly predict two-dimensional gamma distributions by framing them as a deep-learning-based image synthesis problem. For example, Matsuura *et al* [89] used a generative adversarial network (GAN) to predict gamma distribution for EPID-based PSQA using the calculated fluence map as input (figure 12.7). Similarly, Mahdavi *et al* [90] created an artificial neural network (ANN)-based model to convert measured EPID fluences to the equivalent 2D gamma agreement between TPS and 2D array measurement.

There are considerations when training or evaluating the machine-learning-based PSQA models. First, the data (whether GPR or voxels with gamma > 1) the models are trained on are highly skewed towards passing. To address the class imbalance, a large sample size is needed for model training, or remedies such as oversampling (SMOTE) have to be taken. Second, the model should be interpretable so that root causes for poor dose agreement are fed back to the planning or machine QA process as actionable information.

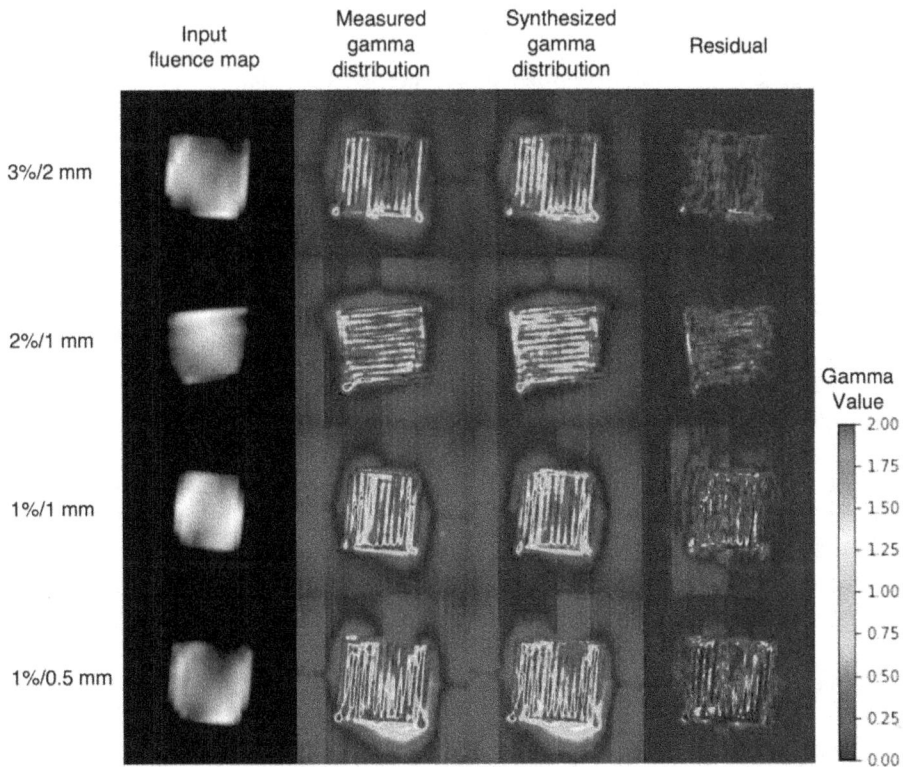

Figure 12.7. Examples of two-dimensional gamma distributions from IMRT QA synthesized by a GAN from an input fluence map. (Reproduced from [89] with permission from John Wiley & Sons. Copyright 2023 American Association of Physicists in Medicine.)

12.2.3 On-treatment QA

A patient undergoing treatment is monitored by physics, typically as weekly chart review. Weekly chart checks involve monitoring of treatment records and documentation which are recorded in the oncology information system (OIS) [91]. The literature is scant on the use of AI to assist in that scope of weekly chart review, apart from the proposed software solutions [92, 93]. Although it is the physician's responsibility, the review of daily imaging and registration accuracy and learning the dose implication of positioning error or anatomical changes is a task that can benefit from AI. Simple models were developed to detect gross alignment error in vertebral bodies [94, 95]. The same group implemented a CNN-based model that can detect not only vertebral body misalignment [96] but also soft tissue changes [97].

In vivo dosimetry is another form of on-treatment monitoring. EPID-based *in vivo* dosimetry, which captures exit radiation through a patient during treatment (transit dose), has drawn much interest due to its convenience and high spatial resolution. The EPID images can be compared to the fluence from the treatment plan in a similar manner to pre-treatment PSQA. Wolfs *et al* built a hidden Markov model [98] and CNN-based [99] prediction system that can detect anatomical or positional change by analysing transit EPID images. Alternatively, EPID can be backprojected into 3D dose in patient geometry, which enables direct comparison of target or OAR dose against planned dose [100]. DL has been applied to enhance the accuracy of the reconstructed dose for an MR-linac to correct for the effect of the magnetic field [101]. The same group modeled the generic deviation in a reconstructed *in vivo* dose using DL in order to increase the sensitivity of *in vivo* dosimetry in patient-related sources of deviations [102] (figure 12.8).

12.3 Treatment delivery systems and instruments

12.3.1 Machine commissioning

Zhao *et al* [103] introduced a machine-learning-based approach to model linac beam data, streamlining the processes of linac commissioning and QA. The model, trained with 43 Varian TrueBeam beam data, sets encompassing PDDs and profiles across various energies and field sizes from different institutions. Figure 12.9 shows the workflow for model building.

Using a 10×10 cm^2 field as the input, a multivariate regression model was developed for predicting beam specific PDDs and profiles for different field sizes. The predictions for PDDs exhibited a mean absolute percent relative error (%RE) ranging from 0.19% to 0.35% across various beam energies, with a maximum mean absolute %RE of 0.93%. In profile prediction, the mean absolute %RE was within the range of 0.66%–0.93%, and the maximum absolute %RE was 3.76%. Figure 12.10 shows the comparison between the ground truth and the predicted PDDs and profiles of 4×4 cm^2 and 30×30 cm^2 fields. Notably, this method showed potential in simplifying the linac commissioning procedure, offering time and resource efficiency while enhancing the accuracy of the commissioning process. It is particularly promising for its ability to address uncertainties, with the largest

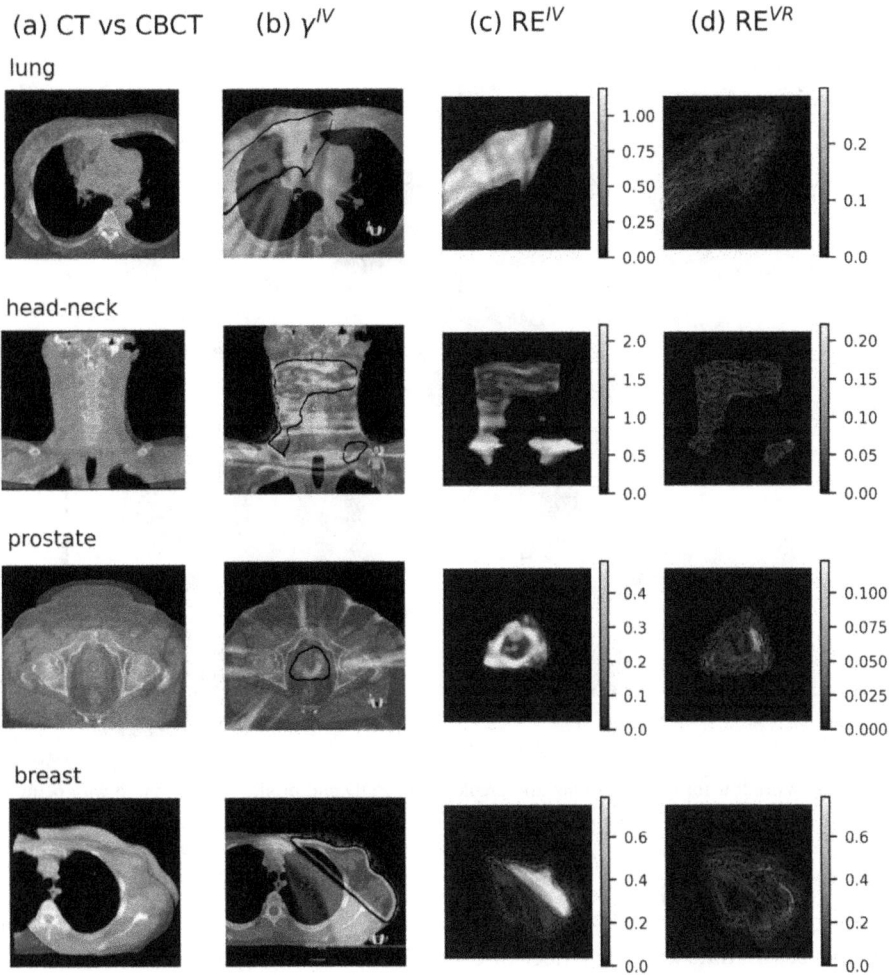

Figure 12.8. Example of anatomical changes that can be detected by 3D-U-Net based *in vivo* dose reconstruction prediction. Column (a): overlay between simulation and cone-beam CT demonstrating anatomical changes. Column (b): dose agreement in a 3D gamma map between *an in vivo* reconstructed dose and TPS. Column (c): U-Net reconstructed gamma map, highlighting patient-specific dose deviations. Column (d): U-Net reconstructed gamma map factoring out patient-specific changes, showing only generic (TPS or detector related) dose deviation. (Reproduced from [102] with permission from John Wiley & Sons. Copyright 2023 American Association of Physicists in Medicine.)

observed in the build-up region for PDD predictions and at the field penumbra for profile predictions.

Liu *et al* [104] from the same research group refined the data acquisition process for linac beam data through the application of implicit neural representation (NeRP) learning, as illustrated in figure 12.11. This aimed to enhance the accuracy of beam data collection verification and streamline the linac commissioning and QA procedure.

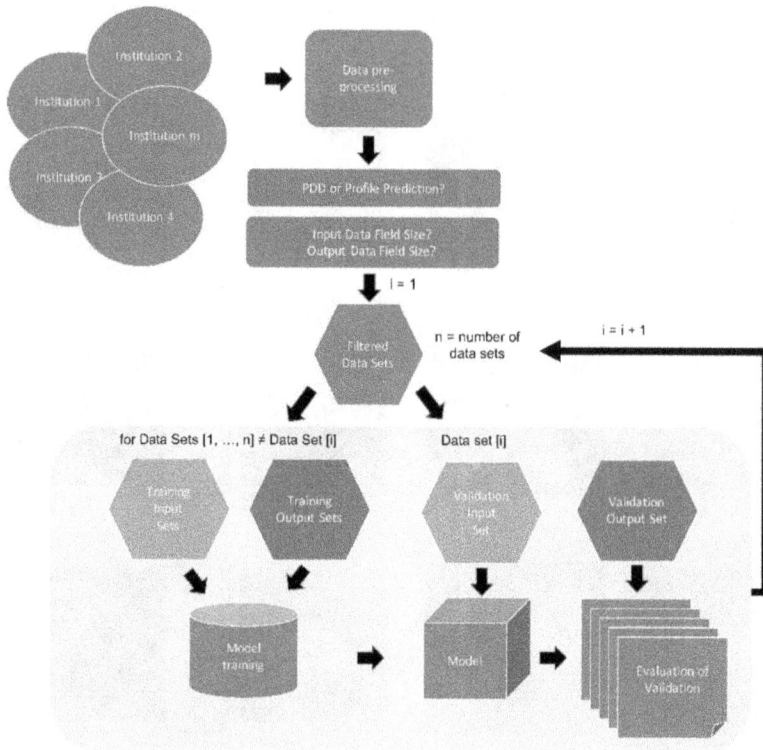

Figure 12.9. Workflow for model training and prediction of PDD and profiles. (Reproduced with permission from [103]. Copyright 2020 Elsevier.)

The authors incorporated prior knowledge of beam data into a multilayer perceptron network, achieved by learning the NeRP from a vendor-provided 'golden' beam dataset. This network underwent training to align with clinical beam data collected at a specific field size. Subsequently, it demonstrated the capability to predict beam data accurately for other field sizes. To assess prediction accuracy, the authors compared the network-predicted beam data with measurements obtained from water tanks across 14 clinical linacs. They found that the linac beam data predicted by the model exhibited strong agreement with water tank measurements (averagely > 95% passing rates at 1%/1 mm criteria and < 0.6% mean absolute errors). Figure 12.12 shows beam profile predictions against the ground truth data. Moreover, the model unveiled instances of measurement errors by identifying inconsistent beam predictions when trained with correct versus erroneous data samples. These discrepancies were characterized by a GPR < 90%. It is concluded that the model verifies beam data collection accuracy and holds promise of simplifying commissioning and QA processes by minimizing the number of required measurements without compromising the quality of medical physics service.

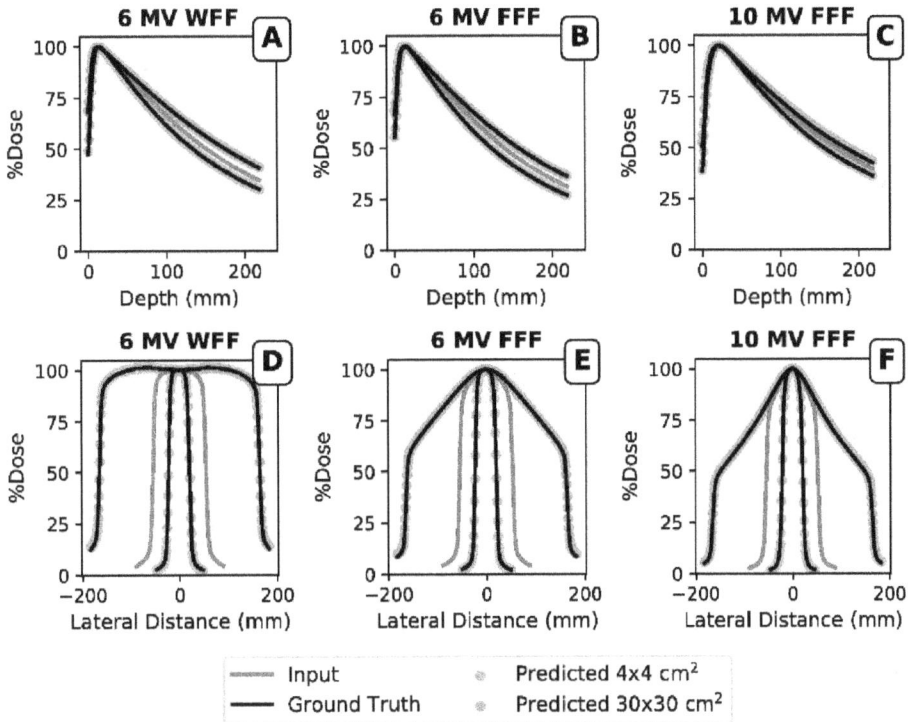

Figure 12.10. Example of PDD (A)–(C) and profile (D)–(F) prediction of a 4 × 4 cm² field (yellow dots) and a 30 × 30 cm² field (blue dots) with 10 × 10 cm² field as input (red line). The measured PDDs and profiles (ground truth) are depicted as black lines. (Reproduced with permission from [103]. Copyright 2020 Elsevier.)

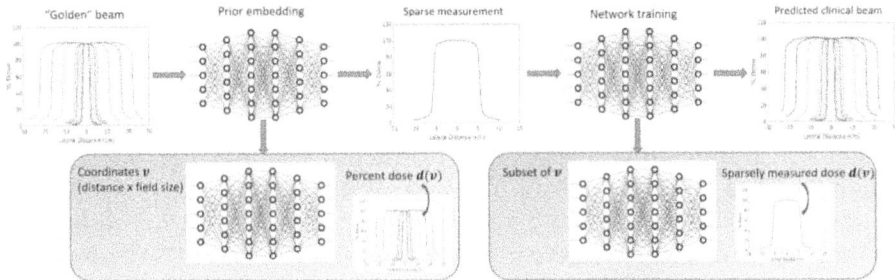

Figure 12.11. Workflow of NeRP learning for linac beam modeling and prediction. (Reproduced from [104] with permission from John Wiley & Sons. Copyright 2023 American Association of Physicists in Medicine.)

Wagner *et al* [105] introduced a machine-learning approach to expedite the modeling process for M6 CyberKnife integrated in Moderato. A machine-learning algorithm was trained to find electron beam parameters for other M6 devices. The algorithm simulated dose curves with varying spot size and energy, optimizing its performance through cross-validation, and validating its accuracy with measurements from other institutions equipped with M6 CyberKnife devices. The agreement

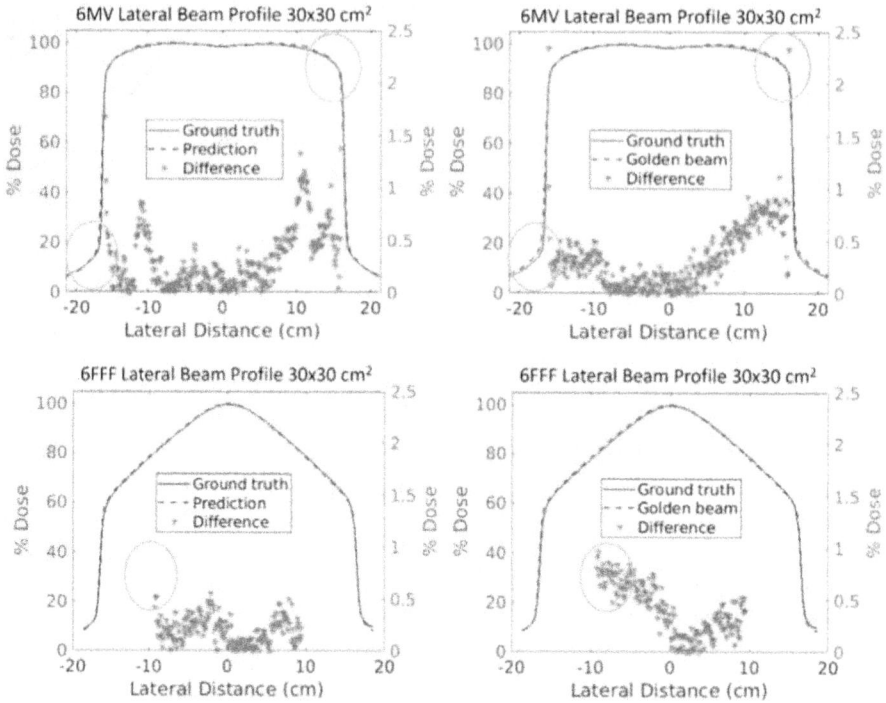

Figure 12.12. Example beam profile predictions for 6 MV and 6FFF beam at 30×30 cm^2 field size. Enhanced consistency in water tank measurements was achieved by fitting the prior-embedded network to sparse beam data, indicated by green circles, rather than using direct 'golden' beam data. (Reproduced from [104] with permission from John Wiley & Sons. Copyright 2023 American Association of Physicists in Medicine.)

in the Monte Carlo model was achieved for a monoenergetic electron beam of 6.75 MeV with a Gaussian spatial distribution of 2.4 mm full-width-at-half-maximum (FWHM). Clinical plan dose distributions from Moderato exhibited an agreement within 2% with the TPS, and film measurements further corroborated the precision of the model. During cross-validation of the prediction algorithm, minimal mean absolute errors of 0.1 MeV and 0.3 mm were observed for beam energy and spot size, respectively. The prediction agreements were within 3% with measurements, except for one device where differences up to 6% were detected. This approach can expedite the modeling of new machines within Monte Carlo systems, offering efficiency and reliability in the intricate process of medical physics modeling.

12.3.2 Machine QA

Numerous investigations have explored the diverse applications of machine learning in linac QA [106, 107]. These studies have delved into various avenues, encompassing models constructed from beam data commissioning, as detailed in the preceding section, to models derived from delivery log files [108–110]. Additionally, machine-learning models have been built using proton fields [111, 112], addressing image artifacts [113], and implementing automated QA through electronic portal imaging

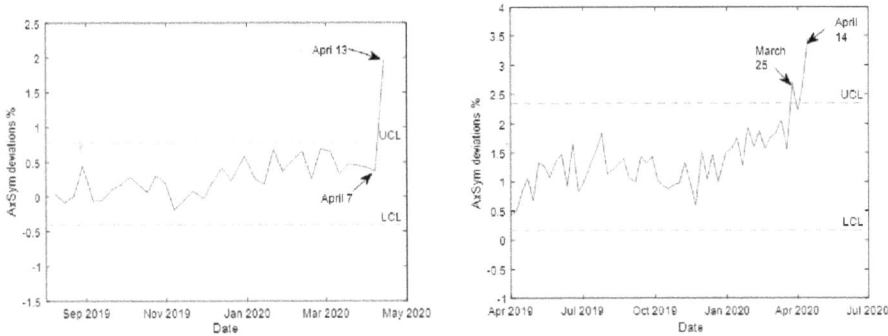

Figure 12.13. Results from SPC using symmetry data from open field beam (left) and EDW data (right). (Reproduced with permission from [117]. Copyright 2023 IOP Publishing Ltd.)

device (EPID) images [114]. This multifaceted exploration underscores the versatility of machine learning across various aspects of linac QA, highlighting its potential to enhance efficiency and accuracy in QA processes.

Chan *et al* [115] utilized five years of daily linac QA data for visual analysis and correlation studies among dosimetric parameters and the researchers gained insights into the intricacies of the data. Subsequently, they developed a convolutional neural network (time-series modeling) to predict beam symmetry using the same daily QA dataset [116]. The same research group further utilized the daily QA data, but to include both open fields and enhanced dynamic wedge (EDW) measurements [117]. They employed statical process control and autoregressive integrated moving average modeling to predict linac target failure. The EDW mechanism, characterized by nonuniform magnification factors within its wedge-directed beam profiles, played a pivotal role in their analysis. This nonuniformity introduced sensitivity to changing beam properties induced by a degrading target. Figure 12.13 illustrates two occurrences of target failures that can be effectively predicted from the daily symmetry data. The comprehensive approach contributes insights into the prediction of linac performance.

12.3.3 Dosimetry tool QA

Chang *et al* [118] presented a deep-learning hierarchical neural network (HNN) method to calibrate the EBT3 film with better calibration accuracy than the conventional R-NOD method. They used the Keras functional application program interface to build an HNN, with the inputs of net optical densities, pixel values, and inverse transmittances to reveal the delivered dose and train the neural network with deep learning. About the aging effect, the percentage error of the HNN method is within 4% and proved to be unaffected, while the averaged percentage error of the conventional R-NOD method is about 6.8% (figure 12.14). This new technique can be improved by updating the new calibration data into the HNN training system whenever physicists perform the recalibration. Based on collecting calibration data

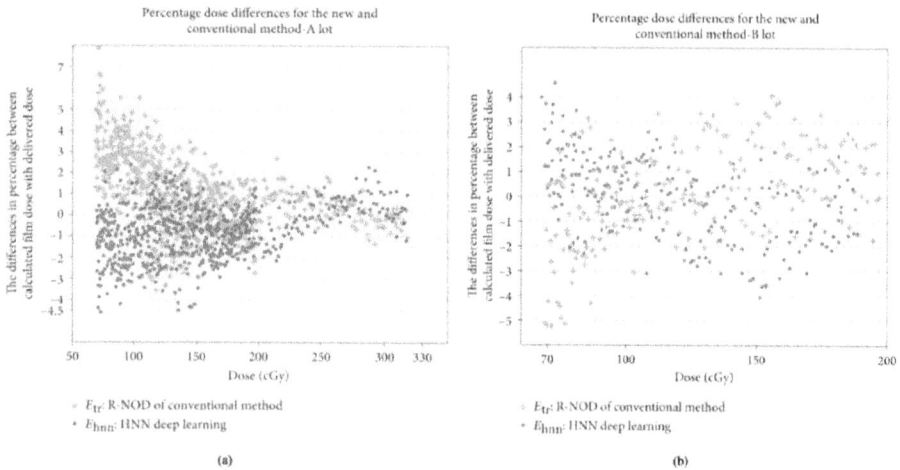

Figure 12.14. Percentage differences between the calculated dose and the delivered dose for the verification test of Lot A and Lot B films. (Reproduced from [118]. CC BY 4.0.)

with the HNN method, physicists could require less calibration time and reduce film usage.

Zhuang *et al* [119] described the development of an ANN approach for processing EBT3 films from various batches without requiring specific calibration for each batch. Utilizing PyTorch, researchers constructed a feed-forward ANN model that transforms pixel values from scanned images across different batches into the corresponding absorbed dose. To facilitate this, films exposed to x-ray doses from different batches were scanned in transmission mode using an Epson 11000XL scanner, serving both for model training and validation. The dose map generated by the TPS was employed as the target output for the ANN model. To assess the method's effectiveness and its adaptability, a cross-validation study was conducted. The ANN model, once trained, was used to convert scanned images into dose maps, demonstrating a high level of consistency with the dose maps calculated by TPS. For films exposed using the sliding window technique, the mean square errors (MSEs) were below 16.0 cGy for the training batches and under 18 cGy for the testing batches. In the case of patient IMRT films, the γ (3%, 3 mm) for comparison between the dose maps from the ANN and TPS exceeded 97.5% for the training set and 97.0% for the testing set. These results indicate the potential of this method to accurately convert pixel values to absorbed doses for EBT3 films without needing batch-specific calibrations, suggesting its applicability to other scenarios.

Avanzo *et al* [120] developed a machine-learning model to forecast skin dose from targeted intraoperative (TARGIT) treatment, facilitating the timely implementation of strategies to mitigate the risk of excessive skin dose. The process involved feature selection of predictors of *in vivo* skin dose, followed by the training of various machine-learning models using *in vivo* dosimetry results. The evaluation was conducted through tenfold cross-validation, with rankings based on both roots mean square error (RMSE) and adjusted correlation coefficient of true versus predicted values (adj-R2). The identified predictors strongly correlated with *in vivo* dosimetry, including factors such as the distance of skin from source, depth-dose in water at the depth of the applicator in the breast, utilization of a replacement source, and irradiation time. Among the models, support vector regression (SVR) emerged as the most effective, achieving an RMSE of 0.746 (95% confidence intervals, 0.737, 0.756) and an adj-R2 of 0.481 (95% CI 0.468, 0.494) during the tenfold cross-validation. This SVR model, trained on *in vivo* dosimetry results, holds significant practicality. The authors concluded that it can be employed to predict skin dose during the patient set-up for TARGIT, enabling the timely adoption of strategies to prevent excessive skin dose, thus enhancing the overall safety and efficacy of the procedure.

12.4 Summary

Quality assurance plays a crucial role in ensuring the accuracy of radiotherapy planning, delivery, and instrumentation within the clinical workflow. This critical process places a substantial demand on clinical physicists' resources. The integration of AI into QA brings forth a twofold enhancement. First, AI serves to accentuate components with heightened susceptibility to failure, enabling physicists to allocate their attention more effectively towards those vulnerabilities. By pinpointing these areas of concern, AI augments the specificity of QA process, facilitating a more targeted and efficient utilization of resources. Second, AI possesses the capability to discover intricate system errors that may elude human detection due to their complexity. The analysis of various influencing factors is a forte of AI, enabling it to discern anomalies that might otherwise remain hidden, reinforcing the overall reliability of the QA process. In summary, the incorporation of AI into QA efforts contributes to an elevated level of efficiency and standardization within the QA program, advancing the precision, safety, and consistency of radiotherapy practices.

References

[1] ASTRO 201 Safety is no accident *Guide* American Society for Radiation Oncology https://astro.org/Patient-Care-and-Research/Patient-Safety/Safety-is-no-Accident

[2] McIntosh C, Svistoun I and Purdie T G 2013 Groupwise conditional random forests for automatic shape classification and contour quality assessment in radiotherapy planning *IEEE Trans. Med. Imaging* **32** 1043–57

[3] Chen H C *et al* 2015 Automated contouring error detection based on supervised geometric attribute distribution models for radiation therapy: a general strategy *Med. Phys.* **42** 1048–59

[4] Hui C B *et al* 2018 Quality assurance tool for organ at risk delineation in radiation therapy using a parametric statistical approach *Med. Phys.* **45** 2089–96

[5] Zhang Y, Plautz T E, Hao Y, Kinchen C and Li X A 2019 Texture-based, automatic contour validation for online adaptive replanning: a feasibility study on abdominal organs *Med. Phys.* **46** 4010–20

[6] Cardenas C E *et al* 2018 Deep learning algorithm for auto-delineation of high-risk oropharyngeal clinical target volumes with built-in Dice similarity coefficient parameter optimization function *Int. J. Radiat. Oncol. Biol. Phys.* **101** 468–78

[7] Rhee D J *et al* 2019 Automatic detection of contouring errors using convolutional neural networks *Med. Phys.* **46** 5086–97

[8] Gooding M J, Boukerroui D, Vasquez Osorio E, Monshouwer R and Brunenberg E 2022 Multicenter comparison of measures for quantitative evaluation of contouring in radiotherapy *Phys. Imaging Radiat. Oncol.* **24** 152–8

[9] Rhee D J *et al* 2022 Automatic contouring QA method using a deep learning-based autocontouring system *J. Appl. Clin. Med. Phys.* **23** e13647

[10] Cha E *et al* 2021 Clinical implementation of deep learning contour autosegmentation for prostate radiotherapy *Radiother. Oncol.* **159** 1–7

[11] Gooding M J *et al* 2018 Comparative evaluation of autocontouring in clinical practice: a practical method using the turing test *Med. Phys.* **45** 5105–15

[12] Yang J, Veeraraghavan H, van Elmpt W, Dekker A, Gooding M and Sharp G 2020 CT images with expert manual contours of thoracic cancer for benchmarking auto-segmentation accuracy *Med. Phys.* **47** 3250–5

[13] Allozi R *et al* 2010 Tools for consensus analysis of experts' contours for radiotherapy structure definitions *Radiother. Oncol.* **97** 572–8

[14] Sherer M V *et al* 2021 Metrics to evaluate the performance of auto-segmentation for radiation treatment planning: a critical review *Radiother. Oncol.* **160** 185–91

[15] Brock K K, Mutic S, McNutt T R, Li H and Kessler M L 2017 Use of image registration and fusion algorithms and techniques in radiotherapy: report of the AAPM Radiation Therapy Committee Task Group No. 132 *Med. Phys.* **44** e43–76

[16] Rong Y *et al* 2021 Rigid and deformable image registration for radiation therapy: a self-study evaluation guide for NRG oncology clinical trial participation *Pract. Radiat. Oncol.* **11** 282–98

[17] Paganelli C, Meschini G, Molinelli S, Riboldi M and Baroni G 2018 Patient-specific validation of deformable image registration in radiation therapy: overview and caveats *Med. Phys.* **45** e908–e22

[18] Nenoff L *et al* 2023 Review and recommendations on deformable image registration uncertainties for radiotherapy applications *Phys. Med. Biol.* **68** 24TR01

[19] Hussein M, Akintonde A, McClelland J, Speight R and Clark C H 2021 Clinical use, challenges, and barriers to implementation of deformable image registration in radiotherapy—the need for guidance and QA tools *Br. J. Radiol.* **94** 20210001

[20] Yuen J *et al* 2020 An international survey on the clinical use of rigid and deformable image registration in radiotherapy *J. Appl. Clin. Med. Phys.* **21** 10–24

[21] Yang D *et al* 2017 A method to detect landmark pairs accurately between intra-patient volumetric medical images *Med. Phys.* **44** 5859–72

[22] Paganelli C, Peroni M, Baroni G and Riboldi M 2013 Quantification of organ motion based on an adaptive image-based scale invariant feature method *Med. Phys.* **40** 111701

[23] Han D, Gao Y, Wu G, Yap P T and Shen D 2015 Robust anatomical landmark detection with application to MR brain image registration *Comput. Med. Imaging Graph.* **46** 277–90

[24] Grewal M, Wiersma J, Westerveld H, Bosman P A N and Alderliesten T 2023 Automatic landmark correspondence detection in medical images with an application to deformable image registration *J. Med. Imaging* **10** 014007

[25] Bender E T and Tomé W A 2009 The utilization of consistency metrics for error analysis in deformable image registration *Phys. Med. Biol.* **54** 5561–77

[26] Varadhan R, Karangelis G, Krishnan K and Hui S 2013 A framework for deformable image registration validation in radiotherapy clinical applications *J. Appl. Clin. Med. Phys.* **14** 4066

[27] Saleh Z H *et al* 2014 The distance discordance metric: a novel approach to quantifying spatial uncertainties in intra- and inter-patient deformable image registration *Phys. Med. Biol.* **59** 733–46

[28] Neylon J, Min Y, Low D A and Santhanam A 2017 A neural network approach for fast, automated quantification of DIR performance *Med. Phys.* **44** 4126–38

[29] Eppenhof K A J and Pluim J P W 2018 Error estimation of deformable image registration of pulmonary CT scans using convolutional neural networks *J. Med. Imaging* **5** 024003

[30] Galib S M, Lee H K, Guy C L, Riblett M J and Hugo G D 2020 A fast and scalable method for quality assurance of deformable image registration on lung CT scans using convolutional neural networks *Med. Phys.* **47** 99–109

[31] Smolders A, Lomax A, Weber D C and Albertini F 2023 Deep learning based uncertainty prediction of deformable image registration for contour propagation and dose accumulation in online adaptive radiotherapy *Phys. Med. Biol.* **68** 245027

[32] Ge Y and Wu Q J 2019 Knowledge-based planning for intensity-modulated radiation therapy: a review of data-driven approaches *Med. Phys.* **46** 2760–75

[33] Tol J P, Dahele M, Delaney A R, Slotman B J and Verbakel W F 2015 Can knowledge-based DVH predictions be used for automated, individualized quality assurance of radiotherapy treatment plans? *Radiat. Oncol.* **10** 234

[34] Cao W *et al* 2022 Knowledge-based planning for the radiation therapy treatment plan quality assurance for patients with head and neck cancer *J. Appl. Clin. Med. Phys.* **23** e13614

[35] Stanhope C *et al* 2015 Utilizing knowledge from prior plans in the evaluation of quality assurance *Phys. Med. Biol.* **60** 4873–91

[36] Fan J, Wang J, Chen Z, Hu C, Zhang Z and Hu W 2019 Automatic treatment planning based on three-dimensional dose distribution predicted from deep learning technique *Med. Phys.* **46** 370–81

[37] Nguyen D *et al* 2019 3D radiotherapy dose prediction on head and neck cancer patients with a hierarchically densely connected U-Net deep learning architecture *Phys. Med. Biol.* **64** 065020

[38] Gronberg M P *et al* 2023 Deep learning-based dose prediction for automated, individualized quality assurance of head and neck radiation therapy plans *Pract. Radiat. Oncol.* **13** e282–e91

[39] Ford E *et al* 2020 Strategies for effective physics plan and chart review in radiation therapy: report of AAPM Task Group 275 *Med. Phys.* **47** e236–e72

[40] Ford E C, Terezakis S, Souranis A, Harris K, Gay H and Mutic S 2012 Quality control quantification (QCQ): a tool to measure the value of quality control checks in radiation oncology *Int. J. Radiat. Oncol. Biol. Phys.* **84** e263–9

[41] Gopan O, Zeng J, Novak A, Nyflot M and Ford E 2016 The effectiveness of pretreatment physics plan review for detecting errors in radiation therapy *Med. Phys.* **43** 5181

[42] Clark B G, Brown R J, Ploquin J and Dunscombe P 2013 Patient safety improvements in radiation treatment through 5 years of incident learning *Pract. Radiat. Oncol.* **3** 157–63

[43] Siochi R A, Pennington E C, Waldron T J and Bayouth J E 2009 Radiation therapy plan checks in a paperless clinic *J. Appl. Clin. Med. Phys.* **10** 43–62

[44] Yang D and Moore K L 2012 Automated radiotherapy treatment plan integrity verification *Med. Phys.* **39** 1542–51

[45] Covington E L *et al* 2016 Improving treatment plan evaluation with automation *J. Appl. Clin. Med. Phys.* **17** 16–31

[46] Holdsworth C *et al* 2017 Computerized system for safety verification of external beam radiation therapy planning *Int. J. Radiat. Oncol. Biol. Phys.* **98** 691–8

[47] Azmandian F *et al* 2007 Towards the development of an error checker for radiotherapy treatment plans: a preliminary study *Phys. Med. Biol.* **52** 6511–24

[48] Kalet A M, Gennari J H, Ford E C and Phillips M H 2015 Bayesian network models for error detection in radiotherapy plans *Phys. Med. Biol.* **60** 2735–49

[49] Kalet A M, Doctor J N, Gennari J H and Phillips M H 2017 Developing Bayesian networks from a dependency-layered ontology: a proof-of-concept in radiation oncology *Med. Phys.* **44** 4350–9

[50] Luk S M H *et al* 2019 Characterization of a Bayesian network-based radiotherapy plan verification model *Med. Phys.* **46** 2006–14

[51] Chang X, Li H H, Kalet A M and Yang D 2019 Development and validation of a Bayesian network method to detect external beam radiation therapy physician order errors *Int. J. Radiat. Oncol. Biol. Phys.* **105** 423–31

[52] Lee S *et al* 2015 Bayesian network ensemble as a multivariate strategy to predict radiation pneumonitis risk *Med. Phys.* **42** 2421–30

[53] Liu S *et al* 2023 Implementation of a knowledge-based decision support system for treatment plan auditing through automation *Med. Phys.* **50** 6978–89

[54] Breiman L 2001 Random forests *Mach. Learn.* **45** 5–32

[55] Chen J H, Alagappan M, Goldstein M K, Asch S M and Altman R B 2017 Decaying relevance of clinical data towards future decisions in data-driven inpatient clinical order sets *Int. J. Med. Inform.* **102** 71–9

[56] Kalet A M, Luk S M H and Phillips M H 2020 Radiation therapy quality assurance tasks and tools: the many roles of machine learning *Med. Phys.* **47** e168–e77

[57] Ruan D *et al* 2012 Evolving treatment plan quality criteria from institution-specific experience *Med. Phys.* **39** 2708–12

[58] Ezzell G A *et al* 2003 Guidance document on delivery, treatment planning, and clinical implementation of IMRT: report of the IMRT Subcommittee of the AAPM Radiation Therapy Committee *Med. Phys.* **30** 2089–115

[59] Low D A, Harms W B, Mutic S and Purdy J A 1998 A technique for the quantitative evaluation of dose distributions *Med. Phys.* **25** 656–61

[60] Miften M *et al* 2018 Tolerance limits and methodologies for IMRT measurement-based verification QA: recommendations of AAPM Task Group No. 218 *Med. Phys.* **45** e53–83

[61] Du W, Cho S H, Zhang X, Hoffman K E and Kudchadker R J 2014 Quantification of beam complexity in intensity-modulated radiation therapy treatment plans *Med. Phys.* **41** 021716

[62] McNiven A L, Sharpe M B and Purdie T G 2010 A new metric for assessing IMRT modulation complexity and plan deliverability *Med. Phys.* **37** 505–15

[63] Chiavassa S, Bessieres I, Edouard M, Mathot M and Moignier A 2019 Complexity metrics for IMRT and VMAT plans: a review of current literature and applications *Br. J. Radiol.* **92** 20190270

[64] Crowe S B *et al* 2015 Examination of the properties of IMRT and VMAT beams and evaluation against pre-treatment quality assurance results *Phys. Med. Biol.* **60** 2587–601

[65] Younge K C, Roberts D, Janes L A, Anderson C, Moran J M and Matuszak M M 2016 Predicting deliverability of volumetric-modulated arc therapy (VMAT) plans using aperture complexity analysis *J. Appl. Clin. Med. Phys.* **17** 124–31

[66] Masi L, Doro R, Favuzza V, Cipressi S and Livi L 2013 Impact of plan parameters on the dosimetric accuracy of volumetric modulated arc therapy *Med. Phys.* **40** 071718

[67] Park S Y, Kim I H, Ye S J, Carlson J and Park J M 2014 Texture analysis on the fluence map to evaluate the degree of modulation for volumetric modulated arc therapy *Med. Phys.* **41** 111718

[68] Park J M, Kim J I and Park S Y 2019 Prediction of VMAT delivery accuracy with textural features calculated from fluence maps *Radiat. Oncol.* **14** 235

[69] Hirashima H *et al* 2020 Improvement of prediction and classification performance for gamma passing rate by using plan complexity and dosiomics features *Radiother. Oncol.* **153** 250–7

[70] Valdes G, Scheuermann R, Hung C Y, Olszanski A, Bellerive M and Solberg T D 2016 A mathematical framework for virtual IMRT QA using machine learning *Med. Phys.* **43** 4323

[71] Valdes G, Chan M F, Lim S B, Scheuermann R, Deasy J O and Solberg T D 2017 IMRT QA using machine learning: a multi-institutional validation *J. Appl. Clin. Med. Phys.* **18** 279–84

[72] Interian Y *et al* 2018 Deep nets vs expert designed features in medical physics: an IMRT QA case study *Med. Phys.* **45** 2672–80

[73] Tomori S *et al* 2018 A deep learning-based prediction model for gamma evaluation in patient-specific quality assurance *Med. Phys.* **45** 4055–65

[74] Ono T *et al* 2019 Prediction of dosimetric accuracy for VMAT plans using plan complexity parameters via machine learning *Med. Phys.* **46** 3823–32

[75] Granville D A, Sutherland J G, Belec J G and La Russa D J 2019 Predicting VMAT patient-specific QA results using a support vector classifier trained on treatment plan characteristics and linac QC metrics *Phys. Med. Biol.* **64** 095017

[76] Lam D *et al* 2019 Predicting gamma passing rates for portal dosimetry-based IMRT QA using machine learning *Med. Phys.* **46** 4666–75

[77] Li J *et al* 2019 Machine learning for patient-specific quality assurance of VMAT: prediction and classification accuracy *Int. J. Radiat. Oncol. Biol. Phys.* **105** 893–902

[78] Yan G, Liu C, Simon T A, Peng L C, Fox C and Li J G 2009 On the sensitivity of patient-specific IMRT QA to MLC positioning errors *J. Appl. Clin. Med. Phys.* **10** 120–8

[79] Kruse J J 2010 On the insensitivity of single field planar dosimetry to IMRT inaccuracies *Med. Phys.* **37** 2516–24

[80] Nelms B E, Zhen H and Tomé W A 2011 Per-beam, planar IMRT QA passing rates do not predict clinically relevant patient dose errors *Med. Phys.* **38** 1037–44

[81] Stasi M, Bresciani S, Miranti A, Maggio A, Sapino V and Gabriele P 2012 Pretreatment patient-specific IMRT quality assurance: a correlation study between gamma index and patient clinical dose volume histogram *Med. Phys.* **39** 7626–34

[82] Kry S F *et al* 2014 Institutional patient-specific IMRT QA does not predict unacceptable plan delivery *Int. J. Radiat. Oncol. Biol. Phys.* **90** 1195–201

[83] Kearney V, Solberg T, Jensen S, Cheung J, Chuang C and Valdes G 2018 Correcting TG 119 confidence limits *Med. Phys.* **45** 1001–8

[84] Nyflot M J, Thammasorn P, Wootton L S, Ford E C and Chaovalitwongse W A 2019 Deep learning for patient-specific quality assurance: identifying errors in radiotherapy delivery by radiomic analysis of gamma images with convolutional neural networks *Med. Phys.* **46** 456–64

[85] Kimura Y, Kadoya N, Tomori S, Oku Y and Jingu K 2020 Error detection using a convolutional neural network with dose difference maps in patient-specific quality assurance for volumetric modulated arc therapy *Phys Med.* **73** 57–64

[86] Kimura Y, Kadoya N, Oku Y, Kajikawa T, Tomori S and Jingu K 2021 Error detection model developed using a multi-task convolutional neural network in patient-specific quality assurance for volumetric-modulated arc therapy *Med. Phys.* **48** 4769–83

[87] Potter N J, Mund K, Andreozzi J M, Li J G, Liu C and Yan G 2020 Error detection and classification in patient-specific IMRT QA with dual neural networks *Med. Phys.* **47** 4711–20

[88] Sakai M *et al* 2021 Detecting MLC modeling errors using radiomics-based machine learning in patient-specific QA with an EPID for intensity-modulated radiation therapy *Med. Phys.* **48** 991–1002

[89] Matsuura T, Kawahara D, Saito A, Yamada K, Ozawa S and Nagata Y 2023 A synthesized gamma distribution-based patient-specific VMAT QA using a generative adversarial network *Med. Phys.* **50** 2488–98

[90] Mahdavi S R *et al* 2019 Use of artificial neural network for pretreatment verification of intensity modulation radiation therapy fields *Br. J. Radiol.* **92** 20190355

[91] Xia P *et al* 2021 Medical Physics Practice Guideline (MPPG) 11.a: plan and chart review in external beam radiotherapy and brachytherapy *J. Appl. Clin. Med. Phys.* **22** 4–19

[92] Hadley S W *et al* 2016 SafetyNet: streamlining and automating QA in radiotherapy *J. Appl. Clin. Med. Phys.* **17** 387–95

[93] Li H H, Wu Y, Yang D and Mutic S 2014 Software tool for physics chart checks *Pract. Radiat. Oncol.* **4** e217–25

[94] Jani S S, Low D A and Lamb J M 2015 Automatic detection of patient identification and positioning errors in radiation therapy treatment using 3-dimensional setup images *Pract. Radiat. Oncol.* **5** 304–11

[95] Lamb J M, Agazaryan N and Low D A 2013 Automated patient identification and localization error detection using 2-dimensional to 3-dimensional registration of kilovoltage x-ray setup images *Int. J. Radiat. Oncol. Biol. Phys.* **87** 390–3

[96] Luximon D C *et al* 2022 Development and interinstitutional validation of an automatic vertebral-body misalignment error detector for cone-beam CT-guided radiotherapy *Med. Phys.* **49** 6410–23

[97] Neylon J, Luximon D C, Ritter T and Lamb J M 2023 Proof-of-concept study of artificial intelligence-assisted review of CBCT image guidance *J. Appl. Clin. Med. Phys.* **24** e14016

[98] Wolfs C J A *et al* 2020 External validation of a hidden Markov model for gamma-based classification of anatomical changes in lung cancer patients using EPID dosimetry *Med. Phys.* **47** 4675–82

[99] Wolfs C J A, Canters R A M and Verhaegen F 2020 Identification of treatment error types for lung cancer patients using convolutional neural networks and EPID dosimetry *Radiother. Oncol.* **153** 243–9

[100] Wendling M, McDermott L N, Mans A, Sonke J J, van Herk M and Mijnheer B J 2009 A simple backprojection algorithm for 3D *in vivo* EPID dosimetry of IMRT treatments *Med. Phys.* **36** 3310–21

[101] Olaciregui-Ruiz I, Torres-Xirau I, Teuwen J, van der Heide U A and Mans A 2020 A deep learning-based correction to EPID dosimetry for attenuation and scatter in the Unity MR-linac system *Phys Med.* **71** 124–31

[102] Olaciregui-Ruiz I, Simões R and Jan-Jakob S 2023 Deep learning-based tools to distinguish plan-specific from generic deviations in EPID-based *in vivo* dosimetry *Med. Phys.* **51** 854–69

[103] Zhao W, Patil I, Han B, Yang Y, Xing L and Schüler E 2020 Beam data modeling of linear accelerators (linacs) through machine learning and its potential applications in fast and robust linac commissioning and quality assurance *Radiother. Oncol.* **153** 122–9

[104] Liu L *et al* 2023 Modeling linear accelerator (linac) beam data by implicit neural representation learning for commissioning and quality assurance applications *Med. Phys.* **50** 3137–47

[105] Wagner A *et al* 2020 Integration of the M6 Cyberknife in the Moderato Monte Carlo platform and prediction of beam parameters using machine learning *Phys. Med.* **70** 123–32

[106] Chan M F, Witztum A and Valdes G 2020 Integration of AI and machine learning in radiotherapy QA *Front. Artif. Intell.* **3** 577620

[107] Simon L, Robert C and Meyer P 2021 Artificial intelligence for quality assurance in radiotherapy *Cancer Radiother* **25** 623–6

[108] Carlson J N, Park J M, Park S Y, Park J I, Choi Y and Ye S J 2016 A machine learning approach to the accurate prediction of multi-leaf collimator positional errors *Phys. Med. Biol.* **61** 2514–31

[109] Osman A F I, Maalej N M and Jayesh K 2020 Prediction of the individual multileaf collimator positional deviations during dynamic IMRT delivery *priori* with artificial neural network *Med. Phys.* **47** 1421–30

[110] Chuang K C, Giles W and Adamson J 2021 A tool for patient-specific prediction of delivery discrepancies in machine parameters using trajectory log files *Med. Phys.* **48** 978–90

[111] Sun B *et al* 2018 A machine learning approach to the accurate prediction of monitor units for a compact proton machine *Med. Phys.* **45** 2243–51

[112] Grewal H S, Chacko M S, Ahmad S and Jin H 2020 Prediction of the output factor using machine and deep learning approach in uniform scanning proton therapy *J. Appl. Clin. Med. Phys.* **21** 128–34

[113] Valdes G, Morin O, Valenciaga Y, Kirby N, Pouliot J and Chuang C 2015 Use of TrueBeam developer mode for imaging QA *J. Appl. Clin. Med. Phys.* **16** 322–33

[114] El Naqa I *et al* 2019 Machine learning for automated quality assurance in radiotherapy: a proof of principle using EPID data description *Med. Phys.* **46** 1914–21

[115] Chan M F *et al* 2015 Visual analysis of the daily QA results of photon and electron beams of a trilogy linac over a five-year period *Int. J. Med. Phys. Clin. Eng. Radiat. Oncol.* **4** 290–9

[116] Li Q and Chan M F 2017 Predictive time-series modeling using artificial neural networks for linac beam symmetry: an empirical study *Ann. N. Y. Acad. Sci.* **1387** 84–94

[117] Li J, Wang D and Chan M 2023 Predictive quality assurance for linear accelerator target failure using statistical process control *Biomed. Phys. Eng. Express* **9** 055018

[118] Chang L, Yeh S A, Ho S Y, Ding H J, Chen P Y and Lee T F 2021 Calibration of the EBT3 Gafchromic film using HNN deep learning *BioMed. Res. Int.* **2021** 8838401

[119] Zhuang Y, Li Y, Zhu J, Chen L and Liu X 2019 A trial for EBT3 film without batch-specific calibration using a neural network *Phys. Med. Biol.* **64** 05NT1

[120] Avanzo M *et al* 2019 Prediction of skin dose in low-kV intraoperative radiotherapy using machine learning models trained on results of *in vivo* dosimetry *Med. Phys.* **46** 1447–54

IOP Publishing

Artificial Intelligence in Adaptive Radiation Therapy

Yi Wang and X. Sharon Qi

Chapter 13

Artificial intelligence empowered response prediction and adaptation

Denis Dudas and Issam El Naqa

Treatment response prediction is an important part of radiation therapy management, as it describes and explains relationships between pre- or on-treatment variables (imaging data, treatment planning data, demographics, clinical, -omics data, etc) and follow-up outcomes (tumor control probability, radiation toxicities, survival time, etc). Such knowledge, combined with advanced imaging techniques, offers a promising opportunity for the adaptation of planning dose distribution, target and organ delineations, and dose prescription to maximize the treatment's benefits while minimizing its side effects.

In the last two decades, adaptive radiotherapy (ART) has mostly been represented by treatment plan modifications based on on-treatment imaging data, combined with simple population-based response models or even no response models. In recent years, more advanced artificial intelligence (AI) techniques, such as neural networks and other deep learning applications, have been adopted and successfully implemented in treatment response modeling. Consequently, treatment adaptation has become more personalized, benefiting from individual-based AI response models. This, together with various explainability methods of machine learning models, has made AI-based ART one of the most promising areas of personalized radiation oncology with great potential in future years.

In this chapter, we provide an overview of the data resources typically utilized in response modeling, a summary and examples of traditional and AI-based response models, and we also discuss current trends and challenges in AI-based response-adaptive radiotherapy.

13.1 Data resources for response modeling in radiotherapy

Response modeling is currently an integral part of radiation oncology. It focuses on relating patient, clinical, and treatment details with specific endpoints, e.g. treatment

doi:10.1088/978-0-7503-6119-4ch13

13-1

outcomes or time to follow-up events [1, 2]. The aim is to extract meaningful insights and provide a reliable prediction of modeled events, which could be effectively used in treatment planning, assessment, and adaptation. Therefore, it can sometimes be thought of as a data science applied in radiotherapy. Consequently, we must first define the data resources typically used in this area before discussing how AI empowers response prediction and treatment adaptation.

13.1.1 Clinical data

Patient demographics and clinical details are often among the first data considered in treatment response modeling and assessment since they are usually easily accessible and considerably impact the final treatment outcome.

Various demographic details can play an essential role in response prediction. One of the most significant factors is age. As shown by several studies, older patients tend to exhibit worse treatment results and are more likely to be non-compliant with radiotherapy treatment [3–5]. Other typical demographic information that is often employed in outcome modeling and can be significant predictors are gender [6], ethnicity and race [7, 8], household income [9], marriage status [10–12], smoking status [13], and many others.

Any oncology disease and its treatment require a thorough consideration of the patient's complete medical condition. Therefore, relevant comorbidities and physiological details (e.g. cardiac function tests, pulmonary function tests, body mass index, etc) might provide an essential insight into a patient's prognosis and possible outcomes. As many studies presented, comorbidities are highly associated with overall clinical outcomes and survival [14–17]. However, in most patients, there are multiple coexisting medical conditions, which makes it difficult for interpretation and complex consideration with respect to the primary condition under investigation. Consequently, it is crucial to have an effective, accurate, and robust method for measuring total comorbidity burden. For this purpose, different comorbidity indices exist. The most typical, with general purpose, are the Elixhauser comorbidity index (EI) and the Charlson comorbidity index (CCI) [18, 19].

Another relevant resource of clinical details is information involving the tumor, whether its biology, site, or stage. One of the most critical factors is the tumor's histology, which can reveal its aggressivity or radiosensitivity. Tumor histology also often predicts the probability of tumor local control (LC) and provides a valuable insight for dose prescription [20–22]. Additionally, larger tumors, in terms of volume and maximum tumor diameter (MTD), show poorer prognosis. Multiple studies identified MTD and tumor volume as significant predictors of LC and progression-free survival (PFS) [23–26]. This indicates a similar association between the patient's prognosis and cancer staging [27–29], since the stage is determined at diagnosis according to the primary tumor's size and its spread to regional or distant nodes.

With the expansion of precision medicine and personalized treatment, a significant effort has been made to find predictors and markers that could be used to design an optimal treatment, while having a reliable outcome prediction. The main idea is to predict tumor's response to radiotherapy before executing it, and adapt the

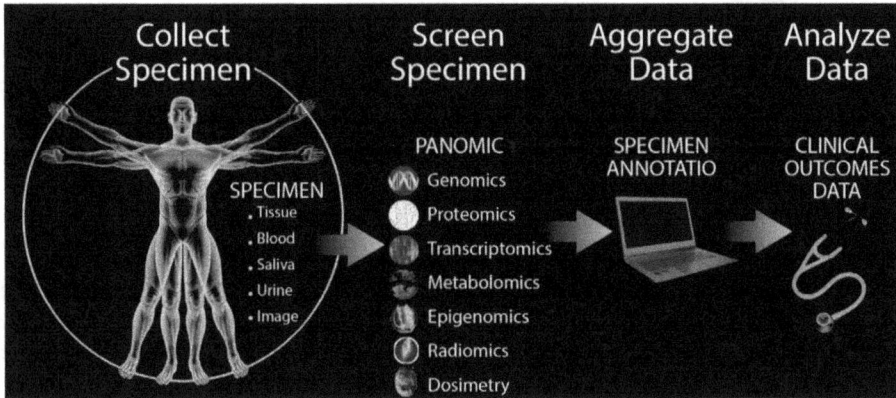

Figure 13.1. The patient is the most valuable source of data and information, that can be used to tailor patient-specific treatment. The usual workflow involves collecting specimens, extracting and annotating various biomarkers and predictors (radiomics, dosiomics, genomics, proteomics, etc), and final data analysis with design and validation of the outcome model. (Reproduced with permission from [92]. Copyright 2017 Institute of Physics and Engineering in Medicine.)

treatment to patient-specific conditions and factors. Precision medicine involves numerous techniques and specimen types (image, tissue, blood, etc), that can generate different biomarkers [30]. There are several groups of biomarkers, depending on the specimen, and some of them are further discussed in subsequent chapters. Integration of information from more specimens and heterogeneous biomarkers is called panomics [31, 32]. Figure 13.1 shows a typical outcome modeling workflow and data-supporting resources.

13.1.2 Imaging (radiomics)

Imaging data is perhaps the most prevalent resource for information in radiotherapy. It is used to plan the treatment and extract numerous biomarkers and features that are highly useful in outcome modeling. It provides patient-specific anatomy and physiology, and thus it is a great contributor to precision medicine. There are multiple imaging modalities in radiotherapy. The most common are CT, MRI, and PET or SPECT. They use different imaging principles and provide different information. Diagnostic modalities, such as CT, are usually used for diagnosis and radiotherapy planning. They show patient anatomy and are used to extract electron densities in the patient's body, which is crucial for subsequent dose calculation. Treatment planning involves localization and delineation of the tumor, delineation of organs at risk (OARs) and final dose calculation [33]. On the other hand, MRI and nuclear medicine modalities (PET and SPECT) can be characterized as not only anatomical, but also biological, molecular, and functional imaging. For example, MRI can be employed to quantify a tumor's proliferation or necrosis [34, 35], while PET is more suitable for assessment of the tumor's metabolism [36, 37] or the overall cancer staging [38, 39]. The advantage of combining data from more modalities gave rise to PET/CT, which is now commonly used for multiple tasks, including diagnosis, planning, and on/post-treatment follow-up [40, 41].

Techniques involving the extraction of a large number of features from imaging data, quantitative analysis, and relating this to treatment outcomes (clinical endpoints) is called *radiomics* [1, 42–44]. There are two basic approaches—feature-based (conventional radiomics) and featureless (deep learning radiomics) [45, 46].

Feature-based methods utilize hand-crafted features, which are analytically predefined and capture characteristics and patterns in the analysed data. Such features are always associated with a specific region of interest (ROI) (i.e. OAR or target volume). Therefore, feature-based radiomics can only be applied on segmented data (2D or 3D) [42, 45]. There are numerous different radiomic features, and they can be divided into histogram-based, shape-based, texture-based, model-based, and transform-based categories. Histogram-based features are standard statistical descriptors in gray-level histograms and are often referred to as first-order features. A typical example of a histogram-based feature in PET images is the standardized uptake value (SUV). Shape-based features describe the ROI in terms of geometrical properties (e.g. maximum diameter, sphericity, compactness, etc). Texture-based features are often referred to as second-order features. They involve descriptors of the relationships between neighboring pixels, such as gradient features, the gray-level co-occurrence matrix (GLCM), the gray-level run-length matrix (GLRLM), and many others. Model-based and transform-based features fall into a group of higher-order features, which usually involve an application of specific mathematical transformations and operations, for example, Gabor filters, Markov random fields, Wavelet transforms, or fractal analysis [42, 45, 47, 48].

There has been a rapid rise of radiomics-related papers in recent years, thanks to the improvement of standardization in radiomics and the development of accessible tools for its implementation. One of the most utilized open-source platforms is PyRadiomics [49].

After extracting hand-crafted features from images, it is usually necessary to apply some dimensionality reduction techniques, since radiomics often leads to hundreds or even thousands of different features to be analysed. The purpose is to select the most significant features concerning the outcome prediction to decrease the complexity of the model and its computational burden. Various techniques are commonly used to tackle this problem. The most straightforward are based on collinearity analysis using, for example, Pearson's correlation coefficient or variance inflation factor (VIF) [50–52]. More advanced approaches may involve feature transformation methods, such as principal component analysis (PCA) or clustering [48, 53–56]. Another option is sensitivity analysis by stepwise forward or backward feature elimination based on one of the model order optimality measures, i.e. Akaike information criteria (AIC) or Bayesian information criteria (BIC) [57–60].

The last step in feature-based methods is the model design. The main factor to be considered is the purpose of the model, i.e. classification (supervised/unsupervised) or time-to-event prediction. For each category, several different architectures can be adopted [45].

Featureless radiomics benefits mainly from advances in the deep learning area, as it works with features that are learnt and extracted by neural networks directly. The process of feature extraction and outcome prediction is then performed simultaneously within one model (see figure 13.2). The typical architecture used for deep learning feature extraction from images is the convolutional neural network (CNN) [61, 62]. Others may include autoencoders (AE) [45] or architectures which are designed explicitly for sequence data, such as RNNs or transformers [63, 64].

13.1.3 Treatment planning (dosiomics)

Radiotherapy is a treatment that uses targeted application of ionizing radiation to eradicate tumor cells. Therefore, it requires a complex planning procedure, including imaging data acquisition and fusion (CT and potentially also PET and MRI), OAR and target volume delineation, and radiation delivery planning. The main result of the whole planning process is a 3D dose distribution and technical details for its delivery in clinics. The dose distribution is a rich resource for information regarding outcome modeling, since it is directly related to tumor local control [65–68], radiation toxicities in OARs [67, 69, 70], and overall survival [71–73]. The approach of extracting features from the planning dose distribution and relating it to specific clinical endpoints is commonly referred to as *dosiomics*.

Traditional dose features associated with outcome modeling are dose–volume metrics (i.e. histogram-based features), which are directly linked to the concept of dose–volume histogram (DVH) describing the frequency distribution of dose levels in the studied ROI. Typical examples are minimum/maximum dose (D_{min}/D_{max}), mean dose (D_{mean}), minimum dose to $x\%$ volume (D_x), and volume receiving at least x Gy (V_x). DVH metrics are currently the key concept for treatment plan quality assessment. Perhaps the most popular frameworks for normal tissues are Quantitative Analysis of Normal Tissue Effects in the Clinic (QUANTEC) [74, 75] and Hypofractionated Treatment Effects in the Clinic (HyTEC) [76].

More advanced traditional metrics involve quantities, such as equivalent uniform dose (EUD) or effective volume (V_{eff}). EUD is defined as a uniform dose delivered to the target volume, with equivalent outcomes as the real 3D dose distribution. The generalized definition for EUD is called generalized equivalent uniform dose (gEUD) [77], and it is applicable to both target volumes and OARs. V_{eff} is defined as a hypothetical portion of the target volume, which if it receives the prescription dose while the rest of the volume receives 0 Gy, produces equivalent outcomes as the actual dose distribution [78]. The motivation for gEUD and V_{eff} was in the reduction of DVH information into more complex and more straightforward quantity for outcome prediction, as the most common models in clinics—tumor control probability (TCP) and normal tissue complication probability (NTCP)—are inapplicable on 3D dose distribution.

Even though DVH metrics can be good predictors of various clinical endpoints, their main drawback is their inability to account for dose–spatial relationships within the ROI, as DVH is basically a 2D reduction of 3D dose distribution. Moreover, using QUANTEC and HyTeC recommendations and population-based

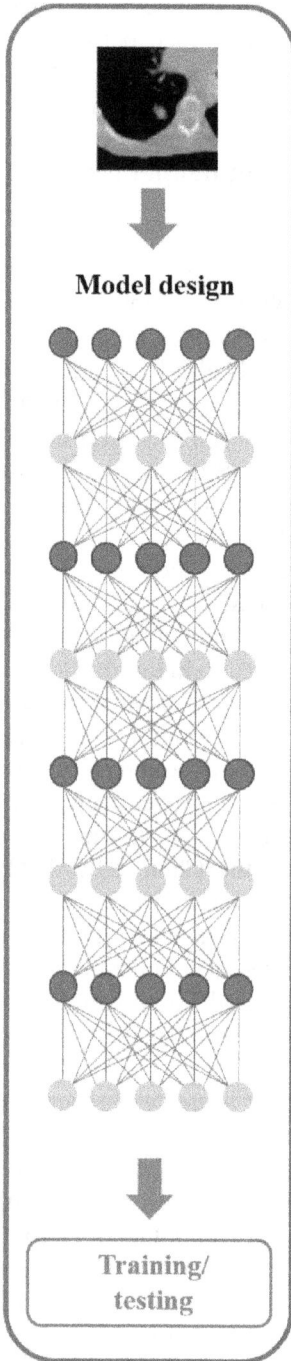

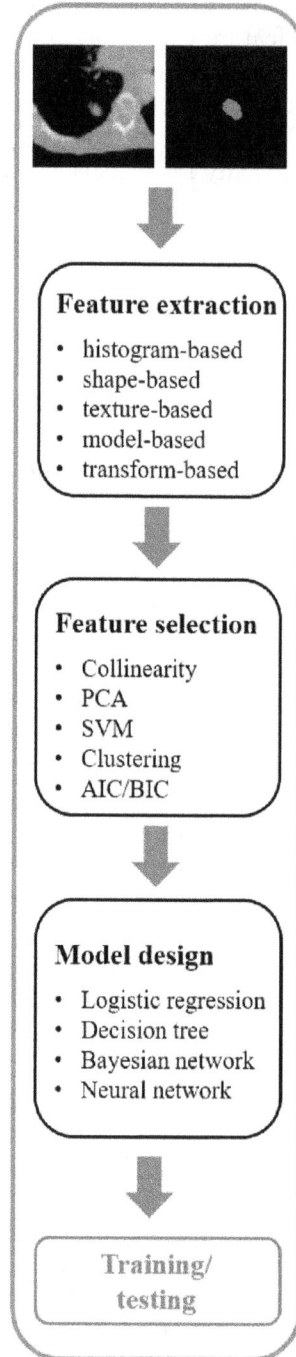

Figure 13.2. Diagrams of feature-based and featureless radiomics workflow.

TCP/NTCP models is limiting for radiotherapy personalization, as they do not reflect patient-specific conditions and factors. Therefore, there has been a great effort in the last few years to apply machine and deep learning techniques in 3D dosiomics. Deeper features, whether extracted as hand-crafted features, similar to those in radiomics (histogram-based, shape-based, texture-based, etc), or using a deep learning approach, can better reflect the real impact of the person-specific dose distribution on clinical outcomes. Many studies have been published on dosiomic predictors of radiation toxicities [79–83] and tumor control [84, 85], and they proved to be promising for clinical application. Moreover, special attention should be paid to models combining dosiomic features with radiomics or even other -omics (see section 13.1.4), which often significantly improves the model's performance [86–88].

13.1.4 Multiomics

The growing field of biotechnology and bioinformatics offers numerous valuable tools and data that can positively contribute towards the accuracy of outcome models, their clinical translation, and precision medicine in general. A wide range of molecular biomarkers can currently be analysed and included in response modeling. Most commonly, they are obtained by analysis of the tumor genome (genomics), its further transcriptions into RNA (transcriptomics), translations into proteins (proteomics), and final metabolites (metabolomics) [89]. Combining all these biomarkers in response models is often referred to as a multiomic approach, due to the combination of different -omic datasets. Furthermore, extending the multiomics approach by radiomics led to the emerge of *radiogenomics* [90–92].

Genomics represents the identification of structural variations in the DNA of the studied specimen. Since there are various classes of genomic variables, it is always important to consider the aim of the analysis and the specimen type before selecting specific genomic biomarkers for modeling. However, the most common classes in radiotherapy are single nucleotide polymorphisms (SNP) and copy number variations (CNV) [93, 94]. Typically, they can be associated with radiation sensitivity, and thus they can, for example, work as prognostic factors of radiation toxicities. There are millions of SNPs and CNVs per 100 nucleotides. Consequently, it is crucial to have large sample sizes to assess the prognostic power of specific SNPs. One of the largest collaborations investigating associations between SNPs and radiation toxicities is the radiogenomics consortium (RGC) [95–97].

Transcriptomics is a quantitative and qualitative sequential analysis of RNA molecules, including their expression levels, functions, and degradations [98, 99]. RNA is a translation between DNA and protein. It carries genes to ribosomes, where proteins are created. However, it also regulates the expression levels of genes and might have structural functions, such as ribosomes. Therefore, transcriptomics can have a major impact on cancer prognosis as it captures extensive and complex information. As is evident from various studies, transcriptomics is a promising part of multiomics in radiotherapy [100–102].

Proteomics involves various analytical techniques to identify the composition, structure, function, and interactions of proteins. It provides another necessary input to the holistic approach of multiomics, as it describes the overall organism reaction to the treatment better than just genomics. Perhaps the most helpful protein expressions in radiotherapy are cytokines, secreted by different immune cells responsible for specific organism responses to radiotherapy, such as radiation toxicities [103–105].

Metabolomics is the profiling of metabolites from collected specimens. Metabolites are final products of gene transcriptions, i.e. metabolism, which conducts essential cell functions, such as energy conversion and metabolic waste management. There is a vast potential for metabolomics in oncology, for example, in hepatocellular carcinoma [106, 107], glioma [108, 109], and non-small cell lung cancer (NSCLC) [110, 111]. In radiotherapy, metabolomics shows promising results in predicting and evaluating treatment outcomes of various diagnoses [112–116].

13.2 Radiotherapy treatment outcome modeling

Radiotherapy outcome modeling historically originated from population-based models, which are often inaccurate due to the lack of individualization of the patient's response. Population-based models use large cohorts of patients to determine relationships between treatment details and clinical endpoints. Consequently, they come up with relationships that describe average trends in the cohort. Typical examples of such models are tumor control probability (TCP) and normal tissue complication probability (NTCP), which were limited to dose response. Currently, with the expansion of machine learning techniques, outcome modeling is becoming a patient-specific task. Therefore, new requirements, such as model's explainability, are usually associated with it [2].

13.2.1 TCP/NTCP in radiotherapy

The most common outcome models in radiotherapy are TCP of the targeted volume and NTCP of surrounding OARs. The goal of radiotherapy is to maximize TCP while minimizing NTCP. Unfortunately, delivering dose to the target volume is always associated with a certain risk of radiation toxicities in normal tissues. Therefore, the main task in radiotherapy is to optimize the trade-off, i.e. the therapeutic ratio (TR) between TCP and NTCP (see figure 13.3) [117, 118].

There are two overarching methods for TCP/NTCP modeling: analytical and data-driven [32]. A more traditional (analytical) approach represents population-based dose response models, that are mostly utilizing the mechanistic radiobiological linear-quadratic (LQ) model [119, 120] and DVH data. The LQ model is a current standard for various clinical calculations and assessments, for example, when clinical outcomes of different treatment regimens need to be compared. It can be expressed as a clonogenic cell survival fraction (SF):

$$SF = e^{-\alpha D - \beta D^2 G(D)}, \tag{13.1}$$

where D denotes total dose, α and β are organ-specific parameters describing lethal damage induced by double and single strand DNA breaks, respectively, and $G(D)$ is

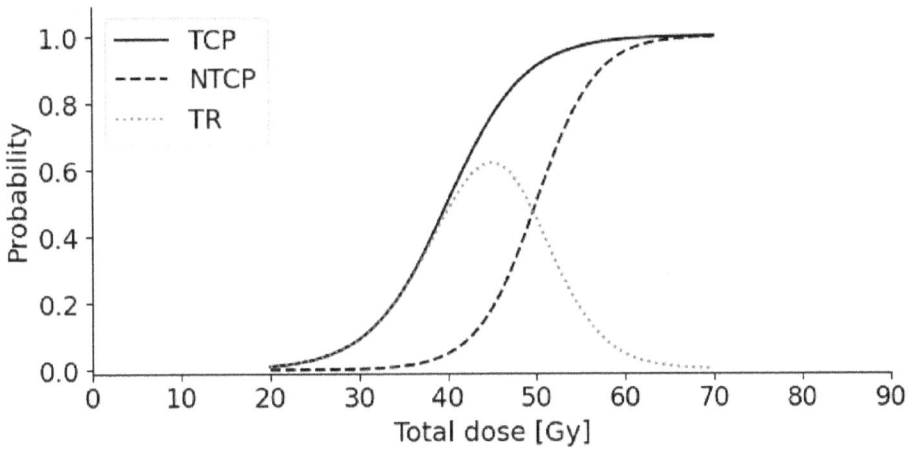

Figure 13.3. Illustration of typical TCP and NTCP curves. Probability of tumor (local) control rises with the dose. However, this also elevates the dose in surrounding organs and thus the probability of radiation toxicity (NTCP) increases as well. The therapeutic ratio refers to a window between TCP and NTCP, defined as the tumor complication-free TR = TCP × (1-NTCP).

the Lea–Catcheside factor accounting for clonogen repopulation between fractions [121, 122].

Analytical TCP models can have different definitions, but one of the most usual follows Poisson distribution and can be described as

$$\text{TCP} = e^{-N \cdot SF}, \tag{13.2}$$

where N is the initial number of tumor cells. A detailed review on the use of TCP models in radiotherapy was published by Zaider and Hanin [123].

Normal tissue complication modeling is similar to TCP, although it is more difficult due to the higher complexity of the problem. Usually, several different OARs are irradiated during the treatment, and their response differs. Moreover, NTCP depends on the spatial dose distribution, which makes the task even more complicated as higher dimensional data are involved. Therefore, published analytical NTCP models often focused on reducing DVH dimensionality into a single or a few metrics, making routine implementation and understanding easier. The most used model involves the Lyman–Kutcher–Burman (LKB) method, which is defined by the following equations:

$$\text{NTCP}\left(D, V\right) = \frac{1}{\sqrt{2\pi}} \int_{-\infty}^{u(D,\ V)} e^{\left(\frac{-x^2}{2}\right)} dx, \tag{13.3}$$

$$u\left(D, V\right) = \frac{D - \text{TD}_{50}(V)}{m \cdot \text{TD}_{50}(V)}, \tag{13.4}$$

$$TD_{50}(V) = \frac{TD_{50}(1)}{V^n}, \tag{13.5}$$

where $TD_{50}(V)$ is the tolerance dose for partial volume V that results in 50% complication probability after 5 years, m is a measure of the slope of the dose response curve (i.e. the standard deviation of $TD_{50}(1)$) and n is a tissue-specific volume effect factor, determining the serial/parallel type of the structure [32, 118].

The most impactful publications of dose–volume responses in various OARs are summarized in QUANTEC review articles [124, 125] and subsequent HyTec for hypofractionation studies [76]. Provided data are nowadays commonly used in clinics as treatment planning criteria, limiting the probability of radiation-induced post-treatment complications.

Another approach to TCP/NTCP modeling involves AI techniques, which can usually provide better accuracy than analytical models, as they can capture the non-linear relationship between input data and clinical endpoints. They create a new opportunity to personalize the outcome and potentially the treatment by including patient-specific data from different resources (see section 13.1) and exploring their underlying interactions [32]. Many different types of machine learning techniques can be effectively utilized in radiotherapy outcome modeling. More details are summarized in following sections.

13.2.2 Clinical outcomes versus PROs

Next to conventionally followed and physician-assessed clinical endpoints, such as tumor control, survival, andr various radiation toxicities, more patient quality of life (QoL) focused endpoints have recently been studied. This typically involves patient reported outcome (PRO) evaluations, which is a systematically prepared question-naire, usually filled in by patient before, during, and after the treatment in follow-up appointments. PRO questions and their evaluation are disease-specific. Therefore, different departments and clinics might use other questionnaires, depending on a patient's needs that are specific in given medical department. One of the most common questionnaires in oncology is the Edmonton Symptom Assessment System (ESAS) [126, 127]. It is routinely used in several oncology clinics for symptom management and patient QoL monitoring [128–132]. However, another potential application is in the prediction of clinical endpoints, for example, the overall survival. Recent studies showed evidence of ESAS PROs as significant predictors of survival in cancer patients [133–135]. This might help with various clinical decisions, such as transitioning from curative to palliative treatment.

The prognostic power of PROs offers a variety of potential applications in outcome modeling. Incorporating time-sequential PROs into outcome models could improve their accuracy and impact. One of the possible applications is outcome models that could be used to optimize treatment plan parameters not only with respect to typical clinical endpoints, but also concerning the patient-specific QoL. An example of effort made in this area is a project led by the H Lee Moffitt Cancer Center and Research Institute (Data Science to Improve Treatment Planning for Advanced Prostate Cancer Patients Treated with Radiotherapy), supported by the

Department of Defense (DoD) Congressional Directed Medical Research Program. The project focuses on using PROs in radiotherapy outcome modeling and predicting patients' QoL after the treatment.

Patient's PROs are sequential data acquired at different time points. Consequently, it has to be dealt with as a data sequence, which represents a specific task regarding suitable machine learning architecture. The inspiration can be taken from natural language processing (NLP) models, which are designed exactly for data sequences, i.e. words and sentences. Typical architectures in this field include recurrent neural networks (RNN), such as long short-term memory (LSTM), and gated recurrent unit (GRU), or recently more advanced and famous transformers.

13.2.3 Machine learning response prediction

As a subcategory of AI, machine learning (ML) technologies influence almost all fields currently. There are numerous possible medical applications, and major benefits are also evident in radiotherapy outcome modeling. Machine learning enables the aggregation of a large amount of data from different resources (i.e. multiomics), allowing for further personalization in outcome prediction, while increasing its accuracy. This can be attributed to AI capabilities in capturing underlying relationships between the provided data and recognizing inter-human cancer-specific differences, which are usually impossible for humans to detect and process. Therefore, in the last decade, machine learning response prediction has dominated over traditional approaches, based on simple TCP/NTCP dose–volume responses. It is further expected that ML-based outcome modeling will play a leading role in the future exploration of cancer biology and personalization of treatment planning/adaptation, where the patient-specific response should always be considered a priority. It is especially envisioned as a key part of future clinical decision-support systems (CDSS), which can assist in several clinical tasks [1, 2]. Initially, it can serve as a decision-support system for determining the optimal treatment procedure. Further, it can guide treatment planning for the optimized outcomes. In the next step, it can be applied during radiotherapy adaptation of an ongoing treatment course. Finally, it can provide an early prediction of recurrence or post-treatment complications, enabling physicians to determine and apply the optimal follow-up treatment. Therefore, there are various data resources and formats that can be employed in the aforementioned tasks. Generally, there are two data formats—structured and unstructured. Structured data are most often tabular, while unstructured data involve images, 3D dose distributions, or unstructured clinician-provided notes.

There are numerous algorithms that can be used for structured data. Typically, they belong to conventional ML algorithms, although artificial neural networks (ANN) can also be used. Typical examples of conventional ML methods used in radiotherapy outcome modeling are logistic regression, support vector machine (SVM), decision tree (DT), random forest (RF), Bayesian network (BN), and various ensemble methods, such as extreme gradient boosting (XGBoost).

Logistic regression is a classification ML technique. Typically, it is used for modeling discrete outcomes by fitting a sigmoid function to extracted features (multivariable logistic regression) [136–138]. The logistic regression requires the features to be uncorrelated and independent. Therefore, a careful feature selection has to be performed before the regression. In dose–volume space, this practically implies using a single summarizing dose–volume metric, as DVH metrics are highly correlated [118].

The support vector machine is a regression/classification ML technique, which uses a kernel function to define a 'hyperplane' separating data points according to their classes, for example, tumor local control/recurrence or survival/death [139, 140]. Depending on the kernel definition, SVM algorithms can be categorized as linear, polynomial, sigmoid, or radial basis.

Another type of conventional ML technique used as a classifier in outcome modeling is the Bayesian network (BN). It is a probabilistic model based on conditional dependencies among input variables. It is a type of directed acyclic graph (DAG), thus it is easily interpretable. Thanks to the probabilistic character of the BN, it can work with partially missing input data. However, some of the drawbacks are the need for larger datasets compared to other methods or poorer identification of causality in the dataset. A simpler alternative to BN is the naïve Bayesian network (NBN), which assumes independence in input features. Therefore, it is more effective and easier to train, even though it does not often correspond to real scenarios. Nevertheless, it is very popular in many applications, including radiotherapy outcome prediction, often outperforming other ML methods [141].

Decision tree is a non-parametric classification/regression ML technique that separates data points based on recursive partitioning analysis. Due to its clear and simple design, it is very convenient for interpretation. A more advanced alternative (random forest) utilizes an ensemble approach, building multiple DTs and averaging their results. It is currently one of the most popular conventional ML techniques due to its accuracy and direct interpretability, and it is usable in time-to-event modeling as well [138, 142–146].

The ensemble technique is a concept combining more ML models to improve the prognostic accuracy. One of the most utilized and popular is the gradient boosting machine (GBM) [147]. It is based on sequentially adding new models focusing on previously misclassified samples. The idea in each step is to create a model that correlates with the negative gradient of the ensemble loss function. There are several implementations of GBM and one of the most utilized is XGBoost [148–150].

Unstructured (raw) data (e.g. dose distributions, images, -omics, etc) are usually processed using deep learning (DL) methods (i.e. deep neural networks (DNN)), which are built by stacking up multiple layers of specifically designed mathematical operations (see the featureless approach in figure 13.2.). This technique is able to identify underlying representations and relationships to learn specific tasks without any prior feature selection. Typically employed architectures are the multilayer perceptron (MLP), convolutional neural networks (CNNs), recurrent neural network (RNNs), autoencoders (AEs), and generative neural networks, such as

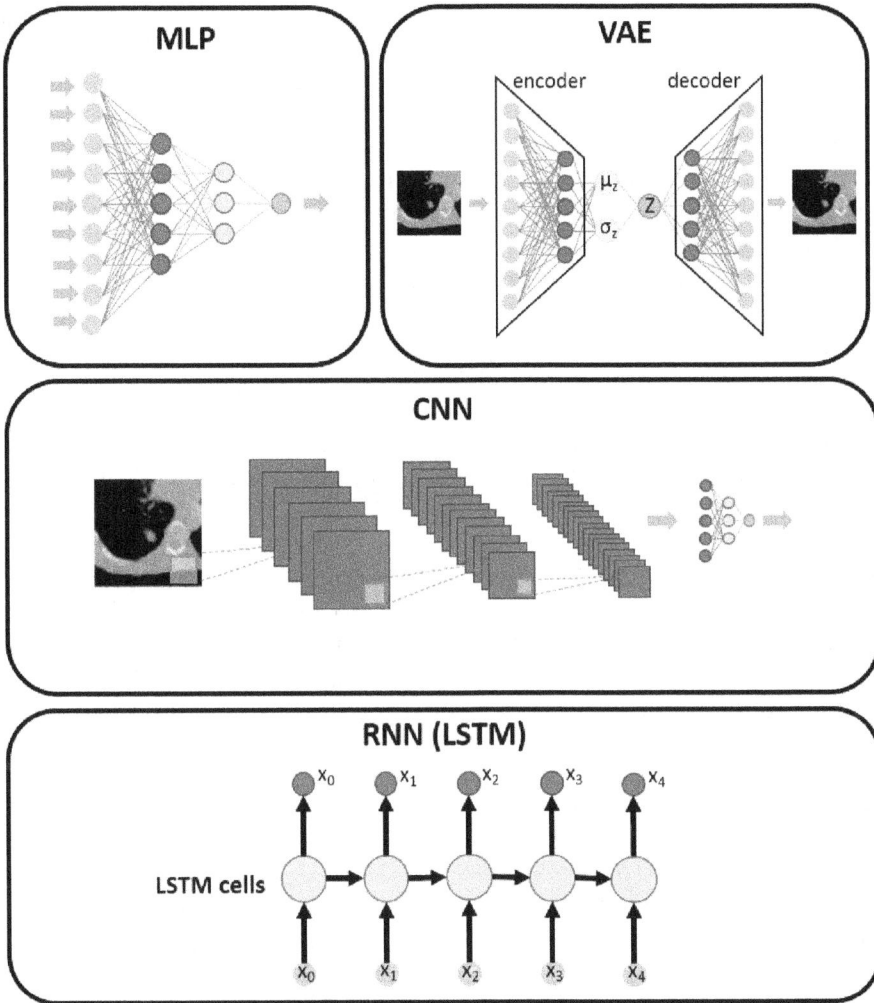

Figure 13.4. Diagrams of basic deep learning architectures. (1) Multilayer perceptron consisting of several fully connected layers; (2) variational autoencoder; (3) convolutional neural network followed by MLP; and (4) recurrent neural network with LSTM units.

generative adversarial networks (GANs) and denoising diffusion probabilistic models (DDPMs).

A multilayer perceptron is a basic neural network consisting of several fully connected layers containing multiple nodes (see figure 13.4). One node is a weighted sum of the nodes from the previous layer, followed by an activation function (e.g. ReLu, SeLu, sigmoid, etc). The aim of outcome modeling is usually predicting an endpoint probability. Therefore, the last layer of MLP is typically followed by a sigmoid activation function to simulate the probability. The MLP works only with 1D data, thus any higher dimensional data has to be flattened before the MLP can be applied [62, 88].

The convolutional neural network is an architecture typically used for 2D and 3D data, although it can also be applied to 1D data. Compared to MLP, the CNN contains fewer parameters, which makes training easier. Consequently, it requires less training data than MLP. The main blocks of the CNN are convolutional layers, which represent a convolution between a specific kernel and the previous layer. The CNN maintains local connectivity and spatial invariance, which is one of its main advantages and also the reason why it is so useful in higher dimensional unstructured data. A typical CNN consists of several layers, each usually followed by a down-sampling using a pooling layer. The output of a CNN is a set of most significant features that can be further used as an input for a small MLP to provide the outcome prediction (see figure 13.4) [62, 151].

An autoencoder is an unsupervised DL technique with many implementations. One of the most popular, due to its continuous latent space described by a probability distribution, is the variational autoencoder (VAE) (see figure 13.4). Even though the VAE cannot be used directly for outcome prediction, since it is an unsupervised technique, it is still a useful approach for feature extraction. Any autoencoder consists of an encoder and a decoder. The encoder extracts features and maps them to a latent space while the decoder learns to reconstruct the original input from the latent space. The latent space representation is often used in outcome modeling for feature extraction and dimensionality reduction. It can also be combined with some supervised techniques, such as MLP, and utilized in outcome modeling directly in an end-to-end approach [152].

Another type of data, common in outcome modeling, is sequential or longitudinal data, such as a time-sequence of images or textual information. For this type of unstructured data, RNNs (see figure 13.4) are commonly used. The main idea behind an RNN is to capture longitudinal associations between the input data. One of the most common and effective architectures is long short-term memory (LSTM) or gated recurrent unit (GRU) [153, 154]. A more recent technique that outperforms traditional RNN methods in many tasks, especially in NLP, is the transformer [155, 156]. It is an architecture utilizing a multi-head attention mechanism, making it faster and more robust than LSTM or GRU.

Generative neural networks represent a category of machine learning frameworks which aims to learn contextual information and underlying representations to generate unique new samples. The most typical examples of such models are GANs and, recently, DDPMs. Previously, most of the generative tasks were assigned to VAEs, which could generate new samples by randomly sampling the latent space. A more recent architecture involves GAN, which trains two neural networks to compete against each other (the generator and discriminator). The discriminator is trained to distinguish between real and synthetic images, while the generator is trained to create synthetic samples to deceive the discriminator. Even though GAN produces more realistic images, it is often associated with a mode collapse [157]. The most recent and highly promising generative architecture, outperforming GANs, is based on denoising diffusion models (DDPM) [157, 158]. Generative models in outcome modeling can be used for data augmentation or addressing the class imbalance in the training dataset, as shown in the study by Dudas *et al* [159].

Deep learning methods are promising alternatives for radiotherapy outcome modeling. They usually exhibit excellent performance and offer a large variability in the input data type. However, their explainability is not as simple and straightforward as in conventional machine learning techniques. Another disadvantage is the amount of data, which has to be big enough, since DL techniques are usually associated with more trainable parameters than conventional ML methods. Consequently, DL models have to be trained cautiously to avoid overfitting. All critical aspects regarding training, validation and testing of outcome models are summarized in the TRIPOD ('Transparent reporting of a multivariable prediction model for individual prognosis or diagnosis') reporting guideline [160]. In general, predictive models should always be cross-validated and tested. The cross-validation can be performed using one of the recommended methods, for example, *k*-fold or leave-one-out. The testing can be done prospectively or retrospectively on a held-out independent dataset [1].

13.2.4 Explainability of ML response models

The ultimate goal of ML outcome models, whether used alone or as a part of a complex clinical system, is to provide decision-making support to clinicians. Therefore, the key part of this human–machine interaction is the machine's explainability. Clinicians must understand the reasoning behind the algorithm's decision [161]. Moreover, explainability allows for better alignment with ethical principles in applications with an impact on individuals. It can also help identify errors, thus facilitating further improvements to the model. Some ML techniques, such as decision trees or Bayesian networks, are inherently well-explainable due to their simple architecture, although their performance is limited. In most cases, models with higher performance usually have poorer explainability. For example, deep learning methods often outperform conventional ML models, but their explainability is complicated, since they work with implicitly learned features, which are abstract to the human mind [1].

Three main explainability techniques are commonly used in outcome modeling. These are local interpretable model-agnostic explanations (LIME), Shapley values, and gradient-weighted class activation mapping (Grad-CAM).

LIME is an agnostic model, which approximates the model with a simple interpretable model locally. Then, it perturbs selected input samples and evaluates its impact on the local model approximation [161, 162]. It can be applied to any outcome model which incorporates a classifier.

The Shapley values method, another agnostic model, arises from a cooperative game theory, where marginal contributions of each input variable towards the model output are evaluated. The most popular implementation, easily applicable to any ML/DL architecture, is Shapley additive explanation (SHAP) [161, 163].

Grad-CAM [164] is a model-specific method, especially suitable for CNNs (figure 13.5). It utilizes gradient information from a specific layer to illustrate the

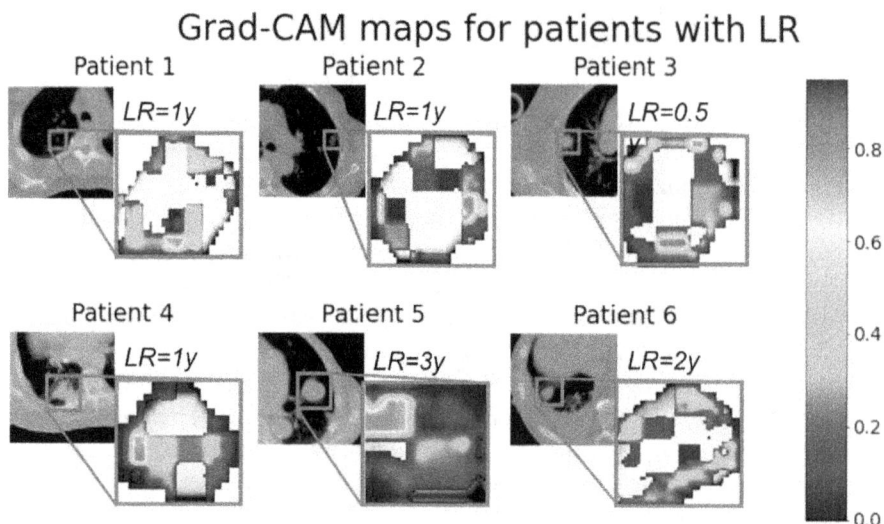

Figure 13.5. Grad-CAM analysis of dose distributions for patients with LR—examples of dose distribution slices with Grad-CAM maps, including the time of local recurrence in years. (Reproduced with permission from [151]. Copyright 2024 Elsevier.)

importance of each neuron in the model behavior. Typically, it is applied to the last convolutional layer, as it has the most significant impact on the model's decision. Its main advantage, and the reason why it is very popular in outcome models using imaging data, is the ability to visualize the model's focus region spatially. See, for example, Grad-CAM applied in the deep learning model, predicting local failures in NSCLC treated with stereotactic body radiation therapy (SBRT) published by Dudas *et al* [151].

13.2.5 Sample use cases

13.2.5.1 Lung cancer—tumor local control prediction

A deep learning outcome model predicting local control in NSCLC patients treated with SBRT was adopted in the study by Dudas *et al* [151] (figure 13.6). The model utilized multi-modality data. It was built from three separate neural networks—two CNNs and one VAE. The CNNs were applied to extract features from planning CT images and planning dose distribution, while the VAE was used to extract underlying features from clinical/demographic patient details. The outputs from all three NN were then concatenated and fed into a discrete-time survival NN, as shown in figure 13.6. The survival neural network predicted the conditional probability of tumor local control.

The dataset was split according to TRIPOD criteria type 2b [160]. The first part, 80% of the data, were used for stratified five-fold cross-validation. The remaining 20% were kept as an independent dataset for final testing.

The explainability technique Grad-CAM was applied to identify the parts of the data which are the most significant with respect to the local control prediction.

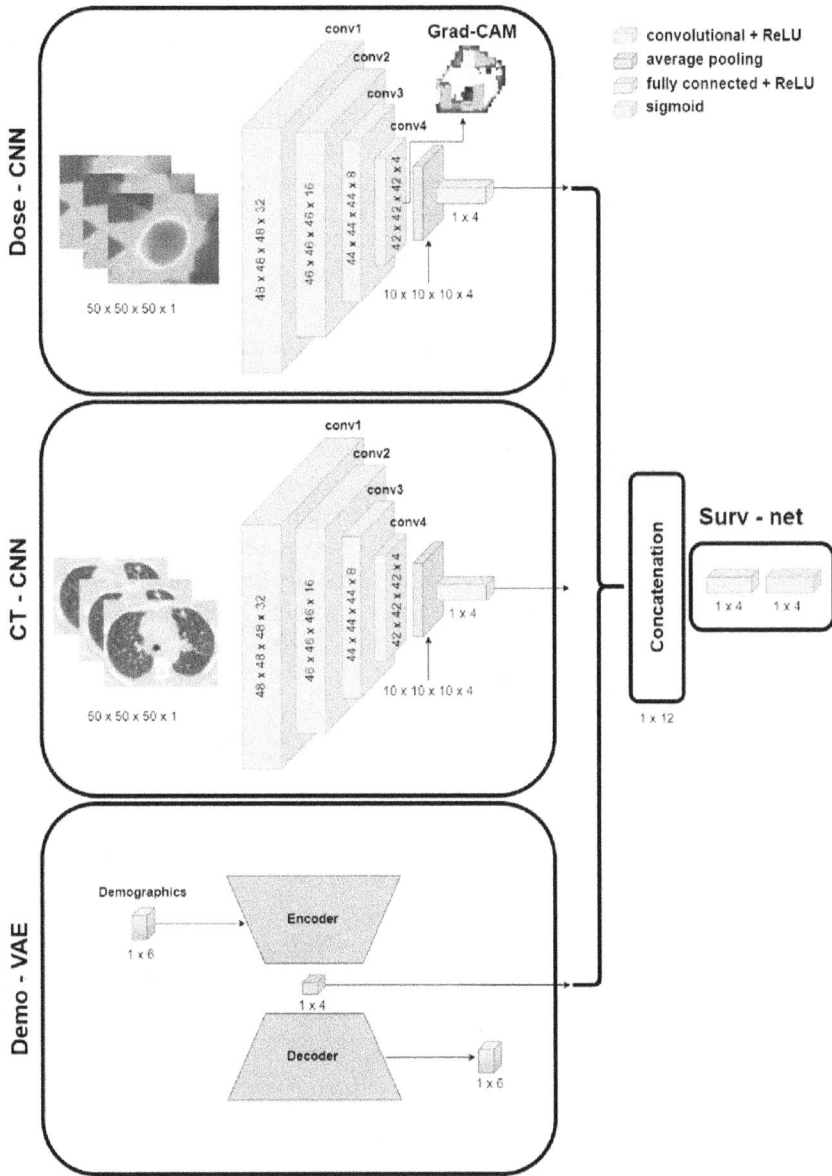

Figure 13.6. Diagram of the DL-based outcome model for prediction of local control in NSCLC patients treated with SBRT. (Reproduced with permission from [151]. Copyright 2024 Elsevier.)

Subsequently, the results were used to guide the design of planning dose criteria to mitigate local failures.

13.2.5.2 Breast cancer—acute skin toxicity prediction

The study by Saednia *et al* [165] presented conventional ML models, based primarily on a random forest approach, to predict acute skin toxicity (radiation dermatitis) after whole-breast RT. The model was trained on quantitative biomarkers, extracted as surface temperature and texture features from thermal images, acquired before and during the treatment (after the fifth, tenth, and fifteenth treatment fractions).

The dataset consisted of 90 patients, split into training (83%) and independent testing (17%) subsets. The model was cross-validated using the leave-one-out methodology. The highest prediction accuracy (testing accuracy = 0.87) was associated with thermal biomarkers obtained after the fifth treatment fraction.

13.2.5.3 Head and neck cancer—loco-regional failure, distant metastasis, and overall survival prediction

About 300 multi-institutional patients from The Cancer Imaging Archive were involved in the study by Diamant *et al* [166] to develop DL-based models predicting loco-regional failures (LRF), distant metastasis (DM), and overall survival (OS). CNNs, followed by MLPs, were applied to extract features from pre-treatment CT images and model the endpoints.

The training/validation dataset included 194 patients, while the independent testing dataset included 106 patients. The AUCs of predicting DM, LRF, and OS were about 0.88, 0.65, and 0.70, respectively. The study also demonstrated the use of explainability techniques (grad-CAM), showing a significant difference in the decision explanation of patients who did or did not develop distant metastasis.

13.2.5.4 Prostate cancer—disease progression prediction

Conventional ML methods were applied in the study by Nayan *et al* [167] to predict a grade progression in very-low and low-risk prostate cancer patients. Various clinical and demographic features, such as age, family history of prostate cancer, tumor stage, PSA level, prostate size, biopsy characteristics, and use of a 5-alpha reductase inhibitor were included in the modeling.

The study investigated several ML approaches, including logistic regression (the traditional and ML versions), SVM, RF, and ANN. Using a stratified random split, the dataset was split in a ratio of 80% (training/validation) and 20% (independent testing). The results showed a superior performance of ML approaches predicting progression on active surveillance for prostate cancer.

13.2.5.5 Liver cancer—overall survival prediction

Three types of patient data (clinical, radiomics, and contrast-enhanced CT images) were used in the study by Wei *et al* [168] for training a multi-modality DL-based outcome model to predict the OS in hepatocellular carcinoma (HCC) patients treated with SBRT.

Three separate models were trained: (i) VAE latent representation of clinical details fed into DeepSurv NN [169]; (ii) VAE latent representation of radiomic features fed into DeepSurv NN; and (iii) CNN-extracted features from CECT fed into DeepSurv NN. Subsequently, all three models were combined in a joint survival model for clinical, radiomic, and CECT features, as shown in figure 13.7. The joint model reported the best performance (c-index 0.650; 95% CI 0.635–0.683).

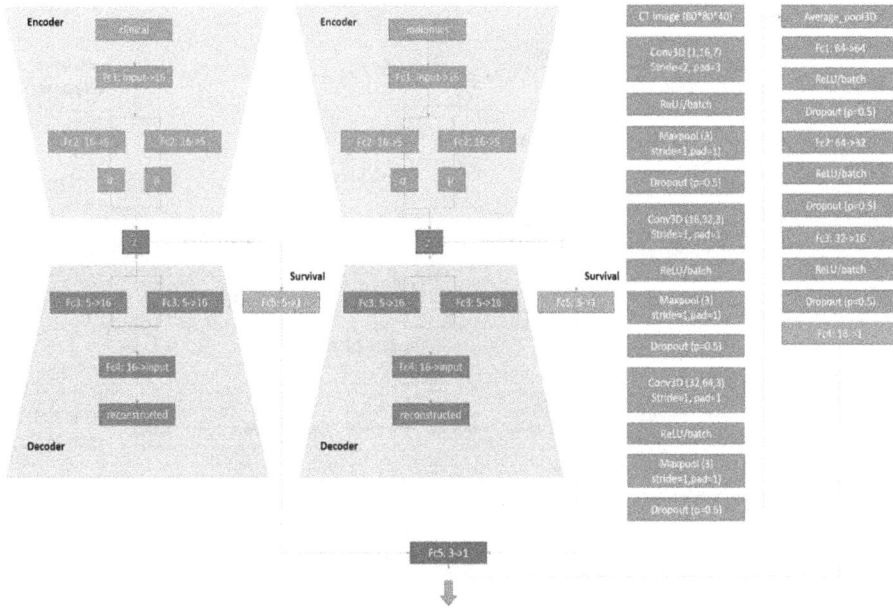

Figure 13.7. VAE-based clinical survival NN, VAE-based radiomics survival NN, and CNN-based CECT survival NN were jointly employed in the OS prediction of HCC patients treated with SBRT. (Reproduced with permission from [168]. Copyright 2021 Elsevier.)

The integrated gradient method provided the interpretation and concluded the increased importance of normal tissue status for the OS.

13.3 AI response-based adaptive radiotherapy

Adaptive radiotherapy (ART) has been advancing since the late 1990s [170]. Typically, it is associated with anatomy-based modifications, requiring new PTV/ OARs delineations, or biology-based modifications using simple population-based response models. However, with the emergence of AI, multi-modality imaging and biotechnology, more advanced and individual-based approaches to response modeling were adopted. Consequently, significant improvements in the personalization of ART can be achieved. Patient-specific response models can accurately predict treatment outcomes while considering the actual state of a patient on treatment. Therefore, it allows for personalized treatment adjustments during the treatment course. This framework is often called knowledge-based response-adapted radiation therapy (KBR-ART) [171]. Its diagram, in the context of current and previous frameworks for ART, is in figure 13.8.

13.3.1 Requirements and challenges

All essential requirements and challenges related to response-based adaptive radiotherapy are encompassed in the acronym KBR-ART. These are knowledge, response, and adaptation. The adaptation process is formulated based on

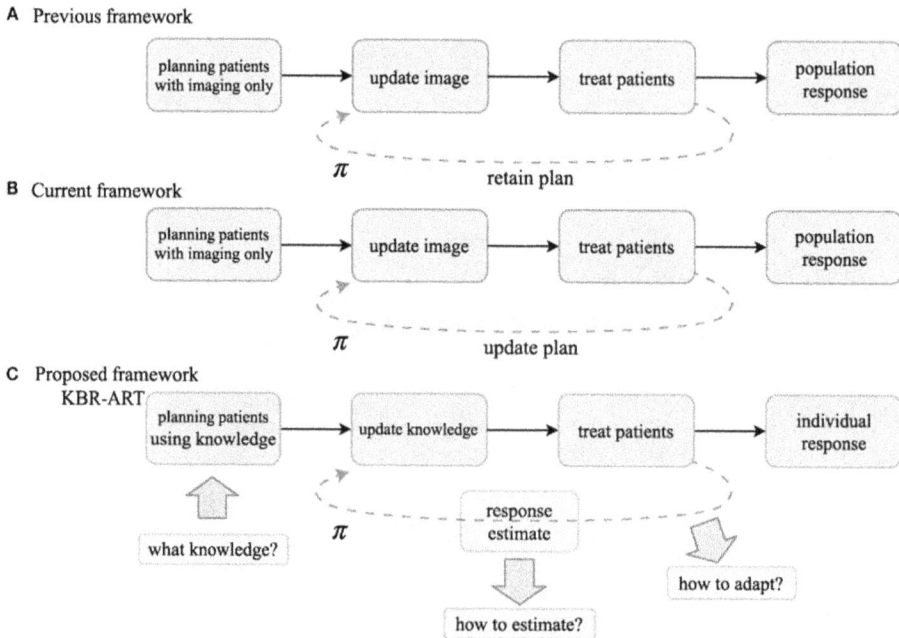

Figure 13.8. Comparison of previous, current and KBR frameworks for ART. (A) Previous framework—treatment planning provided on imaging data, no adaptation during the course, outcomes estimated using population-based response models. (B) Current framework—treatment planning provided on imaging data, anatomy-based adaptation, outcomes estimated using population-based response models. (C) KBR-ART framework—individualized treatment planning utilizing imaging and multiomics data for informed response-based planning, personalized response-based adaptation, outcomes estimated using personalized response models. (Reproduced from [171]. CC BY 4.0.)

predictions from the response model, which, in turn, relies on the availability of comprehensive patient datasets. As is evident, each KBR-ART component is interdependent and cannot work without the rest.

The first requirement is knowledge (i.e. patient data). As introduced in section 13.1, various data resources prove valuable for outcome modeling. Particularly data that capture characteristics of the patient, the patient's disease, and planned treatment. That includes clinical and demographic details (see section 13.1.1), imaging biomarkers (see section 13.1.2), treatment planning data (see section 13.1.3), and multiomic biomarkers (see section 13.1.4).

The second requirement is a suitable and reliable response model. Modeling the treatment response is a key part of modern oncology research, as it enables treatment personalization. Radiotherapy outcomes are typically expressed in terms of TCP and NTCP. Both can be modeled either analytically or via data-driven models. While analytical methods have clear interpretation, ML/DL approaches are often poorly interpretable with limited or no radiobiological understanding. However, ML/DL-based outcome models usually outperform analytical models, since they are capable of finding important underlying data representations. Common outcome modeling approaches were reviewed in section 13.2.

Finally, the third requirement is an adaptation of decision-making, illustrated in figure 13.8 by the adaptation function π. The question is, how can we use outcome models in a strategically optimal manner to adapt a patient's treatment plan? The resolution of this challenge leverages modern AI techniques. Architectures such as reinforcement learning (RL) have a crucial impact in this area, as they are specifically suitable for adaptive systems and sequential decision-making [172–177]. Their primary advantages lies in their ability to explore the effects of decision-making several steps ahead, for example, in dose regimen adaptations between radiotherapy fractions. Other ML methods applicable in KBR-ART involve Bayesian networks [178] or quantum deep RL [174].

The core component of RL is the Markov decision process (MDP), a framework applied in sequential decision-making models. Each step of the MDP can be described as four-tuple (s_t, a_t, R_t, γ'), where s_t denotes the current state of the system ($s_t \in S$), a_t is the action undertaken in step t (i.e. from state s_t to s_{t+1}) ($a_t \in A$), R is the reward function for a given action, and γ is the importance rate, which sets how far in the future the reward is considered. The system assigning actions to states (i.e. $s_t \cdot a_t$) is called the policy. The policy in KBR-ART is called the adaptation function (π) [171, 172]. The ultimate goal of RL, and other MDP methods, is to find a policy that maximizes cumulative reward in the modeled problem. The objective of MDP (the Q function), being maximized, is mathematically expressed by the following equation:

$$Q^\pi(s, a) = \mathrm{E}\left[\sum_{t=0}^{\infty}\gamma^t R(s_t, \pi(s_t))_{\pi, s, a}\right]. \tag{13.6}$$

The optimal policy $Q^{\pi*}$ is determined as $\max_{\pi} Q^\pi$. However, equation (13.6) is impractical for implementation due to the infinite sum. A more effective formulation is called the Bellman equation:

$$\widetilde{Q}_{i+1}^\pi(s, a) = E_{s' \sim P(s, a)}\left\{R(s, a) + \gamma \max_{a' \in A; s' \in S} \widetilde{Q}_i(s', a')\right\}, \tag{13.7}$$

such that $\lim_{i \to \infty} \widetilde{Q}_i = Q^{\pi*}$, and $s' \sim P(s, a)$ denotes the transition probability from state s to state s'. As proved earlier, the convergent point $Q^{\pi*}$ is optimal [179]. The Q function is often solved utilizing deep learning techniques—deep Q-networks (DQNs).

In KBR-ART, MDP simulates the clinical workflow. Each step (i.e. delivery of each fraction) is described by a patient state s_t, reward R_t, and external action a_t to maximize the outcomes. The patient state is commonly characterized by TCP/NTCP models, utilizing various input data (see section 13.2.1). The reward is usually a predefined combination of treatment outcomes, prioritizing maximum TCP and minimum NTCP. The external action may involve, for example, dose escalation, localized radiation boosting, adapting the number of fractions, adapting the target volume or even boosting the treatment with other modalities, such as chemotherapy or immunotherapy. In practical deployment, the only option to change the current patient state and maximize treatment benefits is by actions of the adaptation function. The optimal decision-making for each state is trained in the RL model via numerous trial/error $(s_t \; R_t) \underset{a_t}{\rightarrow} (s_{t+1}, R_{t+1})$ interactions.

13.3.2 Prediction versus treatment optimization

Precision medicine can encompass many tasks in a real clinical environment, such as anatomy-based or outcome-optimized treatment adaptations. Personalized treatment adaptations may be performed before, during, and after the treatment.

The traditional approach involves adaptations as a result of on-treatment changes in the patient's anatomy and geometry (anatomy-based adaptations). Typically, a new treatment plan must be created on new planning CT images when a significant change in the geometry is detected. The adaptation can be offline (between fractions), online (immediately prior to a fraction), or even real-time (during an ongoing fraction) [180]. All three approaches may utilize various ML-empowered tools, such as auto-image registration, auto-contouring, or auto-planning, but no outcome model is necessary in such a framework. However, outcome modeling can be applied to predict ART eligibility based on numerous imaging and multiomic biomarkers [181, 182]. Other applications have demonstrated the promising role of longitudinal CT radiomics in evaluating the point of the tumor's most significant change to trigger the anatomy-based ART [183]. In a study by Forouzannezhad *et al* [184], a promising value of longitudinal CT, FDG-PET, and SPECT radiomics, to predict survival in NSCLC patients for risk-adaptive cancer therapy, was presented.

One of the possible strategies involves treatment optimization prior to the initial fraction. Suitable response models, predicting TCP and NTCP, can guide the dose schedule adaptation to optimize outcomes [185].

Another potential, and perhaps more common, approach involves treatment adaptation during the treatment course, based on actual (mid-treatment) patient data and information. Traditionally, baseline imaging biomarkers (e.g. PET or MRI) would be evaluated before the treatment, followed by mid-treatment evaluation. The adaptation in dose scheduling or target volume definition would then be determined based on the comparison of these two datasets [186, 187].

As discussed in the previous section, the state-of-the-art response-based ART is KBR-ART. This framework is built on advanced AI models, comprising two essential components: (i) the outcome model for predicting clinical outcomes and (ii) the adaptation model optimizing the treatment, typically dose scheduling, based on the outcome model prediction. Both models must work in an effective cooperation, the RL model, where the reward function utilizes the outcome model. Most commonly, the adaptation is not proposed between each fraction, but at a certain point of the treatment, when it is possible to evaluate current outcomes and tailor the adaptation [176].

13.3.3 Sample use cases

13.3.3.1 Response-based dose prescription

In the study by Lou *et al* [185], a deep learning outcome model was applied to individualize the dose prescription in lung cancer patients. The outcome model had an autoencoder-like architecture to extract features from CT images, which were fed into another neural network to predict the probability of tumor local control. Prediction results were combined with other patient's clinical data, in a regression model, to provide a recommendation for personalized dose prescription, that reduced tumor local failure probability below 5%.

Dose recommendations, provided by the model, had a wider range and were more continuous than the actual delivered doses. It also suggested dose de-escalation in a number of patients. Therefore, it provides a more flexible approach to treatment personalization than regular clinical protocol. This framework allows personalizing dose prescription according to the risk prediction, which potentially changes the radiotherapy planning paradigm from binary decisions to response-informed adjustments.

13.3.3.2 Response-based dose schedule adaptation

A framework for dose fractionation adaptation was presented in a study by Tseng *et al* [177]. There were three complementary neural networks: GAN, DNN and DQN. The GAN was used to generate more training data samples as the original number of patients involved in this retrospective study was insufficient. Input characteristics involved clinical, genetic, and imaging features. The DNN was applied to reconstruct a radiotherapy artificial environment (RAE) to simulate transition probabilities, for a given action, between different states (i.e. dose schedule modifications). The last neural network (DQN) was responsible for the evaluation of possible adaptation strategies and recommendation of the optimal one, considering the treatment outcomes modeled by the RAE. This framework was designed to provide dose schedule adaptations at about 2/3 period of the treatment, based on dosimetric variables, clinical details, multiomics features, and PET radiomics, acquired before and after about 1/3 and 2/3 of scheduled fractions. The presented results were benchmarked against real clinical dose adaptations, performed on patients enrolled in a dose-escalation clinical protocol.

A similar approach was adopted in the study by Niraula *et al* [175], which introduced the Adaptive Radiotherapy Clinical Decision Support (ARCliDS) software. They used GAN to generate more training samples, an artificial RT environment (ARTE) to estimate treatment outcomes (TCP/NTCP), and an optimal decision maker (ODM), built on DQN, to recommend an optimal treatment adaptation. The ARTE combined a linear-quadratic-linear response model with graph neural networks (GNNs), developed by Niraula *et al* [174]. The input characteristics for TCP/NTCP modeling were dosimetric, clinical, multiomics, and PET-radiomics features. The system was trained and validated in two different treatment types for two different diseases (NSCLC and HCC). A diagram of the

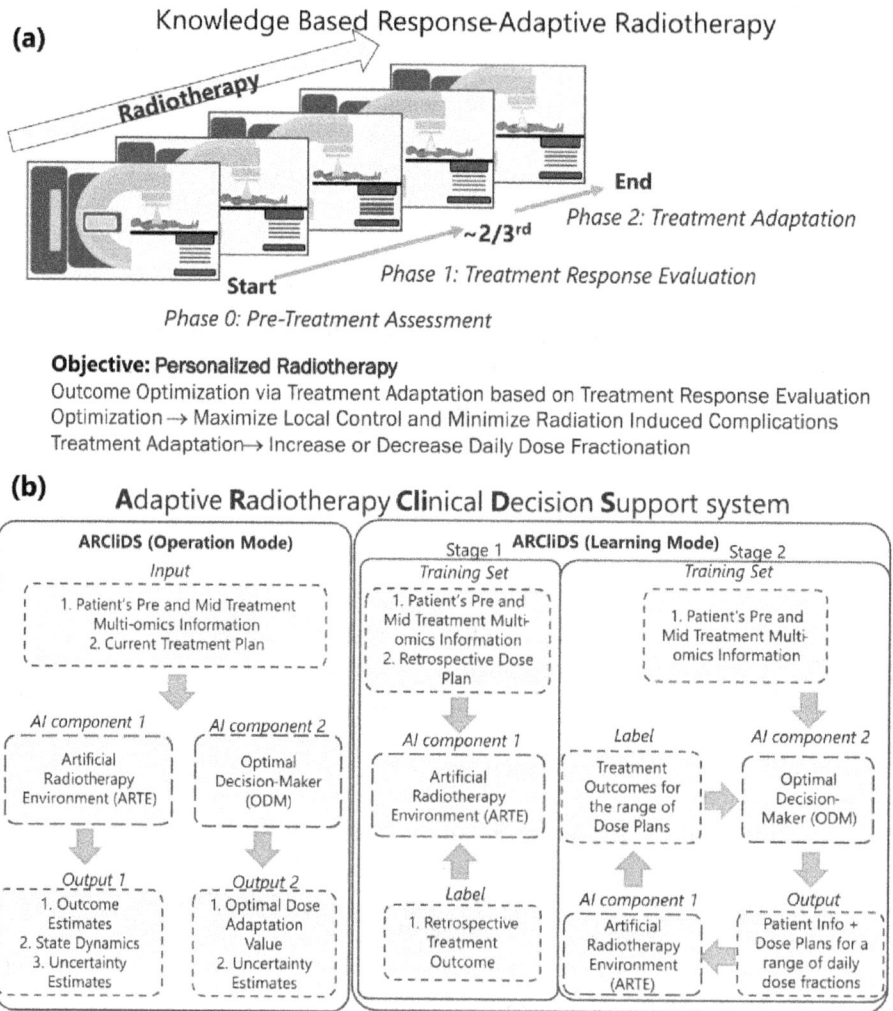

Figure 13.9. (a) Diagram of response-adaptive radiotherapy using the ARCliDS system. A treatment plan is created in phase 0, the patient's treatment response is evaluated in phase 1, treatment adaptation is planned at the end of phase 1, and it is executed in phase 2. (b) ARCliDS consists of two components—ARTE and ODM. In learning mode, ARTE is trained in supervised learning, and its outputs are used in the reinforcement learning of ODM. In operation mode, both components run simultaneously, providing outcome estimates and optimal dose adaptation. (Reproduced with permission from [175]. Copyright 2023 Springer Nature.)

framework and description of the ARCliDS operation/learning modes are shown in figure 13.9.

13.4 Challenges and recommendations

Any AI deployment is generally associated with multiple challenges. However, radiotherapy AI response modeling and response-based adaptations have several specific requirements, in addition to the general ones, of which all developers and researchers in this field have to be aware.

A trustworthy and reliable response model in radiation oncology should always be based on a comprehensive understanding of the biological mechanisms behind disease specifics, progression, and control. Only then can the developer decide whether the available data capture sufficient information for the desired prediction. It is the lack of understanding of the disease biology and, hence, insufficient data representation, which often limits the accuracy and trustworthiness of developed response models. For the same reason, it is sometimes also difficult to select the most indicative features for a given task. Input features are mostly selected based on various statistical methods, not considering their real biological/clinical importance for the modeled endpoint.

Another critical challenge for AI response modeling is the model's architecture. There is no universal architecture that fits all possible scenarios, clinical endpoints, and the variability of input datasets. Therefore, the architecture is heavily influenced by the developer's skills and knowledge. The optimal architecture depends, for example, on the problem definition (classification/regression), data type (structured/unstructured), number of training samples, class imbalance ratio, and so on.

One of the most common issues in radiotherapy outcome modeling regarding dataset quality is the imbalance of modeled endpoints. There are multiple methods to overcome this problem, for example, over-sampling, under-sampling, class weights, and the synthetic minority over-sampling technique (SMOTE) and its variants [188–192]. However, the most effective appears to be generative models, which can be utilized to generate new synthetic data points of any class. The applicability of this concept to radiotherapy outcome modeling was recently showcased in a study by Dudas et al [159].

The ultimate goal of all response and treatment adaptation models is their translation into clinical practice. This can be accomplished only for models which are properly validated and provide a robust explainability. The clinically preferred validation process involves a prospective validation using a randomized controlled trial or clinical trial. The randomized controlled trial is commonly regarded as the optimal choice for prospective validation since it is expected to offer an unbiased tool for causal inferences. An alternative to prospective validation is retrospective validation, which evaluates models in past patients, who were not preselected for the study. There are several scenarios for retrospective validation, and some of them are described in the TRIPOD report [160]. The optimal approach for retrospective validation involves a separate validation dataset, ideally from different institutions. However, retrospective validation can never completely reduce all biases. For example, it may suffer from biases such as clinicians'/patients' treatment preferences or changes in care quality over time. Therefore, this is a drive towards prospective validation via randomized clinical trials [193].

Existing challenges can be diminished if developers adhere to a suitable and standardized checklist [1] (see the example in figure 13.10.

a) **Define clinical end-points and specify input data**

b) **Data pre-processing**

- *Select included/excluded patients and justify*
- *Define how to manage incomplete data*
- *Check the reliability of the data*
- *Standardize input variables*

c) **Training/Validation**

- *Split the data into Training/validation/testing*
- *Feature extraction and selection (if applicable)*
- *Manage class imbalance (if applicable)*
- *Tune architecture and hyperparameters*

d) **Test the model on an independent prospective (ideal) or retrospective dataset**

e) **Explain the model (e.g. Grad-CAM, LIME, SHAP)**

f) **Evaluation of systemic bias**

- *Evaluate the model on under- and over-representation data.*
- *Evaluate the model on edge case patients*
- *Design boundaries for input data which are out of training/testing bounds*

Figure 13.10. Example checklist for AI-based outcome model development.

13.5 Summary

The progress and development in medical imaging, biotechnology, and treatment modalities is an unstoppable process, introducing new data resources for outcome modeling and treatment adaptation. Due to the amount and complexity of the available data, AI technologies are often the only suitable tool for its integration. However, it leverages multiple challenges, primarily associated with data aggregation/sharing/quality, AI architecture, and AI explainability. Poor or missing AI explainability can quickly transform any model from a promising technology to an untrustworthy and unreliable black box. Therefore, all AI-empowered outcome models must be comprehensively validated and concept-proofed according to standardized methodologies to become a viable and reliable decision-support tool in the clinic. As such, it can represent a promising improvement for precision medicine, where the key to success lies in response-based treatment adaptation and personalization. For several decades, it has been the clinical team's role to provide patient response estimation (often utilizing poor population-based models) and recommend treatment adjustments. With the expansion of AI technologies, this task is nowadays transferable to automated systems, which can integrate larger and more complex patient-specific data. This is where the concept of knowledge-based response-adapted radiotherapy reaches its full potential. It integrates comprehensive information, identifies the most important links to patient-specific treatment response, and tailors the optimal adjustments to maximize the benefits.

Acknowledgments

This work was supported by National Institute of Health (NIH) grant R01-CA233487 and Department of Defense (DoD) Congressional Directed Med Res Prog (CDMRP) W81XWH-22-1-0277.

References

[1] Cui S, Hope A, Dilling T J, Dawson L A, Ten Haken R and El Naqa I 2022 Artificial intelligence for outcome modeling in radiotherapy *Semin. Radiat. Oncol.* **32** 351–64

[2] Niraula D *et al* 2022 Current status and future developments in predicting outcomes in radiation oncology *Br. J. Radiol.* **95** 20220239

[3] Osong B, Bermejo I, Lee K C, Lee S H, Dekker A and van Soest J 2022 Prediction of radiotherapy compliance in elderly cancer patients using an internally validated decision tree *Cancers* **14** 6116

[4] Straube C *et al* 2017 Does age really matter? Radiotherapy in elderly patients with glioblastoma, the Munich experience *Radiat. Oncol.* **12** 77

[5] Gao S J *et al* 2023 Prediction of distant metastases after stereotactic body radiation therapy for early stage NSCLC: development and external validation of a multi-institutional model *J. Thorac. Oncol.* **18** 339–49

[6] De Courcy L, Bezak E and Marcu L G 2020 Gender-dependent radiotherapy: the next step in personalised medicine? *Crit. Rev. Oncol. Hematol* **147** 102881

[7] Yap Y-S 2023 Outcomes in breast cancer—does ethnicity matter? *ESMO Open* **8** 101564

[8] Abdelkarem O A I, Choudhury A, Burnet N G, Summersgill H R and West C M L 2022 Effect of race and ethnicity on risk of radiotherapy toxicity and implications for radio-genomics *Clin. Oncol.* **34** 653–69

[9] Panzone J, Wu M S, Chandrasekar T, Basnet A, Bratslavsky G and Goldberg H 2023 The impact of household income on prostate cancer diagnosis, treatment, and outcomes *J. Clin. Oncol.* **41** 5038

[10] Kim M, Schrag D, Li L and Chen A B 2015 Predictors of radiation therapy (RT) use among Medicare patients with metastatic non-small cell lung cancer (NSCLC) *J. Clin. Oncol.* **33** 124

[11] Zhou Y-J *et al* 2020 Marital status, an independent predictor for survival of gastric neuroendocrine neoplasm patients: a SEER database analysis *BMC Endocr. Disord.* **20** 111

[12] Zhang S, Yang Z, Qiu P, Li J and Zhou C 2022 Research on the role of marriage status among women underwent breast reconstruction following mastectomy: a competing risk analysis model based on the SEER database, 1998–2015 *Front. Surg.* **8** 803223

[13] Tang A *et al* 2021 Non-small cell lung cancer in never- and ever-smokers is it the same disease? *J. Thorac. Cardiovasc. Surg.* **161** 1903–17.e9

[14] Fink C A *et al* 2023 Comorbidity in limited disease small-cell lung cancer: age-adjusted Charlson comorbidity index and its association with overall survival following chemo-radiotherapy *Clin. Transl. Radiat. Oncol.* **42** 100665

[15] Guzzo T J, Dluzniewski P, Orosco R, Platz E A, Partin A W and Han M 2010 Prediction of mortality after radical prostatectomy by Charlson comorbidity index *Urology* **76** 553–7

[16] Hjälm-Eriksson M, Ullén A, Johansson H, Levitt S, Nilsson S and Kälkner K-M 2017 Comorbidity as a predictor of overall survival in prostate cancer patients treated with external beam radiotherapy combined with HDR brachytherapy boosts *Acta. Oncol.* **56** 21–6

[17] Dreyer J, Bremer M and Henkenberens C 2018 Comorbidity indexing for prediction of the clinical outcome after stereotactic body radiation therapy in non-small cell lung cancer *Radiat. Oncol.* **13** 213

[18] Sharma N, Schwendimann R, Endrich O, Ausserhofer D and Simon M 2021 Comparing Charlson and Elixhauser comorbidity indices with different weightings to predict in-hospital mortality: an analysis of national inpatient data *BMC Health Serv. Res.* **21** 13

[19] Huang Y-J, Chen J-S, Luo S-F and Kuo C-F 2021 Comparison of indexes to measure comorbidity burden and predict all-cause mortality in rheumatoid arthritis *J. Clin. Med.* **10** 5460

[20] Allen A J, Labella D A, Kowalchuk R O, Waters M R and Kersh C R 2023 Effect of histology on stereotactic body radiotherapy for non-small cell lung cancer oligometastatic pulmonary lesions *Transl. Lung. Cancer Res.* **12** 66–78

[21] Shiue K *et al* 2018 Histology, tumor volume, and radiation dose predict outcomes in NSCLC patients after stereotactic ablative radiotherapy *J. Thorac. Oncol.* **13** 1549–59

[22] Cao C, Wang D, Tian D H, Wilson-Smith A, Huang J and Rimner A 2019 A systematic review and meta-analysis of stereotactic body radiation therapy for colorectal pulmonary metastases *J. Thorac. Dis.* **11** 5187–98

[23] Parsons M *et al* 2021 The effect of maximum tumor diameter on disease control in intermediate and high-risk prostate cancer patients treated with brachytherapy boost *J. Clin. Oncol.* **39** 252

[24] Hutten R *et al* 2022 The clinical significance of maximum tumor diameter on MRI in men undergoing radical prostatectomy or definitive radiotherapy for locoregional prostate cancer *Clin. Genitourin. Cancer* **20** e453–9

[25] Illidge T M *et al* 2020 Maximum tumor diameter is associated with event-free survival in PET-negative patients with stage I/IIA Hodgkin lymphoma *Blood. Adv.* **4** 203–6

[26] Davey A *et al* 2023 Predicting cancer relapse following lung stereotactic radiotherapy: an external validation study using real-world evidence *Front. Oncol.* **13** 1156389

[27] Goorts B *et al* 2017 Clinical tumor stage is the most important predictor of pathological complete response rate after neoadjuvant chemotherapy in breast cancer patients *Breast. Cancer Res. Treat.* **163** 83–91

[28] Talebi A *et al* 2023 Predicting metastasis in gastric cancer patients: machine learning-based approaches *Sci. Rep.* **13** 4163

[29] Inagaki T *et al* 2022 Escalated maximum dose in the planning target volume improves local control in stereotactic body radiation therapy for T1–2 lung cancer *Cancers* **14** 933

[30] Meehan J *et al* 2020 Precision medicine and the role of biomarkers of radiotherapy response in breast cancer *Front. Oncol.* **10** 628

[31] Sandhu C, Qureshi A and Emili A 2018 Panomics for precision medicine *Trends Mol. Med.* **24** 85–101

[32] Coates J T T, Pirovano G and El Naqa I 2021 Radiomic and radiogenomic modeling for radiotherapy: strategies, pitfalls, and challenges *J. Med. Imaging* **8** 031902

[33] Davis A T, Palmer A L and Nisbet A 2017 Can CT scan protocols used for radiotherapy treatment planning be adjusted to optimize image quality and patient dose? A systematic review *Br. J. Radiol.* **90** 20160406

[34] Yee P P *et al* 2022 Temporal radiographic and histological study of necrosis development in a mouse glioblastoma model *Front. Oncol.* **12** 993649

[35] Beddy P *et al* 2014 Tumor necrosis on magnetic resonance imaging correlates with aggressive histology and disease progression in clear cell renal cell carcinoma *Clin. Genitourin. Cancer.* **12** 55–62

[36] Abrantes A M *et al* 2020 Tumour functional imaging by PET *Biochim. Biophys. Acta— Mol. Basis Dis.* **1866** 165717

[37] Lewis D Y, Soloviev D and Brindle K M 2015 Imaging tumor metabolism using positron emission tomography *Cancer J.* **21** 129–36

[38] Kandathil A, Kay F U, Butt Y M, Wachsmann J W and Subramaniam R M 2018 Role of FDG PET/CT in the eighth edition of TNM staging of non-small cell lung cancer *RadioGraphics* **38** 2134–49

[39] Schrevens L, Lorent N, Dooms C and Vansteenkiste J 2004 The role of PET scan in diagnosis, staging, and management of non-small cell lung cancer *Oncologist* **9** 633–43

[40] Bussink J, Kaanders J H A M, van der Graaf W T A and Oyen W J G 2011 PET–CT for radiotherapy treatment planning and response monitoring in solid tumors *Nat. Rev. Clin. Oncol.* **8** 233–42

[41] Zaidi H and El Naqa I 2010 PET-guided delineation of radiation therapy treatment volumes: a survey of image segmentation techniques *Eur. J. Nucl. Med. Mol. Imaging* **37** 2165–87

[42] Mayerhoefer M E *et al* 2020 Introduction to radiomics *J. Nucl. Med.* **61** 488

[43] Sollini M, Cozzi L, Antunovic L, Chiti A and Kirienko M 2017 PET radiomics in NSCLC: state of the art and a proposal for harmonization of methodology *Sci. Rep.* **7** 358

[44] El Naqa I *et al* 2018 Radiation therapy outcomes models in the era of radiomics and radiogenomics: uncertainties and validation *Int. J. Radiat. Oncol. Biol. Phys.* **102** 1070–3

[45] Avanzo M *et al* 2020 Machine and deep learning methods for radiomics *Med. Phys.* **47** e185–202

[46] Sung Y S, Park B, Park H J and Lee S S 2021 Radiomics and deep learning in liver diseases *J. Gastroenterol. Hepatol.* **36** 561–8

[47] Trinh D-L, Kim S-H, Yang H-J and Lee G-S 2022 The efficacy of shape radiomics and deep features for glioblastoma survival prediction by deep learning *Electronics* **11** 1038

[48] Rizzo S *et al* 2018 Radiomics: the facts and the challenges of image analysis *Eur. Radiol. Exp.* **2** 36

[49] van Griethuysen J J M *et al* 2017 Computational radiomics system to decode the radiographic phenotype *Cancer Res.* **77** e104–7

[50] Ruan M *et al* 2022 Radiomics based on DCE-MRI improved diagnostic performance compared to BI-RADS analysis in identifying sclerosing adenosis of the breast *Front. Oncol.* **12** 888141

[51] Marzi C *et al* 2023 Collinearity and dimensionality reduction in radiomics: effect of preprocessing parameters in hypertrophic cardiomyopathy magnetic resonance T1 and T2 mapping *Bioengineering* **10** 80

[52] Koçak B, Durmaz E S, Ateş E and Kılıçkesmez Ö 2019 Radiomics with artificial intelligence: a practical guide for beginners *Diagn. Interv. Radiol.* **25** 485–95

[53] DeLeu A-L *et al* 2022 Principal component analysis of texture features derived from FDG PET images of melanoma lesions *EJNMMI Phys.* **9** 64

[54] Li S *et al* 2018 Use of radiomics combined with machine learning method in the recurrence patterns after intensity-modulated radiotherapy for nasopharyngeal carcinoma: a preliminary study *Front. Oncol.* **8** 648

[55] Rizzo S *et al* 2018 Radiomics of high-grade serous ovarian cancer: association between quantitative CT features, residual tumour and disease progression within 12 months *Eur. Radiol.* **28** 4849–59

[56] Zhang Y, Oikonomou A, Wong A, Haider M A and Khalvati F 2017 Radiomics-based prognosis analysis for non-small cell lung cancer *Sci. Rep.* **7** 46349

[57] El Naqa I *et al* 2006 Multivariable modeling of radiotherapy outcomes, including dose–volume and clinical factors *Int. J. Radiat. Oncol. Biol. Phys.* **64** 1275–86

[58] El Naqa I and Chien J-T 2022 Computational learning theory *Machine and Deep Learning in Oncology, Medical Physics and Radiology* ed I El Naqa and M J Murphy (Cham: Springer International) pp 17–26

[59] Sanchez-Pinto L N, Venable L R, Fahrenbach J and Churpek M M 2018 Comparison of variable selection methods for clinical predictive modeling *Int. J. Med. Inform.* **116** 10–7

[60] Bagherzadeh-Khiabani F, Ramezankhani A, Azizi F, Hadaegh F, Steyerberg E W and Khalili D 2016 A tutorial on variable selection for clinical prediction models: feature selection methods in data mining could improve the results *J. Clin. Epidemiol.* **71** 76–85

[61] Cui S, Ten Haken R K and El Naqa I 2021 Integrating multiomics information in deep learning architectures for joint actuarial outcome prediction in non-small cell lung cancer patients after radiation therapy *Int. J. Radiat. Oncol. Biol Phys.* **110** 893–904

[62] Wei L *et al* 2021 A deep survival interpretable radiomics model of hepatocellular carcinoma patients *Phys. Med. Eu. J. Med. Phys.* **82** 295–305

[63] Bedford J L and Hanson I M 2022 A recurrent neural network for rapid detection of delivery errors during real-time portal dosimetry *Phys. Imaging. Radiat. Oncol.* **22** 36–43

[64] Chen M, Wang K and Wang J 2023 Vision transformer-based multi-label survival prediction for oropharynx cancer radiotherapy using planning CT *Int. J. Radiat. Oncol. Biol. Phys.* **25** 1123–34

[65] Steber C *et al* 2019 Local control after 50 Gy delivered in 5 fractions versus 10 fractions for primary and metastatic lung tumors *Int. J. Radiat. Oncol. Biol. Phys.* **105** E774

[66] Klement R J *et al* 2020 Correlating dose variables with local tumor control in stereotactic body radiation therapy for early-stage non-small cell lung cancer: a modeling study on 1500 individual treatments *Int. J. Radiat. Oncol. Biol. Phys.* **107** 579–86

[67] Stephans K L *et al* 2018 Tumor control and toxicity for common stereotactic body radiation therapy dose-fractionation regimens in stage I non-small cell lung cancer *Int. J. Radiat. Oncol. Biol. Phys.* **100** 462–9

[68] Tateishi Y *et al* 2021 Stereotactic body radiation therapy with a high maximum dose improves local control, cancer-specific death, and overall survival in peripheral early-stage non-small cell lung cancer *Int. J. Radiat. Oncol. Biol. Phys.* **111** 143–51

[69] Liang B *et al* 2020 Prediction of radiation pneumonitis with dose distribution: a convolutional neural network (CNN) based model *Front. Oncol.* **9** 1500

[70] Creach K M *et al* 2012 Dosimetric predictors of chest wall pain after lung stereotactic body radiotherapy *Radiother. Oncol.* **104** 23–7

[71] Moreno A C *et al* 2020 Biologically effective dose in stereotactic body radiotherapy and survival for patients with early-stage NSCLC *J. Thorac. Oncol.* **15** 101–9

[72] Zhang J *et al* 2011 Which is the optimal biologically effective dose of stereotactic body radiotherapy for stage I non-small-cell lung cancer? A meta-analysis *Int. J. Radiat. Oncol. Biol. Phys.* **81** e305–16

[73] Stahl J M *et al* 2016 The effect of biologically effective dose and radiation treatment schedule on overall survival in stage I non-small cell lung cancer patients treated with stereotactic body radiation therapy *Int. J. Radiat. Oncol. Biol. Phys.* **96** 1011–20

[74] Bentzen S M *et al* 2010 Quantitative Analyses of Normal Tissue Effects in the Clinic (QUANTEC): an introduction to the scientific issues *Int. J. Radiat. Oncol. Biol. Phys.* **76** S3–9

[75] Jackson A *et al* 2010 The lessons of QUANTEC: recommendations for reporting and gathering data on dose–volume dependencies of treatment outcome *Int. J. Radiat. Oncol. Biol. Phys.* **76** S155–60

[76] Grimm J, Marks L B, Jackson A, Kavanagh B D, Xue J and Yorke E 2021 High dose per fraction, Hypofractionated Treatment Effects in the Clinic (HyTEC): an overview *Int. J. Radiat. Oncol. Biol. Phys.* **110** 1–10

[77] Søvik Å, Ovrum J, Olsen D R and Malinen E 2007 On the parameter describing the generalised equivalent uniform dose (gEUD) for tumours *Phys. Med.* **23** 100–6

[78] Ten Haken R K *et al* 1993 Use of Veff and iso-NTCP in the implementation of dose escalation protocols *Int. J. Radiat. Oncol. Biol. Phys.* **27** 689–95

[79] Zhen X *et al* 2017 Deep convolutional neural network with transfer learning for rectum toxicity prediction in cervical cancer radiotherapy: a feasibility study *Phys. Med. Biol.* **62** 8246

[80] Ibragimov B, Toesca D, Chang D, Yuan Y, Koong A and Xing L 2018 Development of deep neural network for individualized hepatobiliary toxicity prediction after liver SBRT *Med. Phys.* **45** 4763–74

[81] Ma Z *et al* 2023 Enhanced prediction of postoperative radiotherapy-induced esophagitis in non-small cell lung cancer: dosiomic model development in a real-world cohort and validation in the PORT-C randomized controlled trial *Thorac. Cancer* **14** 2839–45

[82] Huang Y *et al* 2022 Radiation pneumonitis prediction after stereotactic body radiation therapy based on 3D dose distribution: dosiomics and/or deep learning-based radiomics features *Radiat. Oncol.* **17** 188

[83] Liang B *et al* 2019 Dosiomics: extracting 3D spatial features from dose distribution to predict incidence of radiation pneumonitis *Front. Oncol.* **9** 269

[84] Wu A *et al* 2020 Dosiomics improves prediction of locoregional recurrence for intensity modulated radiotherapy treated head and neck cancer cases *Oral Oncol.* **104** 104625

[85] Buizza G *et al* 2021 Radiomics and dosiomics for predicting local control after carbon-ion radiotherapy in skull-base chordoma *Cancers* **13** 339

[86] Zhang Z *et al* 2023 Radiomics and dosiomics signature from whole lung predicts radiation pneumonitis: a model development study with prospective external validation and decision-curve analysis *Int. J. Radiat. Oncol. Biol. Phys.* **115** 746–58

[87] Kraus K M, Oreshko M, Bernhardt D, Combs S E and Peeken J C 2023 Dosiomics and radiomics to predict pneumonitis after thoracic stereotactic body radiotherapy and immune checkpoint inhibition *Front. Oncol.* **13** 1124592

[88] Cui S, Ten Haken R K and El Naqa I 2021 Integrating multiomics information in deep learning architectures for joint actuarial outcome prediction in non-small cell lung cancer patients after radiation therapy *Int. J. Radiat. Oncol. Biol. Phys.* **110** 893–904

[89] Li R 2022 Radiomics and radiogenomics *Machine and Deep Learning in Oncology, Medical Physics and Radiology* ed I El Naqa and M J Murphy (Cham: Springer International) pp 385–98

[90] Anagnostopoulos A K *et al* 2022 Radiomics/radiogenomics in lung cancer: basic principles and initial clinical results *Cancers* **14** 1657

[91] Fu J *et al* 2022 Radiomics/radiogenomics in hepatocellular carcinoma: applications and challenges in interventional management *iLIVER* **1** 96–100

[92] El Naqa I *et al* 2017 Radiogenomics and radiotherapy response modeling *Phys. Med. Biol.* **62** R179

[93] Kang J, Coates J T, Strawderman R L, Rosenstein B S and Kerns S L 2020 Genomics models in radiotherapy: from mechanistic to machine learning *Med. Phys.* **47** e203–17

[94] Schack L M H *et al* 2022 A genome-wide association study of radiotherapy induced toxicity in head and neck cancer patients identifies a susceptibility locus associated with mucositis *Br. J. Cancer* **126** 1082–90

[95] Tobiasz J, Al-Harbi N, Bin Judia S, Majid Wakil S, Polanska J and Alsbeih G 2023 Multivariate piecewise linear regression model to predict radiosensitivity using the association with the genome-wide copy number variation *Front. Oncol.* **13** 1154222

[96] Naderi E *et al* 2023 Large-scale meta-genome-wide association study reveals common genetic factors linked to radiation-induced acute toxicities across cancer types *JNCI Cancer Spectr.* **7** pkad088

[97] Kerns S L, Williams J P and Marples B 2023 Modeling normal bladder injury after radiation therapy *Int. J. Radiat. Biol.* **99** 1046–54

[98] Shyam K P, Ramya V, Nadiya S, Parashar A and Gideon D A 2023 Systems biology approaches to unveiling the expression of phospholipases in various types of cancer—transcriptomics and protein–protein interaction networks *Phospholipases in Physiology and Pathology* ed S Chakraborti (New York: Academic) ch 15 pp 271–307

[99] Liang K-H 2013 Transcriptomics *Bioinformatics for Biomedical Science and Clinical Applications* (Cambridge: Woodhead) ch 3 pp 49–82

[100] Zhang Y *et al* 2023 Single-cell and spatial transcriptomics to analyze radiation therapy-induced tumor microenvironment reshaping in HPV-cervical cancer *J. Clin. Oncol.* **41** e17528

[101] Xu Y *et al* 2022 Prediction of response to radiotherapy by characterizing the transcriptomic features in clinical tumor samples across 15 cancer types *Comput. Intell. Neurosci.* **2022** 5443709

[102] Shukla L, Lee S A, Du M R M, Karnezis T, Ritchie M E and Shayan R 2022 A transcriptomic dataset evaluating the effect of radiotherapy injury on cells of skin and soft tissue *Data Brief.* **41** 107828

[103] Zhao Y *et al* 2021 ICAM-1 orchestrates the abscopal effect of tumor radiotherapy *Proc. Natl Acad. Sci.* **118** e2010333118

[104] Ozgen Z *et al* 2023 Radiation pneumonitis in relation to pulmonary function, dosimetric factors, TGFβ1 expression, and quality of life in breast cancer patients receiving post-operative radiotherapy: a prospective 6-month follow-up study *Clin. Transl. Oncol.* **25** 1287–96

[105] Takahashi S, Anada M, Kinoshita T, Nishide T and Shibata T 2022 Prospective exploratory study of the relationship between radiation pneumonitis and TGF-β1 in exhaled breath condensate *In Vivo* **36** 1485

[106] Ferrarini A *et al* 2019 Metabolomic analysis of liver tissues for characterization of hepatocellular carcinoma *J. Proteome. Res.* **18** 3067–76

[107] Guo W, Tan H Y, Wang N, Wang X and Feng Y 2018 Deciphering hepatocellular carcinoma through metabolomics: from biomarker discovery to therapy evaluation *Cancer Manag. Res.* **10** 715–34

[108] Pienkowski T, Kowalczyk T, Garcia-Romero N, Ayuso-Sacido A and Ciborowski M 2022 Proteomics and metabolomics approach in adult and pediatric glioma diagnostics *Biochim. Biophys. Acta (BBA)—Rev. Cancer* **1877** 188721

[109] Zhao H *et al* 2016 Metabolomics profiling in plasma samples from glioma patients correlates with tumor phenotypes *Oncotarget* **7** 20486–95

[110] Ghini V *et al* 2020 Metabolomics to assess response to immune checkpoint inhibitors in patients with non-small-cell lung cancer *Cancers* **12** 3574

[111] Botticelli A *et al* 2020 Gut metabolomics profiling of non-small cell lung cancer (NSCLC) patients under immunotherapy treatment *J. Transl. Med.* **18** 49

[112] Jelonek K, Pietrowska M and Widlak P 2017 Systemic effects of ionizing radiation at the proteome and metabolome levels in the blood of cancer patients treated with radiotherapy: the influence of inflammation and radiation toxicity *Int. J. Radiat. Biol.* **93** 683–96

[113] Ng S S W, Jang G H, Kurland I J, Qiu Y, Guha C and Dawson L A 2020 Plasma metabolomic profiles in liver cancer patients following stereotactic body radiotherapy *EBioMedicine* **59** 102973

[114] Menon S S *et al* 2016 Radiation metabolomics: current status and future directions *Front. Oncol.* **6** 20

[115] Nalbantoglu S, Abu-Asab M, Suy S, Collins S and Amri H 2019 Metabolomics-based biosignatures of prostate cancer in patients following radiotherapy *OMICS* **23** 214–23

[116] Vicente E, Vujaskovic Z and Jackson I L 2020 A systematic review of metabolomic and lipidomic candidates for biomarkers in radiation injury *Metabolites* **10** 259

[117] Sminia P *et al* 2023 Clinical radiobiology for radiation oncology *Radiobiology Textbook* ed S Baatout (Cham: Springer International) pp 237–309

[118] Gulliford S and El Naqa I 2022 Modelling of radiotherapy response (TCP/NTCP) *Machine and Deep Learning in Oncology, Medical Physics and Radiology* ed I El Naqa and M J Murphy (Cham: Springer International) pp 399–437

[119] McMahon S J 2019 The linear quadratic model: usage, interpretation and challenges *Phys. Med. Biol.* **64** 01TR01

[120] van Leeuwen C M *et al* 2018 The alfa and beta of tumours: a review of parameters of the linear-quadratic model, derived from clinical radiotherapy studies *Radiat. Oncol.* **13** 96

[121] Brenner D J 2008 The linear-quadratic model is an appropriate methodology for determining isoeffective doses at large doses per fraction *Semin. Radiat. Oncol.* **18** 234–9

[122] El Naqa I 2015 Modeling of tumor control probability (TCP) *Machine Learning in Radiation Oncology: Theory and Applications* ed I El Naqa, R Li and M J Murphy (Cham: Springer International) pp 311–23

[123] Zaider M and Hanin L 2011 Tumor control probability in radiation treatment *Med. Phys.* **38** 574–83

[124] Marks L B *et al* 2010 Use of normal tissue complication probability models in the clinic *Int. J. Radiat. Oncol. Biol. Phys.* **76** S10–9

[125] Marks L B, Ten Haken R K and Martel M K 2010 Guest ed's introduction to QUANTEC: a users guide *Int. J. Radiat. Oncol. Biol. Phys.* **76** S1–2

[126] Richardson L A and Jones G W 2009 A review of the reliability and validity of the Edmonton Symptom Assessment System *Curr. Oncol.* **16** 53–64

[127] Chang V T, Hwang S S and Feuerman M 2000 Validation of the Edmonton Symptom Assessment Scale *Cancer* **88** 2164–71

[128] Goyal U D *et al* 2020 Prospective study of use of edmonton symptom assessment scale versus routine symptom management during weekly radiation treatment visits *JCO Oncol. Pract.* **16** e1029–35

[129] Youssef I, Hoogland A I, Chahoud J, Spiess P E, Jim H and Johnstone P A S 2022 Patient reported outcomes in advanced penile cancer *Urol. Oncol.: Semin. Orig. Invest.* **40** 412.e9–412.e13

[130] Darko J, McKenna C B, McKnight K, Osei E and Peters C 2023 Systematic self-reporting of patients' symptoms: improving oncologic care and patients' satisfaction *J. Radiother. Pract.* **22** e55

[131] Palm R F, Jim H S L, Boulware D, Johnstone P A S and Naghavi A O 2020 Using the revised Edmonton Symptom Assessment Scale during neoadjuvant radiotherapy for retroperitoneal sarcoma *Clin. Transl. Radiat. Oncol.* **22** 22–8

[132] Savla B, Venkat P and Yu M 2016 Effect of Edmonton Symptom Assessment Scale (ESAS) on symptom data collection in a radiation oncology department *J. Clin. Oncol.* **34** 83

[133] Wong E *et al* 2016 Correlating symptoms and their changes with survival in patients with brain metastases *Ann. Palliat. Med.* **5** 253–66

[134] Barbera L *et al* 2020 The impact of routine Edmonton Symptom Assessment System (ESAS) use on overall survival in cancer patients: results of a population-based retrospective matched cohort analysis *Cancer Med.* **9** 7107–15

[135] Turner K *et al* 2022 Longitudinal patient-reported outcomes and survival among early-stage non-small cell lung cancer patients receiving stereotactic body radiotherapy *Radiother. Oncol.* **167** 116–21

[136] El Naqa I *et al* 2006 Multivariable modeling of radiotherapy outcomes, including dose-volume and clinical factors *Int. J. Radiat. Oncol. Biol. Phys.* **64** 1275–86

[137] Liu Y, Xu C, Xing C and Chen M 2022 Influencing factors and prediction methods of radiotherapy and chemotherapy in patients with lung cancer based on logistic regression analysis *Sci. Rep.* **12** 21094

[138] Deist T M *et al* 2018 Machine learning algorithms for outcome prediction in (chemo) radiotherapy: an empirical comparison of classifiers *Med. Phys.* **45** 3449–59

[139] Klement R J *et al* 2014 Support vector machine-based prediction of local tumor control after stereotactic body radiation therapy for earlystage non-small cell lung cancer *Int. J. Radiat. Oncol. Biol. Phys.* **88** 732–8

[140] Nam K *et al* 2022 Development of a support vector machine-based tool for survival prediction after stereotactic body radiotherapy for liver metastases using multi-institutional data *Int. J. Radiat. Oncol. Biol. Phys.* **114** e122

[141] Akcay M, Etiz D, Celik O and Ozen A 2020 Evaluation of prognosis in nasopharyngeal cancer using machine learning *Technol. Cancer Res. Treat.* **19** 1533033820909829

[142] Gennatas E D *et al* 2018 Preoperative and postoperative prediction of long-term meningioma outcomes *PLoS One* **13** e0204161

[143] Valdes G, Solberg T D, Heskel M, Ungar L and Simone C B 2016 Using machine learning to predict radiation pneumonitis in patients with stage I non-small cell lung cancer treated with stereotactic body radiation therapy *Phys. Med. Biol.* **61** 6105

[144] Ospina J D *et al* 2014 Random forests to predict rectal toxicity following prostate cancer radiation therapy *Int. J. Radiat. Oncol. Biol. Phys.* **89** 1024–31

[145] Valdes G *et al* 2018 Salvage HDR brachytherapy: multiple hypothesis testing versus machine learning analysis *Int. J. Radiat. Oncol. Biol. Phys.* **101** 694–703

[146] Soares I, Dias J, Rocha H, Khouri L, do Carmo Lopes M and Ferreira B 2018 Predicting xerostomia after IMRT treatments: a data mining approach *Health Technol.* **8** 159–68

[147] Natekin A and Knoll A 2013 Gradient boosting machines, a tutorial *Front. Neurorobot.* **7** 21

[148] Guan X *et al* 2023 Construction of the XGBoost model for early lung cancer prediction based on metabolic indices *BMC Med. Inform. Decis. Mak.* **23** 107

[149] Liu W, Wang S, Ye Z, Xu P, Xia X and Guo M 2022 Prediction of lung metastases in thyroid cancer using machine learning based on SEER database *Cancer Med.* **11** 2503–15

[150] Hage Chehade A, Abdallah N, Marion J-M, Oueidat M and Chauvet P 2022 Lung and colon cancer classification using medical imaging: a feature engineering approach *Phys. Eng. Sci. Med.* **45** 729–46

[151] Dudas D, Saghad P G, Dilling T J, Perez B A, Rosenberg S A and Naqa I E 2024 Deep learning-guided dosimetry for mitigating local failure of non-small cell lung cancer patients receiving SBRT *Int. J. Radiat. Oncol. Biol. Phys.* **119** 990–1000

[152] Cui S, Luo Y, Tseng H-H, Ten Haken R K and El Naqa I 2019 Combining handcrafted features with latent variables in machine learning for prediction of radiation-induced lung damage *Med. Phys.* **46** 2497–511

[153] Huang Y *et al* 2023 Deep learning prediction model for patient durvival outcomes in palliative care using actigraphy data and clinical information *Cancers* **15** 2232

[154] Jalalifar S A, Soliman H, Sahgal A and Sadeghi-Naini A 2022 Predicting the outcome of radiotherapy in brain metastasis by integrating the clinical and MRI-based deep learning features *Med. Phys.* **49** 7167–78

[155] Chen M, Wang K and Wang J 2024 Vision transformer-based multilabel survival prediction for oropharynx cancer after radiation therapy *Int. J. Radiat. Oncol. Biol. Phys.* **118** 1123–34

[156] Fink M A *et al* 2022 Deep learning-based assessment of oncologic outcomes from natural language processing of structured radiology reports *Radiol. Artif. Intell.* **4** e220055

[157] Zhang K 2021 On mode collapse in generative adversarial networks *Artificial Neural Networks and Machine Learning—ICANN 2021* ed I Farkaš, P Masulli, S Otte and S Wermter (Cham: Springer International) pp 563–74

[158] Dhariwal P and Nichol A 2021 Diffusion models beat GANs on image synthesis *Proc. 35th Int. Conf. on Neural Information Processing Systems* pp 8780–94

[159] Dudas D, Dilling T J and El Naqa I 2024 Improved outcome models with denoising diffusion *Phys. Med.* **119** 103307

[160] Collins G S, Reitsma J B, Altman D G and Moons K G M 2015 Transparent reporting of a multivariable prediction model for individual prognosis or diagnosis (TRIPOD): the TRIPOD Statement *BMC Med.* **13** 1

[161] Fuhrman J D, Gorre N, Hu Q, Li H, El Naqa I and Giger M L 2022 A review of explainable and interpretable AI with applications in COVID-19 imaging *Med. Phys.* **49** 1–14

[162] Ribeiro M T, Singh S and Guestrin C 2016 Why should I trust you?' Explaining the predictions of any classifier *Proc. of the 22nd ACM SIGKDD Int. Conf. on Knowledge Discovery and Data Mining* pp 1135–44

[163] Lundberg S M and Lee S-I 2017 A unified approach to interpreting model predictions *Proc. 31st Int. Conf. on Neural Information Processing SystemsPages* pp 4768–77

[164] Selvaraju R R, Cogswell M, Das A, Vedantam R, Parikh D and Batra D 2017 Grad-cam: Visual explanations from deep networks via gradient-based localization *Proc. of the IEEE Int. Conf. on Computer Vision* pp 618–26

[165] Saednia K *et al* 2020 Quantitative thermal imaging biomarkers to detect acute skin toxicity from breast radiation therapy using supervised machine learning *Int. J. Radiat. Oncol. Biol. Phys.* **106** 1071–83

[166] Diamant A, Chatterjee A, Vallières M, Shenouda G and Seuntjens J 2019 Deep learning in head and neck cancer outcome prediction *Sci. Rep.* **9** 2764

[167] Nayan M *et al* 2022 A machine learning approach to predict progression on active surveillance for prostate cancer *Urol. Oncol. Semin. Ori. Investig.* **40** 161.e1–7

[168] Wei L *et al* 2021 A deep survival interpretable radiomics model of hepatocellular carcinoma patients *Phys. Med. Eur. J. Med. Phys.* **82** 295–305

[169] Katzman J L, Shaham U, Cloninger A, Bates J, Jiang T and Kluger Y 2018 DeepSurv: personalized treatment recommender system using a Cox proportional hazards deep neural network *BMC Med. Res. Methodol.* **18** 24

[170] Yan D, Vicini F, Wong J and Martinez A 1997 Adaptive radiation therapy *Phys. Med. Biol.* **42** 123

[171] Tseng H-H, Luo Y, Ten Haken R K and El Naqa I 2018 The role of machine learning in knowledge-based response-adapted radiotherapy *Front. Oncol.* **8** 266

[172] Tseng H-H, Ten Haken R K and El Naqa I 2022 Smart adaptive treatment strategies *Machine and Deep Learning in Oncology, Medical Physics and Radiology* ed I El Naqa and M J Murphy (Cham: Springer International) pp 439–52

[173] Ger R B, Wei L, El Naqa I and Wang J 2023 The promise and future of radiomics for personalized radiotherapy dosing and adaptation *Semin. Radiat. Oncol.* **33** 252–61

[174] Niraula D, Jamaluddin J, Matuszak M M, Haken R K T and El Naqa I 2021 Quantum deep reinforcement learning for clinical decision support in oncology: application to adaptive radiotherapy *Sci. Rep.* **11** 23545

[175] Niraula D *et al* 2023 A clinical decision support system for AI-assisted decision-making in response-adaptive radiotherapy (ARCliDS) *Sci. Rep.* **13** 5279

[176] Sun W *et al* 2022 Precision radiotherapy via information integration of expert human knowledge and AI recommendation to optimize clinical decision making *Comput. Methods Prog. Biomed.* **221** 106927

[177] Tseng H-H, Luo Y, Cui S, Chien J-T, Ten Haken R K and El Naqa I 2017 Deep reinforcement learning for automated radiation adaptation in lung cancer *Med. Phys.* **44** 6690–705

[178] Luo Y *et al* 2018 A multiobjective Bayesian networks approach for joint prediction of tumor local control and radiation pneumonitis in nonsmall-cell lung cancer (NSCLC) for response-adapted radiotherapy *Med. Phys.* **45** 3980–95

[179] Barto A G and Sutton R S 1998 *Reinforcement Learning: An Introduction (Adaptive Computation and Machine Learning)* (Cambridge, MA: MIT Press)

[180] Green O L, Henke L E and Hugo G D 2019 Practical clinical workflows for online and offline adaptive radiation therapy *Semin. Radiat. Oncol.* **29** 219–27

[181] Yu T *et al* 2019 Pretreatment prediction of adaptive radiation therapy eligibility using MRI-based radiomics for advanced nasopharyngeal carcinoma patients *Front. Oncol.* **9** 1050

[182] Lam S-K *et al* 2022 Multi-organ omics-based prediction for adaptive radiation therapy eligibility in nasopharyngeal carcinoma patients undergoing concurrent chemoradiotherapy *Front. Oncol.* **11** 792024

[183] Zhang R, Cai Z, Luo Y, Wang Z and Wang W 2022 Preliminary exploration of response the course of radiotherapy for stage III non-small cell lung cancer based on longitudinal CT radiomics features *Eur. J. Radiol. Open* **9** 100391

[184] Forouzannezhad P *et al* 2022 Multitask learning radiomics on longitudinal imaging to predict survival outcomes following risk-adaptive chemoradiation for non-small cell lung cancer *Cancers* **14** 1228

[185] Lou B *et al* 2019 An image-based deep learning framework for individualising radiotherapy dose: a retrospective analysis of outcome prediction *Lancet Digit. Health* **1** e136–47

[186] Mierzwa M L *et al* 2022 Randomized phase II study of physiologic MRI-directed adaptive radiation boost in poor prognosis head and neck cancer *Clin. Cancer Res.* **28** 5049–57

[187] Kong F-M *et al* 2017 Effect of midtreatment PET/CT-adapted radiation therapy with concurrent chemotherapy in patients with locally advanced non-small-cell lung cancer: a phase 2 clinical trial *JAMA Oncol.* **3** 1358–65

[188] Gameng H A, Gerardo B B and Medina R P 2019 Modified adaptive synthetic SMOTE to improve classification performance in imbalanced datasets *2019 IEEE 6th Int. Conf. on Engineering Technologies and Applied Sciences (ICETAS)* pp 1–5

[189] Sharma A, Singh P K and Chandra R 2022 SMOTified-GAN for class imbalanced pattern classification problems *IEEE Access* **10** 30655–65

[190] Chawla N V, Bowyer K W, Hall L O and Kegelmeyer W P 2002 SMOTE: synthetic minority over-sampling technique *J. Artif. Intell. Res.* **16** 321–57

[191] Dablain D, Krawczyk B and Chawla N V 2023 DeepSMOTE: fusing deep learning and SMOTE for imbalanced data *IEEE Trans. Neural Netw. Learn. Syst.* **34** 6390–404

[192] He H, Bai Y, Garcia E A and Li S 2008 ADASYN: adaptive synthetic sampling approach for imbalanced learning *2008 IEEE Int. Joint Conf. on Neural Networks (IEEE World Congress on Computational Intelligence)* (Piscataway, NJ: IEEE) pp 1322–8

[193] El Naqa I 2021 Prospective clinical deployment of machine learning in radiation oncology *Nat. Rev. Clin. Oncol.* **18** 605–6

Chapter 14

Challenges of artificial intelligence implementation in adaptive radiation therapy

Yi Wang and X. Sharon Qi

The integration of artificial intelligence (AI) into adaptive radiation therapy (ART) holds immense promise for revolutionizing radiation therapy [1]. While the prior chapters in this volume have thoroughly explored the use of AI in each step of the ART workflow, this chapter carefully examines the multifaceted challenges accompanying the research, development, and clinical implementation of AI in ART. Starting with a brief overview of the current landscape of AI-driven ART, the chapter will discuss the challenges in various dimensions, including data, technical, operational, ethical, regulatory, and financial [2, 3]. Developing reliable AI models in clinical practice faces data-related challenges, such as limited availability, privacy concerns, and imbalanced datasets. On the technical front, selecting optimal architectures, managing transfer learning, estimating uncertainties, and ensuring real-time performance add layers of complexity. Equally important is the human factor—building clinician trust in AI recommendations, enhancing interpretability, and training clinicians for AI collaboration demand careful attention. Additionally, rigorous validation and evaluation processes, coupled with navigating regulatory pathways, further complicate AI implementation. This chapter underscores the critical need for model robustness, well-defined performance metrics, and strict adherence to regulatory frameworks to facilitate seamless clinical adoption.

14.1 Overview of challenges in AI-driven ART

ART was first introduced as a closed-loop radiation treatment process that involves modifying the initial treatment plan through systematic feedback from frequent imaging acquisition, typically done on a daily basis [4]. The concept of ART has evolved and emerged as a transformative approach in cancer treatment, allowing for adjustments to treatment plans based on patient-specific anatomic, biological, and/or functional changes during radiation therapy [1, 2]. ART, particularly the online

doi:10.1088/978-0-7503-6119-4ch14

14-1

version, has been widely implemented using various online image-guided radiation therapy (IGRT) modalities, including computed tomography (CT) on-rail [5], cone-beam CT (CBCT) [6], magnetic resonance imaging (MRI) [7], and positron emission tomography (PET) [8]. These highly personalized approaches hold immense promise for improving patient outcomes and minimizing side effects. As described in prior chapters, the current landscape of AI in ART presents exciting possibilities [1, 3]. AI algorithms are already demonstrating their power in various aspects of treatment, from enhancing tumor segmentation and dose prediction to optimizing treatment planning and assessing treatment response [1]. These advancements are driven by the ability of AI to analyze vast amounts of medical data, including imaging, dosimetry, and clinical records, to uncover hidden patterns and relationships that would elude human analysis. However, integrating cutting-edge AI technologies into this complex clinical workflow presents a multifaceted array of challenges that need to be addressed before its full potential can be realized [9].

The path towards seamless AI integration in ART is paved with numerous hurdles, which can be broadly be categorized into several key domains: data, technical, operational, ethical, regulatory, and legal [1]. Moreover, online and real-time ART workflows induce additional challenges. In the following sections, each of these challenges will be discussed in detail, with potential solutions explored. This comprehensive review aims to facilitate safe implementation and smooth operation of AI-ART, fulfilling its full potential to provide personalized radiation therapy.

14.2 Data challenges

One of the most substantial challenges on the path to AI-driven ART is data. This section examines three key data obstacles on the development of robust AI models for ART: data availability, quality, and privacy.

14.2.1 Data availability

While offline ART has many similarities with initial treatment planning, online and real-time ART face additional challenges in data collection due to their unique clinical workflow. Many current ART systems (e.g. Ethos by Varian Medical Systems, Palo Alto, CA) operate as closed-loop environments, tightly integrating data acquisition with adaptive treatment delivery [10]. This can make it difficult for researchers and developers to access the raw data needed for AI training and validation. The data may be locked within proprietary formats or require specific permissions and authorization procedures. While the vendors and their authorized researchers could gain access to the ART imaging and planning data, the obstacles for independent researchers and developers to access these data could slow down AI innovation in ART.

Despite the wide availability of the various ART platforms, e.g. the CBCT-based Varian Ethos system [11], MRI-based ViewRay system [12], and Elekta Unity system [13], the percentage of patients receiving ART treatment remains small and the utilization of ART is limited to a few disease sites and protocols (e.g. gastrointestinal tumors which are subject to daily variation of stomach and bowel fillings, stereotactic body radiation therapy in which a large dose of radiation is delivered in few fractions, and head and neck cancers which can grow or shrink during the treatment course) [14–16]. Due to the lack of proper data, such as labeled target and organs on fractional images (e.g. CBCT), specifically trained and evaluated AI models are generally lacking or inaccurate for clinical ART applications. Despite the efforts of bridging the two modalities with pseudo-CT to enable the use of the CT-based segmentation model, the difference in imaging modality and image quality adds additional uncertainty that may reduce the benefit of online adaptation [17]. With further expansion of ART, more accurate AI models could be trained on intrinsic ART data, eliminating the cross-modality uncertainty.

14.2.2 Data quality

Robust AI models rely on high-quality data. Building reliable and effective AI models requires a robust foundation of accurate, balanced, diverse, and well-annotated data [18]. However, in the context of ART, this presents unique challenges that impede the progress and effectiveness of AI implementation. ART generates a dynamic stream of data, including imaging (e.g. CBCT), segmentation, and dosimetry. The quality of these data might be inferior to those acquired for initial simulation and planning [16]. The quality of the online images (e.g. CBCT) which are used for adaptive re-planning often does not match that of the initial simulation images (e.g. simulation CT), with the exception of the less-common, space-extensive CT-on-rail system [19]. The time that the radiation oncologist or ART team members spend on reviewing and editing the online contours is often much shorter than what they spend during initial planning [20]. In some cases, the online contours may be reviewed and edited by non-physician team members. Finally, online ART requires a quick turn-around, and the capacity of the optimizer of the online planning system (e.g. Varian Ethos) might not match that of its counterpart for initial planning (e.g. Varian Eclipse) [21].

When developing AI models using data acquired in initial simulation and treatment planning, it is generally possible to assemble a large and diverse dataset while avoiding reliance on multiple datasets from the same patient. In contrast, data acquired during online ART are far more limited, with models often trained on fewer patients but multiple datasets from each adaptive fraction. As a result, AI models trained by ART data are less likely to cover the broad diversity of patient characters, such as the size, shape, and location of the tumor, as well as the patient's body size, gender, and race—factors that can affect the patient's normal anatomy [21].

14.2.3 Data privacy

The integration of AI technologies into ART presents substantial data privacy challenges, requiring robust measures to safeguard sensitive patient information and maintain trust. AI tools rely on extensive patient data—such as medical histories, imaging studies, treatment plans, and outcomes—exposing this information to risks such as unauthorized access, data breaches, and misuse [22]. Ensuring data protection is paramount, demanding strict encryption methods, access controls, and AI systems designed with inherent security measures to prevent cyberattacks and ensure data integrity. Regular security updates address emerging vulnerabilities. While anonymizing data for AI applications is crucial, risks of re-identification persist, particularly when anonymized datasets are merged with public information. Enhancing and validating anonymization techniques are essential for reducing identification risks and complying with privacy regulations. Data sharing across institutions, often required for AI model development, raises concerns about patient consent and ethical compliance [18]. Transparent policies must be implemented to inform patients about data usage, sharing, and protection, while explicit consent fosters trust and fulfills legal and ethical obligations. Collaborations with external vendors necessitate stringent data protection agreements and oversight, ensuring adherence to high standards of privacy and security. Comprehensive vendor management policies mitigate the risks associated with third-party involvement, promoting consistent data protection practices.

14.3 Technical challenges

Beyond the data-related hurdles, this section will explore the technical challenges associated with AI models used for ART, such as model accuracy, efficiency, robustness, generalizability, explainability, interpretability, and computation speed.

14.3.1 Model accuracy and efficiency

Choosing the right AI model for a specific ART application is critical for the success of this highly demanding technology [23]. While computation time is not usually critical for AI applications in initial simulation and treatment planning, it becomes mission-critical in online ART when the patient is on the treatment couch and in real-time ART when multiple dynamic components of the treatment delivery system are moving simultaneously. Each AI algorithm has its strengths and limitations in different aspects such as efficiency, accuracy, robustness, and interpretability. For online ART applications, AI models need to be highly efficient to minimize the time between imaging and treatment. The longer the wait time, the more patient motion occurs, reducing the benefits of adaptation. Conversely, since the ART team works under significant time pressure, the AI models need to be highly robust to produce reliable results, reducing the chance of human error or the need for compromise. A prime example is dose prediction. In initial planning, it is generally acceptable for the AI algorithm to complete dose prediction and plan optimization in 10–30 min, as the treatment planner can multitask. However, the same process needs to be completed in a few minutes in online ART and almost in real time in real-time ART [20]. Additionally, in initial planning, the treatment planner, typically a medical dosimetrist or physicist, has more time to identify, analyze, and trouble-shoot any dose discrepancies. In online ART, however, the treatment planner, often a medical dosimetrist or radiation physicist, is under significant time pressure, leaving less time to create and evaluate the adaptive plan [1]. This constraint can potentially compromise plan quality. Online ART follows a different treatment planning workflow than the initial treatment plan, and it is desirable to have specialized AI models to address specific challenges. Ideal solutions should optimize both accuracy and efficiency to facilitate the time-critical decision-making processes, such as contouring and adaptive re-planning [3].

14.3.2 Model robustness and generalizability

Robustness refers to an AI model's ability to maintain its performance and accuracy when subjected to variations in input data or operating conditions [24]. In ART, robustness is paramount due to significant variability in patients under treatment. Factors such as differences in anatomy, tumor characteristics, imaging protocols (e.g. kVp and mA settings in CBCT), equipment, and treatment protocols can all impact AI model performance. A robust AI system in ART must be resilient to these variations and capable of producing consistent results. Achieving robustness requires thorough testing and validation of AI models using diverse datasets encompassing a wide range of patient demographics, imaging techniques, and clinical scenarios. This process helps identify potential weaknesses and refine the models to enhance their resilience.

Generalizability is the ability of an AI model to apply its learned knowledge and perform well on new, unseen data [25]. For ART, this means that an AI system trained on a specific dataset should generalize its predictions and recommendations to patients and clinical settings not included in the initial training data. One of the primary challenges in achieving generalizability is ensuring that the training data are representative of the broader patient population and clinical practices. If the training data are biased or limited to a specific subset of patients or conditions, the AI model may fail to generalize effectively, leading to inaccurate predictions and suboptimal treatment recommendations for patients who differ from the training cohort [18]. To enhance generalizability, AI models must be developed using diverse and representative datasets. Collaboration between multiple institutions and clinical sites can help aggregate data from various sources, ensuring a more comprehensive training dataset. Additionally, techniques such as transfer learning, which involves fine-tuning pre-trained models on new data, can improve the generalizability of AI systems.

Robustness and generalizability are essential for the clinical success of AI in ART. Achieving these attributes requires addressing challenges such as variability in imaging protocols (e.g. kVp and mAs) and equipment (e.g. imagers), as well as differences in patient populations (e.g. age, gender, weight, and medical history). The continuous evolution of medical practices and technologies further necessitates regular updates and validation of AI models. Key strategies to overcome these hurdles include standardizing data collection and preprocessing protocols, diversifying training datasets, and leveraging advanced machine learning techniques to enhance adaptability [25]. Rigorous validation across multiple clinical sites is vital to identify and mitigate limitations, while clinician feedback and expert oversight throughout development ensure that AI models meet the required standards. Ensuring consistent performance across diverse conditions and generalization to new data are critical for reliable ART delivery [18].

14.3.3 Model explainability and interpretability

Explainability refers to the extent to which the internal workings of an AI model can be understood by humans. It involves making the decision-making process of the model transparent so that clinicians can comprehend why a particular recommendation or prediction is made. This is crucial for building trust, as clinicians need to be confident in the AI's outputs to rely on them in critical clinical settings [25].

Interpretability, on the other hand, is the degree to which a human can understand the cause of a decision. It focuses on the clarity with which the AI's predictions can be presented and explained, making it easier for clinicians to grasp the reasoning behind the AI model's outputs. In the context of ART, especially in time-sensitive situations, interpretability ensures that clinicians can quickly and accurately interpret AI recommendations to make informed treatment decisions [25, 26].

Many advanced AI algorithms, such as deep learning neural networks (DLNNs), involve numerous layers and parameters. They often operate as black boxes, where the internal decision-making processes are not readily understandable even to experts. This makes it difficult to trace how specific inputs lead to particular outputs. The lack of clear insights into how AI models arrive at their conclusions can hinder the ART team's ability to understand and trust the AI model's recommendations. Additionally, if the model's outputs are not easily interpretable, there is a risk of misinterpreting the recommendations, potentially leading to errors in treatment decisions. Several strategies can be employed to address these challenges. Designing user-friendly interfaces that present AI outputs in an intuitive manner can facilitate quick interpretation. Interfaces that highlight key information and offer clear, concise explanations enhance the clinicians' ability to make informed decisions efficiently. Implementing visualization tools that graphically represent the AI model's reasoning can help make the internal workings more transparent. Ongoing training and education on how to interpret and utilize AI outputs effectively are also essential for users to understand why specific decisions were made. Finally, collaborative efforts between AI developers and model users can help improve performance, enhance transparency, and promote trustworthiness [27].

14.3.4 Computational efficiency

The unique demands of ART, particularly in online and real-time settings, require AI systems that deliver fast and accurate results without compromising performance [28]. In online ART, where adaptive re-planning occurs while the patient remains on the treatment couch, computation delays can increase patient motion risks and reduce ART's effectiveness. Real-time ART, involving continuous adaptation during treatment delivery, demands even greater computational efficiency, as AI models must provide immediate feedback to dynamic treatment components.

The complexity of AI models, with numerous layers and parameters, often limits computational efficiency. Additionally, processing high-resolution imaging data and performing online plan optimizations are computationally intensive, necessitating significant hardware resources. Seamless integration with existing medical devices and systems, as well as efficient data transfer pipelines, are essential to minimize delays and ensure real-time performance. Optimizing AI algorithms, utilizing specialized hardware, and streamlining clinical workflows are critical to achieving the processing speeds required for online and real-time ART. Addressing these challenges enables AI systems to deliver timely and accurate treatment adaptations, unlocking ART's full potential to improve treatment outcomes [18].

14.4 Challenges associated with online and real-time workflows

The primary benefit of online ART is its ability to optimize the dose distribution based on inter-fractional variations such as daily changes in anatomy, biology, or function. In real-time ART, dose distributions can be dynamically adjusted to account for intra-fractional motion. However, both online and real-time ART workflows introduce new uncertainties that may negate some of their intrinsic advantages. This section explores the uncertainties arising from AI tools in these workflows.

14.4.1 Image quality

CBCT is the most common imaging modality used for online ART, as exemplified by the Ethos system from Varian Medical Systems. However, the image quality of CBCT is often inferior to that of simulation CT, posing significant challenges for accurate contouring and dose calculations. To overcome these challenges, systems such as Ethos utilize synthetic CT (sCT) images generated from CBCT data. This approach allows deep learning (DL)-based deformable image registration (DIR) and auto-segmentation models to generate autocontours on the sCT images. Despite these advancements, synthetic CT cannot fully recover the lost contrast resolution inherent in CBCT images, leading to inaccuracies in Hounsfield unit (HU) values that may compromise the accuracy of online dose calculations. Additionally, current sCT generation algorithms have limited capability in reducing the artifacts present in the original CBCT images, such as metal artifacts or motion artifacts [29]. These artifacts can propagate into the sCT images, affecting the quality of adaptive re-planning. To fully realize the benefits of online ART, further research into hardware improvements, advanced image reconstruction techniques, and artifact reduction methods is necessary to enhance sCT image quality [30].

In MRI-based online ART, the superior soft tissue contrast of MRI allows for more accurate contouring of tumors and organs compared to CT- or CBCT-guided ART [7]. DL algorithms may struggle with regions that exhibit very low signal intensities on MRI. For example, cortical bones have very low signal on MRI but relatively high attenuation on CT, while metal implants may be invisible on MRI but produce high attenuation and artifacts on CT. These discrepancies can lead to mischaracterization of such regions during pseudo CT generation, causing uncertainty in HU values and subsequently affecting the accuracy of dose calculations.

Addressing these challenges necessitates the development of more sophisticated DL models and training strategies capable of accurately representing these problematic areas. Moreover, most MR simulators operate at high magnetic fields of 1.5 tesla (T) or 3 T, such as SIGNA (GE Healthcare), MAGNETOM (Siemens Healthineers), and Ingenia (Philips). While available online MR systems also operate at 1.5 T (Unity from Elekta) [13], others function at much lower field strengths, such as the 0.35 T system (ViewRay from ViewRay Inc.) [12]. Due to the limited availability of low-field MR data, DL-based auto-segmentation algorithms are often trained on pre-treatment MRI acquired from high-field MR scanners. The inconsistency between the training data (high-field strength) and the application (low-field strength) can increase contouring uncertainty, hindering the full benefits for online ART. Addressing this challenge requires either collecting low-field MR data for training or developing DL models that are robust to variations in field strength.

14.4.2 Dose calculation

The use of AI, including machine learning (ML) and deep learning (DL), for dose calculation in ART faces several challenges. One major issue is the computational complexity of these ML and DL algorithms, which needs to conduct pixel-wise dose prediction constrained by dose–volume histogram (DVH) requirements, within tight time limits to enable online adaptation [31]. Variability in imaging protocols and equipment across clinical settings can introduce inconsistencies in input data, affecting the accuracy of dose predictions. Moreover, the diversity in patient anatomy and tumor characteristics requires these models to generalize effectively across different cases, which can be difficult without extensive and diverse training datasets. Furthermore, ensuring the robustness against noise and artifacts in imaging data is another critical challenge, as these factors can compromise dose calculation accuracy. Additionally, integration with existing clinical workflows and treatment delivery systems also poses difficulties, requiring seamless communication between AI algorithms and hardware components. Currently, non-AI-based online dose calculation approaches primarily rely on rapid re-optimization of the pre-adaptation plan (which could be the initial treatment plan or the most recent fraction's plan). For ML- or DL-based dose prediction algorithms, computation speed must be as fast as, if not faster than, the current re-optimization approaches [32]. Additional investigations are needed to find innovative methods to simplify neural network structures to improve computational efficiency, while not compromising the accuracy of pixel and DVH-based dose predictions.

14.4.3 Real-time ART

Real-time ART holds the greatest potential for treating moving tumors that can be visualized through real-time imaging, such as x-ray tracking and cine MRI [33]. In real-time ART, the plan is continuously adapted based on real-time imaging, requiring AI models to rapidly analyse new imaging data, predict future movement, and adjust the radiation beam within milliseconds. This represents a paradigm shift in cancer treatment, enabling dynamical adaptation to intra-fractional anatomical changes [3]. The highly dynamic nature of real-time ART demands AI models that can keep pace with the fast-moving components of the treatment delivery system. Compared to online ART, real-time ART requires far greater performance on AI tools, where even minor delays in image processing, motion predictions, or treatment adaptation could compromise treatment efficacy and patient outcomes. Conquering these real-time performance challenges involves not only speed but also accuracy and robustness. Significant further advancements in neural network architecture, enhanced computational efficiency, and rigorous validation are necessary to ensure the seamless and reliable integration of AI into real-time ART workflows.

14.5 Operational challenges

Integrating AI into ART is a complex undertaking that introduces several operational challenges. These challenges stem from the intricacies involved in incorporating any AI systems into clinical workflows, the requirement for extensive training and education for healthcare professionals, and the necessity to maintain a seamless operation within a high-stakes clinical environment.

14.5.1 Clinical validation

The clinical validation of AI models for ART poses significant challenges, primarily due to the lack of standardized evaluation metrics and criteria [34]. Unlike traditional medical devices and software, AI models require rigorous validation to ensure their safety, efficacy, and reliability. In ART, where online and real-time decisions can directly impact patient outcomes, the stakes are particularly high. The lack of standardization complicates the process of model evaluation across different disease sites, clinical settings, and patient populations. This variability can lead to inconsistencies in evaluation results, making it difficult to determine an AI model's true clinical utility. Moreover, the dynamic nature of ART, which involves continuous adaptation to patient-specific changes (e.g. patient anatomy and tumor characteristics), necessitates that AI models undergo extensive testing in diverse and evolving scenarios. For example, an auto-segmentation model for online ART treating bladder cancer will need to manage varying levels of bladder fillings [2].

To address these challenges, establishing standardized evaluation metrics and criteria is essential. Collaborative efforts involving government agencies (e.g. the US FDA, NIH, NCI), professional societies (e.g. AAPM and ASTRO), clinical users, research investigators, and industrial vendors are essential to establish standardized qualitative and quantitative evaluation metrics and methods [25, 34, 35]. Additionally, creating and sharing large, annotated datasets representative of diverse patient populations can improve the robustness and generalizability of AI models. Implementing rigorous testing protocols that simulate real-world clinical scenarios can further enhance the reliability of AI systems in ART. The streamlined clinical validation process can lead to safer and more effective AI-driven ART.

14.5.2 Workflow integration

Integrating AI into ART is not as simply as adding a new tool into the existing process. Most of the current online ART platforms operate within closed-loop systems using proprietary software, allowing only vendor-approved AI models and their authorized collaborators to integrate into the clinical workflow [12, 17]. As a result, inserting any alternative or new AI tools into the closed-loop workflow is challenging, if not impossible. Data extraction from the online ART system is difficult, and even if access is granted, the data transfer between the ART platform and third-party software is time-consuming and prone to communication errors (e.g. incomplete transfer of DICOM data). This substantial limitation and the associated liability issues discourage researchers and developers from investing in independent AI tools for online ART. The challenge is even more significant for real-time ART, where immediate adjustments to treatment delivery systems are required [1].

It is also technically challenging to integrate the closed-loop online ART platform with existing clinical systems, particularly when they are provided by different vendors. Varian Ethos, as the most popular CBCT-based online ART platform, has been widely implemented in all Varian environments using the Eclipse treatment planning system (TPS) and ARIA record and verification (R&V) system [17]. Such an integration, although not yet seamless, has been thoroughly examined by the vendor during the design, manufacturing, and evaluation processes. While it has been demonstrated that the Ethos system can work with other TPSs (e.g. RayStation by RaySearch Laboratories, Stockholm, Sweden) and R&V systems (e.g. MOSAIQ by Elekta, Stockholm, Sweden), such a non-uniform integration requires special attention for data transfer, and increases the manpower and resources needed for maintenance [29].

14.5.3 Staff training

Providing ART team members with adequate training on basic concepts of AI and the specific AI tools involved in the ART workflow is an essential requirement for successful clinical implementation [36]. First, much of the current workforce in radiation therapy did not receive formal education or training in AI. The introduction of AI into clinical practice represents a significant paradigm shift, requiring the ART team members to acquire new competencies and understand complex AI-driven processes. This gap necessitates substantial investment in training programs designed to bridge the knowledge divide [37]. Effective training should encompass both theoretical understanding of AI concepts and practical skills for operating AI systems. Second, AI is a rapidly evolving field, with new algorithms, techniques, and tools emerging continuously. Practitioners must stay current with the latest advancements to utilize AI effectively and safely in ART. Continuous education is essential to ensure that practitioners are up to date with the latest developments and best practices. This need for ongoing learning requires a commitment to professional development and access to updated educational resources. Institutions and professional organizations play a critical role in facilitating continuous education, ensuring that ART professionals are equipped with the latest knowledge and best practices [38].

Developing and implementing comprehensive training and continuing education programs can be resource-intensive and time-consuming, presenting a significant barrier for individual institutions. Therefore, it is important for professional organizations (e.g. AAPM, ASTRO, and ESTRO) to offer formal AI training through regular workshops, courses, and access to current literature, and provide certificate to demonstrate competency on practicing AI in clinical settings [18]. By tackling these challenges, the ART workforce can harness the full potential of AI in ART, ultimately improving patient outcomes.

14.5.4 User experiences

Successful implementation of AI in ART requires collaboration and coordination among various stakeholders, including radiation oncologists, medical physicists, IT professionals, and administrators. Each group brings a unique perspective and set of expertise to the table, and effective communication and teamwork are essential to address the multifaceted challenges posed by AI integration. Establishing clear roles, responsibilities, and lines of communication can help facilitate smoother collaboration and ensure that all stakeholders are aligned in their goals and objectives [39].

Distinctive from many other RT technologies, ART is mostly executed in a close-looped software environment provided by the vendor of the treatment machine. In such a highly integrated system, it is impractical, if not impossible, to use any AI model trained or refined by institutional data. Despite the variations in clinical practice between different institutions (e.g. contouring, planning), all users of ART need to use the same AI model provided by the vendor [25]. Therefore, this puts additional burden on medical physicists (who often take charge of the clinical implementation of ART) to gain their fellow radiation oncologists' trust in the results provided by the vendor models. While clinicians often appreciate the efficiency gain provided by AI, they may want to maintain clinical consistency between their adaptive and non-adaptive patients. Therefore, when introducing ART, the medical physicists should provide clear guidance on how to facilitate the clinicians to achieve clinical consistency while not losing the efficiency gain [40].

14.5.5 Quality management program

Establishing robust quality assurance (QA) and monitoring processes to continuously track AI model performance, detect potential errors, and ensure ongoing safety and efficacy is essential [39]. This includes developing contingency plans for situations where AI systems fail or produce unexpected results, ensuring that clinicians can seamlessly revert to conventional treatment approaches or seek alternative decision support mechanisms.

Failure mode and effects analysis (FMEA), a systematic approach to identifying and mitigating potential failures, can play a crucial role in ensuring the safe and effective integration of AI into ART workflow. The FMEA framework is documented in the American Association of Physicists in Medicine's (AAPM) Task

Group 100 (TG-100) report [41]. FMEA can identify potential failure modes, analyze their potential impacts on patient safety and treatment outcomes, and prioritizes actions to mitigate those risks. AAPM TG-100 outlined how to develop and implement quality management programs [42]. For an AI-driven ART program, the team should optimize the allocation of resources towards preventing the most substantial risks indicated by the FMEA. Moreover, AAPM TG-100 provided important guidance on how to build effective quality management tools, such as checklists. Once properly implemented, FMEA can safeguard every step in the ART workflow in which AI plays important roles, from data collection and model development to clinical deployment and maintenance. Integration of FMEA as an organic part of AI development in ART will also help foster a culture of safety and trust among different role groups (e.g. physicians, physicists, dosimetrists, and therapists) [42].

The most common AI application in online ART is auto-segmentation of online images, typically CBCT or MR images [43]. FMEA could help identify vulnerabilities in the clinical workflow and provide insights for quality improvements. AAPM TG-275 suggested that errors in target and organ delineation ranked among the highest failure modes, as inaccurate segmentation could jeopardize tumor control and increase the risk of complications [44]. Contouring errors originating from AI-generated contours could go undetected during the planning and review process, despite the required review by physicians and physicists. This risk would become even more significant in online ART, when the clinical team is under enormous pressure to minimize the time interval between imaging and treatment. To mitigate this risk, it is crucial to develop a robust QA tool to catch such errors. Relying on human consciousness in manual checks is not enough to minimize such a risk in online ART [45]. A potential solution is implementing a secondary automated system capable of identifying discrepancies between the physician-edited primary contour and an independently generated secondary auto-contour, thereby enhancing safety and accuracy in online ART.

14.5.6 Financial challenges

ART requires more initial financial investment into hardware, software, personnel training, and other recourses. The highly complex clinical workflow also requires more manpower and treatment machine time. Consequently, each adaptive treatment session is more costly than a conventional, non-adaptive session [46]. However, as of 2025, ART is not assigned a specific Current Procedural Terminology (CPT) code by the US Center for Medicare and Medicaid Services (CMS), meaning there is no dedicated reimbursement mechanism under Medicare, and billing for this technology is considered a 'gray area' with most practices likely including the additional work within existing treatment codes. Essentially, providers are not currently receiving separate payment for the adaptive component of radiation therapy treatment.

The financial implications of AI implementation in ART cannot be overlooked, either. The integration of AI tools into ART workflow significantly reduces the time required for each session, resulting in faster treatment adaptation and potentially better clinical outcomes. Despite these operational advantages, investments in AI technologies, including hardware, software, and training, represent a significant financial commitment. The lack of clear reimbursement guidelines further complicates the financial viability of AI implementation, adding constraints on its adoption, ongoing use, and maintenance within ART workflow. Given the considerable capital and operational costs involved, healthcare institutions must carefully evaluate the cost–benefit ratio to ensure that the expected improvements in treatment precision and workflow efficiency justify the investment. Successfully implementing AI in ART requires strategic planning, securing appropriate funding, and optimizing resource allocation to sustain long-term benefits [47].

14.6 Ethical, regulatory, and legal challenges

The ethical, regulatory, and legal considerations of using AI in ART are complex and multifaceted. Addressing these challenges requires a collaborative approach involving healthcare professionals, AI vendors, professional societies, regulatory agencies, and legal experts. By fostering an environment of transparency, accountability, and innovation, the potential of AI in ART can be harnessed to improve patient outcomes while upholding ethical principles and legal standards.

14.6.1 Ethical issues

A variety of ethical issues must be carefully addressed to ensure responsible and equitable use of the AI technologies in ART. A primary ethical issue is the potential for bias within AI algorithms [48]. AI systems are trained on data that may reflect historical biases or inequities, leading to suboptimal outcomes for under-represented patient populations. For example, prostate cancer is one of the disease sites most frequently treated using ART. Black patients exhibit higher PSA levels and Gleason score > 6 compared to white patients [49]. Addressing these biases requires diligent efforts in the collection, curation, and validation of diverse datasets that accurately represent all patient demographics. Ensuring transparency in the development and deployment of AI systems is crucial to build trust and confidence among both patients and healthcare professionals.

Furthermore, maintaining human oversight on AI under significant time pressure is a unique challenge for online ART [36]. When decisions must be made rapidly, ART practitioners may feel compelled to lower their ethical standards for oversight to expedite the treatment process. This urgency can lead to insufficient scrutiny of AI-generated contours and plans, potentially resulting in errors that could have been avoided with more thorough evaluation. Furthermore, there is a risk that clinicians might favor the adaptive re-plan over the original plan due to financial incentives, even when the re-plan offers no clear clinical advantage. This raises concerns about the integrity of decision-making. Additionally, the reliance on AI systems in time-sensitive scenarios might inadvertently diminish the role of human judgment and expertise, leading to over-reliance on technology. To address these ethical challenges, it is crucial to establish robust guidelines and training programs that emphasize the importance of maintaining high ethical standards in oversight, regardless of time constraints [18]. Transparency in the financial incentives associated with treatment decisions should also be ensured to prevent conflicts of interest.

14.6.2 Regulatory and legal issues

Healthcare institutions must navigate a complex landscape of regulatory requirements related to data privacy, including the Health Insurance Portability and Accountability Act (HIPAA) in the United States, the General Data Protection Regulation (GDPR) in Europe, and other national and international regulations. Compliance with these regulations requires continuous monitoring and adaptation of data protection practices to meet evolving legal standards [25]. In the United States, AI models used in ART workflow may require model-specific approval from the US Food and Drug Administration (FDA). While it is the vendor's responsibility to obtain initial 510(k) clearance and maintain continuing compliance, it is the medical physicist's responsibility to verify the approval and compliance, particularly when preparing for initial commissioning and major model or software upgrades. Moreover, the medical physicists need to establish a quality management program to ensure that the local use of the AI models follows the regulatory approval and vendor recommendation. Any customized use of the integrated AI tools should undergo through evaluation in consultation with the vendor. The use of third-party or research AI tools without approval from the primary vendor may not only pose significant clinical risks, but also jeopardize regulatory compliance. Similarly, research that seeks to alter the standard workflow of the AI solutions also needs to be designed and applied with great caution.

The deployment of AI in ART raises several legal concerns that must be addressed to mitigate risks and ensure compliance with applicable laws and regulations [50]. One prominent legal issue is liability in the event of errors or adverse outcomes. Determining liability can be complex when AI systems are involved in clinical decision-making. Legal frameworks must clarify the responsibilities and accountability of various stakeholders, including AI developers, healthcare providers, and institutions. Establishing clear guidelines for the documentation and reporting of AI-driven decisions is essential to facilitate transparency and accountability in clinical practice. Additionally, legal considerations extend to data protection and privacy laws that govern the collection, storage, and use of patient data in AI systems. Legal frameworks must also address cross-border data transfers and international collaborations, providing guidelines for the secure and compliant exchange of data in a global healthcare landscape.

14.7 Summary

In conclusion, the journey towards the effective implementation of AI in ART is marked by challenges spanning the data, technical, operational, as well as ethical, regulatory, and legal domains. Overcoming these challenges requires a multi-disciplinary approach with strong collaboration among healthcare providers, data scientists, AI vendors, professional societies, and regulatory bodies. As technologies continue to evolve, the synergy between AI and ART is poised to revolutionize radiation therapy paradigms, offering more precise, effective, and personalized cancer care.

References

[1] Wang Y *et al* 2022 Artificial intelligence in adaptive radiation therapy *Artificial Intelligence in Radiation Therapy* (Bristol: IOP Publishing) pp 7-1–20

[2] Dona Lemus O M *et al* 2024 Adaptive radiotherapy: next-generation radiotherapy *Cancers* **16** 1206

[3] Brock K K 2019 Adaptive radiotherapy: moving into the future *Semin. Radiat. Oncol.* **29** 181–4

[4] Yan D *et al* 1997 Adaptive radiation therapy *Phys. Med. Biol.* **42** 123–32

[5] Li X *et al* 2013 A fully automated method for CT-on-rails-guided online adaptive planning for prostate cancer intensity modulated radiation therapy *Int. J. Radiat. Oncol. Biol. Phys.* **86** 835–41

[6] Liu H *et al* 2023 Review of cone beam computed tomography based online adaptive radiotherapy: current trend and future direction *Radiat. Oncol.* **18** 144

[7] Benitez C M *et al* 2024 MRI-guided adaptive radiation therapy *Semin. Radiat. Oncol.* **34** 84–91

[8] Shenker R *et al* 2023 Adaptive positron emission tomography radiation therapy in patients with locally advanced vulvar cancer: a prospective study *Adv. Radiat. Oncol.* **8** 101208

[9] Fu Y *et al* 2022 Artificial intelligence in radiation therapy *IEEE Trans. Radiat. Plas. Med. Sci.* **6** 158–81

[10] Kisling K *et al* 2022 Clinical commissioning of an adaptive radiotherapy platform: results and recommendations *J. Appl. Clin. Med. Phys.* **23** e13801

[11] van de Schoot A J *et al* 2023 Characterization of Ethos therapy systems for adaptive radiation therapy: a multi-machine comparison *J. Appl. Clin. Med. Phys.* **24** e13905

[12] Mutic S and Dempsey J F 2014 The ViewRay system: magnetic resonance-guided and controlled radiotherapy *Semin. Radiat. Oncol.* **24** 196–9

[13] Gupta A *et al* 2022 Online adaptive radiotherapy for head and neck cancers on the MR linear accelerator: introducing a novel modified adapt-to-shape approach *Clin. Transl. Radiat. Oncol.* **32** 48–51

[14] Glide-Hurst C K *et al* 2021 Adaptive radiation therapy (ART) strategies and technical considerations: a state of the ART review from NRG oncology *Int. J. Radiat. Oncol. Biol. Phys.* **109** 1054–75

[15] Kibrom A Z and Knight K A 2015 Adaptive radiation therapy for bladder cancer: a review of adaptive techniques used in clinical practice *J. Med. Radiat. Sci.* **62** 277–85

[16] Lavrova E *et al* 2023 Adaptive radiation therapy: a review of CT-based techniques *Radiol. Imaging Cancer* **5** e230011

[17] Byrne M *et al* 2022 Varian Ethos online adaptive radiotherapy for prostate cancer: early results of contouring accuracy, treatment plan quality, and treatment time *J. Appl. Clin. Med. Phys.* **23** e13479

[18] Landry G, Kurz C and Traverso A 2023 The role of artificial intelligence in radiotherapy clinical practice *BJR Open* **5** 20230030

[19] Nesteruk K P *et al* 2021 CT-on-rails versus in-room CBCT for online daily adaptive proton therapy of head-and-neck cancers *Cancers* **13** 5991

[20] Green O L, Henke L E and Hugo G D 2019 Practical clinical workflows for online and offline adaptive radiation therapy *Semin. Radiat. Oncol.* **29** 219–27

[21] Stanley D N *et al* 2023 A roadmap for implementation of kV-CBCT online adaptive radiation therapy and initial first year experiences *J. Appl. Clin. Med. Phys.* **24** e13961

[22] Murdoch B 2021 Privacy and artificial intelligence: challenges for protecting health information in a new era *BMC Med. Ethics* **22** 122

[23] Mastella E *et al* 2025 A systematic review of the role of artificial intelligence in automating computed tomography-based adaptive radiotherapy for head and neck cancer *Phys. Imaging. Radiat. Oncol.* **33** 100731

[24] Vandewinckele L *et al* 2020 Overview of artificial intelligence-based applications in radio-therapy: recommendations for implementation and quality assurance *Radiother. Oncol.* **153** 55–66

[25] Hurkmans C *et al* 2024 A joint ESTRO and AAPM guideline for development, clinical validation and reporting of artificial intelligence models in radiation therapy *Radiother. Oncol.* **197** 110345

[26] Cui S *et al* 2023 Interpretable artificial intelligence in radiology and radiation oncology *Br. J. Radiol.* **96** 20230142

[27] Wahid K A *et al* 2024 Artificial intelligence uncertainty quantification in radiotherapy applications—a scoping review *Radiother. Oncol.* **201** 110542

[28] Kawamura M *et al* 2023 Revolutionizing radiation therapy: the role of AI in clinical practice *J. Radiat. Res.* **65** 1–9

[29] Olberg S *et al* 2025 Commissioning a standalone adaptive radiotherapy linac in a multi-vendor environment *J. Appl. Clin. Med. Phys.* **26** e70033

[30] Rusanov B *et al* 2022 Deep learning methods for enhancing cone-beam CT image quality toward adaptive radiation therapy: a systematic review *Med. Phys.* **49** 6019–54

[31] Khalifa A *et al* 2024 Machine learning automated treatment planning for online magnetic resonance guided adaptive radiotherapy of prostate cancer *Phys. Imaging Radiat. Oncol.* **32** 100649

[32] Buchanan L *et al* 2023 Deep learning-based prediction of deliverable adaptive plans for MR-guided adaptive radiotherapy: a feasibility study *Front. Oncol.* **13** 939951

[33] Keall P, Poulsen P and Booth J T 2019 See, think, and act: real-time adaptive radiotherapy *Semin. Radiat. Oncol.* **29** 228–35

[34] Sherer M V *et al* 2021 Metrics to evaluate the performance of auto-segmentation for radiation treatment planning: a critical review *Radiother. Oncol.* **160** 185–91

[35] Lee S H, Geng H and Xiao Y 2022 Radiotherapy standardisation and artificial intelligence within the National Cancer Institute's Clinical Trials Network *Clin. Oncol.* **34** 128–34

[36] Wang Y F *et al* 2024 Enhancing safety in AI-driven cone beam CT-based online adaptive radiation therapy: development and implementation of an interdisciplinary workflow *Adv. Radiat. Oncol.* **9** 101399

[37] Almeida N D *et al* 2024 Artificial intelligence potential impact on resident physician education in radiation oncology *Adv. Radiat. Oncol.* **9** 101505

[38] Shepherd M *et al* 2025 Training for tomorrow: establishing a worldwide curriculum in online adaptive radiation therapy *Tech. Innov. Patient. Support. Radiat. Oncol.* **33** 100304

[39] Chetty I J *et al* 2024 Quality and safety considerations for adaptive radiation therapy: an ASTRO White paper *Int. J. Radiat. Oncol. Biol. Phys.* **122** 838–64

[40] Fiagbedzi E, Hasford F and Tagoe S N 2023 The influence of artificial intelligence on the work of the medical physicist in radiotherapy practice: a short review *BJR Open* **5** 20230003

[41] Huq M S *et al* 2016 The report of Task Group 100 of the AAPM: application of risk analysis methods to radiation therapy quality management *Med. Phys.* **43** 4209

[42] Nishioka S *et al* 2022 Identifying risk characteristics using failure mode and effect analysis for risk management in online magnetic resonance-guided adaptive radiation therapy *Phys. Imaging Radiat. Oncol.* **23** 1–7

[43] Chapman J W *et al* 2022 Robustness and reproducibility of an artificial intelligence-assisted online segmentation and adaptive planning process for online adaptive radiation therapy *J. Appl. Clin. Med. Phys.* **23** e13702

[44] Ford E *et al* 2020 Strategies for effective physics plan and chart review in radiation therapy: report of AAPM Task Group 275 *Med. Phys.* **47** e236–72

[45] Claessens M *et al* 2022 Quality assurance for AI-based applications in radiation therapy *Semin. Radiat. Oncol.* **32** 421–31

[46] Bock M 2020 On adaptation cost and tractability in robust adaptive radiation therapy optimization *Med. Phys.* **47** 2791–804

[47] McComas K N *et al* 2023 Online adaptive radiation therapy and opportunity cost *Adv. Radiat. Oncol.* **8** 101034

[48] Hurkmans C *et al* 2024 Assessment of bias in scoring of AI-based radiotherapy segmentation and planning studies using modified TRIPOD and PROBAST guidelines as an example *Radiother. Oncol.* **194** 110196

[49] Lillard J W *et al* 2022 Racial disparities in Black men with prostate cancer: a literature review *Cancer* **128** 3787–95

[50] Cohen E B and Gordon I K 2022 First, do no harm. Ethical and legal issues of artificial intelligence and machine learning in veterinary radiology and radiation oncology *Vet. Radiol. Ultrasound* **63** 840–50

IOP Publishing

Artificial Intelligence in Adaptive Radiation Therapy

Yi Wang and X. Sharon Qi

Chapter 15

Offline computed tomography-based and online cone beam computed tomography-based adaptive radiation therapy

Joel A Pogue, Natalie Viscariello, Dennis N Stanley, Joseph Harms, Richard A Popple and Carlos E Cardenas

Adaptive radiotherapy (ART) encompasses offline and online approaches to adjust treatment plans based on anatomical and physiological changes during the course of radiotherapy. This chapter reviews the clinical considerations, technical workflows, and current limitations of both offline computed tomography (CT)-based and online cone beam computed tomography (CBCT)-based ART (figure 15.1). Offline ART workflows involve re-simulation and re-planning triggered by observed anatomical changes, with dose recalculation aided by deformable registration or synthetic CT generation. Online CBCT-guided ART systems, such as Varian Ethos, Elekta Evo, and United Imaging's uRT-linac, enable real-time plan adaptation with on-board imaging and fast optimization engines. Key challenges include image quality, synthetic CT accuracy, increased workload, and quality assurance (QA) without interrupting clinical throughput. The integration of AI, knowledge-based planning, and adaptive triggers offers new avenues for workflow efficiency and clinical impact. This chapter provides practical guidance for the implementation, patient selection, and QA strategies essential for the successful clinical deployment of both ART paradigms.

15.1 Clinical considerations for CT-based offline ART

Radiation therapy is generally delivered over the course of weeks. During this time, patient anatomy may change, potentially impacting target coverage and delivery of unnecessary dose to surrounding tissues. Common examples of changes that impact the delivered dose distribution include tumor regression, weight loss, changes in swelling, and variable organ filling. In response to these changes, offline adaptive radiation therapy (ART) may be employed to ensure that patients are treated as initially intended. Offline ART consists of taking a repeat CT simulation during the course of an RT course and re-optimizing the treatment plan. The ART

doi:10.1088/978-0-7503-6119-4ch15
15-1

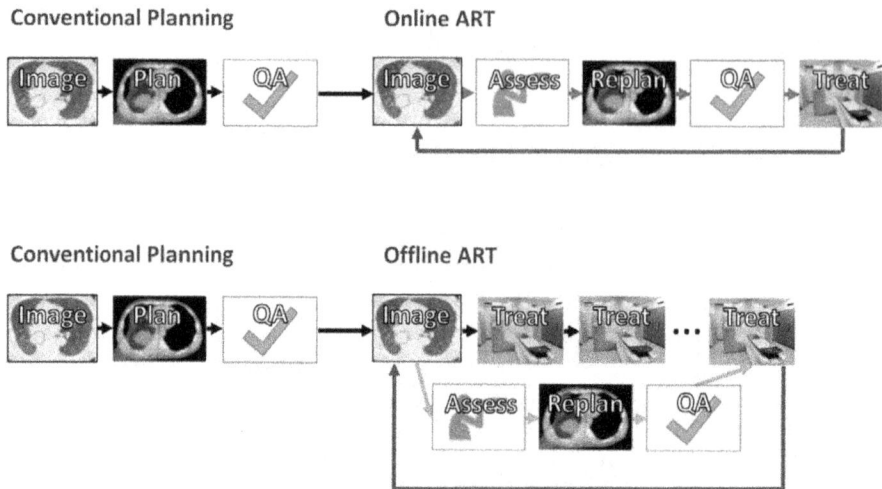

Figure 15.1. Comparison of online and offline ART. (Reproduced with permission from [1]. Copyright 2019 Elsevier.)

process can be initiated either at a planned date/fraction or, more commonly, in response to anatomical changes and/or disease progression/response observed on either image-guided radiation therapy (IGRT) and/or on-treatment diagnostic imaging. The ART process has been shown to provide dosimetric benefit for the head-and-neck [2] and has been investigated to trigger dose escalation for non-small cell lung cancer [3].

While offline ART can be beneficial, the accelerated timeline for treatment planning, as compared to initial treatment planning, produces a burden on staff and can potentially lead to errors [4]. A survey by Krishnatrry *et al* [5] found that while many centers employ offline ART (84% of respondents), there are noted barriers to ART which need to be overcome for increased utilization of ART, most prominently a lack of proper equipment (i.e. delivery systems and planning tools optimized for adaptive radiotherapy) which was reported by 48% of respondents. In a separate survey conducted by Betholet *et al*, 63% of respondents ranked 'human resources' as either the primary or secondary barrier to the implementation/expansion of ART [6]. A majority of respondents also listed technical limitations and equipment/financial resources as highly important.

15.1.1 Patient and site selection

Offline adaptive radiotherapy addresses progressive changes to the treatment volume or organs at risk (OARs), such as patient weight loss or tumor regression. Monitoring for anatomical or physiological changes can be done by the observation of tumor change during image review or by determining thresholds for changes seen in daily CBCT imaging [7–9]. Routine scans (e.g. weekly quality assurance (QA) simulation during proton therapy workflow) may also be used to appreciate changes at regular intervals.

Typical sites for offline adaptive therapy are the head and neck and thorax, although anticipating which patients will have the most dosimetric benefit from adaptation at the time of initial planning is difficult. There have been several studies exploring the ability to predict patients that will exhibit anatomical changes throughout treatment [10]. For example, Lee *et al* [11] used a deep learning model to predict the geometric evolution of lung and esophagus contours throughout treatment, and used weekly CBCTs to update the model's predictions on a patient-specific basis. Wang *et al* [12] built a convolutional neural network (CNN) to predict lung tumor shrinkage using weekly MRIs throughout the course of treatment. Even with these developments, determining which patients will benefit most from offline adaptive therapy is not straightforward at the time of initial planning. Instead, monitoring of tumor or OAR change using routine imaging is typically used.

The process of offline adaptation is employed when visible changes to the tumor or normal tissue are indicated, or functional changes are shown mid-treatment [3]. Daily anatomical changes (e.g. bladder filling) are not appropriate for offline adaptive therapy, given the timeframe for re-simulation and planning. A majority of centers consider adaptation on an ad hoc basis [6], although there have been protocols designed to trigger once dosimetric thresholds have been met [13]. Typically, this process requires registration and contour propagation from the planning CT to CBCT [14] automated contour and recalculation of the planned dose to the current daily anatomy.

Direct plan recalculation and dosimetric evaluation using CBCT alone can lead to erroneous results because the Hounsfield units (HUs) in CBCT may not share a one-to-one correspondence with the HUs in treatment planning CTs. To mitigate this, a synthetic CT (sCT) can be created, either using artificial neural networks or deformable image registration (DIR). In the neural network (NN) approach [15–18] models are typically trained to learn a mapping from the CBCT HU domain to the CT HU domain, allowing for accurate recalculation. In the DIR-based workflow, which is more commonly implemented in clinics [19], the CT numbers from the planning CT are propagated to the anatomy of the day based on the daily CBCT according to the deformation vector fields from the registration [20–22]. While either of these approaches are typically superior to direct calculation on the CBCT, they can both lead to errors and should only be implemented with proper QA and reviewed with clinical judgment [23].

15.1.2 Re-simulation

The re-simulation process for offline adaptive therapy is often the same as the initial CT simulation [1]. For disease sites affected by motion, maintaining the same motion management protocol, such as respiratory gating, as used during initial simulation helps ensure consistency in planning and delivery, when still clinically appropriate. In most cases, the immobilization equipment from the initial radiotherapy course is preserved. However, one potential cause of ad hoc offline adaption is immobilization equipment no longer fitting properly, as can happen when patients undergo significant weight loss during the course of treatment.

Another option for generating a new plan is to use the CBCT for deformable registration, as was done by Bojechko *et al* [24]. Rather than creating a new planning

CT, the Halcyon CBCT was used to create deformed structures on the initial planning CT; this was possible due to the large field-of-view and soft tissue contrast. Theoretically, this workflow could be implemented when changes to the patient's anatomy are apparent and the CBCT has a large enough field-of-view to create an adequate structure deformation map back to the planning CT.

15.1.3 Re-planning

After re-simulation is performed, the planning process begins with either delineating or propagating previous contours. Deformable image registration has been used for the propagation of targets in CBCT-based offline re-planning for patients with oropharyngeal tumors [25]. Mencarelli *et al* [26] found that DIR accuracy for both normal and tumor tissues was < 1 mm, but precision was variable, with precision significantly degrading with larger intervals between the planning CT and follow-up CBCT. DIR for target propagation is an attractive option because of the availability of DIR algorithms within many treatment planning systems, however the accuracy of the registration has been found to be dependent on the registration algorithm or software [27]. AI-based automated contouring has also been demonstrated as a feasible option to expedite re-planning in adaptive settings [28, 29].

15.1.4 Plan summation and evaluation

Offline adaptive summation of dose can be used for the summation of entirely new plans, as described above, or on a regular basis to monitor how the original planned dose compares to what was actually delivered. For re-simulation and re-planning, once a new plan is generated, summation with the initial plan is needed to estimate the total dose in the course of treatment. The accuracy of the combined dose is limited by the uncertainty of the image registration between the initial and new CT scan [30], slice thickness, and dose grid sizes. These limitations are amplified in regions of marked tumor growth or regression, making the resulting plan sum, potentially, less accurate [31]. DIR is commonly used to register images where the shape or size of targets and organs differ between the new planning image and initial CT image. There are many deep learning methods employed in image registration [32], including reinforced learning [33], generative adversarial network mapping [34], and unsupervised transformation prediction [35]. The deformation vector fields from the DIR dictate the dose accumulation, so uncertainty in the DIR process propagates throughout the plan summation [36]. Because of this, validation of image registration algorithms is paramount. The AAPM Task Group 132 [31] provides guidelines on metrics for evaluating the accuracy of an image registration algorithm. The new and initial plans can also be calculated on different grid sizes, leading to differences in interpolation between the grid points. The observed dose summation is based on the alignment of the treatment planning system (TPS) dose calculation matrices from image registration, and the sum is displayed as the interpolation between the two matrices. Care must be taken when interpreting the plan sum in areas with steep dose gradients and for small structures.

Dose summation may also be performed on a daily basis with daily dose mapping. Daily dose mapping relies on remapping the calculated dose to the daily imaging, which is subject to the uncertainties discussed above. Because the dose accumulation is used to monitor delivered dose and incorporate this into decisions about the plan going forward, there is a need for high accuracy. These so-called 'dose of the day' studies that consider dose calculation on deformed CTs found dose calculation errors on the order of 1%–2%, depending on the site considered [21, 22, 37]. The effect of the deformation vector field used for calculation of the daily dose depends on the dose heterogeneity and gradients of the dose distribution, and it relies on the assumption that the dose mapping transformation is valid across the entire registered images [38]. Particularly in regions of anatomical changes (e.g. tumor shrinkage), the direct one-to-one mapping from one image to another is not always straightforward in deformable image registrations. Even so, Murr *et al* [38] recommend using registration algorithms that maintain this mapping strategy when resampling dose. In short, daily dose summation is resource-intensive and prone to additional uncertainties that can complicate interpretation, thus clinical teams must support its use with a robust QA program to guide treatment decisions.

15.1.5 Patient specific quality assurance

For offline ART, treatment plans should go through the same process as any new plan, even if the workflow is slightly compressed compared to initial planning. This workflow includes plan quality review by both the physicist and physician, and typically measurement of the delivered plan. While independent measurement of the dose distribution is the gold standard for patient-specific quality assurance (PSQA) in radiation oncology, the majority of errors in the treatment planning process are not caught by measurement [39].

Because of the added burden of PSQA measurement, there is interest in techniques to eliminate the explicit measurement in lieu of other safety checks. In a prospective study by Wall *et al* [40], a virtual QA system was tested to replace physical dose measurement with predicted dose measurement. In this study, a machine learning model was trained to extract plan complexity features from radiation treatment plans and predict differences between planned and measured dose, based on 579 historical measurements. The model had a mean absolute error of 1% and if used to determine whether PSQA measurement was needed for a given plan, would yield a 69% reduction in QA workload.

Deep learning approaches have also been employed to predict PSQA results. Zeng *et al* employed a self-attention network with a modified U-Net to predict measured dose distributions on a PSQA measurement device [41]. Rather than predicting dose, Kimura *et al* [42] trained a CNN to detect MLC positioning errors during delivery of VMAT plans. Developments such as these, which eliminate the need for machine time to deliver PSQA, could have significant impact for offline adaption because ensuring adequate time for PSQA measurement can add delays to the ART process.

15.1.6 Limitations and future directions

One of the current limitations of offline ART is its ad hoc nature. In the patterns of practice for adaptive and real-time radiation therapy (POP-ART) survey of 177 radiation therapy centers, Bertholet *et al* found that while over half of the surveyed centers performed offline ART, less than a third had specific ART protocols [6]. AI has been shown to be able to predict treatment changes during RT in the head and neck, further studies such as this could be used to develop prospective protocols for offline adaptation, triggering re-simulation and re-planning and specific time points. Integration of AI into the clinic also has high potential for utility in developing thresholds to trigger offline adaption [43]. Examples of AI applications in the offline workflow include automated segmentation on CBCT images, allowing for tracking of target or OAR shrinkage or growth [44]. Using corrected CBCT images, dose prediction based on daily imaging, whether from deep learning or knowledge-based planning algorithms, may also be effective triggers for offline ART, alerting the treatment team when certain dose metrics are exceeded.

Offline ART typically takes 1–3 days to go from re-simulation to treatment commencement of the revised plan. This timescale means offline ART has limited ability to adapt to either rapid or frequent changes in daily anatomy, for example variable rectum or bladder filling in the pelvis. In disease sites that respond rapidly to radiation, for example head-and-neck or lung tumors may shrink over the course of 1–3 days, offline ART can lead to planners 'chasing' anatomical changes because the response time is similar to the time needed to create a new treatment plan [1, 45].

15.2 Clinical considerations for CBCT/CT-based online ART

Online ART is an emerging field with a limited number of commercially available systems. Notable examples include Varian Ethos, Elekta Evo, and United Imaging's uRT-linac 506c.

The Varian Ethos kV-CBCT-guided online ART treatment system is at the time of writing the only Food and Drug Administration (FDA)-cleared commercial system to utilize on-board CBCT imaging for online ART. Ethos consists of a Halcyon O-ring linear accelerator (Varian Medical Systems, Inc., Palo Alto, CA) with integrated online adaptive software capabilities. The accelerator features a 6 MV flattening filter free (FFF) beam with jaw-less collimation via a dual layer and staggered 10 mm multileaf collimator (MLC) banks, enabling 5 mm effective MLC resolution and decreased intra-leaf leakage compared to single layer MLCs. The MLCs allow a maximum exposure area of 28 cm × 28 cm, and the compact accelerator and closed bore design allow four revolutions per minute [46]. These features combined with the 800 MU/min maximum dose rate enable faster treatments compared to flattened beam treatments on C-arm linear accelerators. The online TPS produces both IMRT and VMAT plans, which are calculated using Acuros XB with dose-to-medium "... reporting mode" [47].

The Elekta Evo (Elekta, Stockholm, Sweden) is a CT-guided adaptive radiotherapy (CTgART) system introduced in 2024. It integrates with the Versa HD linear accelerator and Elekta ONE software ecosystem, including the TPS and oncology information system (OIS). The system uses Iris™, an AI-enhanced CBCT solution for direct dose calculation and automated contouring, with planning supported by MIM software and dose calculated using Monte Carlo algorithms with dose-to-medium reporting. Evo supports IMRT (sliding window and step-and-shoot) and VMAT delivery with a 6DoF couch, allowing for non-coplanar arrangements and precise IGRT. The adaptive workflow begins with CBCT acquisition, registration, and AI-generated contours, which users can edit. Plans are recalculated on the daily image and reviewed to determine whether adaptation is needed. If so, optimization goals can be adjusted dynamically. Secondary dose calculation and optional *in vivo* verification are available. A pre-treatment CBCT can verify stability before delivery, and re-adaptation is supported.

Additionally, the uRT-linac 506c (United Imaging Healthcare Co. Ltd, Shanghai, China) is a China Food and Drug Administration (CFDA) certified C-arm linac equipped with fan-beam computed tomography (FBCT) capabilities [48, 49]. The unit boasts a 16 slice helical CT imager coaxially attached to the linac gantry, energies (maximum dose rate) of 6X (600 MU/minute) and 6FFF (1400 MU/minute), dual layer collimating jaws, two opposing banks of 60 MLCs (0.5 cm width MLCs in the central 20 cm and 1.0 cm width MLCs in the outer 20 cm), and a maximum field size of 40 cm × 40 cm. A diagnostic-quality helical CT acquired on the CT-integrated linac feeds VB-Net autosegmentation of the target and OARs, after which a hybrid voxel-based optimizer (U-Net dose-prediction prior + preset objectives) generates a single-arc VMAT plan on-couch. Couch shifts derived from the CT are applied automatically during optimization, and any physician edits to contours or objectives trigger instant re-optimization to create an updated adaptive plan. The approved plan is verified with *in vivo* EPID transit-dose γ-analysis (3%/3 mm) and a low-dose CT (or MV portals) before delivery [73].

15.2.1 Online-ART-specific challenges

Despite the early adoption of CBCT-based online ART by some institutions, many technical challenges remain which prevent more widespread clinical adoption; these challenges include, but are not limited to, uncertainties in dose calculations due to sCT deformation [50–53], contouring limitations caused by suboptimal image quality [54], the inability to perform traditional patient-specific QA [55, 56], and significantly increased resource allocation compared to the standard-of-care [57, 58]. More physician, physicist, and dosimetrist time is required throughout the reference planning process to evaluate the clinical objectives and carefully inspect the contoured target and organ-at-risk structures, as adaptive plans must remain robust to anatomical changes such as target deformation or shifts relative to nearby OARs [25]. Online ART requires an adaptor, a clinical team member trained in organ delineation, who is responsible for reviewing and, if necessary, editing all automatically generated contours of normal tissues and targets that influence plan optimization and evaluation. While often assigned to specific team members, this role can be incorporated into various staffing models [59, 60]. Because these contours directly impact the adapted plan, they must undergo careful and timely offline review by a physician, contributing to a significant increase in image review time compared to standard IGRT workflows. Furthermore, online ART treatment times are substantially longer due to additional treatment processes and safety checks [61–63], significantly minimizing patient throughput and/or extending the treatment day, which subsequently affects hospital costs and staffing needs [58].

15.2.2 Patient and site selection

Because of the increased resource allocation associated with CBCT-based online ART, identifying high-yield treatments is necessary for clinics seeking to implement online CBCT-guided ART. This is made possible by bifurcating patients based on either body site or patient-specific metrics. Body sites typically selected for CT/CBCT-based online ART include those in the pelvic region with variable bladder and rectal filling (e.g. prostate [39, 64–66], gynecological [59, 62, 67, 68], anal/rectal [62, 69–73], and bladder cancers [69, 74–78]), advanced disease where tumor regression is likely (e.g. head-and-neck [79–82], lung cancers [83–86], and seminomas [87]), sites with increased set-up uncertainty and target deformation (e.g. accelerated partial breast irradiation (APBI) [88, 89]), and high dose per fraction treatments near critical OARs (e.g. SBRT for abdominal oligometastases [90], ultracentral thoracic disease [25], and pancreatic cancer [54, 91]).

More recently, multiple groups have focused on identifying higher yield patients within specific treatment sites to further save resources, as some patients receive minimal dosimetric benefit with adaption even if they are receiving treatment to a site that typically benefits from online ART. Moazzezi et al first discussed the rationale for selecting patients for CBCT-guided ART prior to treatment because they observed that certain patients experienced greater adaptive benefit than others for prostate cancer [66]. Yock et al investigated the use of statistically derived adaptive triggers for standard and hypo-fractionated pelvic treatments, allowing patients to be bifurcated as either adaptive or non-adaptive based on the difference between scheduled (initial plan recalculated on daily anatomy) and reference plan metrics [92]. Ghimire et al utilized a LASSO machine learning regularization technique to forecast online ART dosimetric benefit for cervical cancer patients based solely on reference plan dose metrics, enabling a priori bifurcation of patients into adaptive and non-adaptive workflows [93]. Furthermore, Pogue et al utilized multiple supervised and unsupervised machine learning approaches for a priori selection of optimal stereotactic APBI patients based on reference plan metrics, an example of which is shown in figure 15.2 [94, 95]. These studies demonstrate the feasibility of implementing models and techniques to identify patients who would benefit from adaptive therapy, potentially supporting broader adoption of CBCT-guided online ART by enabling more efficient triage of clinical resources.

15.2.3 Simulation

The standard CBCT-based online ART simulation process largely aligns with standard-of-care procedures, with a few exceptions. For example, daily ART auto-contours may erroneously include high-density structures if contrast was

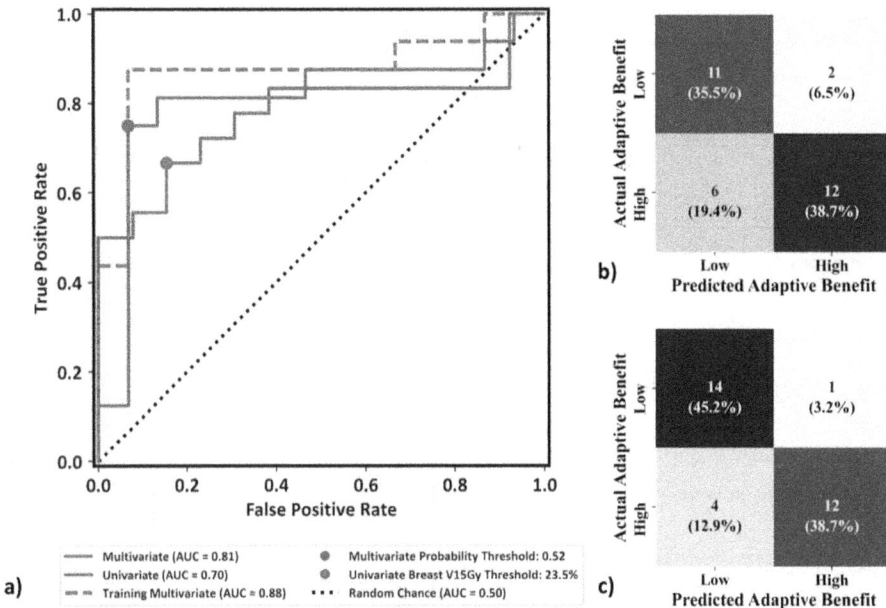

Figure 15.2. (a) Receiver operating characteristic curves when using a univariate model, a multivariate training model using the entire dataset, and using a leave-one-out cross-validation multivariate model. Youden's indices (circles) illustrate the thresholds resulting from maximum differences between true positive and false positive rates. (b) Confusion matrix heat map for the univariate ipsilateral Breast V15Gy model. (c) Confusion matrix heat map of the multivariate validation model. (Reproduced from [95]. Copyright 2024 The Author(s). Published on behalf of Institute of Physics and Engineering in Medicine by IOP Publishing Ltd. CC BY 4.0.)

present in the planning CT scan, thus the clinical team needs to have a deep understanding of the online ART algorithms' performance under different clinical conditions. It is important to note that some online ART platforms offer unique simulation capabilities that are not available in conventional IGRT workflows. Nellissen *et al* and Oldenburger *et al* investigated the feasibility of simulation-free palliative workflows for single visit online adaptive treatments of painful bone metastases [51, 96]. Reference plans were generated using previous high-quality diagnostic CT images, and resulting daily sCT images allowed for highly conformal adaptive plan delivery in single patient visits with acceptable timeframes. Additionally, Price *et al* performed *in silico* analysis of hippocampal-sparing whole brain RT using an atlas based MRI to CT registration technique; the patient-specific MRI was registered with the closest match from a library of CT scans, then both images were imported into Ethos for daily adaptive re-planning [97]. Atlas based simulation resulted in adaptive plans with improved hippocampal sparing and 45 min adaptive sessions. Furthermore, Nelissen *et al* successfully performed simulation-free consultation and palliative treatment for bone metastases with high patient satisfaction scores and two hour timeframes as part of the prospective FAST-METS clinical trial [98]. Lastly, advancements in CBCT technology have

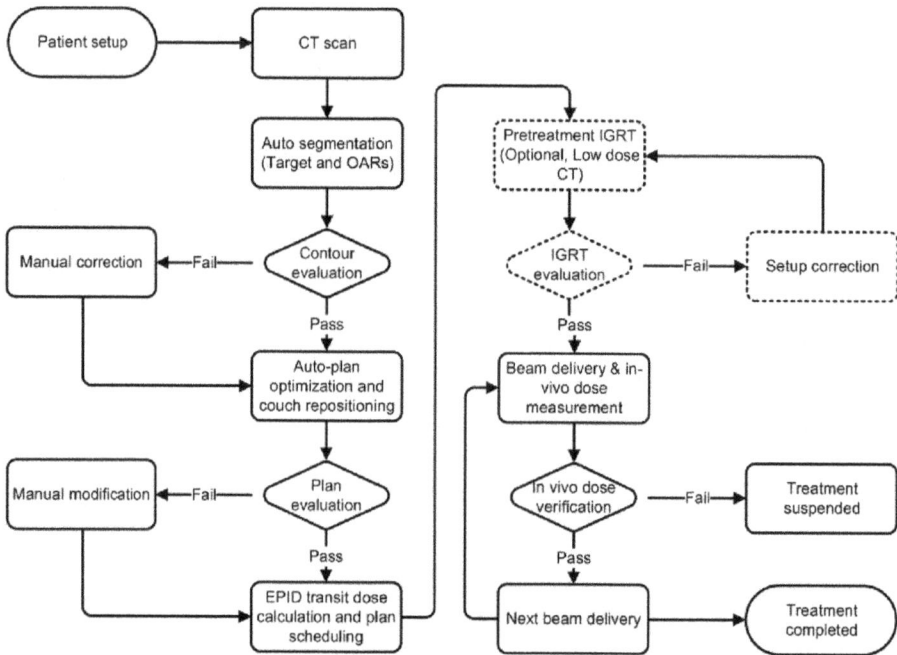

Figure 15.3. Workflow utilized by the 'All-in-One' uRT-linac 506c, illustrating that the entire treatment process (simulation, contouring, planning, and delivery) is performed with the patient on the couch. (Reproduced from [73] with permission from John Wiley & Sons. Copyright 2023 American Association of Physicists in Medicine.)

improved image quality to the point where direct dose calculation is now feasible, potentially eliminating the need for a separate simulation scan [94–97].

Some treatment units integrate diagnostic-quality fan-beam CT scanners, enabling simulation and treatment to occur on the same couch without patient repositioning. These 'all-in-one' systems could streamline workflow, although technical parameters vary by vendor and may influence clinical implementation and image quality considerations. Yu *et al* demonstrated excellent deliverability using an all-in-one treatment unit (uRT-linac 506c) for ten rectal cancer patients, with a maximum time of 30 min from the start of simulation CT to completion of beam delivery and *in vivo* QA; the workflow is illustrated in figure 15.3 [73]. While early online ART systems relied on sCT generation for dose calculation, introducing potential uncertainties, advances in CBCT technology now enable direct dose calculation on CBCT images, reducing reliance on sCTs and improving dosimetric accuracy [23, 85, 99].

15.2.4 Pre-planning review

CBCT-based online ART treatment planning requires workflows and considerations beyond standard practice, including evaluation of sCT generation (if applicable) based on planning CT attributes, assessment of target and structure derivation accuracy, consistency in structure naming, automated management of high-density regions and artifacts, and ensuring plan robustness. Because online ART planning workflows are still evolving, all members of the clinical team require an enhanced understanding of the technical aspects involved in reference plan generation and adaptive planning to ensure safe and effective implementation. Clinic-specific workflows vary, with some teams assigning reference planning to physicists, while others rely on dosimetrists with physicist support [100]. The increase in planning complexity with online ART could lead to more errors, and thus more unintended re-plans. Wegener *et al* performed failure mode and effects analysis of their institutional events relating to treatment with Ethos, finding that the highest number of events occurred in the conceptualization and contouring phase (i.e. creation of prescription, intent, and planning directives) [101]. Because of this, many clinics have implemented intent reviews to reduce error rates and provide physicist technical support earlier in the treatment planning process [61, 102].

Beyond verifying standard prescription details (e.g. treatment site, laterality, dose, number of targets and phases, and treatment frequency), additional technical components specific to online ART platforms should be reviewed to ensure proper workflow performance during the intent review phase. Planning CT images should generally be contrast-free and acquired in a consistent breathing state (e.g. free-breathing or breath-hold), particularly for systems that do not support phase gating. CT datasets should also be of manageable size to support efficient TPS optimization. The accuracy of daily auto-contours is often influenced by both predefined structure classification codes and the quality of planning CT contours; therefore, structure naming, coding, and contour accuracy should be carefully reviewed and corrected when necessary to prevent propagation of errors during online contour generation. Target and optimization structure derivations should be reviewed for accuracy and robustness to interfractional anatomy change, particularly when delivering high dose near critical OARs [25]. Lastly, the planner and/or physicist should ensure that the planning template is consistent with planning goals, and that goals needed for daily ART plan evaluation are in the appropriate priority level to be visualized at the console during treatment delivery.

Rahman *et al* performed fault tree and failure mode and effects analysis, observing a large reduction in risk priority number for many adaptive specific portions of plan preparation (tasks between simulation and plan optimization) when pre-planning reviews were performed [63]. These results, highlighted in figure 15.4, illustrate the increased physics and dosimetry resource requirements compared to standard IGRT workflows.

15.2.5 Reference planning

Online ART workflows require rapid plan generation to fit within the time constraints of same-day adaptive treatment. To meet this demand, modern TPSs incorporate intelligent optimization technologies that automate key components of the planning process. These systems translate clinical goals into optimization objectives, generate supporting structures as needed (e.g. to resolve overlap or

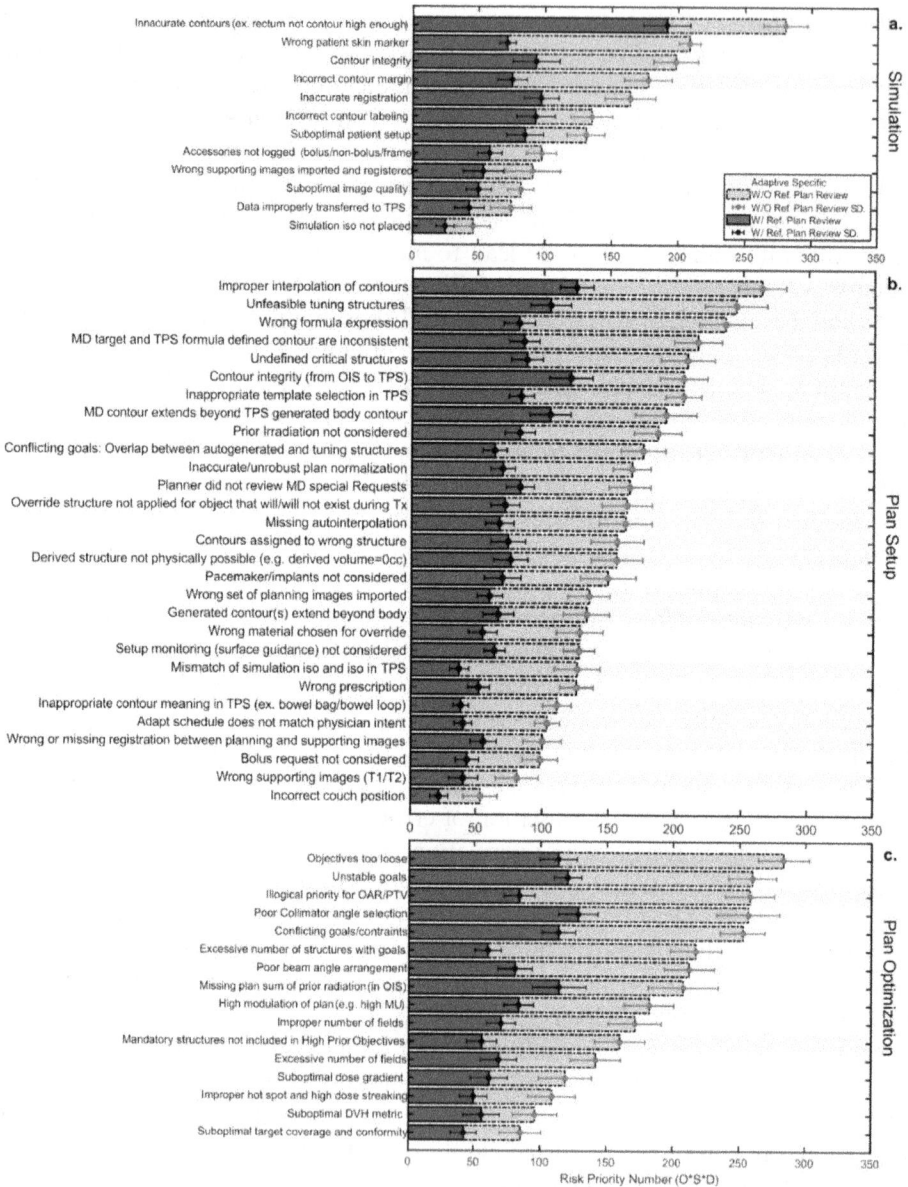

Figure 15.4. Risk priority number (RPN) scoring with and without reference planning review, using failure mode and effects analysis of the faults from (a) simulation, (b) plan set-up, and (c) plan optimization processes. The error bars illustrate the mean and standard deviation risk priority number for each failure mode. (Reproduced with permission from [63]. Copyright 2024 Elsevier.)

enhance dose shaping), and assign objective weights based on planning priorities. Some platforms use quality-monitoring functions to guide iterative optimization and halt refinement once specific clinical goals are satisfied, enabling efficient convergence. These fast optimizers are designed not only to meet planning objectives but also to further improve plan quality when time permits. Because these tools influence both reference and adaptive plan quality, clinical teams must understand their behavior and limitations when designing planning templates and workflows for online ART.

The Ethos kV-CBCT online ART platform utilizes a proprietary intelligent optimization engine (IOE) to automatically generate plans from a planning goal template submitted to the TPS. The IOE is a hands-off 'algorithm that orchestrates the plan optimization' by seeking to 'perform all the actions necessary to generate high-quality dose distributions that meet the clinical expectations for the plan and ensure that the plan is diametrically accurate' [103]. This is made possible by automated creation of helper/optimization structures, deriving non-overlapping structures in the presence of overlapping structures with opposing objectives, and assigning objective weights based on the hierarchy of the planning goal template submitted to the dose preview workspace [104]. The IOE functions by first translating clinical goals into photon optimizer objectives, then generating piecewise quality functions (Q-functions) for monitoring and influencing the optimization process. The form of each function prototype (e.g. target upper/lower dose and organ upper dose) is derived from known features of a good distribution and generated by assigning a goal priority and relative goal value, allowing each function to be placed on a priority–quality plane (P, Q) [103]. The optimizer seeks to iterate until the Q-function meets an individual goal point (P_i, Q_i), then this goal does not contribute to additional optimizations for lower priority functions. Additionally, the IOE is designed to further reduce organ and target upper dose levels once all planning goals are achieved.

For each goal template submitted to the TPS in the dose preview workspace, several preselected IMRT (7, 9, or 12 equidistant fields) and VMAT (two and three full arcs, two partial arcs) plans are automatically optimized and calculated using a collimator rotation of zero, although custom geometries can be exported from Eclipse on a patient-by-patient basis. The superior reference plan geometry, i.e. the plan selected for adaptive treatment, defines the optimization objective template and geometry utilized for daily online ART plan generation. Many groups have investigated the quality and clinical acceptability of Ethos IOE automated plans for multiple beam geometries using standardized planning templates. It has been thoroughly demonstrated that, given a well-designed template, the IOE automatically generates high-quality standard fractionation plans for sites in the male and female pelvis [66, 67, 105] and head and neck [106], with similar and sometimes improved performance compared to manually generated Eclipse plans [69, 104].

Pogue *et al* demonstrated that the IOE can automatically produce plans similar in quality to knowledge-based planning models for locally advanced lung cancer [107]. Furthermore, Visak *et al* and Roberfroid *et al* investigated the feasibility of using U-Net machine learning models to develop IOE head-and-neck and prostate planning goals, respectively, on a patient-by-patient basis; they each observed that AI-guided planning was superior to standard template planning [108, 109]. Additionally, despite the IOE being designed for organ avoidance planning with homogeneous target coverage, multiple groups have effectively developed automated or semi-automated stereotactic planning techniques for APBI [110] and lung and brain tumors [47, 111]. However, Ethos V2.0 offers a 'High-Fidelity' stereotactic planning selection which largely mitigates the need for many of the complex stereotactic planning strategies outlined above, with improved online treatment efficiency observed [112, 113]. It should also be mentioned that several groups observed that the IOE IMRT plan dosimetry and optimization time was superior to VMAT, likely due to increased degrees of freedom when gantry angle is included in the optimization objective function [105, 107]. Given that reference planning defines online ART optimization, daily VMAT treatments require more time than IMRT plans, causing some clinics to exclusively adapt using IMRT [105].

Conversely, the uRT-linac 506c TPS, uRT-TPOIS, utilizes a hybrid voxel-based optimization approach, combining 3D U-Net network dose predictions with a preset list of clinical objectives [73, 114, 115]. Stochastic gradient descent optimization is utilized to obtain an optimal solution to the hybrid objective function, which is the sum of voxel and DVH-based objective functions. This novel, automated treatment planning system predicts the deliverable dose from a structure set containing target and OAR contours via U-Net based deep learning, then minimizes the mean squared error of calculated and predicted dose during optimization, resulting in the generation of accurate plans during delivery. The Elekta Evo system uses a Monte Carlo based treatment planning engine within the Elekta ONE TPS to support adaptive plan generation. Clinical goals—defined through a planning intent—are translated into optimization objectives that guide the generation of IMRT or VMAT treatment plans. During re-optimization, users can interactively modify objective priorities, dose constraints, and normalization values in real time. The system supports iterative re-planning to improve dose distributions, with automated handling of overlapping structures and dose shaping objectives.

15.2.6 Patient specific quality assurance

Patient-specific QA (PSQA) for all online ART reference plans is performed using the same methods as those applied in standard-of-care treatment planning: patient-specific treatment plans are recalculated onto a phantom, then delivered at the machine and measured, followed by three-dimensional analysis of dose agreement between the TPS and measured doses. Zhao *et al* demonstrated that reference plans agree well with measured doses for 16 patients receiving treatment to various sites and with differing fractionations [56]. All ion chamber measurements were within 3% absolute dose difference and all cylindrical diode array measurements were above 95% gamma passing rate (3%/2 mm with 10% threshold). Furthermore, Sibolt *et al* performed measurement-based analysis (Delta4+, ScandiDos AB, Uppsala, Sweden and portal dosimetry) and calculation-based analysis (Mobius3D, Varian Medical Systems) of 32 bladder and rectum reference plans, finding that both agreed excellently with Ethos using 3%/2 mm and 3%/3 mm gamma passing criteria, respectively.

Specialized software platforms have been developed to enable independent, calculation-based dose verification for online adaptive radiotherapy, addressing the limitations of traditional measurement-based QA in time-sensitive adaptive workflows [116]. These tools should incorporate ultra-fast dose calculation engines and support comprehensive 3D dosimetric evaluation, including gamma index analysis and dose–volume histogram comparisons, to ensure the accuracy and safety of delivered adaptive plans across various treatment systems.

15.2.7 Online ART workflow

The CT-based online ART treatment delivery workflow is dynamic and differs from the standard-of-care in many ways, several of which can be visualized through a representative workflow shown in figure 15.5 [61]. In both adaptive and non-adaptive workflows, patients undergo initial CBCT imaging. However, in online ART, the daily CBCT is further used for organ and target segmentation, which informs daily plan optimization, if applicable. After careful review by the clinical team, either the scheduled (non-adaptive) or adaptive plan is selected for treatment. If the adaptive plan is chosen, a secondary dose calculation is often performed for quality assurance purposes. Due to the additional time required for contour review and plan generation in the adaptive workflow, a secondary position verification scan is recommended prior to treatment delivery.

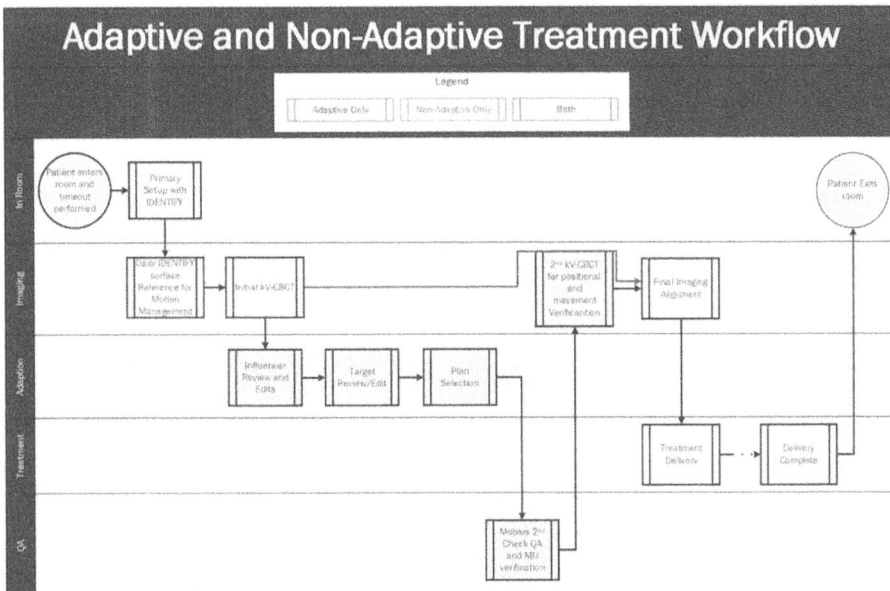

Figure 15.5. Example CBCT-based online ART and non-adaptive treatment workflows utilized by Stanley *et al.* (Reproduced from [61] with permission from John Wiley & Sons. Copyright 2023 The Authors. Journal of Applied Clinical Medical Physics published by Wiley Periodicals, LLC on behalf of The American Association of Physicists in Medicine.)

15.2.7.1 Patient set-up and daily imaging

After the patient has been set up, the appropriate scanning protocol must be selected. This step is critical, as the entire online ART workflow may depend on it. For example, in some systems, the selected algorithm or site determines the influencer structures, i.e. site-specific organs that guide the deformation of target and OAR contours from the reference CT to the daily CBCT. There are two primary reconstruction algorithms offered by Ethos: the analytical and standard Feldkamp–Davis–Kress (FDK) algorithm [117] and the novel iterative CBCT (iCBCT) algorithm, which reduces noise and increases contrast via penalized likelihood statistical analysis [118, 119]. However, iCBCT assumes the patient is static and is thus highly sensitive to anatomic motion [120]. Therefore, iCBCT reconstruction should be utilized in the presence of small amounts of motion (HN, pelvis, brain, thorax/breast/abdomen utilizing breath-hold) and FDK reconstruction should be selected given significant anatomic motion (i.e. free-breathe thorax, abdomen, or breast). Conversely, the uRT-linac 506 allows for kV fan-beam and MV cone-beam CT images to be acquired simultaneously, simplifying image registration and providing image quality sufficient for direct dose calculation, as it is nearly free from image degradation due to photon scatter [48]. Furthermore, the integration of kV and MV imaging enables a significant reduction of artifacts derived from complex metals compared to traditional artifact correction methods [121].

15.2.7.2 Contouring

In online ART workflows, some structures may be automatically contoured using DIR, while others may be segmented using deep learning models such as CNNs [103]. The method of generation often depends on the anatomical site and available system capabilities. Because these auto-generated contours may directly influence downstream processes—such as target propagation, plan optimization, and dose evaluation—it is essential that the clinical team has a strong understanding of how each structure is generated and used. Careful review and editing of these contours are critical to ensure clinical accuracy and safe adaptive plan delivery [103].

15.2.7.3 Plan calculation and selection

In some online ART systems, an sCT is generated by deforming the planning CT to the daily CBCT using DIR, often relying on mutual information-based cost functions and spline-based deformation models [122]. Dose calculation for both scheduled (non-adaptive) and adaptive plans may then be performed on this sCT. In other systems, dose can be calculated directly on the CBCT itself, provided the image quality and HU accuracy are sufficient [23]. For systems using sCTs, rigid alignment between the CBCT and sCT is typically performed prior to dose calculation, sometimes using target-focused similarity metrics. The same planning template used for reference planning is applied during daily adaptation, and the scheduled and adaptive dose distributions are then overlaid on the CBCT anatomy to support plan selection for treatment.

15.2.7.4 Quality assurance

Daily online ART plans differ in MU and fluence compared to reference plans, and should thus be evaluated with PSQA according to traditional professional standards. However, removing the patient from the treatment couch after daily plan generation to perform phantom-based measurements can introduce significant set-up uncertainty, which compromises the use of the reduced planning target volume margins typically employed in online ART. For this reason, PSQA is not typically performed for online adaptive plans prior to delivery.

Instead of performing phantom-based measurements, adapted plans along with the corresponding daily CT and structure sets can be exported to an independent secondary dose calculation system for verification. Prior to adaptive treatment delivery, it is recommended to compare key dosimetric metrics for target coverage and OAR sparing between the primary and secondary calculations, and to evaluate gamma passing rates using clinically appropriate criteria (e.g. 3%/2 mm or 5%/3 mm with a $\geqslant 95\%$ pass rate). Zhao *et al* demonstrated that adapted plan dose calculations on the Ethos system showed good agreement with point dose measurements, patient-specific QA measurements, and independent secondary dose calculations [56]. Furthermore, studies have shown strong correlations between gamma passing rates from secondary dose calculation systems and measurement-based QA across both reference and daily adaptive plans, suggesting that independent dose calculations may serve as an effective QA approach for CBCT-based online ART, particularly when the reference plan has passed initial validation [55].

After secondary dose calculation and evaluation, many clinics will perform a position verification CBCT to account for patient movement and/or anatomy change since the initial CBCT [61, 119], although this may not be required by the delivery system. Once shifts are applied, the patient is ready for treatment. For patients without significant respiratory motion, surface-guided radiotherapy (SGRT) systems can be used to monitor intrafraction motion by tracking the displacement of the surface centroid in real time [123]. In cases requiring breath-hold motion management, the vertical displacement component is often used to monitor chest wall motion and ensure consistency with the planned breath-hold position. In high-precision workflows such as breath-hold CBCT-guided stereotactic adaptive radiotherapy (CT-STAR), deviations beyond a predefined threshold (e.g. 2 mm vertically) can trigger the acquisition of an intrafraction CBCT to verify target alignment [124]. Alternative motion management strategies may include visually guided respiratory training, where patients adjust their breathing to match a predefined amplitude window, supported by either commercial or in-house software solutions. Furthermore, online electronic portal imaging device (EPID) analysis could be used for motion monitoring. Peng *et al* used the EPID panel for monitoring *in vivo* doses from adaptive radiation therapy for cervical cancer. If the global gamma passing rate fell below 88% using a 3%/3 mm threshold, treatments were suspended or terminated pending further investigation [68]. They observed that all plans were at or above a 89% pass rate for six patients, supporting accurate uRT-linac 506c adaptive cervical cancer treatment delivery. The feasibility of this methodology has also been demonstrated for rectal cancer patients [125]. Due to the inability to detect online ART plan deliverability issues without PSQA, Sun *et al* developed a machine learning-based ensemble model for predicting gamma passing rate for uRT-linac 506c SBRT plans. They observed areas under the receiver operator characteristic curve of 0.87 and 0.84 for the 2%/2 mm and 1%/2 mm criteria, respectively, using the ensemble of plan and radiomic models [126].

15.2.8 Offline contour and plan evaluation

Offline contour and plan evaluation in the context of CT-based adaptive radio-therapy extends beyond the initial adaptation process to encompass a comprehensive verification step post-delivery. This phase involves assessing the created plans and contours to ensure concordance with reference plan contour definitions and efficacy in responding to anatomical or physiological changes observed during treatment. Additionally, offline review can be utilized as an opportunity to identify potential changes to the planning directive that can result in an improved plan. Following the delivery of adaptive radiotherapy, the verification process is crucial for confirming the validity of the offline adaptation approach. This involves a detailed analysis of the treated anatomy through comparison with the original treatment plan and the overall objectives of the physician directive. An essential aspect of this verification is the examination of the acquired and created images, where the contours from the planning CT are either propagated or redrawn to the daily anatomy, and the planned dose is recalculated on the current daily anatomy. The goal is to confirm that the adapted plan aligns with the intended treatment goals and adequately addresses any anatomical deviations that may have occurred during the course of treatment. This requires a high level of understanding and communication amongst the treatment team of the goals for the particular patient.

Additionally, with systems that utilize sCT, a pivotal role of the offline assessment is in ensuring the precision and reliability of the generated sCT, particularly in areas of high heterogeneity [99]. The sCT should align closely with the actual patient anatomy, and contours derived from the sCT should accurately represent the target volumes and OARs, as discrepancies in contouring may lead to deviations in dose calculation and subsequent treatment outcomes. While it is not possible to change the sCT with current software versions, evaluation of large discrepancies in sCT can necessitate the need for a re-simulation or changes to the structures and contours.

Lastly, offline dose accumulation review can be used to inform the reviewer of the effects of anatomical variations on the summed, delivered dose. For Ethos, the deformation vector field used in the structure guided DIR is utilized to propagate dose from the sCT to the planning CT. Because of the high-impact that dose mapping and accumulation has on online ART, the results should be closely monitored and methods should be continuously improved [38]. An example of the effects daily adaption may have on dose accumulation, hot and cold spots vary in position daily with adaption, but occur in the same position every day during non-adaptive treatment, leading to greater target homogeneity with online ART [83]. Furthermore, Peng *et al* found good agreement between TPS accumulated adaptive cervical cancer RT dose and three-dimensional dose reconstruction derived from two-dimensional EPID measurements for the uRT-linac 506c [68]. This novel quality assurance step has even been utilized to verify excellent agreement between planned and delivered dose for total bone marrow lymphoid IMRT in the non-adaptive setting [127].

15.2.9 Limitations and future directions

Despite the advancements in offline adaptive strategies, there are inherent limitations and areas for future development. Further integration of clear, site-specific thresholds for determining which patients are the optimal candidates for online ART is needed, and understanding the criteria that warrant adaptive planning is essential for optimizing treatment outcomes. Active offline monitoring and utilization of innovative technologies and artificial intelligence holds promise for allowing detection of subtle anatomical changes that may necessitate adaptation.

Additionally, the exploration of adaptive dose calculation time reduction techniques, particularly with high-quality CBCTs versus sCT, represents a potential avenue for future research. Integrating AI into the dose calculation and evaluation processes may further refine the accuracy of adaptive strategies. Research efforts should focus on developing robust models that can predict dosimetric changes based on patient-specific characteristics and treatment parameters.

15.3 Summary

Offline CT-based ART and online CBCT-based ART represent two complementary strategies for adapting radiotherapy plans in response to patient-specific anatomical changes. Offline ART is typically triggered by anatomical changes observed on routine imaging and involves re-simulation, re-contouring, and re-planning with plan summation to assess cumulative dose. While beneficial, offline ART can be resource-intensive and susceptible to registration uncertainties, requiring robust QA and careful patient selection.

Online ART leverages on-board imaging systems and intelligent optimization platforms to adapt treatment plans in real time, offering precision in daily plan delivery. Clinical adoption remains limited due to challenges in sCT accuracy, resource demands, and workflow complexity. Nevertheless, ongoing advances in AI-based automation, predictive modeling, and integrated QA frameworks are improving feasibility and clinical value.

Together, these approaches highlight the evolving landscape of adaptive radiotherapy, emphasizing the importance of streamlined workflows, reliable image registration, intelligent planning tools, and thoughtful implementation strategies to optimize treatment outcomes.

References

[1] Green O L, Henke L E and Hugo G D 2019 Practical clinical workflows for online and offline adaptive radiation therapy *Semin. Radiat. Oncol.* **29** 219–27

[2] Schwartz D L *et al* 2013 Adaptive radiotherapy for head and neck cancer—dosimetric results from a prospective clinical trial *Radiother. Oncol.* **106** 80–4

[3] Kong F-M *et al* 2017 Effect of midtreatment PET/CT-adapted radiation therapy with concurrent chemotherapy in patients with locally advanced non-small-cell lung cancer: a phase 2 clinical trial *JAMA Oncol* **3** 1358–65

[4] Cai B, Green O L, Kashani R, Rodriguez V L, Mutic S and Yang D 2018 A practical implementation of physics quality assurance for photon adaptive radiotherapy *Z. Für. Med. Phys.* **28** 211–23

[5] Krishnatry R, Bhatia J, Murthy V and Agarwal J P 2018 Survey on adaptive radiotherapy practice *Clin. Oncol.* **30** 819

[6] Bertholet J *et al* 2020 Patterns of practice for adaptive and real-time radiation therapy (POP-ART RT) part II: offline and online plan adaption for interfractional changes *Radiother. Oncol.* **153** 88–96

[7] Brown E *et al* 2015 Predicting the need for adaptive radiotherapy in head and neck cancer *Radiother. Oncol.* **116** 57–63

[8] Brouwer C L, Steenbakkers R J H M, Langendijk J A and Sijtsema N M 2015 Identifying patients who may benefit from adaptive radiotherapy: does the literature on anatomic and dosimetric changes in head and neck organs at risk during radiotherapy provide information to help? *Radiother. Oncol. J. Eur. Soc. Ther. Radiol. Oncol.* **115** 285–94

[9] Heukelom J and Fuller C D 2019 Head and neck cancer adaptive radiation therapy (ART): conceptual considerations for the informed clinician *Semin. Radiat. Oncol.* **29** 258–73

[10] Maniscalco A, Liang X, Lin M-H, Jiang S and Nguyen D 2023 Single patient learning for adaptive radiotherapy dose prediction *Med. Phys.* **50** 7324–37

[11] Lee D *et al* 2022 Deep learning driven predictive treatment planning for adaptive radiotherapy of lung cancer *Radiother. Oncol.* **169** 57–63

[12] Wang C *et al* 2019 Toward predicting the evolution of lung tumors during radiotherapy observed on a longitudinal MR imaging study via a deep learning algorithm *Med. Phys.* **46** 4699–707

[13] Barragán-Montero A M, Van Ooteghem G, Dumont D, Rivas S T, Sterpin E and Geets X 2023 Dosimetrically triggered adaptive radiotherapy for head and neck cancer: considerations for the implementation of clinical protocols *J. Appl. Clin. Med. Phys.* **24** e14095

[14] Liang X *et al* 2021 Automated contour propagation of the prostate from pCT to CBCT images via deep unsupervised learning *Med. Phys.* **48** 1764–70

[15] Liu Y *et al* 2020 CBCT-based synthetic CT generation using deep-attention cycleGAN for pancreatic adaptive radiotherapy *Med. Phys.* **47** 2472–83

[16] Liang X *et al* 2019 Generating synthesized computed tomography (CT) from cone-beam computed tomography (CBCT) using CycleGAN for adaptive radiation therapy *Phys. Med. Biol.* **64** 125002

[17] Chen L, Liang X, Shen C, Jiang S and Wang J 2020 Synthetic CT generation from CBCT images via deep learning *Med. Phys.* **47** 1115–25

[18] Maspero M *et al* 2020 A single neural network for cone-beam computed tomography-based radiotherapy of head-and-neck, lung and breast cancer *Phys. Imaging Radiat. Oncol.* **14** 24–31

[19] Kisling K D *et al* 2018 A snapshot of medical physics practice patterns *J. Appl. Clin. Med. Phys.* **19** 306–15

[20] Yuan Z, Rong Y, Benedict S H, Daly M E, Qiu J and Yamamoto T 2020 Dose of the day' based on cone beam computed tomography and deformable image registration for lung cancer radiotherapy *J. Appl. Clin. Med. Phys.* **21** 88–94

[21] Moteabbed M, Sharp G C, Wang Y, Trofimov A, Efstathiou J A and Lu H-M 2015 Validation of a deformable image registration technique for cone beam CT-based dose verification *Med. Phys.* **42** 196–205

[22] Veiga C *et al* 2014 Toward adaptive radiotherapy for head and neck patients: feasibility study on using CT-to-CBCT deformable registration for 'dose of the day' calculations *Med. Phys.* **41** 031703

[23] Duan J *et al* 2025 Assessing HyperSight iterative CBCT for dose calculation in online adaptive radiotherapy for pelvis and breast patients compared to synthetic CT *J. Appl. Clin. Med. Phys.* **26** e70038

[24] Bojechko C, Hua P, Sumner W, Guram K, Atwood T and Sharabi A 2022 Adaptive replanning using cone beam CT for deformation of original CT simulation *J. Med. Radiat. Sci.* **69** 267–72

[25] Schiff J P *et al* 2023 Prospective *in silico* evaluation of cone-beam computed tomography-guided stereotactic adaptive radiation therapy (CT-STAR) for the ablative treatment of ultracentral thoracic disease *Adv. Radiat. Oncol.* **8** 101226

[26] Mencarelli A *et al* 2014 Deformable image registration for adaptive radiation therapy of head and neck cancer: accuracy and precision in the presence of tumor changes *Int. J. Radiat. Oncol. Biol. Phys.* **90** 680–7

[27] Berenguer R *et al* 2018 The influence of the image registration method on the adaptive radiotherapy. A proof of the principle in a selected case of prostate IMRT *Phys. Med.* **45** 93–8

[28] Rigaud B *et al* 2021 Automatic segmentation using deep learning to enable online dose optimization during adaptive radiation therapy of cervical cancer *Int. J. Radiat. Oncol.* **109** 1096–110

[29] Cardenas C E, Yang J, Anderson B M, Court L E and Brock K B 2019 Advances in auto-segmentation *Semin. Radiat. Oncol.* **29** 185–97

[30] Lowther N J, Marsh S H and Louwe R J W 2020 Quantifying the dose accumulation uncertainty after deformable image registration in head-and-neck radiotherapy *Radiother. Oncol.* **143** 117–25

[31] Brock K K, Mutic S, McNutt T R, Li H and Kessler M L 2017 Use of image registration and fusion algorithms and techniques in radiotherapy: report of the AAPM radiation therapy committee task group no. 132 *Med. Phys.* **44** e43–76

[32] Fu Y, Lei Y, Wang T, Curran W J, Liu T and Yang X 2020 Deep learning in medical image registration: a review *Phys. Med. Biol.* **65** 20TR01

[33] Ghesu F-C *et al* 2019 Multi-scale deep reinforcement learning for realtime 3D-landmark detection in CT scans *IEEE Trans. Pattern. Anal. Mach. Intell.* **41** 176–89

[34] Fu Y *et al* 2020 LungRegNet: an unsupervised deformable image registration method for 4D-CT lung *Med. Phys.* **47** 1763–74

[35] Kearney V, Haaf S, Sudhyadhom A, Valdes G and Solberg T D 2018 An unsupervised convolutional neural network-based algorithm for deformable image registration *Phys. Med. Biol.* **63** 185017

[36] Maintz J B A and Viergever M A 1998 A survey of medical image registration *Med. Image Anal.* **2** 1–36

[37] Guan H and Dong H 2009 Dose calculation accuracy using cone-beam CT (CBCT) for pelvic adaptive radiotherapy *Phys. Med. Biol.* **54** 6239

[38] Murr M *et al* 2023 Applicability and usage of dose mapping/accumulation in radiotherapy *Radiother. Oncol.* **182** 109527

[39] Byrne M *et al* 2022 Varian Ethos online adaptive radiotherapy for prostate cancer: early results of contouring accuracy, treatment plan quality, and treatment time *J. Appl. Clin. Med. Phys.* **23** e13479

[40] Wall P D H, Hirata E, Morin O, Valdes G and Witztum A 2022 Prospective clinical validation of virtual patient-specific quality assurance of volumetric modulated arc therapy radiation therapy plans *Int. J. Radiat. Oncol.* **113** 1091–102

[41] Zeng L *et al* 2023 TransQA: deep hybrid transformer network for measurement-guided volumetric dose prediction of pre-treatment patient-specific quality assurance *Phys. Med. Biol.* **68** 205010

[42] Kimura Y, Kadoya N, Tomori S, Oku Y and Jingu K 2020 Error detection using a convolutional neural network with dose difference maps in patient-specific quality assurance for volumetric modulated arc therapy *Phys. Med.* **73** 57–64

[43] Vandewinckele L *et al* 2020 Overview of artificial intelligence-based applications in radiotherapy: recommendations for implementation and quality assurance *Radiother. Oncol.* **153** 55–66

[44] Schreier J, Genghi A, Laaksonen H, Morgas T and Haas B 2020 Clinical evaluation of a full-image deep segmentation algorithm for the male pelvis on cone-beam CT and CT *Radiother. Oncol.* **145** 1–6

[45] de la Zerda A, Armbruster B and Xing L 2007 Formulating adaptive radiation therapy (ART) treatment planning into a closed-loop control framework *Phys. Med. Biol.* **52** 4137

[46] Kim M M *et al* 2019 Dosimetric characterization of the dual layer MLC system for an O-ring linear accelerator *Technol. Cancer Res. Treat.* **18** 1533033819883641

[47] Byrne M, Archibald-Heeren B, Hu Y, Greer P, Luo S and Aland T 2022 Assessment of semi-automated stereotactic treatment planning for online adaptive radiotherapy in ethos *Med. Dosim.* **47** 342–7

[48] Yu L, Zhao J, Zhang Z, Wang J and Hu W 2021 Commissioning of and preliminary experience with a new fully integrated computed tomography linac *J. Appl. Clin. Med. Phys.* **22** 208–23

[49] Sun W *et al* 2024 The performance of a new type accelerator uRT-linac 506c evaluated by a quality assurance automation system *J. Appl. Clin. Med. Phys.* **25** e14226

[50] Kisling K, Keiper T D, Branco D, Kim G G-Y, Moore K L and Ray X 2022 Clinical commissioning of an adaptive radiotherapy platform: results and recommendations *J. Appl. Clin. Med. Phys.* **23** e13801

[51] Nelissen K J, Versteijne E, Senan S, Hoffmans D, Slotman B J and Verbakel W F A R 2023 Evaluation of a workflow for cone-beam CT-guided online adaptive palliative radiotherapy planned using diagnostic CT scans *J. Appl. Clin. Med. Phys.* **24** e13841

[52] Wegener S, Schindhelm R, Tamihardja J, Sauer O A and Razinskas G 2023 Evaluation of the Ethos synthetic computed tomography for bolus-covered surfaces *Phys. Med.* **113** 102662

[53] Lemus O M D *et al* 2023 Influence of air mapping errors on the dosimetric accuracy of prostate CBCT-guided online adaptive radiation therapy *J. Appl. Clin. Med. Phys.* **24** e14057

[54] Schiff J P *et al* 2022 Simulated computed tomography-guided stereotactic adaptive radiotherapy (CT-STAR) for the treatment of locally advanced pancreatic cancer *Radiother. Oncol.* **175** 144–51

[55] Shen C *et al* 2023 Clinical experience on patient-specific quality assurance for CBCT-based online adaptive treatment plan *J. Appl. Clin. Med. Phys.* **24** e13918

[56] Zhao X, Stanley D N, Cardenas C E, Harms J and Popple R A 2023 Do we need patient-specific QA for adaptively generated plans? Retrospective evaluation of delivered online adaptive treatment plans on Varian Ethos *J. Appl. Clin. Med. Phys.* **24** e13876

[57] Bertholet J *et al* 2020 Patterns of practice for adaptive and real-time radiation therapy (POP-ART RT) part II: offline and online plan adaption for interfractional changes *Radiother. Oncol.* **153** 88–96

[58] Viscariello N N *et al* 2024 Quantitative assessment of full-time equivalent effort for kilovoltage-cone beam computed tomography guided online adaptive radiation therapy for medical physicists *Pract. Radiat. Oncol.* **15** e72–e81

[59] Branco D, Mayadev J, Moore K and Ray X 2023 Dosimetric and feasibility evaluation of a CBCT-based daily adaptive radiotherapy protocol for locally advanced cervical cancer *J. Appl. Clin. Med. Phys.* **24** e13783

[60] Shepherd M *et al* 2021 Pathway for radiation therapists online advanced adapter training and credentialing *Tech. Innov. Patient Support Radiat. Oncol.* **20** 54–60

[61] Stanley D N *et al* 2023 A roadmap for implementation of kV-CBCT online adaptive radiation therapy and initial first year experiences *J. Appl. Clin. Med. Phys.* **24** e13961

[62] Yock A D, Ahmed M, Ayala-Peacock D, Chakravarthy A B and Price M 2021 Initial analysis of the dosimetric benefit and clinical resource cost of CBCT-based online adaptive radiotherapy for patients with cancers of the cervix or rectum *J. Appl. Clin. Med. Phys.* **22** 210–21

[63] Rahman M *et al* 2024 Mitigating risks in cone beam computed tomography guided online adaptive radiation therapy: a preventative reference planning review approach *Adv. Radiat. Oncol.* **9** 101614

[64] Morgan H E *et al* 2023 Preliminary evaluation of PTV margins for online adaptive radiation therapy of the prostatic fossa *Pract. Radiat. Oncol.* **13** e345–53

[65] Zwart L G M *et al* 2022 Cone-beam computed tomography-guided online adaptive radiotherapy is feasible for prostate cancer patients *Phys. Imaging Radiat. Oncol.* **22** 98–103

[66] Moazzezi M, Rose B, Kisling K, Moore K L and Ray X 2021 Prospects for daily online adaptive radiotherapy via ethos for prostate cancer patients without nodal involvement using unedited CBCT auto-segmentation *J. Appl. Clin. Med. Phys.* **22** 82–93

[67] Shelley C E *et al* 2023 Implementing cone-beam computed tomography-guided online adaptive radiotherapy in cervical cancer *Clin. Transl. Radiat. Oncol.* **40** 100596

[68] Peng H, Zhang J, Xu N, Zhou Y, Tan H and Ren T 2023 Fan beam CT-guided online adaptive external radiotherapy of uterine cervical cancer: a dosimetric evaluation *BMC Cancer* **23** 588

[69] Sibolt P *et al* 2021 Clinical implementation of artificial intelligence-driven cone-beam computed tomography-guided online adaptive radiotherapy in the pelvic region *Phys. Imaging Radiat. Oncol.* **17** 1–7

[70] de Jong R, Visser J, van Wieringen N, Wiersma J, Geijsen D and Bel A 2021 Feasibility of conebeam CT-based online adaptive radiotherapy for neoadjuvant treatment of rectal cancer *Radiat. Oncol.* **16** 136

[71] Åström L M, Behrens C P, Storm K S, Sibolt P and Serup-Hansen E 2022 Online adaptive radiotherapy of anal cancer: normal tissue sparing, target propagation methods, and first clinical experience *Radiother. Oncol.* **176** 92–8

[72] Xia X *et al* 2021 An artificial intelligence-based full-process solution for radiotherapy: a proof of concept study on rectal cancer *Front. Oncol.* **10**

[73] Yu L *et al* 2023 Technical note: first implementation of a one-stop solution of radiotherapy with full-workflow automation based on CT-linac combination *Med. Phys.* **50** 3117–26

[74] Åström L M *et al* 2022 Online adaptive radiotherapy of urinary bladder cancer with full re-optimization to the anatomy of the day: initial experience and dosimetric benefits *Radiother. Oncol.* **171** 37–42

[75] Khouya A *et al* 2023 Adaptation time as a determinant of the dosimetric effectiveness of online adaptive radiotherapy for bladder cancer *Cancers* **15** 23

[76] Hotsinpiller W S, Stanley D N, Harms J, Pogue J A, Cardenas C and McDonald A M 2023 Early experience with CBCT-guided online adaptive radiotherapy for muscle invasive bladder cancer *Int. J. Radiat. Oncol. Biol. Phys.* **117** e393–4

[77] Azzarouali S *et al* 2023 Online adaptive radiotherapy for bladder cancer using a simultaneous integrated boost and fiducial markers *Radiat. Oncol.* **18** 165

[78] Pöttgen C *et al* 2023 Fractionation versus adaptation for compensation of target volume changes during online adaptive radiotherapy for bladder cancer: answers from a prospective registry *Cancers* **15** 20

[79] Håkansson K, Giannoulis E, Lindegaard A, Friborg J and Vogelius I 2023 CBCT-based online adaptive radiotherapy for head and neck cancer—dosimetric evaluation of first clinical experience *Acta. Oncol.* **62** 1369–74

[80] All S *et al* 2023 *In silico* analysis of adjuvant head and neck online adaptive radiation therapy *Adv. Radiat. Oncol.* **9** 101319

[81] Guberina M *et al* 2024 Prospects for online adaptive radiation therapy (ART) for head and neck cancer *Radiat. Oncol.* **19** 4

[82] Yoon S W *et al* 2020 Initial evaluation of a novel cone-beam CT-based semi-automated online adaptive radiotherapy system for head and neck cancer treatment—a timing and automation quality study *Cureus* **12** e9660

[83] Mao W *et al* 2022 Evaluation of auto-contouring and dose distributions for online adaptive radiation therapy of patients with locally advanced lung cancers *Pract. Radiat. Oncol.* **12** e329–38

[84] Li R *et al* 2024 Adapt-on-demand: a novel strategy for personalized adaptive radiotherapy for locally advance lung cancer *Pract. Radiat. Oncol.* **14** e395–e406

[85] Duan J *et al* 2024 Enhancing precision in radiation therapy for locally advanced lung cancer: a case study of cone-beam computed tomography (CBCT)-based online adaptive techniques and the promise of HyperSight™ iterative CBCT *Cureus* **16** e66943

[86] Duan J *et al* 2025 Assessing dosimetric benefits of cone beam computed tomography-guided online adaptive radiation treatment frequencies for lung cancer *Adv. Radiat. Oncol.* **10** 101740

[87] Brown M B, Yusuf M B, Harms J M, Pogue J A, Stanley D N and McDonald A 2024 The use of adaptive radiation in a retroperitoneal seminoma patient with poor candidacy for chemotherapy: a teaching case *Appl. Radiat. Oncol.* **13** 49–54

[88] Montalvo S K *et al* 2023 On the feasibility of improved target coverage without compromising organs at risk using online adaptive stereotactic partial breast irradiation (A-SPBI) *J. Appl. Clin. Med. Phys.* **24** e13813

[89] Pogue J A *et al* 2023 Improved dosimetry and plan quality for accelerated partial breast irradiation using online adaptive radiotherapy: a single institutional study *Adv. Radiat. Oncol.* **9** 101414

[90] Schiff J P *et al* 2022 *In silico* trial of computed tomography-guided stereotactic adaptive radiation therapy (CT-STAR) for the treatment of abdominal oligometastases *Int. J. Radiat. Oncol.* **114** 1022–31

[91] Kim M *et al* 2022 The first reported case of a patient with pancreatic cancer treated with cone beam computed tomography-guided stereotactic adaptive radiotherapy (CT-STAR) *Radiat. Oncol.* **17** 157

[92] Yock A D *et al* 2023 Triggering daily online adaptive radiotherapy in the pelvis: dosimetric effects and procedural implications of trigger parameer-value selection *J. Appl. Clin. Med. Phys.* **24** e14060

[93] Ghimire R, Moore K L, Branco D, Rash D L, Mayadev J and Ray X 2023 Forecasting patient-specific dosimetric benefit from daily online adaptive radiotherapy for cervical cancer *Biomed. Phys. Eng. Express* **9** 045030

[94] Pogue J A *et al* 2024 Utilizing unsupervised machine learning to identify an optimal planning target volume size threshold for online adaptive stereotactic partial breast irradiation *Cureus* **16** a1191

[95] Pogue J A *et al* 2024 Unlocking the adaptive advantage: correlation and machine learning classification to identify optimal online adaptive stereotactic partial breast candidates *Phys. Med. Biol.* **69** 115050

[96] Oldenburger E, De Roover R, Poels K, Depuydt T, Isebaert S and Haustermans K 2023 'Scan-(pre)plan-treat' workflow for bone metastases using the ethos therapy system: a single-center, *in silico* experience *Adv. Radiat. Oncol.* **8** 101258

[97] Price A T *et al* 2023 *In silico* trial of simulation-free hippocampal-avoidance whole brain adaptive radiotherapy *Phys. Imaging Radiat. Oncol.* **28** 100491

[98] Nelissen K J *et al* 2023 Same-day adaptive palliative radiotherapy without prior CT simulation: early outcomes in the FAST-METS study *Radiother. Oncol.* **182** 109538

[99] Wegener S, Weick S, Schindhelm R, Tamihardja J, Sauer O A and Razinskas G 2024 Feasibility of Ethos adaptive treatments of lung tumors and associated quality assurance *J. Appl. Clin. Med. Phys.* **25** e14311

[100] Lin M, Kavanaugh J A, Kim M, Cardenas C E and Rong Y 2023 Physicists should perform reference planning for CBCT guided online adaptive radiotherapy *J. Appl. Clin. Med. Phys.* **24** e14163

[101] Wegener S *et al* 2022 Prospective risk analysis of the online-adaptive artificial intelligence-driven workflow using the Ethos treatment system *Z. Für Med. Phys.* **34** 384–96

[102] Iqbal Z *et al* 2025 Establishing a safety net in x-ray-based online adaptive radiation therapy: early detection of planning deficiencies through upstream physics plan review *Int. J. Radiat. Oncol.* **122** 865–72

[103] Archambault Y *et al* 2020 Making on-line adaptive radiotherapy possible using artificial intelligence and machine learning for efficient daily re-planning *Med. Phys. Int. J.* **8** 77–86

[104] Pokharel S, Pacheco A and Tanner S 2022 Assessment of efficacy in automated plan generation for Varian Ethos intelligent optimization engine *J. Appl. Clin. Med. Phys.* **23** e13539

[105] Calmels L *et al* 2022 Evaluation of an automated template-based treatment planning system for radiotherapy of anal, rectal and prostate cancer *Tech. Innov. Patient Support Radiat. Oncol.* **22** 30–6

[106] El-qmache A and McLellan J 2023 Investigating the feasibility of using Ethos generated treatment plans for head and neck cancer patients *Tech. Innov. Patient. Support. Radiat. Oncol.* **27** 100216

[107] Pogue J A *et al* 2023 Benchmarking automated machine learning-enhanced planning with Ethos against manual and knowledge-based planning for locally advanced lung cancer *Adv. Radiat. Oncol.* **8** 101292

[108] Roberfroid B, Barragán-Montero A M, Dechambre D, Sterpin E, Lee J A and Geets X 2023 Comparison of Ethos template-based planning and AI-based dose prediction: general performance, patient optimality, and limitations *Phys. Med.* **116** 103178

[109] Visak J *et al* 2023 Evaluating machine learning enhanced intelligent-optimization-engine (IOE) performance for ethos head-and-neck (HN) plan generation *J. Appl. Clin. Med. Phys.* **24** e13950

[110] Pogue J A *et al* 2023 Leveraging intelligent optimization for automated, cardiac-sparing accelerated partial breast treatment planning *Front. Oncol.* **13** 1130119

[111] Stanley D N *et al* 2024 Suitability of the Ethos treatment planning system for automated SRT planning for large body habitus patients *AAPM 65th Annual Meeting and Exhibition (Houston, TX, July 2023)*

[112] Ram U *et al* 2025 Evaluation of high-fidelity mode for semi-automated multi-met, single-isocenter stereotactic radiosurgery planning using the ethos 2.0 planning system *Cureus* **17** a1420

[113] Pogue J A *et al* 2025 Leveraging high-fidelity planning for improved online adaptive stereotactic partial breast treatment efficacy *Cureus* **17** a1447

[114] Zhong Y *et al* 2021 Clinical implementation of automated treatment planning for rectum intensity-modulated radiotherapy using voxel-based dose prediction and post-optimization strategies *Front. Oncol.* **11** 697995

[115] Sun Z *et al* 2022 A hybrid optimization strategy for deliverable intensity-modulated radiotherapy plan generation using deep learning-based dose prediction *Med. Phys.* **49** 1344–56

[116] Lin J *et al* 2024 ART2Dose: a comprehensive dose verification platform for online adaptive radiotherapy *Med. Phys.* **51** 18–30

[117] Mori S, Endo M, Komatsu S, Kandatsu S, Yashiro T and Baba M 2006 A combination-weighted Feldkamp-based reconstruction algorithm for cone-beam CT *Phys. Med. Biol.* **51** 3953

[118] Lim R, Penoncello G P, Hobbis D, Harrington D P and Rong Y 2022 Technical note: characterization of novel iterative reconstructed cone beam CT images for dose tracking and adaptive radiotherapy on L-shape linacs *Med. Phys.* **49** 7715–32

[119] Wang Y- F *et al* 2023 Enhancing safety in AI-driven cone-beam CT-based online adaptive radiotherapy: development and implementation of an interdisciplinary workflow *Adv. Radiat. Oncol.* **9** 101399

[120] Peterlik I *et al* 2021 Reducing residual-motion artifacts in iterative 3D CBCT reconstruction in image-guided radiation therapy *Med. Phys.* **48** 6497–507

[121] Ni X *et al* 2023 Metal artifacts reduction in kV-CT images with polymetallic dentures and complex metals based on MV-CBCT images in radiotherapy *Sci. Rep.* **13** 8970

[122] Rueckert D, Aljabar P, Heckemann R A, Hajnal J V and Hammers A 2006 Diffeomorphic registration using B-splines *Medical Image Computing and Computer-Assisted Intervention—MICCAI 2006* ed R Larsen, M Nielsen and J Sporring (Berlin: Springer) pp 702–9

[123] Stanley D N, Covington E, Harms J, Pogue J, Cardenas C E and Popple R A 2023 Evaluation and correlation of patient movement during online adaptive radiotherapy with CBCT and a surface imaging system *J. Appl. Clin. Med. Phys.* **24** e14133

[124] Kim T *et al* 2024 Feasibility of surface-guidance combined with CBCT for intra-fractional breath-hold motion management during Ethos RT *J. Appl. Clin. Med. Phys.* **25** e14242

[125] Chen L *et al* 2022 A clinically relevant online patient QA solution with daily CT scans and EPID-based *in vivo* dosimetry: a feasibility study on rectal cancer *Phys. Med. Biol.* **67** 225003

[126] Sun W *et al* 2024 Machine learning-based ensemble prediction model for the gamma passing rate of VMAT-SBRT plan *Phys. Med.* **117** 103204

[127] Jiang D *et al* 2023 Total marrow lymphoid irradiation IMRT treatment using a novel CT-linac *Eur. J. Med. Res.* **28** 463

Chapter 16

Artificial intelligence in MRI-guided adaptive radiation therapy

Lauren Smith, Yao Zhao, Jinzhong Yang and X. Sharon Qi

Adaptive radiation therapy (ART) is a process where a personalized treatment plan may be created for each fraction based on daily imaging information. ART is growing in popularity and has been shown to improve the therapeutic ratio for certain RT sites. In particular, the introduction of MR-linac systems in radiation therapy has allowed for high-quality, real-time MR images to be used to facilitate adaptive treatment. Artificial intelligence (AI) has recently been introduced as a tool in modern radiation therapy and may provide a solution to some challenges that currently burden the efficiency of MR-guided ART. This chapter provides an overview of clinically available MR-guided ART systems and techniques. Further, clinical challenges associated with MR-guided ART, such as synthetic CT generation, auto-segmentation, and image registration, will be introduced and the integration of AI solutions into the MR-guided ART domain will be explored.

16.1 Introduction

Radiation therapy (RT) is currently one of the mainstays of cancer treatment, with approximately 50% or higher of all cancer patients receiving RT during their treatment [1]. Image-guided radiation therapy (IGRT) has become the standard RT practice to enable accurate and precise delivery, leading to the widening of the therapeutic ratio [2, 3]. Various imaging technologies, such as computed tomography (CT), magnetic resonance imaging (MRI), and positron emission tomography (PET), are used to guide RT to precisely deliver the dose to targets while avoiding unnecessary dose to nearby critical structures [3]. CT-guided RT, a type of radiation therapy using CT-based technology, is used to guide the delivery of radiation beams to the tumor, ensuring accurate targeting [3]. The latest development of combining PET-CT and radiotherapy delivery involves using biological markers or characteristics of tumors to guide the delivery of radiation treatment, allowing radiation therapy to be tailored more specifically to the individual characteristics of the tumor and patient to potentially improve treatment outcomes and minimize side effects [4]. Recent development of magnetic resonance-guided radiation therapy (MRgRT) integrates advanced MRI technology with a radiation therapy delivery system, providing a paradigm change in aspects of treatment planning, monitoring, and adaptation. Compared to CT-guided RT, MRgRT provides advantages such as superior soft-tissue contrast, organ motion visualization, and the ability to monitor tumor and tissue physiologic changes [5].

Adaptive radiation therapy (ART) is a closed-loop radiation treatment process where the initial treatment plan may be modified, via frequent imaging acquisition such as daily imaging, using systematic feedback of measurements [6]. ART is expected to maximize the therapeutic ratio by further increasing tumor dose while maintaining or reducing normal tissue complication.

16.2 Overview of MRI-guided ART systems

MRI-guided adaptive therapy is an advanced approach that utilizes real-time MRI during treatment sessions to guide and adapt the delivery of radiation based on changes in the tumor and surrounding anatomy. Real-time MRI provides detailed information about the tumor and surrounding tissues, allowing for adjustments to be made to the radiation treatment plan as needed.

The MRgRT technique allows for precise targeting of tumors while minimizing radiation exposure to healthy tissues, leading to an improved therapeutic ratio. In addition, MRgRT provides superior soft-tissue contrast compared to CT guidance and is capable of providing different contrast based on the sequences used. Unlike CBCT on the linac, MRgRT has the advantage of being able to acquire images while the treatment beam is on, enabling real-time monitoring of organ motion without the need for implanted fiducials or surrogate motion management systems.

16.2.1 High field MRI system

Elekta Unity (Elekta AB, Stockholm, Sweden) is the world's first high-field MR-linac that integrates a 7 MV flattening filter-free (FFF) linear accelerator system with a 1.5 tesla Philips (Philips Healthcare, Best, the Netherlands) MRI system [7]. The system received the CE mark in June 2018 and FDA approval in December 2018 [8]. The Unity system is designed as a bore-type machine with a linac system that rotates around the MRI system and has an inner bore diameter of 70 cm (figure 16.1) [9]. Due to this design, the system has a source axis distance (SAD) of 143.5 cm and a maximum field size of 57.4 cm × 22.0 cm. The radiation beam is perpendicular to the magnetic field orientation. The diaphragms define the cross-plane field size while the multi-leaf collimator (MLC) leaves move in the in-plane direction to shape the field, parallel to the magnet bore. The MLC has 160 leaves with a nominal leaf width of 0.7175 cm. The treatment couch moves in the longitudinal direction only; however, during treatment the couch is not designed to move to adjust treatment iso-center location. Instead, online adaptive planning can be utilized to account for iso-center shifts. The system offers an integrated online adaptive planning workflow implemented with online Moncaco, a Monte Carlo

(a)

(b)

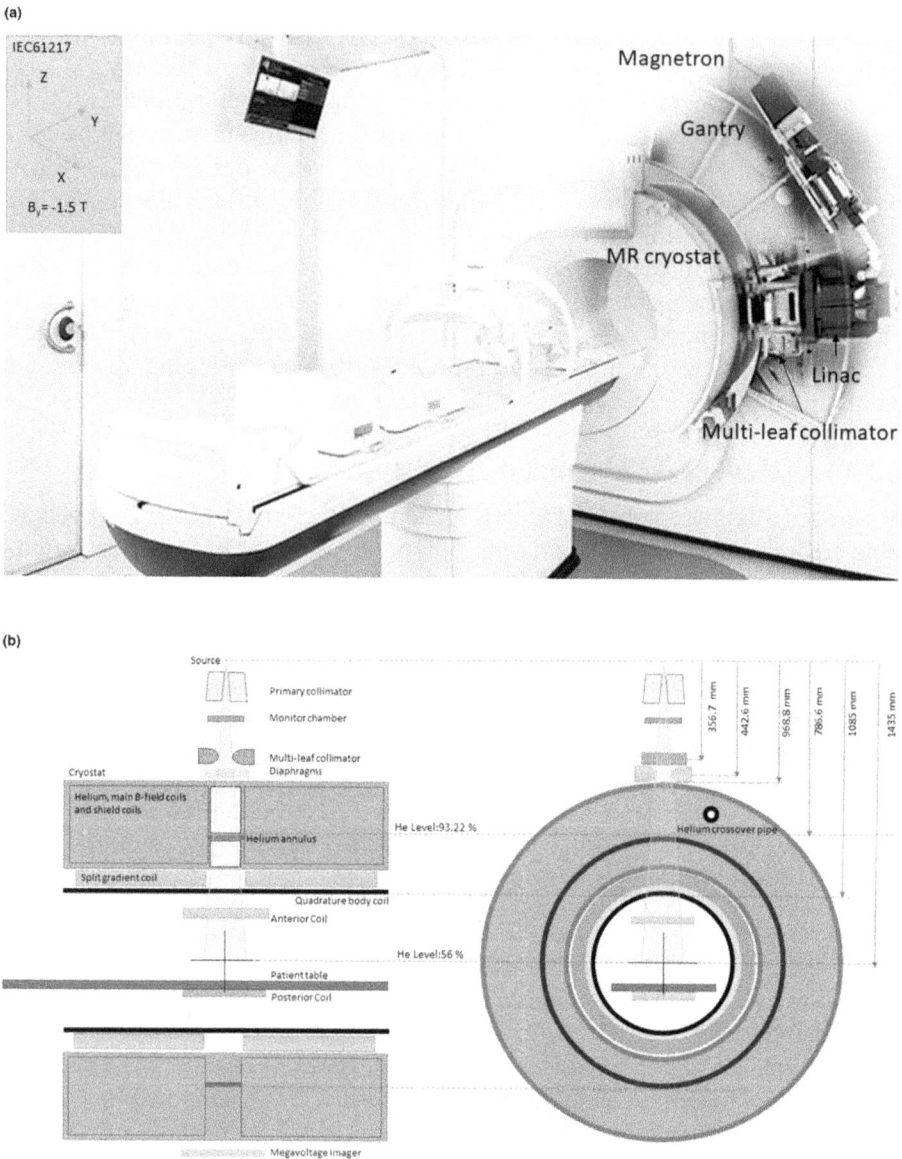

Figure 16.1. (a) Elekta Unity components, IEC61217 coordinate system, and B-field direction. (b) Cross-section of the beam delivery system and the magnet. The main B0 field has its vector directed out of the bore (negative IECY axis). (Reproduced from [9]. CC BY 3.0.)

based treatment planning system (TPS) that optimizes and calculates the dose distribution in the presence of a magnetic field [10]. The system is also capable of real-time tumor tracking, allowing simultaneous MR imagining and treatment delivery. In its first version, the Unity system offered only tumor motion monitoring [11]. In late 2023, Elekta released the comprehensive motion management (CMM) system, allowing for different levels of motion management, including beam gating, for better control of respiratory motion and other motion uncertainty during treatment delivery [12]. It is also worth noting that due to the high strength of the magnetic field, the beam profile is inherently off-central and asymmetric. In addition, the electron return effect (ERE) resulting from the magnetic field causes electrons to change trajectory to 'return' to a higher density material at the interface of exiting a higher density material into a lower density material [13].

16.2.2 Low-field MRI system

The ViewRay MRIdian (Oakwood, Cleveland, OH), shown in figure 16.2, is one of the two currently commercially available MRgRT platforms. In contrast to Elekta's Unity, the ViewRay system makes use of a 0.35 tesla low-field MRI scanner for MRI-guided treatment. This system paved the way for clinical MRgRT, being the first MR-linac device to gain FDA approval in 2012 [14]. The initial system was designed with cobalt-60 sources for irradiation and was later integrated with a linear accelerator, which was cleared by the FDA in 2017 [14]. The MRIdian design consists of a split-bore superconducting magnet with a 70 cm bore diameter perpendicular to a linear accelerator capable of producing 6 MV FFF photon treatment beams [15]. The MRIdian is capable of producing coplanar static IMRT fields and can deliver dose at 650 MU/min with a 0.5 rpm gantry rotation [5]. Currently, the MRIdian uses a balanced steady state free precession pulse sequence for MRI that may be used for treatment planning, set-up verification, and imaging during delivery [5]. Compared to the high-field MR-linac, the 0.35 T MRIdian has the disadvantage of lower image signal–noise ratio (SNR), but the advantages of diminished magnetic susceptibility artifacts, smaller geometric distortion in MR images, and a more minimal electron return effect—resulting in less perturbations to the dose distribution [14]. A significant benefit of the MRIdian system is its ability for real-time imaging during treatment while the radiation beam is on, enabling high-quality monitoring of intrafraction motion during treatment. This feature allows for real-time tracking and automatic gating based on user defined boundaries where the 2D motion is evaluated from a sagittal cine image [5]. Additionally, unlike conventional linacs, the MRIdian has functionality for online adaptive therapy

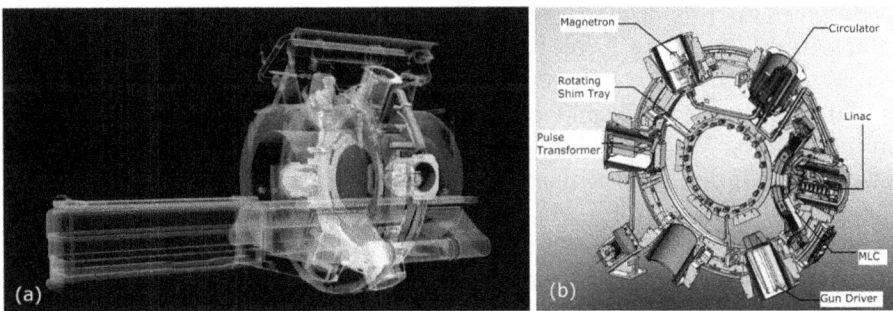

Figure 16.2. (a) Schematic of the Viewray MRIdian system and (b) gantry with linac components. (Reproduced with permission from [16]. Copyright 2019 Elsevier.)

which may be used to adapt the treatment plan while the patient is on the table in cases where there is large interfraction movement or deformation of critical structures. Plan adaption allows for the target and organs at risk (OARs) to be modified or re-contoured and may involve fluence re-optimization using the original objectives or full re-optimization using new planning objectives [16].

Other low-field MR-linac devices are currently in development and, in the future, may become more prevalent in the clinic. One example of such a system is the MagnetTx Aurora-RT which received FDA premarket clearance in 2022 [17] and treated its first patient in 2023 [15]. The Aurora-RT is a 0.5 T MR-linac which utilizes an open bore in-line design to mitigate the electron return effect [15]. The Aurora-RT is starting to image patients as part of an ongoing clinical trial (NCT04358913) [18, 19] and data on clinical experience with this system should become available in the near future. Since there is limited clinical data available on this system, this chapter will focus on the two currently available clinical devices: the high-field Elekta Unity and low-field ViewRay MRIdian MR-linac devices.

16.3 MRI-guided ART workflow

16.3.1 Offline MRI-guided ART workflow

Offline adaptive treatment is possible with MR-linac technology, and the workflow is similar to offline adaptive workflows for conventional linear accelerators where the adaptation takes place between treatment fractions. Imaging acquired at the time of treatment is assessed to determine if adapting the plan would be useful in order to maximize the dose to the target and minimize the dose to surrounding tissue. Typically, the decision for adaptation is based on a pre-defined clinical threshold for plan performance and is dependent on the decision of the treating physician. Assessment of the base plan may be done manually or by using complex automated tools to estimate the cumulative dose that would result from choosing whether to adapt the base plan [20]. The goal of adaptive treatment is to improve clinical outcomes by modifying the plan to account for changes in the target or OAR size, shape, and function or changes due to patient weight loss or gain [20]. Considering MRgRT using an MR-linac, the image acquired at treatment is an MRI which alone cannot be used for planning since it inherently lacks the electron density information necessary for dose calculation. Because of this, the MR-linac planning workflow can be divided into a CT-sim workflow or MRI-sim workflow. The options are to either use a CT-sim image for planning which is registered to secondary MR images (CT-sim workflow), or to create a synthetic CT (sCT) image from the acquired MRI-sim which does not require a CT-sim to be acquired (MRI-sim workflow). If the image acquired during treatment is of sufficient quality, it may be used as the basis for adaptive planning using one of these workflows. Alternatively, a re-simulation CT or MRI may be acquired for the patient.

After an appropriate image for dose calculation is acquired, the target and OAR contours may be adjusted as needed. The base plan may be recalculated on the new image or if the recalculated plan is not deemed clinically acceptable, a newly optimized plan may be created based on the updated image and contours [20]. The optimization process for offline adaptive planning does not differ from conventional treatment planning. Following plan creation, quality assurance (QA) must be performed for that plan, in accordance with standard workflows for plan QA prior to plan delivery. Since this is an entirely new plan compared to the base plan, it should be treated as an independent plan for plan review and QA purposes. The delivery of the offline adapted plan does not differ from the delivery of a conventional plan. Considering the timescale of offline adaptive treatment, it is not suited to correct for anatomical changes that occur at a high frequency (occur within a fraction) but more for gradual changes that may occur once or infrequently over the entire course of treatment [20].

16.3.2 Online MRI-guided ART workflow

The largest difference between online and offline adaptive treatment is the timescale of the process. While offline adaptive plans are adjusted between treatment sessions, over the course of a few days, online adaptive treatments take place entirely during the treatment session, meaning online ART can account for both systematic and random variations in anatomy [21]. Imaging of the patient, assessment of the need for ART, re-planning, and plan QA all occur while the patient is on the table for online ART [20]. Because of this, the workflow is compressed into a short time frame on the scale of minutes. Online ART requires specialized treatment planning systems highly integrated with the treatment delivery unit as well as necessary time allocation to ensure the adaptation can be done during the treatment slot and the availability of physicians, physicists, dosimetrists, and therapists trained in the ART workflow must be accounted for [20]. Since online adaptation has these specific requirements, it is best used in situations where the need to adapt is predictable and known ahead of treatment initiation [20]. For example, sites in the abdomen and pelvis prone to daily anatomic changes are good candidates for online ART [20]. It is likely that online ART will be needed multiple times over the course of treatment and, as such, it is important that the base plan is robust and employs straightforward optimization techniques and structures for efficient re-planning during treatment. For example, optimization structures such as rings and tuning target structures may be avoided and structures far from the target should not be used for plan optimization [22]. Equal importance must be placed on any OARs coplanar to the target as they may move closer to the target and high dose region at the time of treatment [20, 22]. The specifics of online MR ART workflows for high-field and low-field systems are discussed below.

16.3.2.1 High field online ART workflow

A diagram representing the workflow for online ART using the Elekta Unity system is shown in figure 16.3. The online ART workflow begins with daily MR assessment. The patient is first cleared for MR safety, and then set up on the treatment couch, replicating the simulation position. A 3D MR image is acquired for adaptive treatment planning. Upon completion of imaging acquisition, the images are automatically transferred over to the online Monaco treatment planning system.

```
                    ┌─────────────────────────┐
                    │   MR safety Assessment   │
                    └─────────────────────────┘
                                │
                    ┌─────────────────────────┐
                    │      Setup patient       │
                    └─────────────────────────┘
                                │
                    ┌─────────────────────────┐
                    │      Take daily MRI      │
                    └─────────────────────────┘
                                │
                    ┌─────────────────────────┐
                    │ Register daily MRI to ref CT │
                    └─────────────────────────┘
                                │
                    ┌─────────────────────────┐
                    │      Assess anatomy      │
                    └─────────────────────────┘
                                │
                    ┌─────────────────────────┐
                    │ Decide on adaptation method │
                    └─────────────────────────┘
```

Figure depicting flowchart with branches:

- "Adapt to Position"
  - Run optimization
    - Action limit not exceeded
    - Action limit exceeded
      - Physician review
- "Adapt to Shape"
  - Run deformable registration
  - Evaluate contours
  - Re-contour, if needed
  - Re-plan, if needed
  - Run optimization
  - Physician review

Both branches lead to:
- Secondary MU check
- Verification MRI scan, if needed
- Treat and real-time MRI

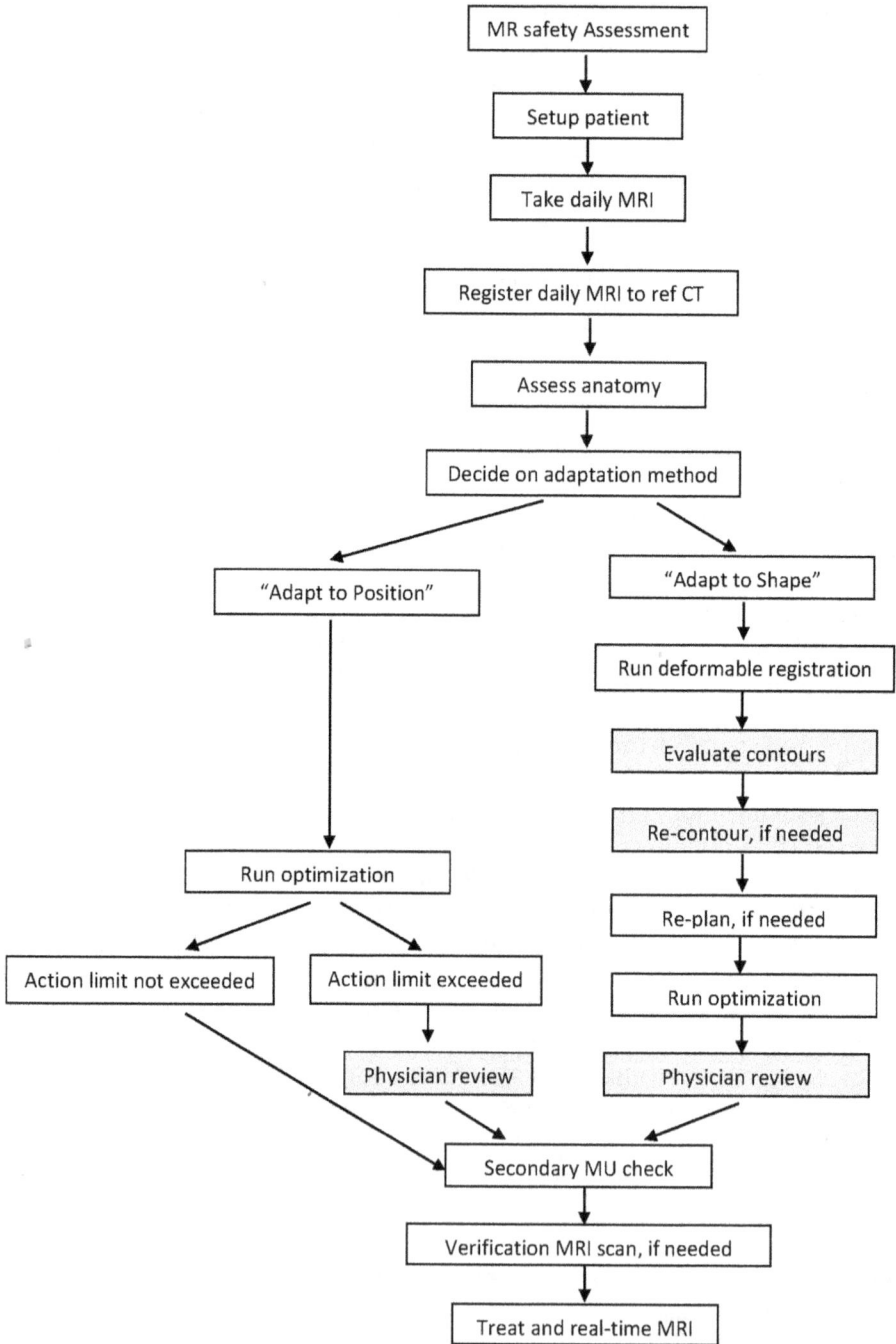

Figure 16.3. Diagram depicting the online adaptive workflow of the Elekta Unity system.

Once the MR image is imported into online Monaco, an automatic rigid registration is initiated, which allows for translation only. Manual registration can be performed to adjust the fusion result. Once the registration has been reviewed and approved, plan adaptation is initiated.

The treatment plan is adapted every fraction. The Elekta Unity system offers two different plan adaptation approaches: adapt to position (ATP) and adapt to shape (ATS) [23]. After image fusion, the physician will choose an adaption workflow based on the anatomical change of that day. The consideration may include tumor size and morphological shape changes, the proximity of OARs to the target compared to simulation, or insufficient ATP plan quality if ATS is not the first choice, etc. In the ATP workflow, the treatment iso-center is moved to a new location (virtual couch shift) based on the image fusion. The treatment plan is then recalculated or re-optimized based on the simulation CT using one of the four different adaptation algorithms provided by the Monaco TPS: original segments, adapt segments, optimize weights, and optimize shapes. This process is equivalent to traditional IGRT approach because the plan adaptation does not consider the daily anatomical variations. Instead of moving the couch, the plan iso-center is moved to the treatment day's position and plan is re-optimized or recalculated based on the anatomy at simulation [24, 25]. In the ATS workflow, a deformable registration between the simulation CT and daily MR scan is performed after the image fusion. All contours are deformed or rigidly mapped from simulation CT scan to the daily MR scan based on the user choice. Contours are then reviewed and edited if needed by the physician. The entire reference plan is then copied to the MR scan, including beam arrangement, IMRT constraints, planning goals, etc. A synthetic CT for dose calculation is created via bulk density override based on the contours on the MR scan and electron density information obtained from the simulation CT scan. The treatment plan is re-optimized either from fluence, in which the segments in the reference plan are discarded and fluence is re-optimized, or from segments based on the reference plan. Compared to optimization from segmentations, optimization from fluence produces a completely new plan with slightly longer plan optimization time. It is recommended for substantial contour changes and/or IMRT constraint updates.

Dosimetric criteria can be customized to each treatment site or treatment template based on planning derivatives and they are initially set during reference planning and adjustable during adaptive planning. Upon the completion of plan adaptation, the dose–volume histogram (DVH) of the adaptive plan will be compared with the original reference plan for evaluation. Once the adaptive plan is approved, the plan will go through an independent secondary monitor unit (MU) verification for plan consistency. A 3D independent dose calculation and gamma comparison is preferred over point dose check [9].

A verification 3D MR scan can be acquired after the adaptive plan is approved. The adaptive plan dose can be overlaid on the new scan to verify that the current patient position is still valid for the adapted plan. Before beam-on, the therapist will verify the MU of each beam and other beam parameters to ensure the plan transfer is completed correctly and the correct plan is being delivered. During beam-on, the motion monitoring system can be turned on to monitor the patient motion qualitatively. Therapists may interrupt the beam-on if significant patient motion is observed. The latest CMM system provides automatic beam gating and intra-fraction drift correction [12].

16.3.2.2 Low-field online ART workflow

The workflow for online ART using the low-field MRIdian system, depicted in figure 16.4, begins with initial set-up of the patient and acquiring a volumetric MRI for patient alignment [22]. Image-guided set-up is based on the daily MR image and couch correction is applied based on registration of the daily MRI with the planning image [26]. Deformable registration is then performed to register the daily MRI to the primary planning image in order to transfer electron density information [16]. The original contours can either be rigidly copied or deformed to the newly acquired MRI [16]. The target structure is rigidly propagated to the new image and may be manually edited by the physician. The adaptive planner can manually edit critical OAR contours and these will be approved by the physician [22]. As this is one of the most time-consuming tasks of the online ART workflow, it is suggested that only contours within a 2–3 cm radius of the target need to be manually re-contoured as this should be the region with the highest dose gradients [27–29]. The planning target

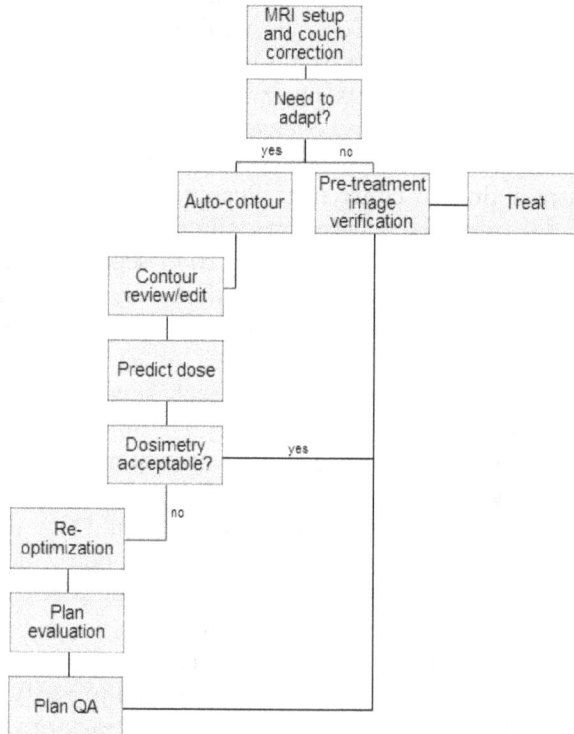

Figure 16.4. Diagram depicting the workflow for online adaptive treatment using the ViewRay system.

volume (PTV) and tuning structures may be automatically generated from the edited contours by applying pre-defined rules for their generation (i.e. a defined rule of expanding the GTV 3 mm isotropically to create the PTV). After contours have been edited and approved by the physician, the dose is recalculated using an electron density image derived via registration of the initial simulation image to the daily MRI [22]. The electron density map can be reviewed during this step and, if necessary, the electron density in specific areas of the image may be overridden using contours to correct for any errors. This recalculated dose is the 'predicted dose' that would be delivered to the newly revised contours by the original treatment plan if there is no adaptation [22]. The physician reviews the predicted dose and daily anatomy to make the clinical decision of whether to treat with the predicted dose or to adapt the plan. If the plan is to be adapted, the TPS performs IMRT optimization using the same beams and optimization weighting as the base plan. If the dosimetry of this adapted plan is not adequate, beam angle and optimization weights may be edited until an acceptable plan is achieved [22]. Note that editing the optimization of the plan adds a significant increase in time to this workflow and it is preferred to make few or no changes to the optimization if possible. A final evaluation of the dosimetry is performed and a decision is made by the physician to treat with the adapted plan, initial plan, or delay treatment [22]. The plan must have QA performed before treatment; however, phantom or EPID measurement-based IMRT QA is not possible as the patient should not be moved from the table during the online ART process [22]. Instead, QA is performed by comparing the TPS dose to the dose calculated using a secondary Monte Carlo tool provided by ViewRay that recalculates the planned dose using the MLC leaf positions and beam-on times of the adapted plan and presents this data as a DVH and gamma analysis [16, 22]. Although this online QA process has some limitations in the fact that it uses the same beam model for both calculations (possibly obscuring errors in the beam model) [22], adaptive plans have shown to be robust when patient-specific QA was retrospectively performed using a multidetector array [30]. After final approval of the plan and plan QA, the treatment is delivered to the patient in the same fashion as a non-adapted plan, using motion management strategies such as automated beam hold if required. After delivery, the MRIdian system generates a report of the delivery record including recorded MUs and MLC leaf positions compared to their planned values and log files may be exported [16].

16.3.3 Challenges in MRI ART workflow

General challenges inherent to MRI adaptive workflows include sCT generation and image registration. Both online and offline adaptive workflows rely on these fundamental steps for dose calculation and large errors in accurate electron density estimation may have a significant impact on dose calculation [31]. The CT-sim workflow introduces challenges associated with error in image registration, including inconsistencies between images due to image quality, artifacts, long durations between CT and MR scans, and dissimilarities in set-up positions [5]. These inconsistencies are especially prevalent if the MRI from time of treatment is being registered to the original CT-sim as a large amount of time has passed between the acquisition of these images. Specifically, regions with inhomogeneities and large variability due to physiological changes such as the abdomen, pelvis, and head and neck present challenges in image registration [5]. Even deformable image registration techniques are associated with uncertainties up to 5 mm [32]. Registration is also important in online ART as the contours are transferred from the planning image to the daily image. Mitigating errors in this registration allows for a more efficient online ART workflow. Meanwhile, the MRI-sim workflow includes challenges related to the creation of the sCT.

In addition to being used to position the patient and evaluate their anatomy at treatment, MRI is used for target delineation in both of the above workflows and, as such, it must be of higher image quality than is usually required for image guidance only. A balance of time efficiency and obtaining images with high resolution and high SNR must be achieved in ART workflows [34]. AI deep learning algorithms can be implemented in MR imaging to reduce scan times by reconstructing images from under-sampled data [34]. Image distortions resulting from the main magnet field inhomogeneities, gradient nonlinearities, motion, and eddy currents degrade image quality and must be corrected [21]. This is particularly important in ART where the MRI is used for re-planning and image quality may affect the accuracy of dose calculation. Mitigating MRI distortion and artifacts may be achieved with careful calibration of the scanner, strategic selection of pulse sequences, and image processing algorithms—which may be accelerated using AI tools [21].

The decision of whether ART is needed and whether the offline or online workflow is appropriate is another challenge of ART. While this is a clinical decision that is ultimately left to the treating physician, guidelines and tools may be implemented to reduce subjectivity in the decision. Factors such as the intent of treatment, dosimetric impact of anatomy deformations, the number of fractions remaining, and patient performance can all influence this decision of if and when to adapt [20]. Defining a set of pre-specified OAR constraints to be the threshold for adaptation may be helpful in reducing additional time for decision making during treatment [20]. AI tools may be able to predict which patients will require adaptation and when it would be ideal to adapt treatment based on extracting key features from existing data [34]. AI models have been used in retrospective studies to predict geometric changes in patients and predict when adapting during the treatment course can maximize tumor control [35–37]. AI-powered automation may also be used to review the cumulative dose impact of adapting a plan and may be a helpful tool in predicting treatment outcomes as a result of ART [20, 34].

Both offline and online adaptive plan workflows suffer from uncertainty in total dose accumulation using multiple plans over the course of treatment. This is an ongoing challenge as both the anatomy and dosimetry change with adaptive treatment. For structures that move considerably between treatments, it is difficult to identify and track point volume doses [20]. Due to this uncertainty, more conservative approaches to dose accumulation may be used, such as summing the max point dose to an OAR over all treatment days and evaluating each new plan as if it were to be delivered for all total fractions to limit OAR dose assuming the 'worst case' scenario [20].

Online adaptive workflows introduce additional challenges, particularly pertaining to the time and resource limitations during treatment. The online ART process is significantly more time consuming than a conventional treatment, with mean total delivery times of 75–90 min reported in the literature [22, 38]. Since the patient is on the table for longer than a typical treatment session, it is important to be mindful of the possibility of large anatomical changes occurring between imaging and delivery. Bladder filling and stomach emptying are examples of processes that may occur within the time it takes to perform online ART and, as such, speeding up the process as much as safely possible may ensure that the delivered plan is still relevant to the anatomy at time of beam-on [20]. Patient comfort should also be considered in initial set-up and custom or non-typical immobilization may be used to increase patient comfort and stability for long adaptive treatment sessions.

Not including treatment delivery, contouring was reported to be the most time-consuming and error-prone step of the online ART workflow [22, 29, 38, 39]. Currently, contours being correctly deformed to daily images are dependent on the accuracy of deformable registration, which was stated as a challenge above. Since this process is not perfect, time must be allocated to manually checking the contour accuracy and integrity. Advanced AI-driven auto-segmentation approaches are promising in minimizing the time allocation for this part of the process to contour both target and OAR volumes [40–43]. AI-based auto-segmentation methods have been shown to perform similarly to manual contours drawn by human experts and to be more accurate than atlas-based methods [34, 44, 45]. Commercial deep learning auto-segmentation solutions have been evaluated in the literature and have been found to provide high-quality contours that agree well with manually drawn contours while offering substantial time savings [44, 46]. Of course, a well-defined and robust QA procedure for any auto-segmentation used would be required for clinical use. AI-based tools may be useful in reducing the time and labor required for QA of auto-segmentation workflows [34]. One example of this is using automated contour refinement to speed up the process of correcting auto-segmented contours [47]. Translation of these approaches into clinical practice faces many challenges including quality of training data and logistical limitations [26].

The second most time-consuming step of the workflow, outside of delivery, is typically re-planning [22, 38]. One approach to increase efficiency in re-planning is using a plan library approach. This plan library would be based on predicable changes in specific OARs that would affect target coverage, for example changes in bladder or rectal filling [20]. Then, at the time of treatment, the most appropriate plan would be chosen to be used for adaption based on the daily anatomy. Monte Carlo dose algorithms must be used to account for the impact of the magnetic field on secondary electrons, and a deep learning dose calculation has been shown to accelerate Monte Carlo for adaptive planning over traditional calculations [48]. Efforts to improve the speed of plan optimization using approaches such as automated beam angle optimization and knowledge-based planning (using databases of prior plan information) may be helpful to increase the efficiency of this step.

AI-based approaches to treatment planning involve predicting the optimal dose distribution and identifying machine parameters that must be used to achieve the optimal distribution [34]. Some studies have demonstrated the ability of deep learning approaches to predict optimal dose distributions and accelerate dose calculations, which would increase the efficiency of ART [49–51]. Auto-planning that can promise consistently high plan quality in a short period of time may become more important for the future of online ART [52].

A limitation of the online ART workflow is the inability for measurement-based IMRT QA while the patient is on the table. The secondary calculation check used by the MRIdian system has a limitation in that it uses the same beam model for the primary and secondary checks [22], therefore considering alternative or additional IMRT QA solutions may enable more confidence in this part of the workflow. Retrospective QA of adaptive plans using film or diode arrays may be performed, particularly during initial clinical adoption of MR ART or for highly complex plans [29, 53, 54]. Offline log-file analysis or EPID measurements during delivery are other methods that can be used to assess plan integrity immediately after treatment [55, 56]. Alternatively, a 'simulated' treatment could be run before delivery without activating the beam to analyse log files to planned patterns before treatment, although these strategies may not detect errors that can occur during delivery [39]. Additional in-house manual and automated checks at this point of the process should be considered [39, 57].

The nature of online ART requires a significant resource burden, with attention from physicians, physicists, dosimetrists, and therapists needed at the time of treatment. The physician present at treatment may not be the attending physician following the patient and may not be familiar with the clinical history. Similarly, the physicist and dosimetrist present at adaptive treatment may not be the same individuals that were involved in the initial plan creation and check. As such, clear communication between these groups is essential to avoid any additional error and confusion. Documentation outlining clear instructions for plan adaptation thresholds and re-creating derived contours for re-optimization should be used in the online ART workflow [22].

MRI has the capability of providing functional and structural data together, using strategies such as dynamic-contrast enhanced imaging and diffusion weighted imaging [5]. This qualitative biological data could potentially be collected with the MR-linac system and incorporated into decision making for adaptive therapy [26]. AI tools may also play a role in this emerging frontier of MRI ART as analysing radiomic trends using AI may provide a more complete picture of tumor sensitivity and behavior during and after adaptive treatment [5].

16.4 AI applications for MRI-guided ART

The implementation of online MR-guided ART has been recognized as a potential advancement in enhancing the precision and efficacy of radiation therapy. The integration of AI into ART aims to enhance precision, efficiency, and outcomes by leveraging data-driven approaches to dynamically modify treatment plans. Despite its promise, the widespread clinical adoption of online MR-guided ART encounters significant barriers, primarily attributed to its operational complexity and the intensive demand for specialized human resources [58, 59]. This challenge under-scores the necessity of AI integration to streamline the MR-guided ART workflow, potentially leading to improved efficiency and cost-effectiveness in clinical applications. Areas of the MRI ART workflow that may benefit from AI-based automation are introduced in the above section. Increasing efficiency and accuracy of these steps has potential to reduce risks as well as the resource and time costs associated with ART. Simulation-free ART may be a next possible avenue for MR-linac technology if these challenges, and challenges associated with MR image quality can be addressed with AI tools. The past decade has witnessed a significant increase of AI applications aimed at augmenting various aspects of the radiotherapy workflow [60, 61]. However, as of the current state of development, a dedicated commercial solution to support MR-guided ART via AI integration is still not commercially available. The principal areas where AI can be applied in MR-guided ART include synthetic CT generation, auto-segmentation, and image registration.

16.4.1 Synthetic CT generation

This section is reproduced with permission from [67].

In the current clinical practice of MR-guided RT, the workflow typically involves a two-step simulation: a CT and subsequent MR simulations. The necessity for CT simulation stems from the inherent limitation of MR imaging to provide electron density maps, which are crucial for accurate dose calculation in treatment planning [62]. Advancing towards an MR-only radiotherapy framework necessitates the development and integration of synthetic CT generation from MR images. This will eliminate the need for conventional CT image in MR-guided RT workflow, thereby reducing the additional radiation exposure and mitigating uncertainties associated with the registration between MR and CT images.

Various methods have been proposed to address this issue, which can be mainly divided into three categories: segmentation-based, atlas-based, and learning-based methods [63–67]. Currently, segmentation-based methods are widely utilized in clinical settings, where sCT images are created by assigning uniform bulk densities to structures identified on MR images. However, these methods heavily rely on the accuracy of organ segmentation and fail to account for heterogeneity within each structure.

In recent years, learning-based methods, including traditional machine learning and deep learning methods, have gained substantial attention for synthetic image generation. These methods exploit self-learning and self-optimizing strategies to learn the MR-CT mapping for sCT generation. Among them, deep learning methods using convolutional neural networks (CNNs) have been demonstrated to have more promising performance in sCT generation without the need for extracting hand-crafted features [68]. For the deep learning methods, generally a model is trained to establish a nonlinear mapping from the MR to CT domain based on a large database of MR and CT pairs. Once the deep learning model has been trained, sCT images can be generated easily in a short amount of time by feeding the new MR image into the model. Han *et al* [69] first developed a U-Net architecture to successfully generate two-dimensional (2D) sCT images of brain patients from T1-weighted MR images. To fully utilize the image information in all dimensions, Nie *et al* [70] proposed a three-dimensional (3D) fully convolution neural network (FCN) to learn the complex translation mapping between MR and CT images. While the CNN method [71] improved the efficiency and quality of sCT generation, its performance is affected by the voxel-wise accuracy of MR-CT registration and might suffer from blurriness during image synthesis [72]. To generate high-quality sCT images with less blurriness, the generative adversarial network (GAN) [73], which consists of a generator and a discriminator, has been proposed. An adversarial loss function was also introduced to simultaneously optimize the generator and discriminator to improve the sCT image quality. Isola *et al* [74] further extended the GAN model and proposed the conditional GAN, in which the output sCT image is constrained by the input MR image. Although the GAN-based methods have achieved great success in generating synthetic images, training a GAN model usually requires perfectly co-registered image pairs, which is especially challenging for inter-modal (MR-CT) images [67, 75]. Nevertheless, the cycle-consistent generative adversarial network (cycleGAN) model proposed by Zhu *et al* [76] could be trained to generate synthetic images without the requirement of spatially aligned image pairs. With the incorporation of cycle-consistency loss, cycleGAN models trained with unpaired CT/MR images could even outperform GAN models trained with paired images in the aspect of the image quality of the generated sCT [72].

Recent investigations conducted by multiple research groups have substantiated the viability of employing deep learning techniques for the generation of synthetic CT for low and high-field MR-linacs [75, 77]. These approaches have been validated for their high dosimetric accuracy across multiple anatomical sites. A notable advantage of this technology is its efficiency, with the generation of synthetic CT images for a single patient being achievable in mere seconds, thanks to advancements in GPU technology [78]. This rapid processing capability, coupled with the demonstrated accuracy, positions synthetic CT technology on the brink of clinical applicability, with Siemens providing the first commercial AI-based sCT solution [5, 33].

16.4.2 Auto-segmentation

MR-guided RT treatment planning begins with the delineation of tumor volumes and surrounding OARs based on the simulation CT and MR images. The accuracy of target and OAR delineation is crucial for effective and safe MRgRT. This process is resource-intensive, the most time-consuming step, and heavily relies on expert knowledge, which may lead to inter- and intra-observer variability [79]. Automated segmentation has been explored for several years, reaching remarkable results especially for OARs on CT and MR images [80–83]. In the case of MR-guided ART applications, automated segmentation not only demands anatomical accuracy but also operational rapidity, ideally generating contours within a few minutes to maintain patient comfort and reduce undesirable intra-fractional patient movement during online adaptive procedures [60].

To address these challenges, deep learning-based methods have emerged as a superior alternative to traditional atlas-based and hand-crafted auto-segmentation techniques. For MR-guided ART, considerable progress has been achieved through the enhancement of deep learning models, particularly those derived from the U-Net architecture. U-Net's architecture, characterized by its convolutional layers in the encoder and transposed convolutional layers in the decoder, linked by long-range skip connections, has been pivotal in improving auto-segmentation tasks. Variants of U-Net, such as Dense U-Net [84] with densely connected convolutional blocks and ResU-Net [85] with residual connections, have been developed to improve feature propagation and facilitate segmentation accuracy. Additionally, Retina U-Net, a two-stage network, and attention mechanisms at skip connections have been integrated to prioritize critical regions within the images for segmentation [86]. nnUNet extends these capabilities by automating preprocessing and optimizing learning parameters, thereby augmenting both efficiency and accuracy [87]. Continuous innovations are leading to more advanced networks for auto-segmentation in MR imaging [47, 88]. There is no dedicated commercial solution for AI-segmentation tools currently available on either MRI-guided ART treatment units.

The performance of these auto-segmentation tools is typically evaluated using similarity metrics, which compare contours generated automatically against those manually contoured by physicians [89]. Recent studies leveraging deep learning for auto-segmentation report faster processing times and enhanced generalizability to novel patient image data [79, 80]. Given the superior soft-tissue contrast offered by MR imaging and the growing implementation of MR-linacs, a clinically approved solution for OAR definition is anticipated in the near future. However, the auto-segmentation of gross target volumes based on MR images, particularly in complex cases, remains a challenge. Further research and expanded datasets are necessary to capture the extensive variability of tumors and to improve delineation precision. Despite these challenges, the auto-segmentation results achieved to date have significant clinical implications. They can either be utilized directly in clinical settings or may require minimal manual revisions. Additionally, patient-specific AI-based auto-segmentation models, utilizing prior images/contours from either the reference plan or previous fractional plans, have demonstrated enhanced auto-segmentation performance [90]. Moreover, semi-automatic/interactive contour editing methods have shown substantial improvement in contour accuracy, thereby reducing the workload for manual editing [47, 91, 92]. It is critical to have online QA programs to continuously monitor performance, detecting malfunctions, outliers, and inaccurate segmentations, triggering necessary contour review and corrections for online ART.

Therefore, AI-driven methodologies are increasingly seen as valuable tools to assist clinicians in online adaptive procedures, promising to augment both the precision and efficiency of MR-guided ART [93].

16.4.3 Image registration

One key step for MR-guided online ART is deformable image registration (DIR) between the simulation CT scan, where the radiation treatment is initially planned, and the daily MRI scans. The DIR establishes the relationship between the CT and MRI scans so that the original treatment plan can be adapted and re-optimized based on daily anatomy to achieve optimal treatment delivery [94, 95]. However, DIR between CT and MRI has long been a difficult task due to significant contrast differences and anatomical variations over time. Traditional DIR methods based on maximizing image similarity between two images is computationally intensive and inefficient in providing accurate and fast contour propagation for online ART [96]

Recently, deep learning (DL)-based approaches have demonstrated superior performance and speed compared to traditional methods [97]. The DL-based DIR methods are broadly categorized into supervised and unsupervised learning methods [97, 98]. In supervised learning methods, the networks are trained with ground-truth deformation vector fields (DVFs) that are usually generated from traditional methods or synthetic data. The registration performance is limited by the quality of the ground-truth DVFs which may be different from the actual anatomical deformation. On the other hand, unsupervised learning methods have been developed to overcome these limitations by training the networks to optimize similarity metrics between deformed and fixed images, like traditional registration methods. VoxelMorph, proposed by Balakrishanan *et al* [99], was a notable example of unsupervised learning methods that utilized a spatial transformer network (STN) [100] to generate the deformed image during training process. Moreover, translation methods using GAN [73] have been proposed to generate sCT from MR images, which are used as a bridge for CT-to-MR registration [101]. However, the CNN-based registration methods with a limited size effective receptive field may suffer from loss of long-range spatial relations in moving and fixed images during registration. Recently, there has been an increase of applying transformers to computer vision tasks. This technique has been demonstrated to have superior performance in image registration because of its self-attention mechanism and ability to build associations between distant parts of images [102, 103].

In addition to contour propagation, DIR has several other important applications in radiation therapy, including dose mapping and accumulation [104]. Specifically, in MR-guided ART, DIR plays an important role in registering daily MR images to the planning CT and enabling the accumulation of dose for plan evaluation and re-planning. This approach allows for a more precise assessment of the accumulated dose distribution in the target volume and surrounding OARs over the course of treatment. Furthermore, in the case of re-treatment, dose mapping is crucial in transforming the previous dose distribution to the new planning images to assess the dose tolerances of OARs and ensure that dose is delivered accurately to the target while minimizing the risk of side effects to surrounding healthy tissue [105]. The ongoing development of more sophisticated deep learning models promises to further enhance the accuracy and efficiency of DIR processes. As these technologies mature, their integration into clinical workflows is anticipated to become more streamlined, enabling real-time adjustments to treatment plans based on patient-specific anatomical changes.

16.4.4 Others

The exploration and application of AI tools has extended beyond synthetic CT generation, auto-segmentation, and image registration to facilitate MR-guided ART workflow [60]. A noteworthy area of ongoing research is the field of automated treatment planning. Extensive reviews, such as the one conducted by Wang *et al* have reported the integration of deep learning techniques across various phases of automated planning, encompassing beam selection, dose prediction, fluence map generation, and the creation of delivery parameters [106]. Concurrently, deep reinforcement learning has emerged as a prospective tool in AI-based auto-planning [107]. These advancements demonstrate the potential of AI in enhancing the efficiency and accuracy of treatment planning processes. Moreover, deep learning methods are being explored to address the challenges of 3D motion trajectory inference and the reconstruction of 3D acquisitions from multi-slice 2D images, which are crucial for managing intrafraction motion in current MR-linac systems [108]. These advancements are pivotal in developing adaptive strategies that dynamically adjust treatment plans based on real-time anatomical information and enhance the precision of MR-guided ART. In addition to these developments, deep learning techniques are also being applied to automate QA processes and outcome prediction in MR-guided RT [109].

16.4.5 Future AI development and implementation

The development and implementation of AI in MR-guided ART is anticipated to significantly enhance clinical efficiency. From reducing treatment times and minimizing intrafraction variability to enabling dynamic treatment adjustments and redefining dosimetric constraints, AI stands at the forefront of advancing the safety, efficacy, and personalization of radiation therapy. As these AI-driven methodologies continue to evolve, they are expected to play an increasingly vital role in optimizing treatment protocols and improving patient outcomes in MR-guided ART.

16.5 Summary

This chapter aims to provide a basis for understanding the clinical need for AI in MRI-guided ART workflows and the unique challenges associated with implementing these solutions. The basic workflow of offline and online ART for clinically available on-board MRI and MR-linac technologies is outlined as necessary background information. Current AI solutions are identified and an overview of clinical implementation of these tools is provided. An analysis of error associated with MRI ART workflow is discussed in order to identify areas for improvement where AI can benefit current workflows. In addition, further areas of improvement and predictions on the future of AI in MRI ART are discussed. Through this text, the reader should have a basic understanding of MRI-guided ART workflows and how AI is implemented in these workflows to improve clinical processes.

References

[1] Baskar R, Lee K A, Yeo R and Yeoh K-W 2012 Cancer and radiation therapy: current advances and future directions *Int. J. Med. Sci.* **9** 193–9

[2] Qi X S, Albuquerque K, Bailey S, Dawes S, Kashani R, Li H, Mak R H, Mundt A J and Sio T T 2023 Quality and safety considerations in image guided radiation therapy: an ASTRO safety white paper update *Pract. Radiat. Oncol.* **13** 97–111

[3] Zelefsky M J, Kollmeier M, Cox B, Fidaleo A, Sperling D, Pei X, Carver B, Coleman J, Lovelock M and Hunt M 2012 Improved clinical outcomes with high-dose image guided radiotherapy compared with non-IGRT for the treatment of clinically localized prostate cancer *Int. J. Radiat. Oncol.* **84** 125–9

[4] Oderinde O M, Shirvani S M, Olcott P D, Kuduvalli G, Mazin S and Larkin D 2021 The technical design and concept of a PET/CT linac for biology-guided radiotherapy *Clin. Transl. Radiat. Oncol.* **29** 106–12

[5] Ng J, Gregucci F, Pennell R T, Nagar H, Golden E B, Knisely J P S, Sanfilippo N J and Formenti S C 2023 MRI-linac: a transformative technology in radiation oncology *Front. Oncol.* **13** 1117874

[6] Yan D, Vicini F, Wong J and Martinez A 1997 Adaptive radiation therapy *Phys. Med. Biol.* **42** 123–32

[7] Raaymakers B W *et al* 2009 Integrating a 1.5 T MRI scanner with a 6 MV accelerator: proof of concept *Phys. Med. Biol.* **54** N229–237

[8] Elekta 2018 Elekta Unity, world's first high field MR-linac, receives FDA 510(k) clearance *Press release* Elekta, Stockholm, Sweden https://ir.elekta.com/investors/press-releases/2018/elekta-unity-worlds-first-high-field-mr-linac-receives-fda-510k-clearance/

[9] Roberts D A *et al* 2021 Machine QA for the Elekta unity system a report from the Elekta MR-linac consortium *Med. Phys.* **48** e67–85

[10] Paudel M R, Kim A, Sarfehnia A, Ahmad S B, Beachey D J, Sahgal A and Keller B M 2016 Experimental evaluation of a GPU-based Monte Carlo dose calculation algorithm in the Monaco treatment planning system *J. Appl. Clin. Med. Phys.* **17** 230–41

[11] Jassar H *et al* 2023 Real-time motion monitoring using orthogonal cine MRI during MR-guided adaptive radiation therapy for abdominal tumors on 1.5 T MR-linac *Med. Phys.* **50** 3103–16

[12] Grimbergen G *et al* 2023 Gating and intrafraction drift correction on a 1.5 T MR-linac: clinical dosimetric benefits for upper abdominal tumors *Radiother. Oncol.* **189** 109932

[13] Raaijmakers A J E, Raaymakers B W and Lagendijk J J W 2008 Magnetic-field-induced dose effects in MR-guided radiotherapy systems: dependence on the magnetic field strength *Phys. Med. Biol.* **53** 909–23

[14] Mutic S and Dempsey J F 2014 The ViewRay system: magnetic resonance-guided and controlled radiotherapy *Semin. Radiat. Oncol.* **24** 196–9

[15] Huang C-Y, Yang B, Lam W W, Geng H, Cheung K Y and Yu S K 2023 Magnetic field induced dose effects in radiation therapy using MR-linacs *Med. Phys.* **50** 3623–36

[16] Klüter S 2019 Technical design and concept of a 0.35 T MR-linac *Clin. Transl. Radiat. Oncol.* **18** 98–101

[17] 510(k) premarket notification *US FDA* https://www.accessdata.fda.gov/scripts/cdrh/cfdocs/cfPMN/pmn.cfm?ID=k092364

[18] LINAC-MR *MagnetTx Oncology Solutions* https://www.magnettx.com/

[19] National Library of Medicine 2025 Northern Alberta Linac-MR Image-Guided Human Clinical Trials—1 *AHS Cancer Control Alberta* https://clinicaltrials.gov/study/NCT05413473

[20] Green O L, Henke L E and Hugo G D 2019 Practical clinical workflows for online and offline adaptive radiation therapy *Semin. Radiat. Oncol.* **29** 219–27

[21] Otazo R, Lambin P, Pignol J-P, Ladd M E, Schlemmer H-P, Baumann M and Hricak H 2021 MRI-guided radiation therapy: an emerging paradigm in adaptive radiation oncology *Radiology* **298** 248–60

[22] Lamb J *et al* 2017 Online adaptive radiation therapy: implementation of a new process of care *Cureus* **9** e1618

[23] Winkel D *et al* 2019 Adaptive radiotherapy: the Elekta Unity MR-linac concept *Clin. Transl. Radiat. Oncol.* **18** 54–9

[24] Yang J, Vedam S, Lee B, Castillo P, Sobremonte A, Hughes N, Mohammedsaid M, Wang J and Choi S 2021 Online adaptive planning for prostate stereotactic body radiotherapy using a 1.5 tesla magnetic resonance imaging-guided linear accelerator *Phys. Imaging Radiat. Oncol.* **17** 20–4

[25] Lakomy D S *et al* 2022 Clinical implementation and initial experience with a 1.5 tesla MR-linac for MR-guided radiation therapy for gynecologic cancer: an R-IDEAL stage 1 and 2a first in humans feasibility study of new technology implementation *Pract. Radiat. Oncol.* **12** e296–305

[26] Keall P J *et al* 2022 ICRU Report 97: MRI-guided radiation therapy using MRI-linear accelerators *J. ICRU* **22** 1–100

[27] Kurz C *et al* 2020 Medical physics challenges in clinical MR-guided radiotherapy *Radiat. Oncol.* **15** 93

[28] Bohoudi O, Bruynzeel A M E, Senan S, Cuijpers J P, Slotman B J, Lagerwaard F J and Palacios M A 2017 Fast and robust online adaptive planning in stereotactic MR-guided adaptive radiation therapy (SMART) for pancreatic cancer *Radiother. Oncol.* **125** 439–44

[29] Garcia Schüler H I *et al* 2021 Operating procedures, risk management and challenges during implementation of adaptive and non-adaptive MR-guided radiotherapy: 1-year single-center experience *Radiat. Oncol.* **16** 217

[30] Bessieres I, Lorenzo O, Bertaut A, Petitfils A, Aubignac L and Boudet J 2023 Online adaptive radiotherapy and dose delivery accuracy: a retrospective analysis *J. Appl. Clin. Med. Phys.* **24** e14005

[31] Nobah A, Moftah B, Tomic N and Devic S 2011 Influence of electron density spatial distribution and x-ray beam quality during CT simulation on dose calculation accuracy *J. Appl. Clin. Med. Phys.* **12** 80–9

[32] Ishida T, Kadoya N, Tanabe S, Ohashi H, Nemoto H, Dobashi S, Takeda K and Jingu K 2021 Evaluation of performance of pelvic CT-MR deformable image registration using two software programs *J. Radiat. Res.* **62** 1076–82

[33] Gonzalez-Moya A, Dufreneix S, Ouyessad N, Guilleminet C and Autret D 2021 Evaluation of a commercial synthetic computed tomography generation solution for magnetic resonance imaging-only radiotherapy *J. Appl. Clin. Med. Phys.* **22** 191–7

[34] Huynh E, Hosny A, Guthier C, Bitterman D S, Petit S F, Haas-Kogan D A, Kann B, Aerts H J W L and Mak R H 2020 Artificial intelligence in radiation oncology *Nat. Rev. Clin. Oncol.* **17** 771–81

[35] Guidi G *et al* 2016 A machine learning tool for re-planning and adaptive RT: a multicenter cohort investigation *Phys. Med.* **32** 1659–66

[36] Varfalvy N, Piron O, Cyr M F, Dagnault A and Archambault L 2017 Classification of changes occurring in lung patient during radiotherapy using relative γ analysis and hidden Markov models *Med. Phys.* **44** 5043–50

[37] Jöhl A, Ehrbar S, Guckenberger M, Klöck S, Meboldt M, Zeilinger M, Tanadini-Lang S and Schmid Daners M 2020 Performance comparison of prediction filters for respiratory motion tracking in radiotherapy *Med. Phys.* **47** 643–50

[38] Güngör G *et al* 2021 Time analysis of online adaptive magnetic resonance-guided radiation therapy workflow according to anatomical sites *Pract. Radiat. Oncol.* **11** e11–21

[39] Noel C E, Santanam L, Parikh P J and Mutic S 2014 Process-based quality management for clinical implementation of adaptive radiotherapy *Med. Phys.* **41** 081717

[40] Mackay K, Bernstein D, Glocker B, Kamnitsas K and Taylor A 2023 A review of the metrics used to assess auto-contouring systems in radiotherapy *Clin. Oncol.* **35** 354–69

[41] Liang F *et al* 2018 Abdominal, multi-organ, auto-contouring method for online adaptive magnetic resonance guided radiotherapy: an intelligent, multi-level fusion approach *Artif. Intell. Med.* **90** 34–41

[42] Fu Y *et al* 2018 A novel MRI segmentation method using CNN-based correction network for MRI-guided adaptive radiotherapy *Med. Phys.* **45** 5129–37

[43] Eppenhof K A J, Maspero M, Savenije M H F, de Boer J C J, van der Voort van Zyp J R N, Raaymakers B W, Raaijmakers A J E, Veta M, van den Berg C A T and Pluim J P W 2020 Fast contour propagation for MR-guided prostate radiotherapy using convolutional neural networks *Med. Phys.* **47** 1238–48

[44] Chen W, Wang C, Zhan W, Jia Y, Ruan F, Qiu L, Yang S and Li Y 2021 A comparative study of auto-contouring softwares in delineation of organs at risk in lung cancer and rectal cancer *Sci. Rep.* **11** 23002

[45] Zabel W J *et al* 2021 Clinical evaluation of deep learning and atlas-based auto-contouring of bladder and rectum for prostate radiation therapy *Pract. Radiat. Oncol.* **11** e80–9

[46] Doolan P J, Charalambous S, Roussakis Y, Leczynski A, Peratikou M, Benjamin M, Ferentinos K, Strouthos I, Zamboglou C and Karagiannis E 2023 A clinical evaluation of the performance of five commercial artificial intelligence contouring systems for radio-therapy *Front. Oncol.* **13** 1213068

[47] Ding J, Zhang Y, Amjad A, Xu J, Thill D and Li X A 2022 Automatic contour refinement for deep learning auto-segmentation of complex organs in MRI-guided adaptive radiation therapy *Adv. Radiat. Oncol.* **7** 100968

[48] Neph R, Lyu Q, Huang Y, Yang Y M and Sheng K 2021 DeepMC: a deep learning method for efficient Monte Carlo beamlet dose calculation by predictive denoising in magnetic resonance-guided radiotherapy *Phys. Med. Biol.* **66** 035022

[49] Xing Y, Nguyen D, Lu W, Yang M and Jiang S 2020 Technical note: a feasibility study on deep learning-based radiotherapy dose calculation *Med. Phys.* **47** 753–8

[50] Campbell W G, Miften M, Olsen L, Stumpf P, Schefter T, Goodman K A and Jones B L 2017 Neural network dose models for knowledge-based planning in pancreatic SBRT *Med. Phys.* **44** 6148–58

[51] Nguyen D, Long T, Jia X, Lu W, Gu X, Iqbal Z and Jiang S 2019 A feasibility study for predicting optimal radiation therapy dose distributions of prostate cancer patients from patient anatomy using deep learning *Sci. Rep.* **9** 1076

[52] Raaymakers B W *et al* 2017 First patients treated with a 1.5 T MRI-linac: clinical proof of concept of a high-precision, high-field MRI guided radiotherapy treatment *Phys. Med. Biol.* **62** L41

[53] Bertelsen A S *et al* 2019 First clinical experiences with a high field 1.5 T MR linac *Acta Oncol.* **58** 1352–7

[54] Werensteijn-Honingh A M *et al* 2019 Feasibility of stereotactic radiotherapy using a 1.5 T MR-linac: multi-fraction treatment of pelvic lymph node oligometastases *Radiother. Oncol.* **134** 50–4

[55] Torres-Xirau I, Olaciregui-Ruiz I, van der Heide U A and Mans A 2019 Two-dimensional EPID dosimetry for an MR-linac: proof of concept *Med. Phys.* **46** 4193–203

[56] Acharya S *et al* 2016 Online magnetic resonance image guided adaptive radiation therapy: first clinical applications *Int. J. Radiat. Oncol.* **94** 394–403

[57] Cai B, Green O L, Kashani R, Rodriguez V L, Mutic S and Yang D 2018 A practical implementation of physics quality assurance for photon adaptive radiotherapy *Z. Für Med. Phys.* **28** 211–23

[58] Benitez C M, Chuong M D, Künzel L A and Thorwarth D 2024 MRI-guided adaptive radiation therapy *Semin. Radiat. Oncol.* **34** 84–91

[59] Garcia Schüler H I, Pavic M, Mayinger M, Weitkamp N, Chamberlain M, Reiner C, Linsenmeier C, Balermpas P, Krayenbühl J and Guckenberger M 2021 Operating procedures, risk management and challenges during implementation of adaptive and non-adaptive MR-guided radiotherapy: 1-year single-center experience *Radiat. Oncol.* **16** 1–10

[60] Cusumano D, Boldrini L, Dhont J, Fiorino C, Green O, Güngör G, Jornet N, Klüter S, Landry G and Mattiucci G C 2021 Artificial Intelligence in magnetic resonance guided radiotherapy: medical and physical considerations on state of art and future perspectives *Phys. Med.* **85** 175–91

[61] Eidex Z, Ding Y, Wang J, Abouei E, Qiu R L, Liu T, Wang T and Yang X 2023 Deep learning in MRI-guided radiation therapy: a systematic review arXiv:2303.11378

[62] Edmund J M and Nyholm T 2017 A review of substitute CT generation for MRI-only radiation therapy *Radiat. Oncol.* **12** 28

[63] Hsu S-H, Cao Y, Huang K, Feng M and Balter J M 2013 Investigation of a method for generating synthetic CT models from MRI scans of the head and neck for radiation therapy *Phys. Med. Biol.* **58** 8419

[64] Huynh T, Gao Y, Kang J, Wang L, Zhang P, Lian J and Shen D 2015 Estimating CT image from MRI data using structured random forest and auto-context model *IEEE Trans. Med. Imaging* **35** 174–83

[65] Andreasen D, Van Leemput K and Edmund J M 2016 A patch-based pseudo-CT approach for MRI-only radiotherapy in the pelvis *Med. Phys.* **43** 4742–52

[66] Cao X, Yang J, Gao Y, Guo Y, Wu G and Shen D 2017 Dual-core steered non-rigid registration for multi-modal images via bi-directional image synthesis *Med. Image Anal.* **41** 18–31

[67] Zhao Y, Wang H, Yu C, Court L E, Wang X, Wang Q, Pan T, Ding Y, Phan J and Yang J 2023 Compensation cycle consistent generative adversarial networks (Comp-GAN) for synthetic CT generation from MR scans with truncated anatomy *Med. Phys.* **50** 4399–414

[68] Boulanger M, Nunes J-C, Chourak H, Largent A, Tahri S, Acosta O, De Crevoisier R, Lafond C and Barateau A 2021 Deep learning methods to generate synthetic CT from MRI in radiotherapy: a literature review *Phys. Med.* **89** 265–81

[69] Han X 2017 MR-based synthetic CT generation using a deep convolutional neural network method *Med. Phys.* **44** 1408–19

[70] Nie D, Cao X, Gao Y, Wang L and Shen D 2016 Estimating CT image from MRI data using 3D fully convolutional networks *Deep Learning and Data Labeling for Medical Applications: First Int. Workshop, LABELS 2016, and Second Int. Workshop, DLMIA 2016, Held in Conjunction with MICCAI 2016 (Athens, Greece, 21 October 2016)* (Berlin: Springer) pp 170–8

[71] Dinkla A M, Florkow M C, Maspero M, Savenije M H, Zijlstra F, Doornaert P A, van Stralen M, Philippens M E, van den Berg C A and Seevinck P R 2019 Dosimetric evaluation of synthetic CT for head and neck radiotherapy generated by a patch-based three-dimensional convolutional neural network *Med. Phys.* **46** 4095–104

[72] Wolterink J M, Dinkla A M, Savenije M H, Seevinck P R, van den Berg C A and Išgum I 2017 Deep MR to CT synthesis using unpaired data *Simulation and Synthesis in Medical Imaging: 2nd Int. Workshop, SASHIMI 2017, Held in Conjunction with MICCAI 2017 (Québec City, QC, Canada, 10 September 2017)* (Berlin: Springer) pp 14–23

[73] Goodfellow I, Pouget-Abadie J, Mirza M, Xu B, Warde-Farley D, Ozair S, Courville A and Bengio Y 2014 Advances in neural information processing systems *Curran Assoc. Inc.* **27** 2672–80

[74] Isola P, Zhu J-Y, Zhou T and Efros A A 2017 Image-to-image translation with conditional adversarial networks *Proc. of the IEEE Conf. on Computer Vision and Pattern Recognition* pp 1125–34

[75] Cusumano D, Lenkowicz J, Votta C, Boldrini L, Placidi L, Catucci F, Dinapoli N, Antonelli M V, Romano A and De Luca V 2020 A deep learning approach to generate synthetic CT in low field MR-guided adaptive radiotherapy for abdominal and pelvic cases *Radiother. Oncol.* **153** 205–12

[76] Zhu J-Y, Park T, Isola P and Efros A A 2017 Unpaired image-to-image translation using cycle-consistent adversarial networks *Proc. of the IEEE Int. Conf. on Computer Vision* pp 2223–32

[77] Maspero M, Savenije M H, Dinkla A M, Seevinck P R, Intven M P, Jurgenliemk-Schulz I M, Kerkmeijer L G and van den Berg C A 2018 Dose evaluation of fast synthetic-CT generation using a generative adversarial network for general pelvis MR-only radiotherapy *Phys. Med. Biol.* **63** 185001

[78] Largent A, Barateau A, Nunes J-C, Mylona E, Castelli J, Lafond C, Greer P B, Dowling J A, Baxter J and Saint-Jalmes H 2019 Comparison of deep learning-based and patch-based methods for pseudo-CT generation in MRI-based prostate dose planning *Int. J. Radiat. Oncol. Biol. Phys.* **105** 1137–50

[79] Cardenas C E, Yang J, Anderson B M, Court L E and Brock K B 2019 Advances in auto-segmentation *Semin. Radiat. Oncol.* **29** 185–97

[80] Zhao Y, Rhee D J, Cardenas C, Court L E and Yang J 2021 Training deep-learning segmentation models from severely limited data *Med. Phys.* **48** 1697–706

[81] Yu C, Anakwenze C P, Zhao Y, Martin R M, Ludmir E B, Niedzielski J S, Qureshi A, Das P, Holliday E B and Raldow A C 2022 Multi-organ segmentation of abdominal structures from non-contrast and contrast enhanced CT images *Sci. Rep.* **12** 19093

[82] Chen X, Mumme R P, Corrigan K L, Mukai-Sasaki Y, Koutroumpakis E, Palaskas N L, Nguyen C M, Zhao Y, Huang K and Yu C 2023 Deep learning-based automatic segmentation of cardiac substructures for lung cancers *Radiother. Oncol.* **191** 110061

[83] Gay S S, Cardenas C E, Nguyen C, Netherton T J, Yu C, Zhao Y, Skett S, Patel T, Adjogatse D and Guerrero Urbano T 2023 Fully-automated, CT-only GTV contouring for palliative head and neck radiotherapy *Sci. Rep.* **13** 21797

[84] Cai S, Tian Y, Lui H, Zeng H, Wu Y and Chen G 2020 Dense-UNet: a novel multiphoton *in vivo* cellular image segmentation model based on a convolutional neural network *Quant. Imaging Med. Surg.* **10** 1275

[85] Diakogiannis F I, Waldner F, Caccetta P and Wu C 2020 ResUNet-a: a deep learning framework for semantic segmentation of remotely sensed data *ISPRS J. Photogramm. Remote Sens.* **162** 94–114

[86] Alom M Z, Hasan M, Yakopcic C, Taha T M and Asari V K 2018 Recurrent residual convolutional neural network based on U-Net (r2U-Net) for medical image segmentation arXiv:1802.06955

[87] Isensee F, Jaeger P F, Kohl S A, Petersen J and Maier-Hein K H 2021 nnU-Net: a self-configuring method for deep learning-based biomedical image segmentation *Nat. Methods* **18** 203–11

[88] Kawula M, Hadi I, Nierer L, Vagni M, Cusumano D, Boldrini L, Placidi L, Corradini S, Belka C and Landry G 2023 Patient-specific transfer learning for auto-segmentation in adaptive 0.35 T MRgRT of prostate cancer: a bi-centric evaluation *Med. Phys.* **50** 1573–85

[89] Baroudi H, Brock K K, Cao W, Chen X, Chung C, Court L E, El Basha M D, Farhat M, Gay S and Gronberg M P 2023 Automated contouring and planning in radiation therapy: what is 'clinically acceptable'? *Diagnostics* **13** 667

[90] Li Z, Zhang W, Li B, Zhu J, Peng Y, Li C, Zhu J, Zhou Q and Yin Y 2022 Patient-specific daily updated deep learning auto-segmentation for MRI-guided adaptive radiotherapy *Radiother. Oncol.* **177** 222–30

[91] Ding J, Zhang Y, Amjad A, Xu J, Thill D and Li A 2021 Guided deep learning auto-correction of suboptimal auto-segmentation of complex structures for MRI-guided adaptive radiotherapy *Int. J. Radiat. Oncol. Biol. Phys.* **111** e90

[92] Zhang Y, Amjad A, Ding J, Ahunbay E E and Li A 2021 A deep learning-based automatic contour quality assurance pipeline for complex anatomy on MRI *Int. J. Radiat. Oncol. Biol. Phys.* **111** e509

[93] Guckenberger M, Andratschke N, Chung C, Fuller D, Tanadini-Lang S and Jaffray D A 2024 The future of MR-guided radiation therapy *Semin. Radiat. Oncol.* **34** 135–44

[94] Owrangi A M, Greer P B and Glide-Hurst C K 2018 MRI-only treatment planning: benefits and challenges *Phys. Med. Biol.* **63** 05TR01

[95] Raaymakers B W, Lagendijk J J W, Overweg J, Kok J G M, Raaijmakers A J E, Kerkhof E M, Van Der Put R W, Meijsing I, Crijns S P M and Benedosso F 2009 Integrating a 1.5 T MRI scanner with a 6 MV accelerator: proof of concept *Phys. Med. Biol.* **54** N229

[96] Brock K K, Mutic S, McNutt T R, Li H and Kessler M L 2017 Use of image registration and fusion algorithms and techniques in radiotherapy: report of the AAPM radiation therapy committee task group No. 132 *Med. Phys.* **44** e43–76

[97] Fu Y, Lei Y, Wang T, Curran W J, Liu T and Yang X 2020 Deep learning in medical image registration: a review *Phys. Med. Biol.* **65** 20TR01

[98] Haskins G, Kruger U and Yan P 2020 Deep learning in medical image registration: a survey *Mach. Vis. Appl.* **31** 8

[99] Balakrishnan G, Zhao A, Sabuncu M R, Guttag J and Dalca A V 2019 VoxelMorph: a learning framework for deformable medical image registration *IEEE Trans. Med. Imaging* **38** 1788–800

[100] Jaderberg M, Simonyan K and Zisserman A 2015 Spatial transformer networks arXiv: 1506.02025

[101] McKenzie E M, Santhanam A, Ruan D, O'Connor D, Cao M and Sheng K 2020 Multimodality image registration in the head-and-neck using a deep learning-derived synthetic CT as a bridge *Med. Phys.* **47** 1094–104

[102] Zhao Y, Chen X, McDonald B, Yu C, Mohamed A S, Fuller C D, Court L E, Pan T, Wang H and Wang X 2023 A transformer-based hierarchical registration framework for multimodality deformable image registration *Comput. Med. Imaging Graph.* **108** 102286

[103] Chen J, Frey E C, He Y, Segars W P, Li Y and Du Y 2022 Transmorph: transformer for unsupervised medical image registration *Med. Image Anal.* **82** 102615

[104] Lim S Y, Tran A, Tran A N K, Sobremonte A, Fuller C D, Simmons L and Yang J 2022 Dose accumulation of daily adaptive plans to decide optimal plan adaptation strategy for head-and-neck patients treated with MR-linac *Med. Dosim.* **47** 103–9

[105] Boman E, Kapanen M, Pickup L and Lahtela S-L 2017 Importance of deformable image registration and biological dose summation in planning of radiotherapy retreatments *Med. Dosim.* **42** 296–303

[106] Wang M, Zhang Q, Lam S, Cai J and Yang R 2020 A review on application of deep learning algorithms in external beam radiotherapy automated treatment planning *Front. Oncol.* **10** 580919

[107] Shen C, Nguyen D, Chen L, Gonzalez Y, McBeth R, Qin N, Jiang S B and Jia X 2020 Operating a treatment planning system using a deep-reinforcement learning-based virtual treatment planner for prostate cancer intensity-modulated radiation therapy treatment planning *Med. Phys.* **47** 2329–36

[108] Paganelli C, Whelan B, Peroni M, Summers P, Fast M, van de Lindt T, McClelland J, Eiben B, Keall P and Lomax T 2018 MRI-guidance for motion management in external beam radiotherapy: current status and future challenges *Phys. Med. Biol.* **63** 22TR03

[109] Chen X, Ahunbay E, Paulson E S, Chen G and Li X A 2020 A daily end-to-end quality assurance workflow for MR-guided online adaptive radiation therapy on MR-linac *J. Appl. Clin. Med. Phys.* **21** 205–12

Chapter 17

Functional imaging-guided adaptive radiation therapy

Bin Han and Yu Gao

Conventional adaptive radiation therapy (ART) mainly adjusts treatment plans based on daily anatomical changes, such as the shape and position variations of organs at risk (OARs). However, different tumors and patients can exhibit diverse responses to treatment, which can impact the effectiveness of radiation treatment. Functional imaging techniques, such as positron emission tomography (PET) and functional magnetic resonance imaging (MRI), provide crucial insights into the tumor's metabolism, physiology, and molecular characteristics, offering a more comprehensive understanding than anatomy-based imaging alone. By integrating functional imaging into radiation therapy, we can more precisely tailor treatment plans to individual response. This holds great promise for enhancing treatment effectiveness and improving patient outcomes. This chapter delves deeply into the crucial role of functional imaging in refining ART, with a spotlight on PET and MRI's significant contributions and breakthroughs. Our analysis will showcase how PET and MRI not only form the cornerstone for creating individualized treatment protocols but also pave the way for groundbreaking oncological research and innovation. We aim to illuminate the significant strides in functional imaging, marking a new era in the precision, efficacy, and patient outcomes within radiation therapy's rapidly advancing domain. Sections 17.1 and 17.2 will specifically focus on PET and MRI applications in ART, respectively.

17.1 Functional PET-guided ART

PET imaging has become a pivotal tool in the realm of adaptive radiation therapy [1, 2], primarily due to its unmatched capability in visualizing the metabolic activities of tumors. This functional imaging technique allows for a highly detailed assessment of a tumor's response to radiation therapy, making it possible to tailor treatment plans with unparalleled precision. By highlighting areas of increased

doi:10.1088/978-0-7503-6119-4ch17

17-1

metabolic activity, positron emission tomography (PET) imaging aids in the accurate delineation of tumors, ensuring that radiation doses are optimally targeted to cancerous tissues while sparing adjacent healthy structures.

The application of PET imaging in adaptive radiation therapy (ART) extends to monitoring the effectiveness of treatment over time. Clinicians utilize PET scans to evaluate changes in a tumor's size and metabolic activity during the course of therapy, providing critical insights that can prompt adjustments to the treatment plan [3]. This dynamic approach enables the adaptation of radiation doses, optimizing therapy based on the tumor's real-time response. Furthermore, PET imaging facilitates dose painting [4], where varying radiation doses are applied to different tumor regions based on their metabolic activity, thereby enhancing the efficacy of treatment and minimizing damage to healthy tissues.

Moreover, PET imaging plays a crucial role in the post-treatment phase, serving as a sensitive tool for early detection of cancer recurrence [5]. Its ability to identify metabolic changes offers a significant advantage in monitoring patients for signs of tumor regrowth, ensuring prompt intervention when necessary. Through these applications, PET imaging in adaptive radiation therapy represents a significant stride toward personalized cancer care, offering hope for improved treatment outcomes and reduced side effects for patients undergoing radiation therapy.

17.1.1 PET-based functional imaging overview

PET-based functional imaging leverages PET to visualize the metabolic activities within the body, offering crucial insights beyond what is possible with traditional anatomical imaging techniques. By injecting radiotracers, which are substances designed to target specific biochemical processes, PET can illuminate areas of increased metabolic activity, such as tumors with high glucose consumption. This allows for the precise detection and monitoring of various diseases, particularly in oncology, by providing detailed images of how tissues and organs function at a molecular level. As a result, PET imaging has become an indispensable tool in diagnosis, treatment planning, and the evaluation of therapeutic responses, paving the way for personalized medicine through its ability to reveal the unique functional characteristics of diseases within the body.

17.1.1.1 Principles of PET imaging

The process of generating PET images is a fascinating intersection of physics, chemistry, and medical science, providing a window into the body's functional processes. This journey begins with the careful administration of a radiotracer, a specially designed molecule tagged with a radioactive isotope. These radiotracers are ingeniously crafted to seek out specific biological activities or cell types, with fluorodeoxyglucose (FDG), a glucose analog, being among the most commonly used. Once injected, this compound circulates through the bloodstream, distributing itself across various tissues but preferentially accumulating in areas with high metabolic demand, such as rapidly growing tumors.

Upon reaching its target, the radiotracer undergoes radioactive decay, emitting positrons. These subatomic particles travel a short distance within the tissue before encountering electrons, their negatively charged counterparts. This meeting results in a phenomenon known as annihilation, where the mass of the positron and electron is converted into energy in the form of two gamma rays, ejected in nearly opposite directions. This release of energy is a critical moment, marking the point where invisible biological activities start to translate into visible signals.

The PET scanner plays a crucial role in capturing these signals. Encircling the patient, its ring of detectors is finely tuned to detect the high-energy gamma rays emerging from the annihilation events. By registering the precise timing and location of these rays, the scanner reconstructs a detailed 3D-map of where the radiotracer has accumulated. Advanced algorithms then process these raw data, piecing together a comprehensive three-dimensional image. This image not only reveals the physical structure of the scanned area but, more importantly, highlights the variations in biological activities across different tissues. Bright spots in the image indicate regions of high radiotracer concentration, often correlating with areas of disease, such as cancerous growths. Through this detailed visual representation, PET imaging offers an unparalleled view into the body's inner workings, providing crucial information for the diagnosis, treatment planning, and monitoring of various diseases, thereby embodying a remarkable blend of scientific innovation and clinical utility.

17.1.1.2 Radiotracers used in PET

Common radiotracers used in PET imaging play a crucial role in visualizing different physiological and biochemical processes within the body. Each radiotracer is designed to target specific functions or tissues, enabling the detailed study of various diseases and conditions. The following describes some of the most frequently used radiotracers in PET.

18F-fluorodeoxyglucose (FDG) [6] is the most widely used radiotracer in PET imaging. FDG is a glucose analog that is taken up by cells with high glucose metabolism, making it particularly useful for identifying cancerous tumors, as cancer cells often have higher rates of glucose uptake than normal cells. FDG-PET is also used in the evaluation of brain disorders such as Alzheimer's disease [7] and in cardiology to assess myocardial viability [8].

11C-choline is used primarily for imaging prostate cancer [9] and brain tumors [10]. Choline is a nutrient that is involved in building cell membranes, and prostate cancer cells tend to take up more choline than normal cells due to their increased need for membrane synthesis as they grow and multiply. By labeling choline with carbon-11, doctors can use PET scans to detect areas of increased choline uptake in the body, which may indicate the presence of tumors.

Prostate-specific membrane antigen (PSMA) tracers are used in PET imaging for prostate cancer [11]. They target the PSMA, a protein abundantly expressed on prostate cancer cells. 68Ga-PSMA-11 and 18F-DCFPyL are common examples. 68Ga-DOTATATE (or DOTATOC/DOTANOC) targets somatostatin receptors, which are often overexpressed in neuroendocrine tumors. The use of 68Ga-labeled peptides allows for the precise detection and localization of neuroendocrine tumors. 18F-DCFPyL is marked with the radioactive isotope fluorine-18, which allows for detection of prostate cancer cells due to their expression of PSMA. This tracer has been particularly useful for identifying prostate cancer metastases and is valuable in both initial staging and the detection of recurrence. The high affinity of 18F-DCFPyL for PSMA-expressing cells leads to more accurate imaging results, which can significantly impact the treatment decisions and management of prostate cancer. PSMA tracers have significantly improved the detection of prostate cancer metastases and recurrence, offering high sensitivity and specificity. This advancement aids in accurate staging and treatment planning, enhancing personalized therapy approaches for prostate cancer patients.

18F-sodium fluoride (NaF) is used for bone scanning [12]. When injected into the body, 18F-sodium fluoride binds to areas of bone remodeling, which is indicative of bone growth or repair. Due to its high affinity for areas of calcification, it is particularly effective for detecting bone metastases in cancer patients. 18F-NaF PET scans offer higher sensitivity and resolution compared to traditional bone scintigraphy, providing valuable information for the diagnosis and management of skeletal diseases.

18F-fluciclovine (FACBC) is an amino acid analog used primarily for imaging prostate cancer [13]. It is useful for detecting recurrent prostate cancer, particularly in cases where standard imaging has been inconclusive.

These radiotracers, each with their specific targeting mechanisms, underscore the versatility of PET imaging in diagnosing and monitoring a wide range of conditions. The development and application of new radiotracers continue to expand the capabilities of PET, offering more detailed insights into disease processes and enhancing personalized treatment strategies.

17.1.1.3 Advantages of PET as a functional imaging modality

PET offers unparalleled insight into cellular activity and metabolic processes. Its ability to differentiate between active and dormant cells enhances radiation therapy's precision and effectiveness. PET distinguishes itself in the landscape of functional imaging by its exceptional sensitivity to minute changes in metabolic processes, a trait not as pronounced in other functional imaging techniques such as SPECT [14], which, while functional, cannot match the resolution or quantitative precision of PET. Unlike fMRI, which tracks blood flow as a surrogate for neural activity, PET measures cellular metabolism directly, offering insights into a broader spectrum of diseases, including cancer, beyond the scope of fMRI's primarily neurological applications. MR spectroscopy [15], which offers chemical composition data of tissue, provides a localized spectrum but lacks the whole-body metabolic mapping that PET delivers. Thus, in the functional imaging sphere, PET stands out for its comprehensive metabolic profiling, which, when integrated with anatomical imaging from CT or MRI, provides a holistic view of a patient's condition, crucial for personalized medicine and targeted treatment strategies.

17.1.2 From anatomy to function: the power of PET in radiation therapy

17.1.2.1 Differentiating between anatomical and functional imaging

Anatomical imaging, such as regular MRI and CT scans, excels in providing detailed visualizations of the body's structures, showcasing the physical form, size, shape, and position of organs and tissues. These modalities are particularly adept at detecting structural abnormalities, such as tumors, fractures, or anatomical malformations, by producing high-resolution images that delineate the intricate details of the body's anatomy.

In contrast, functional imaging techniques, such as PET, delve into the biochemical and physiological processes occurring within tissues and organs. PET scans, for instance, track the distribution of radiotracers to reveal metabolic activity, offering insights into cellular function that can indicate the presence of disease even before structural changes become apparent. This differentiation between anatomical and functional imaging underscores their complementary roles in medical diagnosis and treatment planning. While anatomical imaging offers a static picture of what is present, functional imaging provides a dynamic view of how the body operates, enabling early detection of diseases based on metabolic changes and aiding in the assessment of treatment efficacy. Together, these imaging modalities furnish a comprehensive understanding of both the form and function of the human body, facilitating precise diagnoses and tailored therapeutic approaches.

17.1.2.2 Role of PET imaging in detecting and targeting tumor heterogeneity and treatment response

Tumors are not uniform; they possess areas of varied metabolic activity. PET imaging can identify these active zones [16], enabling precise targeting during radiation treatment. PET imaging significantly influences the planning and execution of radiation therapy by illuminating the metabolic heterogeneity within tumors. This advanced imaging technique identifies areas within the tumor that exhibit higher metabolic activity, indicative of aggressive cancer cells. By precisely targeting these hotspots with tailored radiation doses, clinicians can optimize treatment efficacy, sparing surrounding healthy tissues. Furthermore, PET's capability to monitor the tumor's metabolic response to treatment over time provides invaluable feedback, allowing for the dynamic adjustment of radiation plans [17]. This adaptability ensures that therapy remains aligned with the evolving nature of the tumor, enhancing the potential for personalized treatment strategies that directly address the unique characteristics of the cancer. Such a focused approach not only aims to improve therapeutic outcomes but also minimizes the risk of side effects, contributing to an overall enhancement in patient care and prognosis in the battle against cancer.

Regular PET scans during treatment allow clinicians to monitor tumor response, adjusting radiation plans as necessary. This adaptive approach ensures optimal radiation delivery while preserving healthy tissues. PET imaging is pivotal in monitoring the evolution of tumors over the course of treatment by meticulously assessing the metabolic activity within the tumor at various stages prior to the initiation of therapy, during the treatment period, and following the conclusion of therapy. This is achieved through the measurement of fluctuations in the uptake of specific radiotracers, such as FDG, which are indicative of the tumor's metabolic rate. A discernible reduction in the uptake of these radiotracers over successive scans generally signals a favorable response to the treatment, manifesting the therapy's effectiveness in curtailing the tumor's metabolic activity. Conversely, a consistent or escalating uptake could denote the tumor's resistance to the current treatment regimen or the advancement of the disease. This capability of PET imaging to non-invasively track these metabolic changes offers a dynamic insight into the tumor's response, enabling clinicians to tailor treatment plans more accurately and make informed decisions regarding the patient's therapeutic strategy, thereby significantly impacting the overall management and prognosis of the disease.

17.1.3 Practicalities and clinical implications of PET-guided adaptive radiation therapy

17.1.3.1 Treatment planning: incorporating PET information

In the treatment planning phase, PET data can be invaluable. It aids in delineating tumor boundaries, understanding metabolic hotspots, and designing precise radiation beams. Incorporating PET information into daily radiation treatments significantly enhances the personalization and precision of therapy strategies. By utilizing the detailed metabolic activity and tumor extent data provided by PET scans, clinicians can more accurately define the target areas for radiation, differentiating between cancerous and healthy tissues with greater precision than conventional imaging allows. This detailed insight enables the meticulous adjustment of radiation dose distributions, focusing on eradicating cancer cells while minimizing exposure to surrounding healthy tissues. Furthermore, the concept of ART comes into play, wherein PET imaging is repeatedly used to monitor the tumor's response to treatment over time. Adjustments to the radiation plan are made dynamically, based on these sequential PET scans, to address changes in tumor size, shape, or metabolic activity. Such an adaptive approach not only aims to improve the accuracy of radiation delivery but also holds the promise of enhancing patient outcomes by reducing treatment-related side effects. Through this integration of PET data, radiation therapy is tailored to the unique characteristics of each patient's tumor, ensuring a highly individualized treatment process that adapts to the evolving nature of the disease.

17.1.3.2 PET-based biology-guided adaptive radiation therapy

The SCINTIX® biology-guided radiotherapy (BgRT) represents a cutting-edge advancement that merges real-time PET imaging with radiotherapy, enhancing the precision of tumor targeting and the efficacy of treatments. The RefleXion X1 system (RefleXion Medical, Inc., Hayward, CA) is a novel PET-guided radiation therapy machine [18, 19] featuring an 85 cm O-ring gantry linear accelerator (linac) capable of rotating at 60 revolutions per minute (rpm). It incorporates fan-beam kilovoltage computed tomography (kVCT) for precise image guidance in intensity-modulated radiation therapy (IMRT) and stereotactic body radiation therapy (SBRT). Additionally, it utilizes PET imaging for real-time tumor tracking in BgRT. The design of the X1 system is highlighted by its two symmetrically opposing 90-degree arcs of PET detectors seamlessly integrated into the ring gantry's architecture, to direct therapeutic radiation beams in real time, utilizing the tumor as a natural marker to guide and adapt the radiation dose dynamically during treatment. For real-time guidance, the system performs high-speed computations to generate limited time-sample PET images at 100-millisecond intervals, drawing on 500 milliseconds worth of accumulated line of response data.

This sophisticated system is specially tailored for providing comprehensive, real-time, BgRT for the treatment of bone and lung tumors, ensuring precise targeting and treatment delivery. The BIOGUIDE-X study [20] conducted sequential cohorts of participants to ascertain the optimal FDG dosage for SCINTIX therapy application, and to validate that the emulated radiation dose distribution corresponds with the physician-endorsed radiotherapy scheme. This forward-looking study enrolled individuals who presented with at least one FDG-avid tumor that was primary or metastatic, targetable, and measured between 2 and 5 cm, located in the lung or bone. Cohort I employed a modified $3 + 3$ scheme to identify the FDG dose necessary for SCINTIX therapy to produce an adequate signal. In cohort II, PET imaging was utilized on the X1 system to acquire data before the commencement and after the conclusion of the initial and final sessions of conventional stereotactic body radiotherapy. The SCINTIX therapy dose distributions were emulated using patient-specific CT anatomy and the acquired PET data for each treatment fraction. These were then compared against the physician-sanctioned plan.

The findings from cohort I showing sufficient FDG activity in all six evaluable participants following the administration of an initial dose level of 15 mCi FDG. In cohort II, the study saw the enrollment of four patients with lung tumors and five with bone tumors, from which data points for 17 treatment fractions were collected and evaluated. Out of these, 16 emulated deliveries yielded SCINTIX dose distributions that aligned accurately with the authorized SCINTIX therapy plan. Notably, all emulated fluences were found to be feasible for delivery. Furthermore, no adverse effects were ascribed to the repeated administrations of FDG. In essence, SCINTIX therapy presents a pioneering approach in radiotherapy where the radiolabeled tumor inherently serves as a fiducial marker for targeting.

As it stands, FDG is the sole radionuclide that has received FDA approval for use in BgRT. However, the scope of BgRT is set to broaden with the exploration of additional promising radionuclides such as PSMA and [89]Zr-labeled Panitumumab [21]. The incorporation of these new radionuclides into BgRT practices aims to enhance the specificity with which radiation targets tumor biology. This advancement has the potential to extend BgRT applicability across a wider spectrum of diseases and clinical contexts, particularly in improving the targeting of challenging tumors with more precise radionuclide-tumor binding. The SCINTIX radiotherapy system stands out due to its consistent accuracy and replicability in dose delivery. Such reliability, particularly under static conditions, marks SCINTIX as a significant technological development poised to push the boundaries of current radiotherapy modalities.

17.1.4 Artificial intelligence in PET-guided adaptive radiation therapy

17.1.4.1 Role of AI in enhancing image interpretation

Artificial intelligence can significantly enhance the analysis and interpretation of PET images [22, 23]. Machine learning algorithms can detect patterns or anomalies that might be overlooked by human observers, ensuring a more accurate diagnosis and treatment planning. AI algorithms can analyse complex imaging data with high precision and speed, identifying patterns and anomalies that may be subtle or invisible to the human eye. This capability significantly improves diagnostic accuracy and efficiency, enabling earlier and more accurate detection of diseases. AI can also learn from vast datasets to continuously improve its diagnostic capabilities, supporting radiologists in making more informed decisions. By reducing the potential for human error and increasing the consistency of image interpretations, AI ultimately contributes to better patient outcomes and streamlined workflows in healthcare settings.

17.1.4.2 Predictive modeling for treatment outcomes

AI, combined with PET imaging, can predict patient-specific responses to radiation therapy. These predictive models utilize vast amounts of data to estimate how a tumor might react, allowing for more personalized treatments [24]. It enhances the ability to predict patient-specific responses to radiation therapy by analysing metabolic and physiological data from PET scans. AI algorithms can identify patterns in the data that correlate with treatment outcomes, enabling personalized treatment plans that are more likely to be effective for individual patients. This predictive capability allows for the optimization of radiation doses, minimizing exposure to healthy tissues while targeting tumors more precisely. AI-driven analysis of PET imaging data can lead to better treatment decisions, reduced side effects, and potentially improved survival rates for patients undergoing radiation therapy.

17.1.4.3 AI-driven real-time treatment adjustments

With the assistance of AI, real-time adjustments during radiation sessions become feasible [25]. By analysing the ongoing PET data, AI systems can suggest immediate modifications to the treatment plan if deviations or unexpected responses are detected. It is a pivotal advancement in adaptive radiation therapy by enabling highly personalized and dynamic treatment protocols. By continuously analysing data from diagnostic images, patient responses, and other relevant clinical information, AI algorithms can detect subtle changes in tumor size, shape, and metabolic activity. This capability allows for the immediate adjustment of radiation doses and targeting strategies to reflect the tumor's current state and the patient's unique response to treatment. Consequently, treatments can be optimized on-the-fly, enhancing efficacy while minimizing damage to surrounding healthy tissues. This approach not only improves the precision and adaptability of radiation therapy but also opens up new possibilities for individualized patient care, potentially leading to better outcomes and reduced side effects.

17.1.5 Conclusions and future prospects

After exploring PET's role in adaptive radiation therapy and AI's promising potential, it is evident that these technologies are revolutionizing oncology treatments. Their convergence offers better patient outcomes with increased precision. The use of PET in oncology treatments is revolutionizing the field due to its ability to provide detailed metabolic insights into tumors, beyond what conventional imaging offers. PET's capacity to visualize the biological activity of tumors allows for earlier detection, precise staging, and monitoring of treatment responses, leading to more personalized and effective therapy strategies. This improved diagnostic accuracy and treatment monitoring enhance patient outcomes, making PET a cornerstone in the advancement of oncology care.

The synergistic combination of PET and adaptive radiation therapy can lead to innovations such as time-of-flight PET. Using PET functional images in radiation therapy offers potential benefits such as precise tumor targeting, enhanced treatment personalization, and the ability to adapt therapy based on real-time tumor responses. Innovations include more accurate dose distribution, minimizing exposure to healthy tissues, and improved detection of treatment-resistant tumor areas. These advancements lead to better patient outcomes and reduced side effects, marking a significant leap forward in the precision and effectiveness of cancer treatment. Such advancements, along with integration possibilities with other modalities, promise even more accurate and effective treatments in the future.

As technology evolves, so will the landscape of adaptive radiation therapy. Future research should delve into refining techniques, improving patient comfort, and reducing costs while maximizing outcomes. The use of PET in adaptive radiation therapy is poised for significant growth, with future research focusing on enhancing tumor characterization, treatment personalization, and real-time monitoring of therapy effectiveness. Advancements in PET technology and AI integration are expected to improve the precision of radiation dose delivery, reduce side effects, and facilitate the development of novel therapeutic strategies. These trends underscore PET's pivotal role in evolving adaptive radiation therapy towards more targeted, efficient, and patient-specific approaches, promising substantial improvements in cancer care and outcomes.

17.2 Functional MRI-guided ART

MRI has been routinely used in the clinic to facilitate target and OAR delineation owing to its superior soft-tissue contrast. Recent advancements in engineering have led to the successful integration of MR scanners with linear accelerators (linacs) for radiation treatment [26–28]. This integration opens up exciting possibilities for online MRI-based treatment adaptation to account for inter-fraction anatomy variations as well as real-time MRI-based gating to minimize the effect of intra-fraction motion on the delivered dose. There have been promising clinical trial data that demonstrate the potential benefits of MRI-guided ART [29–31].

Nevertheless, the current approach to treatment adaptation in MR-linac systems primarily relies on anatomical information to accommodate inter-fractional ana-tomical changes. It is important to note that the tumor response to radiation may take several weeks or even months to manifest anatomically [32]. This time delay presents a critical challenge in optimizing treatment plans using anatomical MRI. Functional MRI, on the other hand, has the potential to detect early tumor responses to radiation by assessing functional changes in the tumor microenviron-ment. This early detection capability opens a critical window for timely treatment adaptation [33, 34].

In this chapter, we will examine different functional MRI techniques for radiation treatment guidance, discuss current progress and practicalities of integrating func-tional MRI into the treatment adaptation, and explore the potential opportunity of incorporating AI to enhance the ability to optimize radiation treatment strategy.

17.2.1 From anatomy to function: the power of functional MRI in radiation therapy

17.2.1.1 Diffusion-weighted imaging
Diffusion-weighted imaging (DWI) stands as one of the most extensively employed functional MRI techniques. It uses dephasing and rephasing gradient pulses of various strengths (quantified as b-values) to cause signal attenuation. The degree of signal attenuation is related to the strength of gradient pulses as well as the diffusion of water molecules within tissues. By fitting images acquired with different b-values, an apparent diffusion coefficient (ADC) map is generated, which reflects the magnitude of water molecule diffusion within the tissue. Regions with restricted water diffusion, such as cellular structures or tumor, will display lower ADC values, while regions with more free water diffusion will have higher ADC values. DWI's ability to capture cellularity information has made it a pivotal tool in the detection, characterization, and monitoring of tumor response. DWI has shown great success in response prediction for various disease sites including the brain, head and neck, prostate, rectum, etc [34–36]. For most of the studies, it is observed that responders will have an increase in ADC compared to non-responders [34]. Yang *et al* demonstrated that the DWI images acquired on the low-field MR-linac had sufficient quality to capture potential radiation treatment effects [37] (figure 17.1).

17.2.1.2 Dynamic contrast-enhanced MRI
Dynamic contrast-enhanced MRI (DCE-MRI) is a semi-quantitative measurement to study blood flow and vascular permeability in tissues. It involves injecting a contrast agent, usually a gadolinium (Gd)-based contrast agent, into the blood-stream followed by the acquisition of a series of T1-weighted images. These images provide a time-series visualization of how the contrast agent disperses and washes out from the tissue, allowing for quantitative analysis of tissue characteristics such as tissue vascularization, perfusion, capillary permeability, and composition of the interstitial space. In general, malignant and aggressively growing tumors tend to

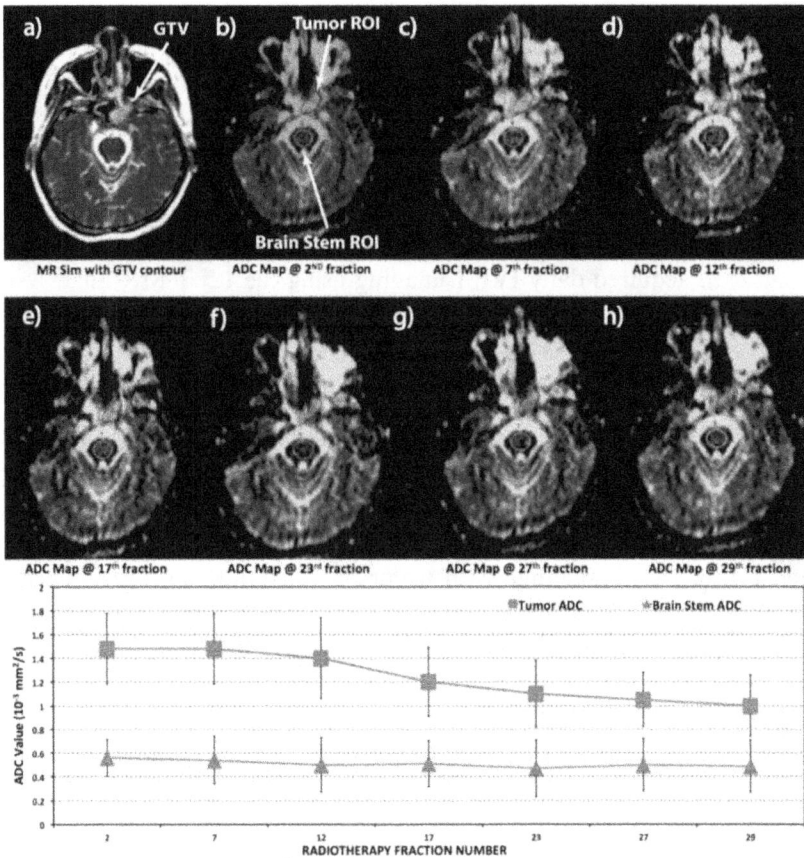

Figure 17.1. Longitudinal diffusion data of a 51 year old head and neck cancer patient. The error bars indicate standard deviations within the ROI. The average tumor ADC was relatively constant ($\sim 1.5 \times 10^{-3}$ mm^2 s^{-1}) during the first three weeks of radiotherapy, and decreased to 1×10^{-3} mm^2 s^{-1} from week 4 until the end of treatment. The ADC of the brainstem was relatively constant throughout the treatment with a nonsignificant linear fit slope of -0.001×10^{-3} mm^2 s^{-1} per day. (Reproduced from [37] with permission from John Wiley & Sons. Copyright 2016 American Association of Physicists in Medicine.)

exhibit a greater degree of vascularity to supply nutrients to the rapidly proliferating cells. Therefore, DCE-MRI has been used as a promising tool for tumor diagnosis and treatment response assessment for many sites such as the brain, breast, rectal, and cervix [36, 38, 39]. In a phase 2 study, DWI and DCE-MRI were combined to identify hypercellular and hyperperfused tumor volumes for dose intensification in GBM patients [40]. They found patients treated with functional boost had promising outcomes.

17.2.1.3 Intravoxel incoherent motion imaging

Unlike DCE-MRI, which relies on contrast injection to obtain tissue perfusion information, intravoxel incoherent motion imaging (IVIM) is one special technique that evaluates perfusion, or microcirculatory blood flow, without a contrast agent

[41]. IVIM imaging is essentially a variant of DWI that incorporates multiple low b-values (< 200 s mm^{-2}). In the IVIM model, the microcirculation of the blood in the capillary network would mimic a pseudo-diffusion process, and this perfusion effect predominantly contributes to the overall signal loss at the low b-value region. Therefore, bi-exponential fitting can be carried out for concurrent estimation of diffusion and perfusion. Although IVIM faces several technical challenges, its capability to concurrently assess diffusion and perfusion without an external contrast agent makes it an appealing technique in the research setting [42, 43]. Kooreman *et al* acquired daily IVIM imaging using the 1.5 T MR-linac system on 43 prostate cancer patients [44]. Despite high repeatability coefficients, IVIM parameter changes caused by radiation were found on a group level.

17.2.1.4 Other functional MRI

There are many other functional MRI techniques that have shown promise in assessing treatment response. One such technique is chemical exchange saturation transfer (CEST) MRI. In CEST imaging, a frequency-specific saturation pulse was first applied to selectively saturate protons on molecules of interest. These saturated protons will exchange with water protons and cause a signal decrease in the detected signal. By measuring the signal change in MRI, information on the molecules of interest can be obtained. There have been promising early results showing the capability of early treatment response assessment using CEST MRI for glioblastoma and nasopharyngeal carcinoma [45, 46]. Blood oxygenation level-dependent (BOLD) MRI measures the changes in bold oxygenation as oxygenated hemoglobin is less magnetic (diamagnetic) compared to deoxygenated hemoglobin (paramagnetic). Therefore, it has been used to assess tumor oxygenation, hence treatment response [47, 48]. MR spectroscopy diverges from traditional MRI by focusing on the spectral profiles of specific isotopes, such as ^{1}H, ^{13}C, or ^{31}P, within the specific voxel. As each metabolite has a unique spectral fingerprint, MR spectroscopy can identify and quantify various metabolites in the tissue. While it has been primarily utilized in the study of brain tumors [49, 50], MR spectroscopy is also being explored for its applicability in other areas such as the head and neck, and breast [51, 52]. Despite the potential of CEST, BOLD, and MR spectroscopy to enhance our understanding of cancer and its microenvironment, their use is primarily confined to research settings. This is mainly due to the technical complexity of these techniques and a pressing need for further validation to establish their clinical utility.

17.2.2 Practicalities and clinical implications of functional MRI-guided adaptive radiation therapy

While functional MRI has demonstrated significant potential benefits for the diagnosis and prognosis of various diseases, its routine clinical application to enhance patient outcomes necessitates further validation through randomized clinical trials. In a randomized phase 3 trial with 571 patients with prostate cancer (NCT01168479), multiparametric MRI (T2-weighted, DWI, and DCE) was used in initial treatment planning to design intraprostatic focal boost [53]. This trial reported that patients receiving focal boosts experienced improved biochemical disease-free survival without an increase in toxicity or a decrease in quality of life.

Treatment adaptation during the course of treatment is resource-intensive and time-consuming. Validating the clinical benefits and identifying the optimal time point for treatment adaptation is important to justify the associated cost. The advent of commercial MR-linac systems has simplified the logistics of treatment adaptation, which is now being explored across a wide range of disease sites including the brain, head and neck, lung, liver, pancreas, prostate, rectum, etc [54, 55]. Evidence from several completed phase 2 and phase 3 clinical trials underscores the potential advantages of using MR-linac for patient treatment. In pancreatic cancer, despite data suggesting dose escalation may improve the local control and overall survival [56, 57], it is usually not employed due to the association with increased gastrointestinal (GI) toxicity. In a multi-institutional phase 2 trial involving 136 patients (NCT03621644), a dose escalation strategy of 50 Gy in five fractions was employed for treating inoperable pancreatic ductal adenocarcinoma with the MR-linac system [30]. Online treatment adaptation was found dosimetric beneficial and was performed on 93.1% of the treatment fraction. Acute grade 3 or higher toxicity possibly or probably attributed to radiation treatment was observed in 8.8% of cases, with no cases definitively linked to the radiation, meeting the trial's primary endpoint. In a randomized phase 3 clinical trial involving 156 patients with prostate cancer (NCT04384770), patients treated on the MR-linac with a reduced planning margin had significantly reduced acute GI and genitourinary (GU) toxicity, although this trial did not implement treatment adaptation [29]. The potential benefits of incorporating treatment adaptation and simultaneous boost are currently being explored in several other phase 2 clinical trials (NCT04845503, NCT05183074).

However, most ART clinical trials on MR-linac systems have primarily focused on anatomical MRI information, with functional data often under-utilized in study designs. In an ongoing MR-ADAPTOR trial (NCT03224000) to study dose adaptation in HPV-positive oropharyngeal cancer, weekly DWI is acquired on the MR-linac to correlate the ADC changes with the final patient outcome [58]. Outside MR-linac, a randomized phase 2 study for head and neck cancer with poor prognosis (NCT02031250) utilized pre-treatment and mid-treatment DCE-MRI on a diagnostic MRI system to identify tumor subregions with poor perfusion for targeted focal boost.

While functional MRI holds significant promise for enhancing clinical treatment adaptation, the integration of functional MRI into clinical treatment adaptation workflows faces several significant challenges. These include the requirement for optimized and standardized imaging sequences, the need for thorough evaluation and validation of imaging biomarkers, and the imperative to develop accurate predictive models. These challenges will be discussed in section 17.2.4.

17.2.3 Artificial intelligence in functional MRI-guided adaptive radiation therapy

AI has emerged as a transformative tool in medicine and has the potential to optimize functional MRI acquisition, improve MRI imaging and parameter map generation, automate tumor segmentation, and provide valuable insights for treatment response prediction.

17.2.3.1 AI for improved imaging

One big disadvantage of function MRI is its prolonged acquisition times. In DWI, a large number of averages is usually needed for high b-value images to maintain a good signal-to-noise ratio (SNR) for diagnosis. AI holds the promise to accelerate the acquisition and improve the imaging efficiency. For example, AI can enable image reconstruction from significantly fewer repetitions. Variational networks have successfully reconstructed images for prostate and liver scans using only half or a third of the typical data [59, 60]. The quality of AI-reconstructed images, despite fewer averages, matches that of conventional acquisitions. Another strategy for acceleration involves denoising images that have been reconstructed with a minimal number of repetitions [61, 62]. Different denoising networks have been developed for different organs demonstrating that the image quality from 1 to 2 repetitions can be comparable to that of traditional DWI protocols, which generally need 10–16 repetitions. Additionally, Hong *et al* introduced a novel approach using a graph convolutional neural network for super-resolution (SR) in the slice direction [63]. This method enables faster acquisition by allowing slice-undersampling without compromising image quality.

Some other issues associated with DWI include its low SNR, low resolution, and strong spatial distortion associated with the single-shot echo-planar imaging (EPI) readout. AI can play a significant role in enhancing the image quality for improved image interpretation. Studies have shown that using deep learning could significantly boost image SNR and contrast-to-noise ratio (CNR) without impacting the ADC value [64]. To improve the image resolution, different SR networks have been proposed to reconstruct higher-resolution images from lower-resolution inputs [65, 66]. To mitigate spatial distortion, Hu *et al* proposed a 2D U-Net based network to correct DWI distortion, which showed reduced distortion compared to conventional methods such as field-mapping or top-up [67]. Their group later proposed a generative adversarial network to simultaneously improve the image resolution as well as reduce the spatial distortion [68].

17.2.3.2 AI for enhanced quantitative mapping

AI's impact extends to the estimation of functional MRI parameters, offering a more accurate and reliable analysis. In DCE-MRI, a parametric pharmacokinetic (PK) model is typically used to fit the time-series MRI and extract physiological parameters related to perfusion. However, the fitting is usually time-consuming and the obtained parameter maps may be noisy due to non-convexity of the cost function. To address these challenges, neural network models have been deployed to streamline the estimation process, achieving faster speeds and greater accuracy [69–72]. In particular,

Ottens *et al* implemented and compared several neural networks in analysing DCE data, and demonstrated the proposed gated recurrent unit (GRU) method had the best performance considering test–retest repeatability and robustness of avoiding potential systematic errors [72].

In IVIM imaging, voxel-wise non-linear least square fitting is the most common method for parameter fitting. Similar to DCE-MRI, the parameter fitting suffers from poor precision and noise. Simple artificial neural networks (ANNs), deep neural networks (DNNs), and convolutional neural networks (CNN) have been explored to achieve more robust parameter estimation [73–76]. In addition, IVIM imaging also presents the challenge of requiring a substantial number of *b*-value images for accurate fitting, compounded by the lack of a clear scheme for selecting optimized *b*-values. Lee *et al* introduced a DNN framework designed to optimize *b*-values and generate IVIM parameter maps simultaneously [77]. Their research revealed that the selection of optimized *b*-values is influenced by the level of noise present in the images.

17.2.3.3 AI for streamlined ART workflow

AI can streamline the adaptation process by automating image segmentation. Numerous studies have explored the application of AI models to automate segmentation processes using DWI [78–80] and DCE-MRI [81, 82], demonstrating the technology's potential to match, and in some cases, surpass human-level accuracy. For example, Trebeschi *et al* showed that combining DWI with other multiparametric MRI techniques enables more accurate rectal cancer segmentation using CNN [78]. Chen *et al* showed that the deep learning based model could detect and segment lesion that may potentially be missed by human expert [80] (figure 17.2).

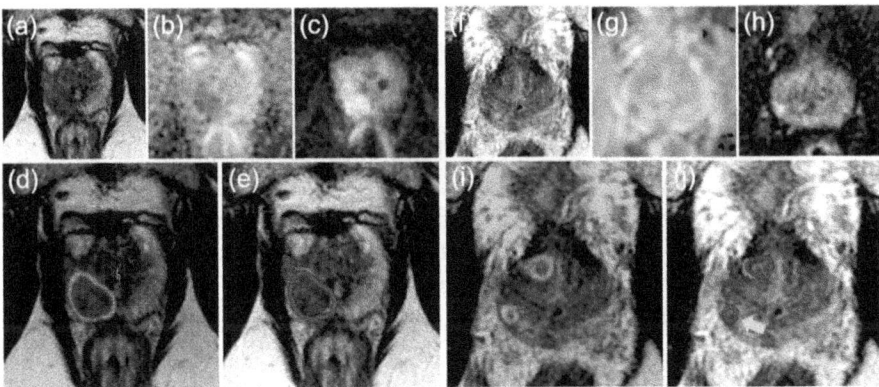

Figure 17.2. MB-U-Net segmentation of intraprostatic lesions in two cases in the testing set (shown in (a)–(e) and (f)–(j), respectively). (a) and (f): T2W; (b) and (g): ADC; (c) and (h): DWI ($b = 1200$ s mm^{-2}); (d) and (i): T2W images overlaid with output probability maps of the MB-U-Net for the lesion class; (e) and (j): T2W images overlaid with contours of the lesion (the red is ground truth, and the blue is predicted by the MB-U-Net). The lower lesion in figure (j) indicated by an orange arrow was not identified in the radiology report and thus not manually contoured as the ground truth, but it was predicted by the MB-U-Net and agreed with the corresponding pathological biopsy result. (Reproduced from [80] with permission from John Wiley & Sons. Copyright 2020 American Association of Physicists in Medicine.)

Liang *et al* developed a square-window based architecture for pancreatic GTV segmentation based on DCE-MRI acquired on a 1.5 T MR-linac, and showed the model performance was comparable to human expert [81].

17.2.3.4 AI for treatment response modeling

Lastly, the combination of AI with functional MRI offers substantial potential in predicting patient-specific responses and is another crucial domain to which AI can significantly contribute. Various deep learning models have been employed to predict treatment responses for different diseases using DWI, DCE-MRI, or other multiparametric MRI techniques [83–85]. Research by Jie *et al* demonstrated that pre-treatment DWI imaging features obtained from deep learning had superior prediction capability than handcrafted features for locally advanced rectal cancer radiation response [86]. In one particular study conducted on a low-field MR-linac, longitudinal DWI was acquired pre-, mid-, and post-treatment course for sarcoma patients [87]. A deep learning network was developed for predicting treatment response and achieved 97.1% accuracy for patient-based prediction. Yoon *et al* investigated the added value of DCE-MRI for local recurrence prediction for grade 4 adult-type diffuse glioma [88]. Their findings revealed that incorporating DCE-MRI data significantly enhanced the model's sensitivity, without affecting specificity.

17.2.4 Conclusion and future prospects

In summary, functional MRI offers a non-invasive method to capture early physiological changes within tumors long before these alterations manifest anatomically. This attribute renders functional MRI an invaluable asset in adaptive radiotherapy, offering the prospect of personalized radiation treatment.

Despite its potential, the transition of functional MRI into routine clinical ART practice is at a nascent stage, necessitating extensive groundwork to validate its efficacy and reliability. One first important step is imaging protocol standardization and optimization. This involves not only refining the protocols to improve the quality but also ensuring that biomarkers are reproducible across studies and institutions [89]. Such efforts require a concerted push towards standardization, which would not only bolster the accuracy of treatment response monitoring but also enhance collaborative opportunities among research institutions globally. Second, a key element in the successful integration of functional MRI into ART is the precise identification and timing of imaging biomarkers. Determining which biomarkers most accurately reflect the tumor's response to therapy, and pinpointing the optimal time points for the acquisition, are crucial steps in ensuring that monitoring is both efficient and impactful. Furthermore, the development of robust predictive models based on functional MRI, along with other imaging or clinical data, is paramount. Such models could significantly enhance the ability of clinicians to foresee treatment outcomes, enabling proactive adjustments to treatment plans. This predictive capacity is essential for the realization of truly adaptive radiotherapy. Finally, the formulation of adaptive treatment strategies must be rigorously evaluated through clinical trials. Such trials are vital for confirming the clinical benefits of ART, setting the stage for its broader implementation.

Artificial intelligence could play a pivotal role in enhancing various aspects of this process, including improving image quality and biomarker generation, selecting the best biomarkers, optimizing imaging schedules, developing accurate response prediction models, and automating the treatment adaptation process. By leveraging AI, the process of integrating functional MRI into ART can be significantly accelerated, paving the way for a more personalized approach to cancer treatment.

17.3 Summary

This chapter delves into the transformative role of AI in refining adaptive radiation therapy through advanced functional imaging techniques, specifically PET and MRI. AI's integration into PET and MRI has unlocked new dimensions in treatment planning and execution, allowing for unprecedented precision in targeting tumors while sparing healthy tissue. AI algorithms excel in analysing the rich, complex data provided by PET and MRI, facilitating adaptations to therapy plans based on the metabolic and biological changes within tumors. This synergy enhances the capability to predict treatment responses, tailor interventions to individual patient needs, and ultimately improve clinical outcomes. The confluence of AI with PET and MRI imaging signifies a major leap towards personalized, dynamic cancer care, promising a future where radiation therapy is not only more effective but also significantly safer.

References

[1] Gouw Z A R, La Fontaine M D, Vogel W V, van de Kamer J B, Sonke J-J and Al-Mamgani A 2020 Single-center prospective trial investigating the feasibility of serial FDG-PET guided adaptive radiation therapy for head and neck cancer *Int. J. Radiat. Oncol. Biol. Phys.* **108** 960–8

[2] Mäurer M *et al* 2022 PET/CT-based adaptive radiotherapy of locally advanced non-small cell lung cancer in multicenter yDEGRO ARO 2017-01 cohort study *Radiat. Oncol. Lond. Engl.* **17** 29

[3] Zaidi H and El Naqa I 2010 PET-guided delineation of radiation therapy treatment volumes: a survey of image segmentation techniques *Eur. J. Nucl. Med. Mol. Imaging* **37** 2165–87

[4] Shi X, Meng X, Sun X, Xing L and Yu J 2014 PET/CT imaging-guided dose painting in radiation therapy *Cancer Lett.* **355** 169–75

[5] Israel O and Kuten A 2007 Early detection of cancer recurrence: 18F-FDG PET/CT can make a difference in diagnosis and patient care *J. Nucl. Med. Off. Publ. Soc. Nucl. Med.* **48** 28S–35S

[6] Ell P J, Kayani I and Groves A M 2006 18F-fluorodeoxyglucose PET/CT in cancer imaging *Clin. Med.* **6** 240–4

[7] Chételat G *et al* 2020 Amyloid-PET and ^{18}F-FDG-PET in the diagnostic investigation of Alzheimer's disease and other dementias *Lancet. Neurol.* **19** 951–62

[8] Skali H, Schulman A R and Dorbala S 2013 ^{18}F-FDG PET/CT for the assessment of myocardial sarcoidosis *Curr. Cardiol. Rep.* **15** 352

[9] Reske S N *et al* 2006 Imaging prostate cancer with 11C-choline PET/CT *J. Nucl. Med. Off. Publ. Soc. Nucl. Med.* **47** 1249–54

[10] Giovannini E, Lazzeri P, Milano A, Gaeta M C and Ciarmiello A 2015 Clinical applications of choline PET/CT in brain tumors . *Curr. Pharm. Des.* **21** 121–7

[11] Maurer T, Eiber M, Schwaiger M and Gschwend J E 2016 Current use of PSMA-PET in prostate cancer management *Nat. Rev. Urol.* **13** 226–35

[12] Araz M, Aras G and Küçük Ö N 2015 The role of 18F-NaF PET/CT in metastatic bone disease *J. Bone. Oncol.* **4** 92–7

[13] Gusman M, Aminsharifi J A, Peacock J G, Anderson S B, Clemenshaw M N and Banks K P 2019 Review of ^{18}F-fluciclovine PET for detection of recurrent prostate cancer *Radiogr. Rev. Publ. Radiol. Soc. N. Am. Inc.* **39** 822–41

[14] Rahmim A and Zaidi H 2008 PET versus SPECT: strengths, limitations and challenges *Nucl. Med. Commun.* **29** 193–207

[15] Pathak A P, Gimi B, Glunde K, Ackerstaff E, Artemov D and Bhujwalla Z M 2004 Molecular and functional imaging of cancer: advances in MRI and MRS *Methods Enzymol.* **386** 3–60

[16] Bailly C *et al* 2019 Exploring tumor heterogeneity using PET imaging: the big picture *Cancers* **11** 1282

[17] Avril N E and Weber W A 2005 Monitoring response to treatment in patients utilizing PET *Radiol. Clin. North. Am.* **43** 189–204

[18] Shirvani S M *et al* 2021 Biology-guided radiotherapy: redefining the role of radiotherapy in metastatic cancer *Br. J. Radiol.* **94** 20200873

[19] Oderinde O M, Shirvani S M, Olcott P D, Kuduvalli G, Mazin S and Larkin D 2021 The technical design and concept of a PET/CT linac for biology-guided radiotherapy *Clin. Transl. Radiat. Oncol.* **29** 106–12

[20] Vitzthum L K *et al* 2024 BIOGUIDE-*X*: a first-in-human study of the performance of positron emission tomography-guided radiation therapy *Int. J. Radiat. Oncol. Biol. Phys.* **118** 1172–80

[21] Natarajan A *et al* 2023 Preclinical evaluation of 89Zr-panitumumab for biology-guided radiation therapy *Int. J. Radiat. Oncol. Biol. Phys.* **116** 927–34

[22] Liu J, Malekzadeh M, Mirian N, Song T-A, Liu C and Dutta J 2021 Artificial intelligence-based image enhancement in PET imaging: noise reduction and resolution enhancement *PET Clin.* **16** 553–76

[23] Reader A J and Pan B 2023 AI for PET image reconstruction *Br. J. Radiol.* **96** 20230292

[24] Wei L and El Naqa I 2021 Artificial intelligence for response evaluation with PET/CT *Semin. Nucl. Med.* **51** 157–69

[25] Archambault Y *et al* 2020 Making on-line adaptive radiotherapy possible using artificial intelligence and machine learning for efficient daily re-planning *Med. Phys. Int. J.* **8** 77–86

[26] Mutic S and Dempsey J F 2014 The ViewRay system: magnetic resonance-guided and controlled radiotherapy *Semin. Radiat. Oncol.* **24** 196–9

[27] Raaymakers B W *et al* 2009 Integrating a 1.5 T MRI scanner with a 6 MV accelerator: proof of concept *Phys. Med. Biol.* **54** N229

[28] Fallone B G 2014 The rotating biplanar linac–magnetic resonance imaging system *Semin. Radiat. Oncol.* **24** 200–2

[29] Kishan A U *et al* 2023 Magnetic resonance imaging-guided vs computed tomography-guided stereotactic body radiotherapy for prostate cancer: the MIRAGE randomized clinical trial *JAMA Oncol.* **9** 365–73

[30] Parikh P J *et al* 2023 A multi-institutional phase 2 trial of ablative 5-fraction stereotactic magnetic resonance-guided on-table adaptive radiation therapy for borderline resectable and locally advanced pancreatic cancer *Int. J. Radiat. Oncol. Biol. Phys.* **117** 799–808

[31] Ma T M *et al* 2023 Quality-of-life outcomes and toxicity profile among patients with localized prostate cancer after radical prostatectomy treated with stereotactic body radiation: the SCIMITAR multicenter phase 2 trial *Int. J. Radiat. Oncol.* **115** 142–52

[32] Thoeny H C and Ross B D 2010 Predicting and monitoring cancer treatment response with DW-MRI *J. Magn. Reson. Imaging JMRI* **32** 2–16

[33] Matuszak M M *et al* 2019 Functional adaptation in radiation therapy *Semin. Radiat. Oncol.* **29** 236–44

[34] van Houdt P J, Yang Y and van der Heide U A 2020 Quantitative magnetic resonance imaging for biological image-guided adaptive radiotherapy *Front. Oncol.* **10** 615643

[35] Lee M K, Choi Y and Jung S-L 2021 Diffusion-weighted MRI for predicting treatment response in patients with nasopharyngeal carcinoma: a systematic review and meta-analysis *Sci. Rep.* **11** 18986

[36] Padhani A R and Khan A A 2010 Diffusion-weighted (DW) and dynamic contrast-enhanced (DCE) magnetic resonance imaging (MRI) for monitoring anticancer therapy *Target. Oncol.* **5** 39–52

[37] Yang Y *et al* 2016 Longitudinal diffusion MRI for treatment response assessment: preliminary experience using an MRI-guided tri-cobalt 60 radiotherapy system *Med. Phys.* **43** 1369–73

[38] Zahra M A, Hollingsworth K G, Sala E, Lomas D J and Tan L T 2007 Dynamic contrast-enhanced MRI as a predictor of tumour response to radiotherapy *Lancet. Oncol.* **8** 63–74

[39] Dijkhoff R A P, Beets-Tan R G H, Lambregts D M J, Beets G L and Maas M 2017 Value of DCE-MRI for staging and response evaluation in rectal cancer: a systematic review *Eur. J. Radiol.* **95** 155–68

[40] Kim M M *et al* 2021 A phase 2 study of dose-intensified chemoradiation using biologically based target volume definition in patients with newly diagnosed glioblastoma *Int. J. Radiat. Oncol. Biol. Phys.* **110** 792–803

[41] Le Bihan D, Breton E, Lallemand D, Aubin M L, Vignaud J and Laval-Jeantet M 1988 Separation of diffusion and perfusion in intravoxel incoherent motion MR imaging *Radiology* **168** 497–505

[42] Noij D P *et al* 2017 Intravoxel incoherent motion magnetic resonance imaging in head and neck cancer: a systematic review of the diagnostic and prognostic value *Oral Oncol.* **68** 81–91

[43] Marzi S *et al* 2017 The prediction of the treatment response of cervical nodes using intravoxel incoherent motion diffusion-weighted imaging *Eur. J. Radiol.* **92** 93–102

[44] Kooreman E S *et al* 2019 Feasibility and accuracy of quantitative imaging on a 1.5 T MR-linear accelerator *Radiother. Oncol.* **133** 156–62

[45] Mehrabian H, Myrehaug S, Soliman H, Sahgal A and Stanisz G J 2018 Evaluation of glioblastoma response to therapy with chemical exchange saturation transfer *Int. J. Radiat. Oncol. Biol. Phys.* **101** 713–23

[46] Qamar S *et al* 2019 Amide proton transfer MRI detects early changes in nasopharyngeal carcinoma: providing a potential imaging marker for treatment response *Eur. Arch. Oto-Rhino-Laryngol.* **276** 505–12

[47] Kim C H, Lee J H, Lee J W, Kim E and Choi S-H 2022 Introducing a new biomarker named R2*-BOLD-MRI parameter to assess treatment response in osteosarcoma *J. Magn. Reson. Imaging JMRI* **56** 538–46

[48] Jiang L, Weatherall P T, McColl R W, Tripathy D and Mason R P 2013 Blood oxygenation level-dependent (BOLD) contrast magnetic resonance imaging (MRI) for prediction of breast cancer chemotherapy response: a pilot study *J. Magn. Reson. Imaging JMRI* **37** 1083–92

[49] Muruganandham M *et al* 2014 3-dimensional magnetic resonance spectroscopic imaging at 3 tesla for early response assessment of glioblastoma patients during external beam radiation therapy *Int. J. Radiat. Oncol. Biol. Phys.* **90** 181–9

[50] Nelson S J *et al* 2016 Serial analysis of 3D H-1 MRSI for patients with newly diagnosed GBM treated with combination therapy that includes bevacizumab *J. Neurooncol.* **130** 171–9

[51] Bezabeh T *et al* 2005 Prediction of treatment response in head and neck cancer by magnetic resonance spectroscopy *AJNR Am. J. Neuroradiol.* **26** 2108–13

[52] Bolan P J *et al* 2017 MR spectroscopy of breast cancer for assessing early treatment response: results from the ACRIN 6657 MRS trial *J. Magn. Reson. Imaging* **46** 290–302

[53] Kerkmeijer L G W *et al* 2021 Focal boost to the intraprostatic tumor in external beam radiotherapy for patients with localized prostate cancer: results from the FLAME randomized phase III trial *J. Clin. Oncol.* **39** 787–96

[54] Keall P *et al* 2022 ICRU REPORT 97: MRI-guided radiation therapy using MRI-linear accelerators *J. ICRU* **22** 1–100

[55] Bryant J M *et al* 2023 Stereotactic magnetic resonance-guided adaptive and non-adaptive radiotherapy on combination MR-linear accelerators: current practice and future directions *Cancers* **15** 2081

[56] Krishnan S *et al* 2016 Focal radiation therapy dose escalation improves overall survival in locally advanced pancreatic cancer patients receiving induction chemotherapy and consolidative chemoradiation *Int. J. Radiat. Oncol. Biol. Phys.* **94** 755–65

[57] Reyngold M *et al* 2021 Association of ablative radiation therapy with survival among patients with inoperable pancreatic cancer *JAMA Oncol.* **7** 735–8

[58] Bahig H *et al* 2018 Magnetic resonance-based response assessment and dose adaptation in human papilloma virus positive tumors of the oropharynx treated with radiotherapy (MR-ADAPTOR): an R-IDEAL stage 2a-2b/Bayesian phase II trial *Clin. Transl. Radiat. Oncol.* **13** 19–23

[59] Johnson P M *et al* 2022 Deep learning reconstruction enables highly accelerated biparametric MR imaging of the prostate *J. Magn. Reson. Imaging JMRI* **56** 184–95

[60] Afat S *et al* 2023 Acquisition time reduction of diffusion-weighted liver imaging using deep learning image reconstruction *Diagn. Interv. Imaging* **104** 178–84

[61] Kawamura M *et al* 2020; Accelerated acquisition of high-resolution diffusion-weighted imaging of the brain with a multi-shot echo-planar sequence: deep-learning-based denoising *Magn. Reson. Med. Sci.* **20** 99–105

[62] Kaye E A *et al* 2020 Accelerating prostate diffusion-weighted MRI using a guided denoising convolutional neural network: retrospective feasibility study *Radiol. Artif. Intell.* **2** e200007

[63] Hong Y, Chen G, Yap P-T and Shen D 2019 Multifold acceleration of diffusion MRI via deep learning reconstruction from slice-undersampled data *Inf. Process. Med. Imaging Proc. Conf.* **11492** 530–41

[64] Ueda T *et al* 2022 Deep learning reconstruction of diffusion-weighted MRI improves image quality for prostatic imaging *Radiology* **303** 373–81

[65] Albay E, Demir U and Unal G 2018 Diffusion MRI spatial super-resolution using generative adversarial networks *Predictive Intelligence in Medicine* ed I Rekik, G Unal, E Adeli and S H Park (Cham: Springer International) pp 155–63

[66] Chatterjee S *et al* 2021 ShuffleUNet: super resolution of diffusion-weighted MRIs using deep learning arXiv: 2102.12898

[67] Hu Z *et al* 2020 Distortion correction of single-shot EPI enabled by deep-learning *NeuroImage* **221** 117170

[68] Ye X *et al* 2023 Simultaneous superresolution reconstruction and distortion correction for single-shot EPI DWI using deep learning *Magn. Reson. Med.* **89** 2456–70

[69] Ulas C *et al* 2019 Convolutional neural networks for direct inference of pharmacokinetic parameters: application to stroke dynamic contrast-enhanced MRI *Front. Neurol.* **9** 1147

[70] Bliesener Y, Acharya J and Nayak K S 2020 Efficient DCE-MRI parameter and uncertainty estimation using a neural network *IEEE Trans. Med. Imaging* **39** 1712–23

[71] Zou J, Balter J M and Cao Y 2020 Estimation of pharmacokinetic parameters from DCE-MRI by extracting long and short time-dependent features using an LSTM network *Med. Phys.* **47** 3447–57

[72] Ottens T *et al* 2022 Deep learning DCE-MRI parameter estimation: application in pancreatic cancer *Med. Image. Anal.* **80** 102512

[73] Bertleff M *et al* 2017 Diffusion parameter mapping with the combined intravoxel incoherent motion and kurtosis model using artificial neural networks at 3 T *NMR Biomed.* **30** e3833

[74] Barbieri S, Gurney-Champion O J, Klaassen R and Thoeny H C 2020 Deep learning how to fit an intravoxel incoherent motion model to diffusion-weighted MRI *Magn. Reson. Med.* **83** 312–21

[75] Vasylechko S D, Warfield S K, Afacan O and Kurugol S 2022 Self-supervised IVIM DWI parameter estimation with a physics based forward model *Magn. Reson. Med.* **87** 904–14

[76] Kaandorp M P T *et al* 2021 Improved unsupervised physics-informed deep learning for intravoxel incoherent motion modeling and evaluation in pancreatic cancer patients *Magn. Reson. Med.* **86** 2250–65

[77] Lee W, Kim B and Park H 2021 Quantification of intravoxel incoherent motion with optimized *b*-values using deep neural network *Magn. Reson. Med.* **86** 230–44

[78] Trebeschi S *et al* 2017 Deep learning for fully-automated localization and segmentation of rectal cancer on multiparametric MR *Sci. Rep.* **7** 5301

[79] Gurney-Champion O J, Kieselmann J P, Wong K H, Ng-Cheng-Hin B, Harrington K and Oelfke U 2020 A convolutional neural network for contouring metastatic lymph nodes on diffusion-weighted magnetic resonance images for assessment of radiotherapy response *Phys. Imaging Radiat. Oncol.* **15** 1–7

[80] Chen Y, Xing L, Yu L, Bagshaw H P, Buyyounouski M K and Han B 2020 Automatic intraprostatic lesion segmentation in multiparametric magnetic resonance images with proposed multiple branch UNet *Med. Phys.* **47** 6421–9

[81] Liang Y *et al* 2020 Auto-segmentation of pancreatic tumor in multi-parametric MRI using deep convolutional neural networks *Radiother. Oncol. J. Eur. Soc. Ther. Radiol. Oncol.* **145** 193–200

[82] Nalepa J *et al* 2020 Fully-automated deep learning-powered system for DCE-MRI analysis of brain tumors *Artif. Intell. Med.* **102** 101769

[83] Mazaheri Y *et al* 2022 Evaluation of cancer outcome assessment using MRI: a review of deep-learning methods *BJR|Open* **4** 20210072

[84] Gao Y, Pham J, Yoon S, Cao M, Hu P and Yang Y 2021 Recent advances in functional MRI to predict treatment response for locally advanced rectal cancer *Curr. Colorectal Cancer Rep.* **17** 77–87

[85] Gurney-Champion O J, Landry G, Redalen K R and Thorwarth D 2022 Potential of deep learning in quantitative magnetic resonance imaging for personalized radiotherapy *Semin. Radiat. Oncol.* **32** 377–88

[86] Fu J *et al* 2020 Deep learning-based radiomic features for improving neoadjuvant chemo-radiation response prediction in locally advanced rectal cancer *Phys. Med. Biol.* **65** 075001

[87] Gao Y *et al* 2021 A preliminary study of deep learning-based treatment response prediction for soft tissue sarcoma using longitudinal diffusion MRI *Med. Phys.* **48** 3262–372

[88] Yoon J *et al* 2024 Added value of dynamic contrast-enhanced MR imaging in deep learning-based prediction of local recurrence in grade 4 adult-type diffuse gliomas patients *Sci. Rep.* **14** 2171

[89] Shukla-Dave A *et al* 2019 Quantitative imaging biomarkers alliance (QIBA) recommendations for improved precision of DWI and DCE-MRI derived biomarkers in multicenter oncology trials *J. Magn. Reson. Imaging JMRI* **49** e101–21

IOP Publishing

Artificial Intelligence in Adaptive Radiation Therapy

Yi Wang and X. Sharon Qi

Chapter 18

Artificial intelligence in proton adaptive radiation therapy

Brian Winey

Adaptive proton therapy workflows are being investigated by multiple institutions and research groups. While both photon and proton adaptive therapy workflows must overcome numerous challenges, the unique aspects of proton interactions resulting in energy deposition in tissue and the limited availability of image guidance with accurate tissue composition information make adaptive proton therapy workflow development a more challenging translational endeavor. Much work has contributed to the clinical deployment of adaptive proton therapy workflows, mostly using in-room CT imaging which achieves the most accurate tissue decomposition. To address the outstanding challenges of adaptive proton therapy, AI tools are being developed to address most of the components of an adaptive workflow, including image correction, contour propagation, treatment planning, dose calculations, and QA of both imaging and treatment plans.

18.1 Proton ART

18.1.1 Clinical context and necessity

Proton therapy uses the Bragg peak physical depth dose to increase the therapeutic ratio of dose to target versus dose to normal tissue. While the clinical significance remains a topic of clinical trials and biological studies, the physical depth dose is well defined in water, dependent on the initial proton kinetic energy, and multiple Bragg peaks can be combined to deliver a prescribed dose to a volume of tissue, either from a single beam angle or multiple beams with individualized beamlet weights.

Given the well-defined relationship between the initial kinetic energy and range of the proton in water [1], there remain multiple sources of uncertainty of the proton range when modeling and delivering protons of a specific energy to a patient or phantom [2]. Some of the range uncertainties are systematic and addressed with more precise CT stopping power ratio (SPR) image calibration, accelerator

doi:10.1088/978-0-7503-6119-4ch18

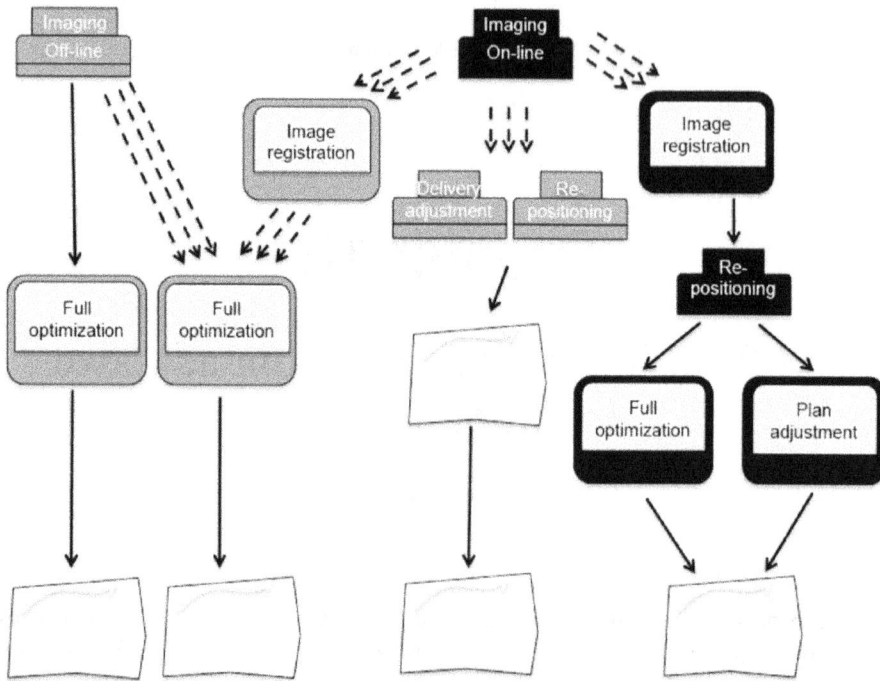

Figure 18.1. A diagram of adaptive proton therapy workflows. AI tools are being developed for Image registration, contour propagation, dose calculation, and online image corrections. (Adapted with permission from [3]. Copyright 2021 Institute of Physics and Engineering in Medicine.)

commissioning, Monte Carlo dose calculations, and treatment planning margins. For other non-systematic range uncertainties, there are proposed methods to reduce the impacts on the dose delivery, namely margins and *in vivo* imaging, but adaptive proton therapy workflows can identify changes in the patient that impact the proton range [3]. Set-up uncertainties and anatomic changes during the course of treatment, either daily or slower anatomic changes, can be detected in daily volumetric imaging. There have been multiple studies of *in vivo* and 4D imaging to detect higher frequency changes in the patient anatomy due to breathing motion and other intrafractional changes [4]. Figure 18.1 provides an illustration of the adaptive workflows being investigated for proton therapy.

Adaptive proton therapy workflows have three primary aims:

1. Detect and measure anatomic changes and set-up changes in the patient geometry.
2. Calculate and quantify any dose differences in the target and surrounding organs, particularly range differences.
3. Generate a new treatment plan or determine the original plan satisfies all clinical goals.

Much work continues in all the above aims, even more so when considering real time imaging for 4D or other intrafractional anatomic changes. Before discussing the roles of artificial intelligence (AI) in adaptive proton therapy, it is important to summarize briefly the patient populations along with the respective changes in the patient anatomy and the current state of adaptive proton therapy workflows.

18.1.2 Patient populations

While there are some patient populations that are more likely to be treated with proton therapy than other external beam or internal radiation therapy, the primary focus of this section will be the different patient populations classified by the geometric changes and the associated need for imaging and adaptation.

18.1.2.1 Set-up uncertainties

The daily set-up uncertainties of patient populations can vary from sub-milli-meter in cranial treatments [5, 6] to larger magnitudes for targets in more challenging locations, especially more deformable soft tissue targets. For patient populations that have reproducible set-up with limited (< 1–2 mm) uncertainties, including anatomic changes, there is generally not a need for adaptive workflows. The initial planning CT is most likely a representative image of the daily patient geometry and small uncertainties can be incorporated into the initial planning target, either with a planning target volume (PTV) or beam specific PTV. Most proton treatment facilities incorporate set-up and range uncertainties into the initial treatment plan and reproducible set-ups can be taken into account in the initial treatment plan.

Set-up uncertainties can become larger and vary with daily positioning for different reasons. Some soft tissue targets such as sarcomas can be set up with high reproducibility using bony anatomy or implanted fiducials as surrogates for the target geometry including shape and location in the patient anatomy. Improved imaging techniques such as in-room CT and the latest CBCT technologies can provide visualization of soft tissue targets but the set-up uncertainties are generally larger for soft tissue targets, particularly those in the thoracic and abdominal regions.

An additional reason for increased set up uncertainties is the size of the target. Proton therapy is often used for craniospinal irradiation (CSI) and heck and neck (H&N) primary lesions with larger nodal volumes which involve large treatment fields covering anatomic regions that can move relative to each other. The set-up uncertainties can be reduced with multiple isocenters and repeated imaging but the motion of one part of the target relative to another component can increase the set-up uncertainties.

In both previous patient populations, soft tissue and large targets, there is a potential need for adaptive proton therapy to improve the target doses and reduce the risk of extra dose in the neighboring OARs. The following section will begin to unpack the implications of anatomic changes, including the impact on set-up uncertainties.

18.1.2.2 Daily or slower anatomic changes

For some patient populations, there can be slow changes in the patient anatomy, for example weight loss, that can reduce the efficacy of the immobilization device and give rise to larger variations in the daily patient position. While rigid 3D and 6D shifts can be applied to the patient position to minimize the impacts of the patient geometry changes, the set-up uncertainties can be increased, for example in the H&N patient population where the cranial immobilization might remain reproducible, but the neck nodal region can have increased set-up uncertainties where the mask is less tight after patient weight loss. Not all patients within a specific primary treatment site are subject to the same slow anatomic changes [7] but the implications of the anatomic changes can be challenging to incorporate into the initial plan, even when using robust optimization [8, 9], thus giving rise to the need for daily or weekly adaptive proton therapy.

18.1.2.3 Real time anatomic changes

Real time anatomic changes are a challenge for all external beam radiation therapy but especially impactful for proton therapy. Most common are the real time changes due to respiratory motion. Compounding the respiratory motion with the target moving outside the treatment volume, proton therapy also encounters changes in tissue density as well as interplay for dynamic deliveries such as scanning deliveries. While photon external beam treatments also encounter the same real time anatomic changes for thoracic and abdominal targets, the impacts on proton dose distributions are more sensitive to the real time changes. At this time, there are limited options for proton delivery systems to adaptively address the impacts of real time anatomic changes. Interventions that have been found to be most effective include rescanning, gating, and breath-hold, in increasing patient intervention. For systems that include an in-room CT, there is the ability to also perform a 4D CT or other respiratory motion analysis in the treatment position and use this information for an adaptive workflow. CBCT reconstruction methods are being developed to address the respiratory motion and AI can be a helpful tool to address the CBCT motion artifacts.

Aside from respiratory motion, other real time anatomic changes can include swallowing, eye movements, bowel changes, and bladder filling. Eye movements during proton therapy are typically gated with direct imaging of the eye but other real time anatomic changes during proton therapy are not regularly detected or measured. To fully extend adaptive workflows to real time anatomic changes will require developments of more imaging options to both detect and measure the real time patient anatomy.

18.1.3 Imaging and adaptive workflows

18.1.3.1 Offline workflows

Imaging for radiation therapy can be divided into two categories, offline and online. Much work has studied the role of offline imaging for adaptive proton therapy. Some patient studies and clinical workflows recommend or require offline CT, MRI, or PET imaging during the course of treatment to evaluate the clinical impact of the radiation treatment as well as anatomic changes in the patient. Depending upon the disease site, changes can include tumor growth or shrinkage, weight loss or gain, and fluid buildup or drainage. When using offline imaging, the time required to process the three steps of the adaptive workflow is less critical.

18.1.3.2 Online workflows

Online adaptive workflows for proton therapy are becoming more common as more online imaging technologies are deployed in clinical proton therapy facilities. Online imaging can either be immediately before the treatment is delivered or during the treatment delivery. Historically, most online imaging was 2D planar imaging until in-room or nearby CTs were deployed in some facilities such as the Paul Scherrer Institute (PSI). Additionally, real time imaging of the PET signal was developed at Gesellschaft für Schwerionenforschung, Helmholtz Centre for Heavy Ion Research, and Heidelberg Ion Beam Therapy Center [4, 10–14]. These earliest measurements of the patient anatomy and beam delivery were not used for complete online adaptive workflows due to the time required for contour propagation, plan creation, and dose calculations. Online adaptive workflows require rapid software applications to process the three adaptive steps.

Currently, CBCT and in-room CT imaging are available in a majority of proton therapy facilities [15, 16], thus allowing for adaptive proton therapy workflows based upon the available 3D imaging of the patient in the treatment position and at isocenter for many CBCT systems. Along with the increased availability of in-room volumetric imaging, the adaptive steps of contour propagation through rigid and deformable registration, plan optimization, and dose calculations have each seen tremendous improvements in speed. Still, there remains a need for improvements in each of the steps of an adaptive proton therapy workflow which gives rise to the opportunity for AI in adaptive proton therapy.

18.1.4 Rationale for AI in proton ART

Other chapters in this book will explore some of the common applications of AI in radiation therapy, including applications that directly impact adaptive proton therapy. Some of the most necessary AI developments for adaptive proton therapy address the workflow steps that require additional time using analytic or brute force methods. Many of the tools for adaptive proton therapy workflows are mature and ready for clinical use but often require minutes to hours for processing. AI can dramatically decrease the time needed for these processes. AI tools for adaptive proton therapy workflows can be classified broadly into imaging, registration, and dose calculations.

Compared to applications of AI in adaptive photon therapy, the dosimetric properties of the Bragg peak can impose greater constraints on the accuracy and precision of the AI tools. For example, the image pixel accuracies for AI generated synthetic CTs will have a greater impact on the proton dose calculations than the photon dose calculations. Additionally, proton therapy can be used for anatomic arrangements where a sharp gradient will spare a critical organ. The accuracy of the relative stopping powers, the registration, the contouring, and the dose calculation can have more pronounced impacts on the proton therapy plan optimization and delivery. The use of AI in adaptive proton therapy workflows can greatly improve the proton therapy delivery and it requires additional quality assurance checks to generate confidence in the AI tools.

18.2 AI in proton ART

18.2.1 Imaging

The most development of AI for adaptive proton therapy has been focused on the improvement of the volumetric imaging for online dose calculations. While the current diagnostic CT quality of in-room CT imaging is generally accepted as sufficient for proton dose calculations, the image quality of CBCT is insufficient for dose calculations without substantial improvements. Historically, the image quality of CBCT was addressed with simple scatter models and hardware modifications, namely anti-scatter grids. These software and hardware modifications improved the image quality such that registrations could be performed more accurately but the image quality was still insufficient for dose calculations.

Analytic models were proposed to address the scatter contamination in the CBCT projections. Such projections could more accurately predict scatter components and mitigate the impact of scatter contamination on the reconstructed CBCT Hounsfield units [17]. While the analytic models could improve the image quality, even to a level sufficient for proton dose calculations [18], the time required for such analytic model-based corrections was prohibitive for online adaptive proton therapy workflows. Additionally, the analytic models typically functioned in the projection space, requiring access to the CBCT projection data, data that are not easily accessible in all imaging systems.

There have been other correction methods proposed to improve the CBCT image quality, including look up table (LUT), deformed CT, and histogram matching. The LUT and histogram matching can be performed rapidly but fail to address all scatter artifacts, particularly when the images have large amounts of cupping and streak artifacts. Deformation of the CT can generate highly accurate corrected CBCT image intensities when there are few artifacts or anatomic differences between the floating and reference images. Deforming the CT can require a large amount of time and fails in the presence of large artifacts and anatomic differences, particularly air pockets [19]. To address the time required for deformation of volumetric imaging, AI can be employed as discussed in chapter 9.

The current uses of AI can be broadly separated into image domain and projection domain models. The advantages of the image domain corrections include more readily accessible data and the ability to correct both the artifacts from the scatter and the reconstruction algorithm, typically an FDK backprojection. The projection domain corrections can more directly the patient and image specific scatter components in the projection space. Specifically, for each unique combination of patient geometry and image system (source and panel) position, the scatter component in the projection space will change based on the underlying physical

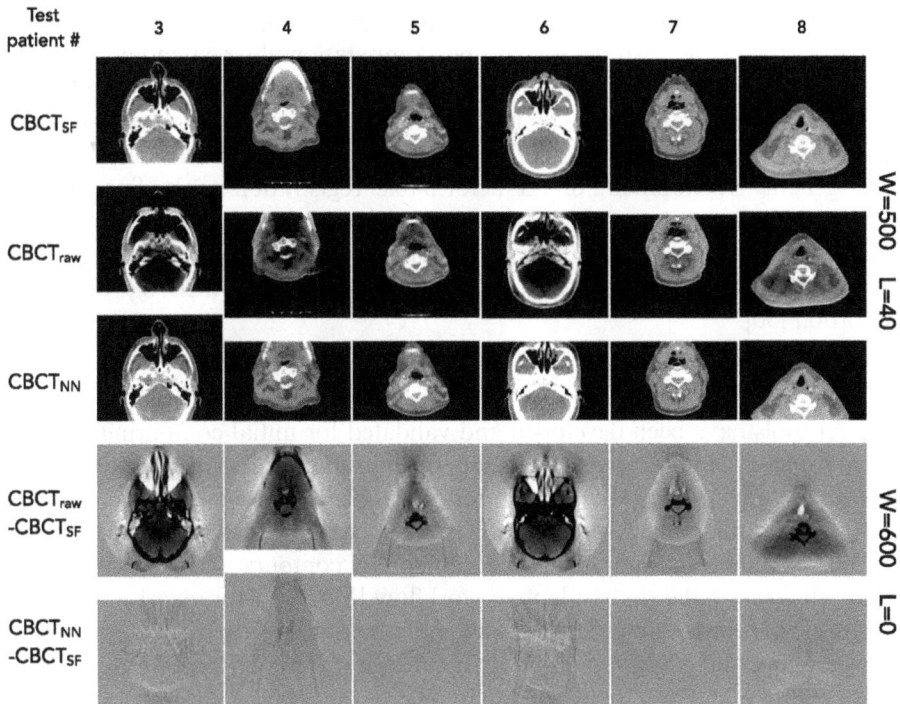

Figure 18.2. The use of AI to correct the online CBCT imaging is demonstrated in this image. (Adapted with permission from [21]. Copyright 2020 Institute of Physics and Engineering in Medicine.)

conditions. Such image and patient specific variability is not as easily determined after reconstruction.

When considering AI applications for CBCT corrections in proton therapy, Hansen *et al* [20] first published a CNN named SCATTERNET which demonstrated significant and rapid image quality improvements. Subsequent studies have further developed, tested, and validated CNNs for the improvement of CBCT image quality [21], as seen in figure 18.2. More recent studies have iterated with different imaging systems, treatment sites, and projection domain. A CNN has been demonstrated to be a rapid and reliable AI tool for CBCT image correction [22].

In addition to CNN models, other groups have used other AI models to correct the CBCT image quality with GANS and cycleGANs, using both paired and unpaired image sets. More recently, additional models such as transformers have been translated into adaptive therapy [23]. Outside of adaptive proton therapy research studies, there are numerous groups developing AI tools for CBCT image quality improvements in a more diagnostic context. The proton RT groups have many more potential models to test and validate for proton dose calculations.

18.2.2 Deformable and rigid registration

As stated above, deformable and rigid registrations are essential for adaptive proton therapy workflows when generating deformed CTs as a surrogate for the insufficient

CBCT or when propagating contours from one volumetric image to a new volumetric image. Registrations can be computationally demanding, requiring much time to perform, and lead to delays in the adaptive proton workflow. AI can significantly reduce the time required for performing the registrations [24]. Chapter 9 looks at the use of AI for deformable and rigid registration as it pertains to the general development of AI deformable registration tools. Specifically to proton therapy, some groups have begun to develop tools to evaluate the robustness of the deformable registration, performed with or without AI assistance [25–29], or used expert analysis to evaluate the contours propagated with the deformable registration [30].

18.2.3 Contour propagation

While AI tools have been developed and validated for initial contouring of patient anatomy and treatment targets (chapter 9), the same tools can be used for daily adaptive therapy. Since other AI contouring tools are designed to generate new contours without a patient specific prior, a recent study focused on adaptive proton therapy workflows incorporated the planning CT contours and generated patient specific models for the daily adaptive workflow [31, 32]. More work is needed to develop more robust, rapid, and reliable daily contouring tools for daily adaptive proton therapy, including rapid quality assurance reviews of the contours [25].

18.2.4 Dose calculations

The third computationally demanding step in the adaptive proton therapy workflow is the dose calculation. While the pencil beam and, more recently, the Monte Carlo, dose calculations can be performed in less than 1 min [33], there are opportunities to use AI as a secondary dose check, refine the pencil beam dose calculation in the local scatter inaccuracies, or perform a full dose model [1, 34–39]. There is significant overlap between the dose calculation and plan optimization, given that each scenario of an analytic plan optimization requires at least an estimate of the dose distribution. The use of AI for proton dose calculations is at an early stage but multiple groups are developing AI tools to increase the speed of the dose calculations and potentially improve the final plan through more optimal plan generation.

18.2.5 Plan optimization

Plan optimization for proton therapy can be a computationally demanding process, with some current commercial optimization algorithms requiring minutes to hours for the creation of multiple potential plans used for the calculation of Pareto optimal solutions. While there is extensive work ongoing to develop AI tools for rapid plan optimization, few studies have looked specifically at the area of online proton plan optimization/reoptimization with AI algorithms [40]. The issue of rapid plan optimization for adaptive proton therapy has been addressed with other analytic tools (plan libraries) or approximations (limiting spots or using prior beam arrangements) [41]. The same AI tools being developed for general plan optimization in chapter 10 can be explored for online adaptive proton therapy.

18.2.6 Other developments

There remain other issues in adaptive proton therapy for which AI will provide additional improvements. Currently, the use of CBCT has been extensively studied and validated for static anatomy. Motion artifacts are particularly challenging for CBCT imaging. As noted in chapter 8, AI can be a powerful tool to correct the motion artifacts in CBCT imaging [42, 43]. Such developments in the imaging of moving anatomy will be important for proton therapy workflows.

Second, current imaging for proton therapy typically focused on the use of CT or CBCT which are not able to provide the same soft tissue or biological information of MRI or PET. Following the work described in chapter 8, the use of AI to provide synthetic MR or biological information in the context of CT based workflows can potentially provide critical information to aid the adaptation or triaging of proton therapy workflows [44, 45].

18.3 Implementation of adaptive proton therapy

As with any adaptive radiotherapy workflow, the daily changes in the patient contours and, when required, the treatment plan must be reviewed with appropriate quality assurance. The need to verify any updated contours was discussed above and remains an area of research, in particular considering AI tools to increase the speed and accuracy of the contour reviews. In addition, there is need to perform secondary verification of the updated plan, as noted above with respect to secondary dose calculations.

There have been recent reports of quality assurance methods for adaptive proton therapy [3, 46, 47]. The current publications have not explicitly included AI tools in the online quality assurance checks but the need for rapid, robust, and reliable QA presents a strong case for incorporating AI tools in the implantation of adaptive proton therapy workflows. Additionally, there are multiple groups deploying adaptive proton therapy workflows including PSI in Switzerland and a collaboration between IBA, Raystation, UC Leuven, and UMCG (ProtonART). The collaborative model allows for the deployment of commercially developed tools in Raystation combined with vendor support from IBA and clinical experts.

18.4 Summary

Proton therapy might provide clinically superior dose distributions for some treatment locations as a result of the Bragg peak depth dose distribution which allows for sparing of distal tissues. Due to the sensitivity of the Bragg peak location in the patient, the precision of the dose distribution requires knowledge of the integral tissue composition, density, and magnitude. Daily set-up uncertainties, motion due to bowels or breathing, and weight or tumor changes can all contribute to variations in the proton Bragg peak locations resulting in dose delivery differences in the target as well as other organs in close proximity to the target. To maximize the advantages of the proton dose distribution, adaptive workflows have been proposed to measure the changes of the integral tissues and adjust the position of the Bragg peak to stop at the intended position more precisely. The current adaptive proton therapy workflows can require significant time and computational resources to image, measure, adjust, and recalculate the optimal dose distribution for the current patient anatomy. Artificial intelligence can provide dramatic reductions in time and improved image quality to detect the anatomic variations.

References

[1] Bortfeld T 1997 An analytical approximation of the Bragg curve for therapeutic proton beams *Med. Phys.* **24** 2024–33

[2] Paganetti H 2012 Range uncertainties in proton therapy and the role of Monte Carlo simulations *Phys. Med. Biol.* **57** R99–117

[3] Paganetti H, Botas P, Sharp G C and Winey B 2021 Adaptive proton therapy *Phys. Med. Biol.* **66** 22TR01

[4] Knopf A C and Lomax A 2013 *In vivo* proton range verification: a review *Phys. Med. Biol.* **58** R131–60

[5] Liebl J, Paganetti H, Zhu M and Winey B A 2014 The influence of patient positioning uncertainties in proton radiotherapy on proton range and dose distributions *Med. Phys.* **41** 091711

[6] Winey B, Daartz J, Dankers F and Bussiere M 2012 Immobilization precision of a modified GTC frame *J. Appl. Clin. Med. Phys.* **13** 3690

[7] Kim J, Park Y K, Sharp G, Busse P and Winey B 2017 Water equivalent path length calculations using scatter-corrected head and neck CBCT images to evaluate patients for adaptive proton therapy *Phys. Med. Biol.* **62** 59–72

[8] Lalonde A, Bobic M, Sharp G C, Chamseddine I, Winey B and Paganetti H 2023 Evaluating the effect of setup uncertainty reduction and adaptation to geometric changes on normal tissue complication probability using online adaptive head and neck intensity modulated proton therapy *Phys. Med. Biol.* **68** 115018

[9] Lalonde A, Bobic M, Winey B, Verburg J, Sharp G C and Paganetti H 2021 Anatomic changes in head and neck intensity-modulated proton therapy: comparison between robust optimization and online adaptation *Radiother. Oncol.* **159** 39–47

[10] Espana S, Zhu X, Daartz J, El Fakhri G, Bortfeld T and Paganetti H 2011 The reliability of proton–nuclear interaction cross-section data to predict proton-induced PET images in proton therapy *Phys. Med. Biol.* **56** 2687–98

[11] Knopf A C *et al* 2011 Accuracy of proton beam range verification using post-treatment positron emission tomography/computed tomography as function of treatment site *Int. J. Radiat. Oncol. Biol. Phys.* **79** 297–304

[12] Min C H *et al* 2013 Clinical application of in-room positron emission tomography for *in vivo* treatment monitoring in proton radiation therapy *Int. J. Radiat. Oncol. Biol. Phys.* **86** 183–9

[13] Parodi K *et al* 2007 Patient study of *in vivo* verification of beam delivery and range, using positron emission tomography and computed tomography imaging after proton therapy *Int. J. Radiat. Oncol. Biol. Phys.* **68** 920–34

[14] Zhu X *et al* 2011 Monitoring proton radiation therapy with in-room PET imaging *Phys. Med. Biol.* **56** 4041–57

[15] Bolsi A *et al* 2018 Practice patterns of image guided particle therapy in Europe: a 2016 survey of the European particle therapy network (EPTN) *Radiother. Oncol.* **128** 4–8

[16] Liu W *et al* 2024 NRG oncology and PTCOG patterns of practice survey and consensus recommendations on pencil-beam scanning proton stereotactic body radiation therapy and hypofractionated radiation therapy for thoracic malignancies *Int. J. Radiat. Oncol. Biol. Phys.* **119** 1208–21

[17] Niu T, Sun M, Star-Lack J, Gao H, Fan Q and Zhu L 2010 Shading correction for on-board cone-beam CT in radiation therapy using planning MDCT images *Med. Phys.* **37** 5395–406

[18] Park Y K, Sharp G C, Phillips J and Winey B A 2015 Proton dose calculation on scatter-corrected CBCT image: feasibility study for adaptive proton therapy *Med. Phys.* **42** 4449–59

[19] Kurz C *et al* 2015 Comparing cone-beam CT intensity correction methods for dose recalculation in adaptive intensity-modulated photon and proton therapy for head and neck cancer *Acta. Oncol.* **54** 1651–7

[20] Hansen D C *et al* 2018 ScatterNet: a convolutional neural network for cone-beam CT intensity correction *Med. Phys.* **45** 4916–26

[21] Lalonde A, Winey B, Verburg J, Paganetti H and Sharp G C 2020 Evaluation of CBCT scatter correction using deep convolutional neural networks for head and neck adaptive proton therapy *Phys. Med. Biol.* **65** 245022

[22] Thummerer A *et al* 2020 Comparison of CBCT based synthetic CT methods suitable for proton dose calculations in adaptive proton therapy *Phys. Med. Biol.* **65** 095002

[23] Chen X *et al* 2022 A more effective CT synthesizer using transformers for cone-beam CT-guided adaptive radiotherapy *Front. Oncol.* **12** 988800

[24] Xiao H *et al* 2021 A review of deep learning-based three-dimensional medical image registration methods *Quant. Imaging Med. Surg.* **11** 4895–916

[25] Nenoff L *et al* 2022 Integrating structure propagation uncertainties in the optimization of online adaptive proton therapy plans *Cancers* **14** 3926

[26] Amstutz F *et al* 2021 An approach for estimating dosimetric uncertainties in deformable dose accumulation in pencil beam scanning proton therapy for lung cancer *Phys. Med. Biol.* **66** 105007

[27] Nenoff L *et al* 2023 Review and recommendations on deformable image registration uncertainties for radiotherapy applications *Phys. Med. Biol.* **68** 24TR01

[28] Nenoff L *et al* 2021 Dosimetric influence of deformable image registration uncertainties on propagated structures for online daily adaptive proton therapy of lung cancer patients *Radiother. Oncol.* **159** 136–43

[29] Nenoff L *et al* 2020 Deformable image registration uncertainty for inter-fractional dose accumulation of lung cancer proton therapy *Radiother. Oncol.* **147** 178–85

[30] Xu Y *et al* 2024 Cone beam CT-based adaptive intensity modulated proton therapy assessment using automated planning for head-and-neck cancer *Radiat. Oncol.* **19** 13

[31] Smolders A, Lomax A, Weber D C and Albertini F 2023 Deep learning based uncertainty prediction of deformable image registration for contour propagation and dose accumulation in online adaptive radiotherapy *Phys. Med. Biol.* **68** 245027

[32] Smolders A, Lomax A, Weber D C and Albertini F 2023 Patient-specific neural networks for contour propagation in online adaptive radiotherapy *Phys. Med. Biol.* **68** 095010

[33] Lee H *et al* 2022 MOQUI: an open-source GPU-based Monte Carlo code for proton dose calculation with efficient data structure *Phys. Med. Biol.* **67** 174001

[34] Alaka B G, Bentefour E H, Teo B K K and Samuel D 2023 A comparative study of machine-learning approaches in proton radiography using energy-resolved dose function *Phys. Med.* **106** 102525

[35] Borderias-Villarroel E *et al* 2023 Machine learning-based automatic proton therapy planning: impact of post-processing and dose-mimicking in plan robustness *Med. Phys.* **50** 4480–90

[36] Mentzel F *et al* 2022 Small beams, fast predictions: a comparison of machine learning dose prediction models for proton minibeam therapy *Med. Phys.* **49** 7791–801

[37] Grewal H S, Chacko M S, Ahmad S and Jin H 2020 Prediction of the output factor using machine and deep learning approach in uniform scanning proton therapy *J. Appl. Clin. Med. Phys.* **21** 128–34

[38] Wu C *et al* 2021 Improving proton dose calculation accuracy by using deep learning *Mach. Learn. Sci. Technol.* **2** 015017

[39] Nomura Y, Wang J, Shirato H, Shimizu S and Xing L 2020 Fast spot-scanning proton dose calculation method with uncertainty quantification using a three-dimensional convolutional neural network *Phys. Med. Biol.* **65** 215007

[40] Qiu Z, Olberg S, den Hertog D, Ajdari A, Bortfeld T and Pursley J 2023 Online adaptive planning methods for intensity-modulated radiotherapy *Phys. Med. Biol.* **68** 10TR01

[41] Botas P, Kim J, Winey B and Paganetti H 2018 Online adaption approaches for intensity modulated proton therapy for head and neck patients based on cone beam CTs and Monte Carlo simulations *Phys. Med. Biol.* **64** 015004

[42] Schmitz H *et al* 2023 ScatterNet for projection-based 4D cone-beam computed tomography intensity correction of lung cancer patients *Phys. Imaging Radiat. Oncol.* **27** 100482

[43] Thummerer A *et al* 2022 Deep learning-based 4D-synthetic CTs from sparse-view CBCTs for dose calculations in adaptive proton therapy *Med. Phys.* **49** 6824–39

[44] Baumer C *et al* 2022 Adaptive proton therapy of pediatric head and neck cases using MRI-based synthetic CTs: initial experience of the prospective KiAPT study *Cancers* **14** 2616

[45] Burigo L N and Oborn B M 2022 Integrated MRI-guided proton therapy planning: accounting for the full MRI field in a perpendicular system *Med. Phys.* **49** 1853–73

[46] Bobic M *et al* 2023 Optically stimulated luminescence dosimeters for simultaneous measurement of point dose and dose-weighted LET in an adaptive proton therapy workflow *Front. Oncol.* **13** 1333039

[47] Neppl S *et al* 2021 Measurement-based range evaluation for quality assurance of CBCT-based dose calculations in adaptive proton therapy *Med. Phys.* **48** 4148–59

Chapter 19

Artificial intelligence in clinical trials

Sang Ho Lee, Huaizhi Geng and Ying Xiao

Artificial intelligence (AI) is transforming clinical trials, making them more efficient, flexible, and focused on patient needs. Clinical trials have always been essential to medical progress, providing the strong evidence needed to ensure that new treatments, drugs, and medical devices are safe and effective. However, traditional trials can be costly, time-consuming, and sometimes difficult to organize, especially when it comes to finding and enrolling the right participants. AI offers new ways to address these challenges by making trials more adaptive and data-driven, allowing researchers to adjust plans based on patient-specific information and ongoing results. This chapter discusses the importance of clinical trials in healthcare, explains key trial methods, and explores how AI is changing the way trials are designed and run. From improving participant selection to using digital twin (DT) technology for personalized trial plans, AI is making trials more accurate and responsive. The chapter also covers important ethical and regulatory issues to consider when applying AI in clinical research. With these advances, AI has the potential to improve the speed, quality, and impact of clinical trials, leading to faster and more reliable medical discoveries.

19.1 Designing clinical trials with AI

19.1.1 The essential role of clinical trials

Clinical trials are research studies conducted to evaluate new medical treatments, drugs, or devices. Clinical trials are pivotal in advancing healthcare technology, serving as the foundation for evaluating new medical innovations. These trials are instrumental in assessing the safety, efficacy, and overall benefit of emerging medical products, including drugs, devices, and health system interventions [1–3]. They offer a critical platform for understanding the mechanisms, therapeutic effects, and potential adverse impacts of new technologies, thus playing a key role in their development.

doi:10.1088/978-0-7503-6119-4ch19
19-1

Particularly in the field of medicine, clinical trials facilitate the testing and validation of novel technologies such as biomedical imaging, digital data management, and online software solutions [4–6]. These trials integrate patient engagement, data science, and technological advancements to forge innovative care pathways [7]. The incorporation of electronic health records, mobile applications, and wearable devices is revolutionizing clinical trials, making them more efficient and pragmatic [8].

Furthermore, clinical trials are crucial for generating evidence that shapes clinical practices and drug development [9]. They enable the comparison of new advancements to conventional treatments using rigorous scientific methods [10], thereby establishing their value and efficacy. The evolving nature of clinical trials, influenced by regulatory and technological advancements, continually refines their designs and capabilities [11].

Clinical trials contribute to the optimization of current clinical procedures and ensure that novel treatments meet the safety and efficacy standards required for FDA approval. Clinical trials are essential in developing and implementing new technologies in healthcare, providing critical evidence-based data to support their application in clinical practice.

19.1.2 Trial protocols and methodologies

Clinical trial design methodologies encompass a range of statistical and practical considerations. Chow [12] and Onken [13] both emphasized the importance of randomization, blinding, and sample size determination in ensuring the validity and reliability of trial results. Sverdlov [14] and Hee [15] further expanded on these principles, with Sverdlov focusing on optimal designs for different stages of drug development and Hee discussing the application of Bayesian decision theory in small trials and pilot studies. Collectively, these methodologies aimed to enhance the efficiency and quality of clinical trials.

Clinical trial design methodologies include various approaches such as single-arm, placebo-controlled, crossover, factorial, noninferiority, and diagnostic device validation designs [16]. Bayesian clinical trial design methodology is used for evaluating the effect of an investigational product on both recurrent event and terminating event processes [17]. Another method involves enrolling patient candidates based on the predicted progression of a condition and analysing subsets of clinical trial data to generate measures of efficacy [18]. Optimal designs are used for different stages of clinical drug development, including phase I dose–toxicity studies, phase I/II studies, phase II dose–response studies, phase III randomized controlled multi-arm multi-objective clinical trials, and population pharmacokinetics–pharmacodynamics experiments [19]. Randomized and controlled clinical trials are considered the gold standard, but the design should be tailored to the specific research question and objectives [20].

A good clinical trial protocol should include a clear research question, a detailed methodology, and a study schedule and costing [21, 22]. It should also address potential bias through blinding and random allocation of subjects [13].

Furthermore, it must adhere to ethical principles, such as respect for persons, beneficence, and justice, as well as good clinical practice guidelines [23].

A good clinical trial protocol should include key elements such as a rationale for the study, a clear method description, measures to ensure subject safety, information about research funders and organizational details, and a plan for monitoring the trial [24]. Additionally, protocols should align with routine clinical techniques and standard clinical processes to increase the likelihood of successful execution [25]. They should also incorporate principles of good clinical practice (GCP) to ensure rigor, reproducibility, and transparency in scientific research [26]. Other important elements include predefined analysis plans, standardization of procedures across sites, assurance of staff competence, transparent data coding and entry, regular quality assurance, and open publication of data [27]. Furthermore, guideline protocols should be prepared and published to clarify the purpose and scope of the guideline, facilitate the development process, ensure integrity and quality, and avoid duplication [28]. Overall, a good clinical trial protocol should be comprehensive, transparent, and aligned with established standards and guidelines.

19.1.3 AI-driven clinical trial design and execution

AI has the potential to significantly impact clinical trial design and execution. It can be used to reshape key steps of trial design, such as patient cohort selection and monitoring, leading to increased success rates [29]. AI can also accelerate clinical testing by automating tasks and optimizing patient selection [30]. The opportunities are significant. AI can create efficiencies in various aspects of clinical trials, such as reducing sample sizes, improving enrollment, and conducting faster and more optimized adaptive trials [3]. AI technologies such as deep learning, neural networks, and natural language processing have been applied in disease diagnosis, personalized treatment, drug discovery, and forecasting epidemics or pandemics [31]. AI-driven platforms can efficiently identify potential trial patients by applying clinical trial criteria to real-world data, reducing patient recruitment timelines by months [32]. However, AI presents both challenges and opportunities in clinical trial design and execution. The challenges include ethical concerns, data availability, and lack of regulatory guidance, which hinder the acceptance of AI tools in drug development [33]. The implementation of AI in clinical practice is still at an early stage, and more research is needed to assess its benefits and challenges [34]. However, as regulators provide more guidance, its scope of use is expected to broaden rapidly [35].

19.1.4 Incorporation of digital twins (DTs) in clinical trials

DT technology represents a transformative approach to enhancing clinical trials, offering a revolutionary means of understanding and predicting the outcomes of medical interventions. At its core, this technology involves creating a virtual replica of each patient, meticulously crafted using advanced AI methods. This DT integrates a comprehensive array of data, encompassing the patient's real-world medical history, physiological and molecular characteristics, and baseline health information [36, 37]. Such an intricate synthesis allows for a deeper, more personalized analysis of clinical trials.

The application of DTs extends across various medical disciplines, with notable impacts in fields such as oncology and cardiology. In oncology, for instance, DTs facilitate the simulation of diverse dosing regimens. This enables researchers to delve into the nuances of dose–response relationships and uncover key determinants that influence a patient's response to treatment. Such detailed insights are invaluable in tailoring more effective, individualized treatment strategies.

Cardiac *in silico* clinical trials is an area where DTs are making significant strides. By generating personalized cardiac models based on individual clinical data, these trials allow for the meticulous assessment of various therapies. This not only enhances the understanding of treatment efficacy but also paves the way for more customized therapeutic approaches [38].

A critical aspect of DT technology in clinical trials is the incorporation of blockchain technology. By embedding these advanced cryptographic systems, the integrity of trial data is significantly bolstered, ensuring its authenticity and reliability. This integration also plays a crucial role in safeguarding participant safety, a paramount concern in any clinical trial [37].

Matched pair analysis emerges as a powerful tool in this context. Researchers can compare the outcomes of a patient undergoing a clinical trial with those predicted for their DT. This comparison allows for a more nuanced evaluation of the treatment's effectiveness, providing a clearer picture of its benefits and potential risks [39].

Moreover, the fusion of AI with *in silico* trials—simulated trials conducted digitally—is set to revolutionize clinical trial design. AI's capability to expand case group sizes, automate and optimize trial designs, and even predict success rates, heralds a new era of efficiency and effectiveness in clinical research. The result is a more streamlined, accurate, and predictive trial process, potentially accelerating the development of new treatments and therapies [40].

19.2 Implementation of AI in ongoing clinical trials

19.2.1 Integration with existing clinical trial frameworks

The key components of a clinical trial infrastructure (figure 9.1) include the performance site, which can be academic medical centers, multi-specialty groups, or clinical trial companies, and the staff involved such as investigators, coordinators, raters/neuropsychologists, and managers. Other important elements are access to study participants for enrollment, appropriate training of staff, regulatory oversight through investigational review boards, and ancillary services. Different types of studies, such as therapeutic, longitudinal observational, and imaging, have varying requirements for staff and infrastructure. Efficient trial development and participant accrual can be facilitated by parallel processing of trial approval steps, a physician-led research team, and regular meetings to foster research accountability. Centralizing resources and expertise, providing training for clinical research staff,

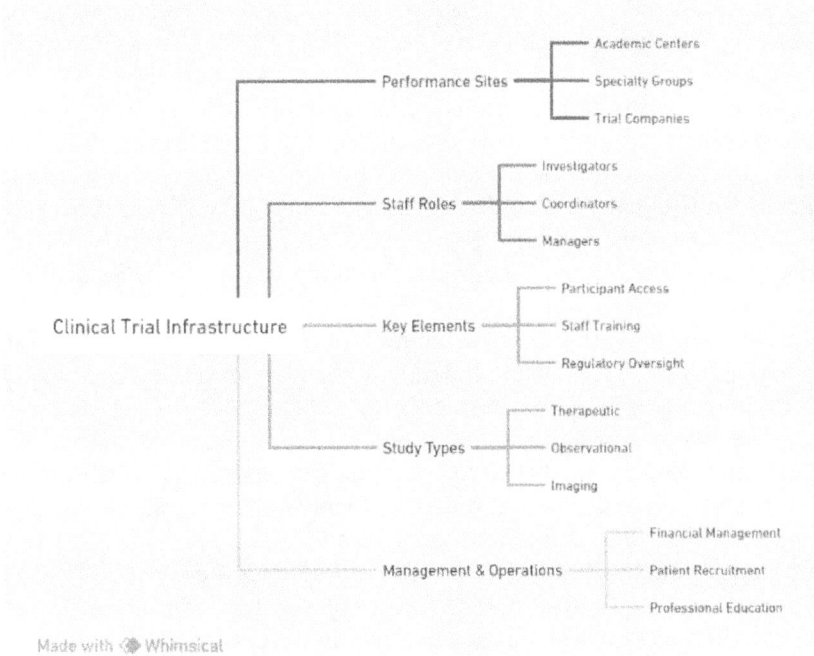

Figure 19.1. Clinical trial infrastructure overview, illustrating core components: performance sites, staff roles, key elements, study types, and management and operations, each detailing essential elements for trial support.

developing common data elements, and evaluating effectiveness are recommended strategies to strengthen clinical trial infrastructure [24].

Additional key components of clinical trial infrastructure include strong hospital administrative support, clinical research staff, site-specific tumor boards, patient care navigators, and integration of translational research infrastructure and capabilities, which is crucial in cancer trials. Financial and organizational management, new trial feasibility assessment, standardization of procedures, compliance and safety monitoring, pharmacy support, patient recruitment, effective marketing, institutional support, building diverse teams, clinician engagement, and continuing professional education are also essential for the success of clinical trials. Information technology infrastructure and human coordinating processes facilitate sponsor/CRO collaboration on international trials. Developing this infrastructure functions as a quality improvement intervention, particularly in low- and middle-income countries, and increasing efficiency in trial development is crucial [41].

The fundamental principles of trial design are also key components, summarized from the previous section, including *a priori* formulation of a specific research question, precise description of the study population, and limitation of potential bias. Randomization and blinding of investigators and participants are critical techniques to reduce bias, and the structure of modern trials, designed to protect patient safety while generating safety and efficacy data, is shaped by regulations and international standards [23].

We illustrate with an example. The National Clinical Trials Network (NCTN), an initiative by the National Cancer Institute (NCI), stands as a cornerstone in the United States' comprehensive cancer research efforts (figure 19.2). Designed to conduct extensive, multi-institutional clinical trials, the NCTN significantly enhances patient care and propels our understanding of cancer forward. The network comprises five principal groups, with four focusing on adult oncology— the Alliance for Clinical Trials in Oncology, the ECOG-ACRIN Cancer Research Group, NRG Oncology, and the Southwest Oncology Group (SWOG) Cancer Research Network—and the Children's Oncology Group (COG) dedicated to pediatric cancer research [42].

Central to the network's efficacy in radiation oncology is the Imaging and Radiation Oncology Core (IROC). IROC's mandate is to ensure quality and uniformity in imaging and radiation therapy across the NCTN's clinical trials. This involves standardizing imaging protocols, harmonizing radiation therapy techniques, and assuring quality across various trial sites. This standardization is crucial in trials where imaging and radiation therapy are integral, ensuring reliable and comparable data across different study locations.

Complementing the role of IROC in NRG Oncology is the Center for Innovation in Radiation Oncology (CIRO). CIRO focuses on the development and integration of novel radiation therapy techniques and technologies in clinical trials. It serves as a hub for innovation, driving advancements in radiation therapy by fostering research collaborations and implementing cutting-edge treatment approaches in clinical settings. The work of CIRO is instrumental in pushing the boundaries of radiation oncology, aligning with NRG Oncology's mission to integrate radiation therapy with other treatment modalities [43, 44].

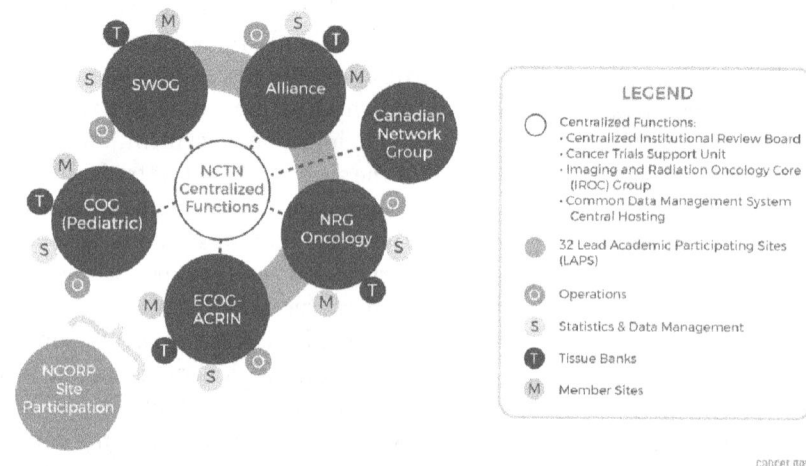

NCI National Clinical Trials Network Structure

Figure 19.2. Use of DTs for simulation, analysis, and monitoring. (Image credit: National Cancer Institute https://www.cancer.gov/research/infrastructure/clinical-trials/nctn/nctn-clinical-trials-network.)

The NCTN is also supported by the Lead Academic Participating Sites (LAPS), the NCI Community Oncology Research Program (NCORP), the Clinical Trials Support Unit (CTSU), and various biorepositories. These resources collectively enhance the network's research capabilities, extending the reach of clinical trials and ensuring the management of biological specimens.

The NCTN's objectives include conducting essential phase II and III clinical trials, integrating cancer biology studies within these trials, and advancing personalized medicine through biomarker research. The network's impact on cancer research is significant, leading to new treatment strategies, the development of innovative drugs, and a deeper understanding of cancer biology. For professionals in radiation oncology and clinical trials, such as those at Penn Medicine, the NCTN's focus on quality assurance in imaging and radiation therapy, bolstered by IROC and CIRO, is of paramount importance.

The NCTN represents a comprehensive and forward-thinking approach to cancer research. Its collaborative model, enhanced by the meticulous standards upheld by IROC in imaging and radiation oncology and the innovative contributions of CIRO, exemplifies a commitment to excellence in cancer treatment and research.

DTs have the potential to be incorporated into the infrastructure of clinical trials by acting as virtual representations of patients. They can integrate various types of data, including clinical, molecular, and therapeutic parameters, as well as sensor data and living conditions. These virtual models are created using artificial intelligence and real-world data, allowing for a comparison between the patient in the clinical trial and their DT. Researchers can use DTs to analyse the outcomes of patients receiving experimental treatments and compare them to their DTs, which could potentially be significant for drug approval trials. Furthermore, the inclusion of DTs in clinical trials can help generate real-world evidence and enhance participant safety through efficient data integration and knowledge management. There is also a proposal for the development and validation of a Virtual Human Twin infrastructure to support the implementation of new DTs in healthcare solutions [36, 45].

19.2.2 Quality assurance, compliance, and standardization

For nearly half a century, the NCI's NCTN has financed practice-altering randomized clinical trials. The stringent requirement for quality assurance, particularly in the fields of radiotherapy and imaging, plays a vital role in this network of clinical trials. Failure to adhere to the prescribed parameters for radiotherapy protocols has been linked to suboptimal clinical outcomes, including an elevated incidence of toxicity, treatment failure, and overall mortality in clinical studies that involve multiple institutions. Upon conducting a comprehensive assessment, discrepancies from the established radiotherapy standards were identified, such as inadequate identification and treatment of target areas, excessive radiation doses administered to normal structures, and prolonged radiotherapy treatments that surpass the recommended durations. In cases where the anticipated distinction between the experimental and conventional groups is minimal, reducing the uncertainty in radiotherapy dosage can lead to a significant decrease in the number of patients required for a randomized clinical study. The accuracy of measurements and the responsiveness of imaging metrics to genuine changes have an impact on the sample size in studies that evaluate the effectiveness of therapy. When the precision of positron emission tomography declines from 10% to 40% during a complete measurement, the sample size can increase by a factor of 15 [43, 46–48]. The establishment of the IROC as part of the NCTN was intended to ensure the quality of imaging and radiotherapy. Likewise, the NRG Oncology CIRO was created as a crucial component dedicated to radiotherapy advancements. IROC and CIRO collaborate in the development of methodologies and exploration of research topics. The functions of IROC and CIRO complement one another by guaranteeing the quality of radiotherapy and the accompanying imaging, as CIRO provides stringent guidelines that are strictly enforced through IROC's core functions. The standardization of procedures, which is an essential aspect of IROC/CIRO's quality assurance program, also contributes to the reduction of variations in the collection of radiation and imaging data, thereby allowing for the broader adoption and application of artificial intelligence tools that have been developed using datasets from a limited number of institutions [43, 44].

19.3 Case studies of AI in adaptive radiotherapy trials

19.3.1 Overview of guidance for advanced radiotherapy in clinical trials

Adaptive radiotherapy (ART) offers the capability to account for anatomical and biological changes during radiation therapy. ART approaches include offline adaptations between fractions, online adaptations prior to delivery, and real-time adaptations during delivery [49]. These target systematic changes, daily variations, and intrafraction changes, respectively. ART may also be anatomically or biologically guided based on imaging findings.

Several key technological components underlie ART implementation. Imaging considerations include contrast, resolution, artifacts, field-of-view, and other properties that differ across modalities such as CT, CBCT, MVCT, MRI, and PET [49]. Deformable image registration enables structure and dose mapping between image sets but requires extensive validation [49, 50]. Dose needs to be accumulated across multiple image sets, which relies on accurate deformation vector fields [49]. For online ART, rapid re-planning necessitates efficient recontouring, fast plan optimization, and real-time quality assurance [49].

Comprehensive quality assurance guidelines for ART are provided across NRG Oncology CIRO publications. Critical areas requiring credentialing include deformable image registration, dose accumulation, end-to-end workflow testing, and adaptive treatment plan quality assurance [49, 51]. Multi-institutional clinical trials, such as those investigating FLASH radiotherapy delivered at ultrahigh dose rates, have specific QA needs for consistent and safe implementation [51].

For clinically implementing ART, clear physician directives should determine adaptations based on metrics such as target coverage violations or organs-at-risk overdosing relative to protocol-defined constraints. Online ART requires substantial physician involvement, including target and organ delineation, plan approval, and QA. Practical considerations such as offline versus online optimization and plan adaptation frequency balance adaptiveness with efficiency. Across disease sites, the greatest ART benefits occur when substantial daily anatomical variations happen adjacent to steep dose gradients [49].

The integration of ART as primary or secondary objectives in clinical trials should be clearly defined. To ensure protocol compliance, central review processes are recommended for physician recontouring and plan quality assurance. ART credentialing should review hardware, software, workflows, and decision-making capacity at each institution. For example, credentialing templates and adaptive radiotherapy physics language for protocols are provided for consistent trial implementation [49].

19.3.2 AI in the radiotherapy clinical trial quality assurance processes

One of the AI applications to radiotherapy is to guide treatment planning with a knowledge-engineering-based plan prediction approach. Knowledge-based radiotherapy planning employs machine learning algorithms to analyse a large dataset of previous radiation therapy treatments [52]. This method leverages patterns found in past successful treatments to guide the dose distribution for new patients, thereby optimizing treatment effectiveness while minimizing exposure to healthy tissues. The process involves training a model, often a neural network or a decision tree, on historical treatment data, including patient anatomy, disease characteristics, and successful dose distributions. This model then predicts an ideal treatment plan for new patients based on their unique clinical features. One of the implementations of knowledge-based planning, the RapidPlan (Varian Inc.), was utilized for three main radiotherapy treatment planning activities related to several clinical trials.

The first activity focused on feasibility studies to establish dose constraints and evaluate treatment planning solutions against protocol criteria. Studies were performed for the NRG-GY006 (cervical cancer), RTOG1308 (lung cancer), and NRG-HN002 (head and neck cancer) trials [53–55]. For NRG-GY006, an atlas-based active bone marrow-sparing model was built to ensure quality assurance for intensity-modulated radiation therapy (IMRT) planning as part of the pre-treatment review process. The model demonstrated the ability to generate plans meeting trial objectives and consistency across institutions. For RTOG1308, a RapidPlan model assessment showed that stringent dose constraints were achievable across patient datasets from two institutions. Recommendations were made to optimize the NRG-HN002 trial launch based on a feasibility study across multiple planning systems and delivery techniques using benchmark patient cases. With minor modifications to spinal cord maximum dose criteria, compliance was demonstrated across institutions.

The second major activity was the use of RapidPlan models to enable online and offline quality reviews of treatment plans submitted to trials [56–59]. Models were trained on high-quality historical plans and used to evaluate and re-optimize new patient plans. This improved protocol compliance, target coverage consistency, and organ-at-risk sparing compared to the originally submitted plans across trials, including spine stereotactic radiosurgery (SRS) (RTOG0631) and lung cancer (RTOG1308, photons, and protons). For head and neck cancer patients on the NRG-HN001 trial, re-optimization with a multi-institutional model showed improved organ-at-risk sparing in 33 out of 50 cases. Similar quality improvements were demonstrated for proton plans relative to institution-submitted plans.

Finally, comparisons were made between RapidPlan and alternative knowledge-based planning solutions. Plan quality metrics and dose–volume histogram predictions generated by RapidPlan models versus PlanIQ models were equivalent for RTOG0631 and RTOG0522 trials. For NRG-HN002 across planning systems, protocol dosimetric compliance was achieved, confirming consistency [60]. In the case of RTOG1308 lung cancer treatment, mean dose deviations up to 14 Gy were observed between model predictions, suggesting superior performance of model-based planning for challenging geometries.

The studies demonstrate multi-pronged utilities of RapidPlan models for radiotherapy trial quality assurance across disease sites, treatment modalities, and phases of trial execution. The knowledge-based planning approach enables assessments of planning consistency and protocol deviations with automated re-planning capabilities.

High-quality data in radiotherapy clinical trials are crucial, requiring protocol-compliant contours. Traditional manual contour reviews are time-intensive and subjective. The AI-based algorithm was implemented to enhance the quality assurance workflow, offering a more objective and efficient process. Utilizing deep active learning, the developed system employs convolutional neural network models trained on high-quality contours for automated evaluation, employing metrics such as the Dice score and Hausdorff distance for decision-making. Results showed high consistency, accuracy, and sensitivity across multiple organs. This automated system is implemented across various disease sites through collaborations with AI segmentation commercial solutions [44, 61].

AI is applied to obtain outcome-driven quality assurance criteria using interpretable machine learning strategies, such as the explainable boosting machine (EBM). EBM is a transparent, tree-based model that simplifies understanding individual feature impacts on predictions. EBM was adapted for survival analysis in radiotherapy, modeling survival as a classification or regression task to identify critical dose–volume constraints for cardiopulmonary structures affecting survival outcomes in advanced non-small cell lung cancer cases [44, 62].

19.4 Ethical and regulatory considerations

19.4.1 Patient consent and data privacy

Obtaining patient consent and safeguarding privacy in clinical trials involves navigating ethical, legal, and practical terrain. At the core lies respect for patient autonomy through informed consent, upholding dignity as active participants rather than passive subjects. Meticulously designed consent processes convey comprehensive yet comprehensible information on study purpose, methods, risks, and benefits.

The documented agreement serves as a testament to patients' understanding and willingness.

Consent and confidentiality are legal imperatives, too, with regulations such as HIPAA enforcing privacy standards. Non-compliance risks significant consequences for individuals and institutions. This legal framework actualizes ethical ideals into enforceable duties. Breaches erode patient trust and transparency, foundational to accurate data collection. Rigorous protocols anonymize data and restrict access to maintain integrity.

Navigating valid consent poses challenges, including disabilities impeding communication, fluctuating capacity, and emergencies precluding engagement [63]. Pragmatic trial consent waivers balance ethical rigor with feasibility and risk mitigation across patients, clinicians, and systems [64]. Cross-disciplinary collaboration is imperative to update guidance and address research gaps. Human-centered solutions such as consent mechanisms, privacy assistants, and dynamic consent platforms further uphold ethical ideals.

Training requirements ensure all personnel adhere to exacting privacy and confidentiality standards. Review boards scrutinize protocols, serving as an oversight layer reinforcing patient rights and autonomy. Complex, ethical, legal, and practical vigilance is essential for consent and privacy to enable advancement through research while minimizing patient risk and maximizing agency in participation.

This framework of multifaceted standards aims to shift clinical trials from a paradigm of patients as passive subjects to one of active collaboration built on trust, transparency, and mutual understanding. Truly informed consent respects participant dignity while propelling scientific progress. Although navigating regulatory, ethical, and communication terrain poses challenges, solutions grounded in human values offer paths to uphold safety and autonomy at once. Overall, the clinical trials ecosystem must reinforce patient centeredness—from reviewing protocol to analysing data to translating findings to practice. Through consent built on education rather than obfuscation and rigorous privacy standards, advancement and ethics intersect rather than conflict. The result, research with the participant rather than research on the participant, offers a blueprint for progress reflecting core human values.

19.4.2 Bias, fairness, and transparency

Bias, fairness, and transparency in clinical trials raise significant validity and ethical concerns requiring comprehensive solutions.

Bias manifests in the selection of non-representative participants, systematically skewed measurements, and selective reporting that misrepresents outcomes. Core strategies to mitigate bias include randomization to minimize the confounding influence variables, double-blinding studies so neither participants nor researchers know the treatment versus control group, and pre-registering trial protocols to prevent manipulating reporting [65].

Fairness in clinical trials involves equitable selection and treatment of participants. Historically, certain groups such as women, minorities, and the elderly were underrepresented, lacking data on how treatments affect them differently. Solutions include proactive diverse recruitment, so results apply more broadly, equity-focused protocols addressing inclusion, and community engagement to understand needs.

Transparency issues arise from insufficient disclosure of methodologies, changes, conflicts of interest, and data management. This erodes public and scientific trust. Solutions encompass open access to protocols and results for scrutiny, independent review boards, and requiring conflict of interest disclosures.

In radiotherapy and imaging, ensuring the techniques evaluated are free from bias and fair across patient demographics is critical. Maintaining transparency in testing and reporting establishes research credibility and ethics. Solutions such as diverse recruitment, rigorous protocols, and transparent reporting are instrumental.

Addressing multifaceted bias, fairness, and transparency issues requires a comprehensive approach targeting research culture, reporting biases and methodological shortcomings [66, 67]. The EU Clinical Trials Regulation improved interventional drug trial result transparency, but a 'two-class system' emerged to distinguish these from other studies [68]. Institutions, funders, and ethics committees should improve transparency across all clinical studies. The EU Portal Clinical Trials Information System also aims to make study documents more transparent for independent analysis of consent and harm–benefit assessment [69]. Ultimately transparency entails publicly sharing information on trial design, conduct, results, and data.

Progress notwithstanding, continued vigilance is essential from multiple stakeholders, wielding an array of transparency tools to uphold ethical, unbiased clinical research.

19.4.3 Regulatory guidelines and compliance

Major regulations are crucial to ensure clinical trials uphold safety, efficacy, and ethical standards. Key guidelines include the International Conference on Harmonization (ICH) Good Clinical Practice (GCP) standards, mandating credible, accurate reporting with subject protections [70]. The Declaration of Helsinki details ethical imperatives such as informed consent, letting participants withdraw, prioritizing welfare, and requiring independent committee reviews [71].

For US trials, Food and Drug Administration (FDA) regulations cover Investigational New Drug applications, protecting subjects, Institutional Review Board (IRB) rules, and reporting adverse events [72]. The European Medicines Agency (EMA) oversees European Union trials, regulating authorization, conduct, and reporting [73].

Navigating complex, detailed regulations poses compliance challenges. With multifaceted protocols, organizations may struggle to fully implement every requirement. Global trials must reconcile varied or conflicting country-level rules. Managing voluminous quality data while upholding accuracy, security, and confidentiality strains resources. Obtaining informed consent and ethical approvals grows more complex with diverse, vulnerable groups.

Solutions include comprehensive training to ensure staff understand relevant guidelines, standardized operating procedures aligning with regulations, independent ethics committees providing guidance, quality assurance audits early addressing non-compliance, and advanced data systems aiding management.

This intricate landscape demands vigilance from sponsors, investigators, and reviewers so trials uphold the most rigorous scientific and ethical standards. With human health at stake, even minor non-compliance could undermine safety or efficacy findings. Yet complex regulations also safeguard against exploitation, preserving rights and welfare consistent with research ethics principles. Although advancing medical knowledge through trials may serve public health aims, the imperative of monitoring standards helps ensure this progress also aligns with public ethical priorities.

Through multifaceted checks-and-balances—extensive guidelines, intensive training, and oversight systems—the clinical trials ecosystem seeks to foster advancement with accountability. By upholding consistency across geographies and populations, regulators enable generalizing insights more responsibly. And by upholding informed consent, subject welfare and data ethics, they reinforce research alignment with participant-centered values. The intent is to catalyze progress and protection in equal measure. While no framework fully eliminates ethical breaches, an infrastructure prioritizing safety and dignity from study design through result dissemination aims to advance science grounded in conscience.

19.5 Future directions and challenges

19.5.1 Emerging technologies and techniques

Emerging radiotherapy technologies such as radiopharmaceutical therapy, FLASH, and MR-guided radiotherapy offer opportunities to advance cancer treatment through enhanced tumor targeting and normal tissue sparing. However, optimizing clinical integration requires rigorous trials evaluating dosimetry, fractionation, disease site dependencies, and long-term impacts [49, 51, 74]. Spatially fractionated regimens may augment immunogenic response when combined with immunotherapy, but consensus guidelines are lacking on appropriate applications [75].

Proton therapy trials should collect comprehensive data on dose, linear energy transfer (LET), and outcomes to inform LET-based treatment planning and models of relative biological effectiveness (RBE), which likely exceeds the standard value of 1.1 in some tissues. Re-irradiation trials warrant meticulous cumulative dose assessment through prior record completeness, image registration for anatomical changes, and biological correction models [76].

Quantum sensing and computing technologies promise future transformations in imaging, treatment planning, and research [77]. Integrating artificial intelligence can facilitate accuracy, efficiency, and quality assurance across radiotherapy trials but requires addressing inherent biases and lack of transparency [78]. Opportunities include knowledge-based and biological image-guided treatment planning, automated segmentation, motion management, and predictive modeling [62, 79, 80].

Advancing radiotherapy hinges on carefully designed prospective trials to optimize modality-specific protocols while collecting comprehensive data on treatment factors, response, and toxicity. Multidisciplinary collaboration and infrastructure modernization, paired with diligent quality assurance, are imperative to firmly establish safety and maximize therapeutic potential. AI-driven tools may accelerate this mission but require thoughtfully crafted validation studies to ensure robust performance and clinician trust.

19.5.2 Alternative strategies

DTs represent an emerging technology with the potential to advance biomedical research and personalized medicine. When paired with clinical trial data, DTs of patients could help optimize and individualize therapies. However, several challenges must be addressed [81].

A key challenge is model complexity—embracing complexity risks models becoming too computationally intensive while oversimplifying risks and losing critical details. Approaches must balance fidelity and feasibility. There were successes in applying high-resolution gene-level models to animal systems and patient cells to determine optimal drug therapies. However, validating predictions remains difficult without human trials.

Capturing spatial and temporal considerations with imaging, molecular simulations, and mathematical models enables key insights, such as predicting chemotherapy delivery and treatment responses. Yet a mismatch persists between measurable biological data and computational capability. Strategies are needed to integrate or generate missing measurements across timescales.

The diversity of models and data is also an obstacle. While benchmark digital patients and populations offer promise in evaluating medical devices or running *in silico* trials, integrating mechanism-based physiological models with sparse, heterogeneous patient data is an open challenge. Techniques leveraging optimal experimental design could strengthen predictive performance from population to individual.

Connecting data across biological scales to build robust multiscale DTs remains an active research gap. Opportunities exist to interface models rather than data directly but communicating across scales and ensuring model composability and reproducibility is nontrivial. Iterative, modular approaches accounting for uncertainties may help bridge insights from molecular simulations toward eventual clinical application.

Privacy and ethical concerns abound regarding access, control, and transparency surrounding patient data used to develop, update, and enrich medical DTs. Engaging participants in managing privacy risks and communication of uncertainties linked to model predictions is paramount, as is ensuring equitable access to emerging DT technologies.

While much potential exists for medical DTs to enhance decision-making, prediction, and optimization of interventions across the clinical trial ecosystem, solving complex data integration, modeling, validation, and ethical challenges remains imperative to eventual real-world implementation. Focused efforts on priority gaps could unlock this nascent technology's full translational power [81].

19.6 Conclusion

In conclusion, AI promises to profoundly enhance clinical trials across myriad facets, from protocol design to data analysis to safety monitoring. AI-based solutions can optimize patient recruitment, reduce costs, accelerate timelines, and extract deeper insights from multifaceted data. Technologies such as DTs and virtual modeling further expand capabilities, enabling sophisticated simulation and prediction unachievable through conventional methodologies.

However, thoughtfully crafted validation frameworks and ethical guidelines are imperative to guide AI integration responsibly. Models must demonstrate reliable, unbiased performance across diverse demographics before influencing high-stakes medical decision-making. Patient privacy, transparency, and autonomy require ongoing safeguarding as data sharing and analytics expand.

Nevertheless, the potential advantages of judiciously incorporating AI are substantial. Personalized, predictive, and dose-optimized treatment plans can be formulated through AI-assisted knowledge. Automated segmentation, registration, and motion management streamline workflows. Risk models calibrated on population data may inform individual risk assessments with greater accuracy.

Ultimately, AI in clinical trials aims not to supplant physicians but to augment human intelligence—equipping practitioners to base recommendations on comprehensive perspectives while retaining experience-driven nuances. This fusion of computational power with clinical acumen may propel more precise, effective, and democratized research, unlocking scientific insights at unprecedented scale and speed. The path ahead undoubtedly entails obstacles, but the promise of ameliorating patient outcomes through data-enlightened understanding compels persistent, collaborative progress. With ethical vigilance and visionary drive, AI-empowered clinical trials can catalyze a new epoch of evidence-based care and scientific discovery benefitting all.

19.7 Summary

AI is reshaping clinical trials by enhancing efficiency, precision, and personalization in research processes. AI-driven tools streamline patient recruitment, optimize trial protocols, and enable adaptive monitoring, resulting in faster timelines and improved outcomes. Technologies such as DTs allow for the creation of virtual patient models that simulate treatment responses, facilitating personalized therapy optimization while minimizing risks. These advancements significantly contribute to improving safety, efficacy, and cost-effectiveness in medical research. However, the integration of AI into clinical trials presents challenges, including concerns around data privacy, transparency, ethical use, and potential biases in decision-making.

Addressing these issues requires robust validation studies, adherence to ethical guidelines, and the development of comprehensive regulatory frameworks. Emerging innovations, such as AI-powered adaptive radiotherapy and quantum computing, further expand the potential of clinical trials, offering transformative opportunities for precision medicine. By combining computational intelligence with rigorous scientific standards, AI is set to revolutionize evidence-based healthcare, enabling more effective and patient-centered clinical research.

References

[1] Kandi V, Vadakedath S, Addanki P S, Godishala V and Pinnelli V B 2023 Clinical trials: the role of regulatory agencies, pharmacovigilance laws, guidelines, risk management, patenting, and publicizing results *Borneo. J. Pharm.* **6** 93–109

[2] Trigueiros B A F D S, Ávila A R and Pimenta F P 2022 An examination of the use of clinical trials as a source of information in scientific research *Transinformação* **34** e210065

[3] Bhattamisra S K, Banerjee P, Gupta P, Mayuren J, Patra S and Mayuren C 2023 Artificial intelligence in pharmaceutical and healthcare research *Big. Data. Cogn. Comput.* **7** 10–0

[4] Robbins W 1994 Rapporteur summary: role of technology in clinical trials—validation of information *Health Care Technology Policy I: The Role of Technology in the Cost of Health Care* (Piscataway, NJ: IEEE)

[5] Max M 1994 Rapporteur summary: role of technology in the cost of health care *Health Care Technology Policy I: The Role of Technology in the Cost of Health Care* (Bellingham, WA: SPIE) pp 134–48

[6] Bleicher P 2003 Clinical trial technology: at the inflection point *BIOSILICO* **1** 163–8

[7] Royle J K, Hughes A, Stephenson L and Landers D 2021 Technology clinical trials: turning innovation into patient benefit *Digit. Health.* **7** 205520762110121

[8] Marquis-Gravel G *et al* 2019 Technology-enabled clinical trials *Circulation* **140** 1426–36

[9] Turner J R and Hoofwijk T J 2013 Clinical trials in new drug development *J. Clin. Hypertens.* **15** 306–9

[10] Ying A J 2023 The importance of the clinical trialing process in the development of modern-day drugs *Proc. SPIE* **12611** 1261166–16

[11] Raber-Johnson M L, Gallwitz W E, Sullivan E J and Storer P 2019 Innovation in clinical trial design and product promotion: evolving the patient perspective with regulatory and technological advances *Ther. Innov. Amp. Regul. Sci.* **54** 519–27

[12] Chow S and Pei Liu J 1998 *Design and Analysis of Clinical Trials: Concept and Methodologies* (Hoboken, NJ: Wiley)

[13] Onken J E and Brazer S R 1994 Clinical trials: how should they be designed? *Gastrointest. Endosc. Clin. N. Am.* **4** 423–34

[14] Sverdlov O, Ryeznik Y and Wong W K 2019 On optimal designs for clinical trials: an updated review *J. Stat. Theory Pract.* **14** 10

[15] Hee S W *et al* 2015 Decision-theoretic designs for small trials and pilot studies: a review *Stat. Methods Med. Res.* **25** 1022–38

[16] Sverdlov O, Ryeznik Y and Wong W K 2020 On optimal designs for clinical trials: an updated review *J. Stat. Theory Pract.* **14** 10

[17] Hung H M J and Wang S-J 2014 Emerging challenges of clinical trial methodologies in regulatory applications *Clinical Trial Biostatistics and Biopharmaceutical Applications* (Boca Raton, FL: CRC Press) pp 39–76

[18] Xu J, Psioda M A and Ibrahim J G 2022 Bayesian design of clinical trials using joint models for recurrent and terminating events *Biostatistics* **24** 866–84

[19] David L E, Albert A T, Danielle B and Keymer Michael A 2020 Systems and methods for designing clinical trials *Justia Patents Patent* # 11,139,051; https://patents.justia.com/patent/11139051

[20] Phadnis M A, Wetmore J B and Mayo M S 2017 A clinical trial design using the concept of proportional time using the generalized gamma ratio distribution *Stat. Med.* **36** 4121–40

[21] Silverman R and Kwiatkowski T 1998 Research fundamentals: III. Elements of a research protocol for clinical trials *Acad. Emerg. Med.* **5** 1218–23

[22] Holloway P J and Mooney J A 2004 What's a research protocol? *Health Educ. J.* **63** 374–84

[23] Karsh L I 2012 A clinical trial primer: historical perspective and modern implementation *Urol. Oncol. Semin. Orig. Investig.* **30** S28–32

[24] Hess A S and Abd-Elsayed A 2019 Components of clinical trials *Pain* ed A Abd-Elsayed (Cham: Springer) pp 83–5

[25] Reddy P and Bhadauria U S 2019 Integral elements of a research protocol *J. Indian Acad. Oral Med. Radiol.* **31** 167

[26] Xun Y *et al* 2022 Protocols for clinical practice guidelines *J. Evid.-Based Med.* **16** 3–9

[27] An M-W, Duong Q, Le-Rademacher J and Mandrekar S J 2020 Principles of good clinical trial design *J. Thorac. Oncol.* **15** 1277–80

[28] Park J-S *et al* 2020 An interactive retrieval system for clinical trial studies with context-dependent protocol elements *PLoS One* **15** e0238290

[29] Harrer S 2020 Artificial intelligence for clinical trial design *2020 IEEE Signal Processing in Medicine and Biology Symposium (SPMB)* (Piscataway, NJ: IEEE)

[30] Woo M 2019 An AI boost for clinical trials *Nature* **573** S100–2

[31] Miyasato G, Kasivajjala V, Kumar K, Kadam A S and Friedman H S 2023 AI-driven real-time patient identification for randomized controlled trials *J. Clin. Oncol.* **41** e13565–5

[32] Askin S, Burkhalter D, Calado G and El Dakrouni S 2023 Artificial intelligence applied to clinical trials: opportunities and challenges *Health Technol.* **13** 203–13

[33] Tsuchiwata S and Tsuji Y 2023 Computational design of clinical trials using a combination of simulation and the genetic algorithm *CPT Pharmacomet. Syst. Pharmacol.* **12** 522–31

[34] Yin J, Ngiam K Y and Teo H H 2021 Role of artificial intelligence applications in real-life clinical practice: systematic review *J. Med. Internet Res.* **23** e25759

[35] Anran Wang X X, Shengyu Liu Q Q and Zhu Wu S i 2022 Characteristics of artificial intelligence clinical trials in the field of healthcare: a cross-sectional study on ClinicalTrials.gov *Int. J. Environ. Res. Public. Health* **19** 13691

[36] Herson J 2023 Digital twins: a futuristic artificial intelligence methodology for design and analysis of clinical trials *Ann. Biostat. Biom. Appl.* **5**

[37] Vatankhah Barenji R and Ebrahimi Hariry R 2023 Blockchain-enabled quality improvement digital twin for clinical trials *Preprint*

[38] Susilo M E *et al* 2023 Systems-based digital twins to help characterize clinical dose–response and propose predictive biomarkers in a phase I study of bispecific antibody, mosunetuzumab, in NHL *Clin. Transl. Sci.* **16** 1134–48

[39] Camps J *et al* 2023 Digital twinning of the human ventricular activation sequence to clinical 12-lead ECGs and magnetic resonance imaging using realistic Purkinje networks for *in silico* clinical trials *Med. Image Anal.* **94** 103108

[40] Wang Z, Gao C, Glass L M and Sun J 2022 Artificial intelligence for *in silico* clinical trials: a review arXiv: 2209.09023

[41] Baer A R, Bridges K D, O'Dwyer M, Ostroff J and Yasko J 2010 Clinical research site infrastructure and efficiency *J. Oncol. Pract.* **6** 249–52

[42] NCI's National Clinical Trials Network (NCTN) *NCI* https://www.cancer.gov/research/ infrastructure/clinical-trials/nctn (Accessed: 15 January 2024)

[43] Zou W, Geng H, Teo B K, Finlay J and Xiao Y 2018 NCTN clinical trial standardization for radiotherapy through IROC and CIRO *Med. Phys.* **45** e850–3

[44] Lee S H, Geng H and Xiao Y 2022 Radiotherapy standardisation and artificial intelligence within the National Cancer Institute's Clinical Trials Network *Clin. Oncol.* **34** 128–34

[45] Viceconti M, De Vos M, Mellone S and Geris L 2023 From the digital twins in healthcare to the virtual human twin: a moon-shot project for digital health research arXiv: 2304.06678

[46] Ohri N, Shen X, Dicker A P, Doyle L A, Harrison A S and Showalter T N 2013 Radiotherapy protocol deviations and clinical outcomes: a meta-analysis of cooperative group clinical trials *J. Natl. Cancer Inst.* **105** 387–93

[47] Doot R K *et al* 2012 Design considerations for using PET as a response measure in single site and multicenter clinical trials *Acad. Radiol.* **19** 184–90

[48] Xiao Y, Rosen M, Xiao Y and Rosen M A 2017 The role of imaging and radiation oncology core for precision medicine era of clinical trial *Transl. Lung Cancer Res.* **6** 621–4

[49] Glide-Hurst C K *et al* 2021 Adaptive radiation therapy (ART) strategies and technical considerations: a state of the ART review from NRG oncology *Int. J. Radiat. Oncol. Biol. Phys.* **109** 1054–75

[50] Nie K *et al* 2019 NCTN assessment on current applications of radiomics in oncology *Int. J. Radiat. Oncol. Biol. Phys.* **104** 302–15

[51] Zou W *et al* 2023 Framework for quality assurance of ultrahigh dose rate clinical trials investigating FLASH effects and current technology gaps *Int. J. Radiat. Oncol. Biol. Phys.* **116** 1202–17

[52] Ge Y and Wu Q J 2019 Knowledge-based planning for intensity-modulated radiation therapy: a review of data-driven approaches *Med. Phys.* **46** 2760–75

[53] Li N, Carmona R and Sirak I 2017 Highly efficient training, refinement, and validation of a knowledge-based planning quality-control system for radiation therapy clinical trials *Int. J. Radiat. Oncol. Biol. Phys.* **97** 164–72

[54] Giaddui T 2016 A feasibility study of the dosimetric compliance criteria of the NRG-HN002 head and neck clinical trial across different radiotherapy treatment planning systems and delivery techniques: a model for optimizing initial trial launch *J Cancer Prev. Curr. Res.* **5** 341–5

[55] Giaddui T, Chen W and Yu J 2016 Establishing the feasibility of the dosimetric compliance criteria of RTOG 1308: phase III randomized trial comparing overall survival after photon versus proton radiochemotherapy for inoperable stage II-IIIB NSCLC *Radiat. Oncol.* **11** 66

[56] Yusufaly T, Miller A and Medina-Palomo A 2020 A multi-atlas approach for active bone marrow sparing radiation therapy: implementation in the NRG-GY006 trial *Int. J. Radiat. Oncol. Biol. Phys.* **108** 1240–7

[57] Younge K C, Marsh R B and Owen D 2018 Improving quality and consistency in NRG oncology radiation therapy oncology group 0631 for spine radiosurgery via knowledge-based planning *Int. J. Radiat. Oncol.* **100** 1067–74

[58] Geng H, Liao Z and Nguyen Q N 2023 Implementation of machine learning models to ensure radiotherapy quality for multicenter clinical trials: report from a phase III lung cancer study *Cancers* **15** 1–11

[59] Giaddui T, Geng H and Chen Q 2020 Offline quality assurance for intensity modulated radiation therapy treatment plans for NRG-HN001 head and neck clinical trial using knowledge-based planning *Adv. Radiat. Oncol.* **5** 1342–9

[60] Geng H *et al* 2021 A comparison of two methodologies for radiotherapy treatment plan optimization and QA for clinical trials *J. Appl. Clin. Med. Phys.* **22** 329–37

[61] Men K *et al* 2020 Automated quality assurance of OAR contouring for lung cancer based on segmentation with deep active learning *Front. Oncol.* **10** 986

[62] Lee S H *et al* 2023 Interpretable machine learning for choosing radiation dose-volume constraints on cardio-pulmonary substructures associated with overall survival in NRG oncology RTOG 0617 *Int. J. Radiat. Oncol. Biol. Phys.* **117** 1270–86

[63] Russell A M *et al* 2023 Complex and alternate consent pathways in clinical trials: methodological and ethical challenges encountered by underserved groups and a call to action *Trials* **24** 151

[64] Doan X, Florea M and Carter S E 2023 Legal-ethical challenges and technological solutions to e-health data consent in the EU *Front. Artif. Intell. Appl.* **368** 243–53

[65] Dietz H P 2006 Bias in research and conflict of interest: why should we care? *Int. Urogynecol. J.* **18** 241–3

[66] Meerpohl J J *et al* 2015 Evidence-informed recommendations to reduce dissemination bias in clinical research: conclusions from the OPEN (Overcome failure to Publish nEgative fiNdings) project based on an international consensus meeting *BMJ Open* **5** e006666–e6

[67] Shabani M and Obasa M 2019 Transparency and objectivity in governance of clinical trials data sharing: current practices and approaches *Clin. Trials* **16** 547–51

[68] Strech D 2022 Transparenz in der klinischen Forschung: welchen Beitrag leistet die neue EU-Verordnung 536/2014? *Bundesgesundheitsbl* **66** 52–9

[69] DeVito N J and Goldacre B 2023 New UK clinical trials legislation will prioritise transparency *Brit. Med. J.* **382** 1547–7

[70] ICH 2016 ICH harmonised guideline: integrated addendum to ICH E6(R1): guideline for good clinical practice E6(R2) https://ich.org/page/efficacy-guidelines

[71] World Medical Association 2025 WMA Declaration of Helsinki: Ethical Principles for Medical Research Involving Human Subjects *Declaration* World Medical Association https://wma.net/policies-post/wma-declaration-of-helsinki-ethical-principles-for-medical-research-involving-human-subjects/

[72] National Archives 2025 Title 21—Food and Drugs *Code of Federal Regulations* www.ecfr.gov/current/title-21

[73] Clinical Trials Regulation *European Medicines Agency* https://ema.europa.eu/en/human-regulatory/research-development/clinical-trials/clinical-trials-regulation

[74] Xiao Y *et al* 2021 Toward individualized voxel-level dosimetry for radiopharmaceutical therapy *Int. J. Radiat. Oncol. Biol. Phys.* **109** 902–4

[75] Li H *et al* 2023 Overview and recommendations for prospective multi-institutional clinical trials of spatially fractionated radiation therapy (SFRT) *Int. J. Radiat. Oncol.* 737–49

[76] Paganetti H 2014 Relative biological effectiveness (RBE) values for proton beam therapy. Variations as a function of biological endpoint, dose, and linear energy transfer *Phys. Med. Biol.* **59** R419–72

[77] Subcommittee on Quantum Information Science 2018 National strategic overview for quantum information science *Strategic Overview* National Science and Research Council https://quantum. gov/wp-content/uploads/2020/10/2018_NSTC_National_Strategic_Overview_QIS.pdf

[78] Vandewinckele L *et al* 2020 Overview of artificial intelligence-based applications in radiotherapy: recommendations for implementation and quality assurance *Radiother. Oncol.* **153** 55–66

[79] Maspero M *et al* 2018 Dose evaluation of fast synthetic-CT generation using a generative adversarial network for general pelvis MR-only radiotherapy *Phys. Med. Biol.* **63** 235007

[80] Chapman J W, Lam D, Cai B and Hugo G D 2022 Robustness and reproducibility of an artificial intelligence-assisted online segmentation and adaptive planning process for online adaptive radiation therapy *J. Appl. Clin. Med. Phys.* **23** e13702

[81] Casola L (ed) 2023 *Opportunities and Challenges for Digital Twins in Biomedical Research: Proceedings of a Workshop-in Brief* (Washington, DC: National Academies Press)

IOP Publishing

Artificial Intelligence in Adaptive Radiation Therapy

Yi Wang and X. Sharon Qi

Chapter 20

Safety and training considerations in the clinical implementation of artificial intelligence adaptive radiation therapy

Kelly Nealon and Jennifer Pursley

In the rapidly evolving landscape of radiation therapy, the integration of artificial intelligence (AI) in adaptive radiation therapy (ART) brings unprecedented advancements but also necessitates a comprehensive understanding of the associated risks and safety considerations that must be made. When implementing new technology into clinical practice, the departmental risk management and staff training program must be re-evaluated to accommodate the changing workflow [1]. The process of utilizing AI ART methods for patient treatment differs substantially from standard linac-based external beam workflows [2, 3]. Specifically, real-time plan adaptation requires an in-depth understanding of patient anatomy, contour quality, and treatment planning. This dynamic adaptation process introduces distinct roles for therapists, physicists, and physicians that may differ from their prior practice. The intricacies of real-time plan adaptation necessitate specialized training to ensure that healthcare professionals have the expertise required to navigate the nuances of patient-specific anatomy and optimize treatment plans effectively. Therefore, to safely and effectively implement AI ART, updates should be made to the risk management and staff training programs, and appropriate end-to-end testing should be performed before clinical deployment.

20.1 Risk management

Risk management programs are used to identify and correct points of weakness in a workflow that could introduce risk to patients and staff. While there are many possible components of an effective risk management program, both prospective and reactionary techniques should be included to ensure that the safety and efficiency of the workflow is optimized.

doi:10.1088/978-0-7503-6119-4ch20

20.1.1 Prospective risk assessments

Prior to introducing ART into clinical practice, a series of prospective risk assessments should be performed in order to proactively anticipate and mitigate issues before they occur. These risk assessments should be performed by a multidisciplinary team. To determine the appropriate specialties that should be represented on the team, the process should first be examined from start to end to identify all role groups that lend a hand to the process. For example, successful implementation of AI ART requires contributions from radiation therapists, both during CT simulation and at the treatment machine, dosimetrists, medical physicists, and radiation oncologists [3]. Therefore, a representative should be nominated from each role group to participate in the risk assessment process. At a minimum, we recommend that a failure mode and effects analysis and hazard testing of the major components of the ART workflow be performed prior to go-live. Each of these methods will be discussed in the following sections.

20.1.1.1 Failure mode and effects analysis

One type of prospective risk assessment that is used in many industries to anticipate and limit risk is called failure mode and effects analysis (FMEA). FMEA is a systematic approach that can be used to ensure that potential weaknesses have been identified and mitigated before their occurrence in a workflow [4]. During FMEA, a multidisciplinary team of representatives from all participating role groups is assembled. This team then creates a process map, during which each step of the workflow is identified and visually mapped out. An example of the steps that would be included in a process map detailing a person's daily drive to work is shown in figure 20.1. For a workflow to be completed correctly, each step of the process map must be completed without error.

Within a radiation oncology department, process maps should be created that encompass the entirety of the workflow, from the patient's first appointment at CT simulation to their final treatment fraction. When implementing AI ART, it is important to create additional process maps that focus on how the updated workflow differs from the standard clinical procedure.

For each step identified in the process map, the team then attempts to predict any potential error, or failure mode, that could occur while completing each given task. These failure modes should include any action that leads to an undesired outcome, including both large-scale issues that could potentially impact final patient treatment and small issues that may only temporarily inconvenience staff. For each failure mode, a fault tree is then created. Fault trees are visual diagrams used to identify potential causes for each given error. For example, if the failure mode identified is someone running a red light while driving, potential causes could include distracted

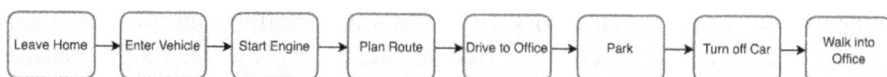

Figure 20.1. An example process map, created to detail the steps involved in commuting to work by car.

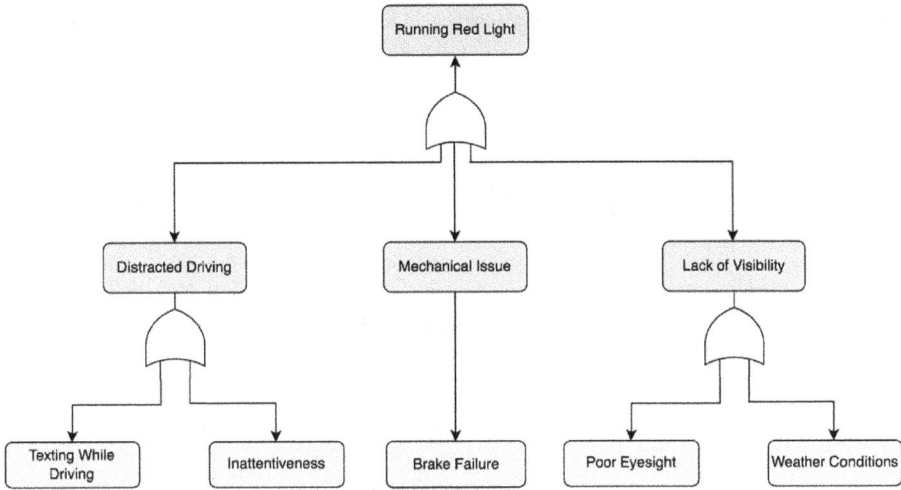

Figure 20.2. An example of a fault tree, generated to identify causes associated with the failure mode of running a red light while driving (red). Identified causes are shown in blue, with possible contributing factors to each cause are shown in yellow.

driving, mechanical issues, and lack of visibility (figure 20.2). Failure modes should be evaluated independently for each identified cause of the error, as some causes are more likely to lead to an event occurring than others.

To maximize the safety of this process, each of these causes should be appropriately addressed prior to the driver returning to the roads.

To quantify the risk, each failure mode is then assigned three numerical scores. First, occurrence (O), which describes the likelihood of that error occurring. Next, severity (S) describes how dangerous or detrimental the effect would be if that error were to occur without being detected. Finally, detectability (D), describes the likelihood that the failure mode will not be detected in time to prevent an event from occurring. It is important to note that scoring for FMEA is a subjective process and can be based on a combination of participant's clinical experience, as well as examples of error occurrence in the literature. By instructing all members of the FMEA team to follow a clear set of scoring guidelines throughout the evaluation, some subjectivity can be eliminated and consistency can be expected. An example of scoring guidelines, similar to those recommended by TG-100, that could be used is shown in table 20.1 [4].

All three scores are then multiplied together to obtain a metric called the risk priority number (RPN), which is a surrogate for the amount of risk that the given error poses to patients. A higher RPN indicates higher risk, and therefore mitigating failure modes with higher scores should be prioritized.

By performing an FMEA prior to the clinical implementation of a new tool or process, the workflow can be designed with proper quality control process steps to eliminate the risk that could be passed down to patients undergoing treatment. Staff training can also be tailored to highlight points of potential risk and limit the

Table 20.1. Example of FMEA scoring guidelines that could be used to create consistency in scoring across all participants.

Score	Occurrence (O)		Severity (S)	Detectability (D)
	Qualitative	Frequency	Impact	Probability of failure mode going undetected
1	Failure unlikely	0.1%	No effect	0.01%
2		0.02%	Inconvenience	0.2%
3	Failure infrequent	0.04%		0.5%
4		0.1%	Minor dosimetric error	1.0%
5		< 0.2%	Limited toxicity or tumor	2.0%
6	Occasional failure	< 0.5%	underdose	5.0%
7		< 1%	Potentially serious toxicity	10%
8	Frequent failure	< 2%	or tumor underdose	15%
9		< 5%	Potentially very serious toxicity or tumor underdose	20%
10	Failure inevitable	> 5%	Catastrophic	> 20%

likelihood of these errors occurring. By prospectively identifying and mitigating points of risk, a culture of safety can be created among the clinical team.

20.1.1.2 Example of improvements made to workflow based on FMEA results

In radiation oncology, FMEA has been proven effective at eliminating points of risk prior to impacting patient care when introducing technologies such as auto-contouring, Gamma Knife and the Halcyon into the clinical workflow [5–8]. Similarly, several groups have also identified the benefits of applying FMEA to evaluate the deployment of AI ART tools [2, 9, 10].

One group that has shown the benefits of using FMEA to limit risk in AI ART processes is Liang *et al* who performed an FMEA to evaluate the proposed workflow for an MR-linac being deployed into a clinic that had previously only made use of standard, non-adaptive, treatment machines [2]. The authors noted that the workflow for the adaptive system was radically different than the conventional treatment workflow, and therefore additional quality management resources were needed. An online reference form was created to guide clinical team members through the treatment planning, quality assurance, and delivery processes. The FMEA revealed that while this reference guide was useful for new users, a more concise checklist should be developed to be completed by physics staff for each fraction of patient treatment. The checklist was made to comply with recommendations from AAPM and contains essential information to be checked before, during, and after treatment to ensure the treatment was delivered as intended and to mitigate several identified high-risk failure modes.

20.1.1.3 Hazard analysis

Another type of prospective risk assessment that can be used to optimize safety when implementing an AI ART workflow into the clinic is hazard analysis, as recommended by IEC 62 366: 'Application of usability engineering to medical devices' [11]. A hazard scenario refers to a potentially dangerous or risky situation that may occur when an error is introduced into a workflow. If this error goes unnoticed by members of a radiation therapy team, it could heighten the risk and jeopardize patient safety. Conducting a hazard analysis allows the identification of the root causes of these scenarios, enabling the implementation of additional safeguards to mitigate and address potential risks. An illustration of hazard analysis is evident in the research conducted by Pawlicki *et al* where they employed a tool known as system theoretic process analysis (STPA) to pinpoint and mitigate potential hazards within clinical radiation therapy workflows [12]. Other studies demonstrated the advantages of applying hazard analysis to evaluate the clinical safety associated with the use of the Halcyon and an automated contouring and treatment planning tool [13, 14].

In order to perform a hazard analysis, errors that are likely to occur in a given workflow should be simulated to evaluate their detectability. When performed in conjunction with an FMEA, the list of high RPN failure modes can be used to inform which errors, or hazard scenarios, should be inserted into the workflow. An end-to-end test of the workflow should then occur during which all members of the clinical team complete their corresponding task, with the hazard present in the process to determine if or when the error hazard is detected. If the hazard is detected and corrected prior to impacting the final output, such as high-quality patient treatment, then the process is working as designed and intended.

If undetected, feedback should be requested from participants to inform what changes in the process or quality management steps should be made to increase detectability. Following changes to the workflow, the testing should be repeated with a new, blinded, set of participants to confirm that the changes made were effective in reducing risk.

20.1.2 Root cause analysis

To maximize the effectiveness of a quality management program, retrospective or reactionary evaluation techniques should also be utilized. Root cause analysis (RCA) is one retrospective risk assessment technique that should be incorporated into radiation therapy programs, including those that utilize AI ART systems [15]. RCA is a process used to identify the cause of a safety event, or failure mode, that has occurred in clinical practice. Performing an RCA requires users to step backward through a process, originating from the safety event until the decision point is identified which causes the workflow to divert from the intended outcome, i.e. successful patient treatment. To successfully perform an RCA, members of all subgroups of the clinical team must participate in order to represent all perspectives of the event that occurred. The team must then work to identify both what happened at each step in the process, and also why each decision was made that allowed the error to perpetuate further into the workflow. By identifying the cause of the error, as well as any weak points in the quality management and quality assurance processes that the error passed through undetected, areas of the workflow requiring improvement can be found [4].

One example of when RCA could be used is the identification of a low-quality AI-generated bladder contour in the clinical plan, after delivering three fractions of an adaptive prostate treatment. The therapist who identified this clinical abnormality would report the failure to the department's safety committee, and an RCA would begin. In this scenario, the cause could be attributed to a failure of the AI model, which inaccurately delineated the bladder. If the AI failed due to the presence of an artifact, a corrective action could be to limit the use of AI to only scans free of artifact. If no artifact was present but the patient anatomy deviated from the standard case, the contouring model could also be retrained to encompass a wider variety of patient anatomy in an attempt to limit the occurrence of this error. After the cause was identified and mitigated, the team would then examine how it was able to go undetected until after the patient began treatment. Perhaps an additional layer of contour QA could be added to the workflow, manual or automated, to add redundancy and increase the detectability. A quality management tool, such as a checklist, could also be added to guide the review of contours to ensure each organ is thoroughly examined. These error mitigation techniques would then be implemented into the clinical workflow to prevent poor-quality AI contours from impacting future patient treatments.

To effectively implement retrospective risk management techniques, there must be a non-punitive culture that allows errors to be freely reported and discussed without fear of punishment. When errors occur, it should be emphasized that the cause was a failure of the process, not any individual member of the team.

20.2 Staff training

To ensure accurate and consistent usage of AI during ART procedures, it is important for each member of the staff to have role group specific training which includes all the information staff need to perform their duties. While the attending radiation oncologist is ultimately responsible for a patient's care, physicians must work closely with and provide oversight for a trained ART support team of therapists, dosimetrists, and physicists. Many ART workflows rely on trained support staff as physician-extenders; for example, in an advanced radiation therapist model, therapists receive training in contouring and make edits to AI-generated contours before the physician arrives [3, 16–18]. Whichever staffing model is chosen for ART, the duties of staff should be clearly established, documented with written policies and procedures, and communicated to staff. Team members should feel comfortable with their duties and be encouraged to voice concerns if they feel certain tasks are outside their scope of practice or training. All team members should understand that completing adaptive treatments in a timely manner is a priority for high-quality online ART, as the internal anatomy is more likely to change from the initial daily volumetric image as the adaptive workflow time increases. The goal of training is to enable staff to perform fast, safe, high-quality online ART with the use of AI.

The first step in designing staff training for a new procedure is to establish the workflows that will be followed and designate duties to specific role groups. Then training programs can be designed to supplement the training and knowledge each role group already maintains as part of their standard practice. All adaptive staff members should be experienced with non-adaptive treatments on the same treatment equipment and devices, including general operational aspects and safety considerations.

20.2.1 Process mapping of AI ART workflow

Process mapping is a tool that graphically shows the inputs, actions, and outputs of a process or workflow using a step-by-step map [4]. The process must be well-defined, with a clear start and end. The graphical representations should be detailed enough for team members to understand each step in the process, identify potential weaknesses in current staff training related to that step, and identify which staff member(s) will be responsible for completing each task. While the hardware and software components of a commercial ART system may be identical between institutions, the workflows that institutions develop to perform ART will be highly dependent on institutional culture and other infrastructure in the department. Therefore, each institution should individually perform process mapping of its ART workflows, although it would be beneficial to start from published analyses of similar systems when available.

Figure 20.3 shows an example of a high-level process map for online ART treatment. Once a graphical process map has been created, it can be beneficial to create a spreadsheet for tracking specific details of the process. Each step in the graphical process map can be numbered, and the spreadsheet can detail for each step number what systems and staff are involved in the step sub-processes. This type of process map can be helpful as input for a hazard analysis in addition to designing staff training programs.

ART-specific process maps can help identify steps in adaptive workflows which utilize AI and differ from conventional RT workflows. Process maps should be considered for CT simulation, treatment planning, plan quality checks, treatment delivery, and post-treatment checks. A detailed process map will include all the systems and staff involved in transferring data, information, and decisions during the process. It would be beneficial to review process maps with a multi-disciplinary group to ensure that all steps are captured accurately. Process maps should be developed prior to starting an ART program and then continually updated as workflows or technology change.

20.2.2 Role-specific training processes

Online ART is complex, resource-intensive, and time-sensitive, as intrafraction changes in the anatomy can render a newly adapted plan obsolete. All adaptive staff should understand the overall adaptive workflow and the time-sensitive nature of

Bring patient into room → Verify identity / Set up to lasers → Acquire pre-treatment image

Adjust patient setup

Adjust segmentations

Remove patient from room

Document adaptive treatment decision

Decide whether to restart adaptive procedure

Image acceptable for adaptation? — NO / YES

Daily image segmentation

Synthetic CT generation

Segmentations acceptable? — NO / YES

Deliver treatment

Is anatomy still aligned for treatment? — NO / YES

Acquire new pre-treatment image and perform shifts

Treat with adapted plan? — NO / YES

Daily plan optimization

Reference plan recalculation

Perform quality assurance checks

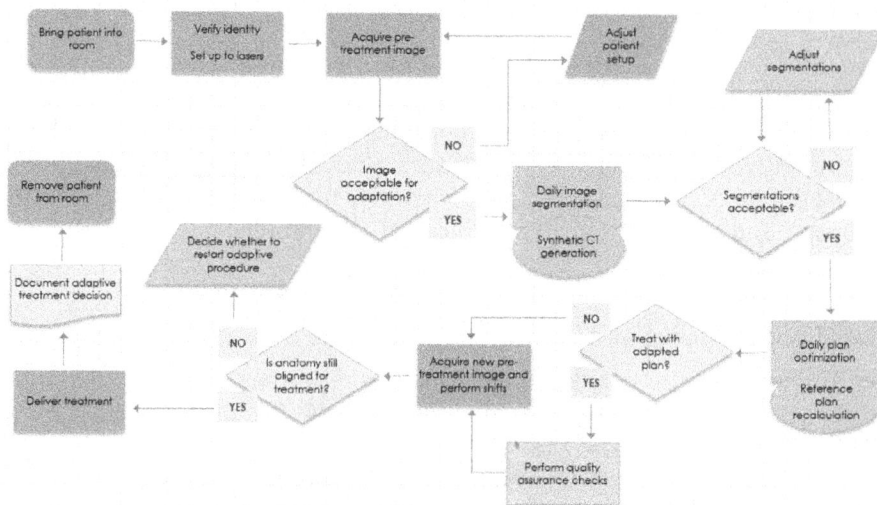

Figure 20.3. A high-level graphical process map for a generic online adaptive treatment workflow. Steps in the workflow are color-coded to indicate staff expected to participate in each step (orange for therapists; yellow for multiple role groups; blue for physicians or physician-extenders; green for often AI-automated steps; gray for physicists). An institutional process map should contain more details specific to its adaptive workflows.

online ART. Responsibility for steps in the process should be clearly assigned so staff know their duties and can perform them without hesitation. When AI is involved, staff must also understand the actions and limitations of AI so that they can adequately check AI outputs.

Institutions should develop standard operating procedures (SOPs) and protocols specific to their adaptive workflow, as documented by process mapping. Staff should be trained specifically on these SOPs using the institution's adaptive equipment and devices; some training, particularly related to contouring and planning, may be disease-site specific. External resources should be utilized when available and may include materials or courses provided by the adaptive system vendor, external teaching courses, and site visits to other institutions performing ART. If the AI used in the adaptive process was developed by the institution in-house, then internally developed training resources will be required. Internally developed training resources require effort to prepare but are essential and may include anonymized patients used for contouring practice, ART emulators used for *in silico* workflow practice, policies and procedures documentation, and lectures or discussions with peers. Suggested topics for training of each role group are shown in table 20.2.

Training should be formally documented with records maintained for all staff participating in adaptive treatments. Implementing an internal credentialing or competency assessment process is strongly advised, and completed credentialing should be documented. Competencies should be reviewed periodically, with refresher training offered as needed. Policies, procedures, documentation, and training should be updated when there are hardware or software changes that

Table 20.2. Recommended training topics are summarized for each role group.

Role group	Recommended training topics
Radiation therapists	Use of the online adaptive system with a focus on image registration. Contouring of normal anatomy and edits to AI contours. Impacts of contours on automated/AI treatment plan optimization. Recognition of dosimetrically significant anatomical changes. Patient safety considerations.
Medical dosimetrists	Use of the online adaptive system with a focus on plan optimization. Robust plan optimization considerations. Contouring of normal anatomy and edits to AI contours. Automated/AI adaptive treatment plan optimization considerations. Recognition of dosimetrically significant anatomical changes.
Medical physicists	Use of the online adaptive system with a focus on AI properties. Robust plan optimization considerations. Contouring considerations for a variety of different disease sites. Automated/AI adaptive treatment plan optimization considerations. Recognition of dosimetrically significant anatomical changes. Adaptive plan quality assurance (QA) checks. Offline plan review.
Radiation oncologists	Use of the online adaptive system with a focus on contouring. Contouring considerations for a variety of different disease sites. Impacts of contours on automated/AI treatment plan optimization. Recognition of dosimetrically significant anatomical changes. Offline plan review.

impact ART processes; given the rapid development of AI, there may be a frequent need for updates. If new AI processes are added, additional credentialing may be needed. The institution should decide how training will be coordinated for each role group, whether internally by the leaders of that role group, or by an ART QA oversight committee.

20.2.2.1 Radiation therapists

Radiation therapists are often primarily responsible for image registration review during online ART, as this is part of their standard practice for IGRT. Therapists should be able to evaluate daily volumetric image quality and identify artifacts that may arise from using AI to improve image reconstruction. If registrations during the ART workflow are performed by AI, therapists should receive training on how to evaluate AI registrations and adjust registrations with the tools available.

In many online ART workflows, radiation therapists also play a role as physician-extenders. As image segmentation is not part of standard therapy practice in most countries, therapists require substantial training on the contouring of normal anatomy. A physician experienced in the online ART workflow should lead contouring training, which should include formal instruction on normal anatomy, offline practice of contouring, and online training [17, 18]. Commercial products are available to guide refresher training and to enable formal evaluation of competency [19]. Both offline and online contour training should, if possible, be performed in the adaptive treatment planning system (TPS) using the same tools available during online ART. This is important because tools in the adaptive TPS often differ from those available in a conventional TPS; it is particularly beneficial to start from AI contours generated by the clinical system [20]. Training should include an understanding of how all contours are generated, whether by AI, deformable image registration, or rigid image registration. Known weaknesses of the AI model should be discussed, such as an inability to differentiate large and small bowel or a model for prostate cancer that does not include a rectal hydrogel spacer so its performance will be suboptimal on patients with such a spacer. It is also beneficial if the contour training uses realistic daily volumetric images from the adaptive system, rather than CT simulation scans. Most adaptive systems use either MRI or CBCT for on-treatment imaging, and contouring on these images will be different from a CT. There is no required minimum number of contouring cases that must be completed under physician supervision; however, the supervising physician should attest by the end of training that the individual has reached an appropriate level of proficiency and is credentialed to contour clinically [21].

While therapists may not be directly involved in adaptive plan optimization, contour edits have a significant impact on adaptive plan optimization and therefore some knowledge of the adaptive planning process is required as part of the contour training. To reduce the treatment time, contours should only be edited in the clinically relevant regions near the target; it may be possible to generate ring structures around the target to guide the user on the region requiring edits [22, 23]. The user should also understand what contours are most important for adaptive plan optimization and how they are used in the optimization, such as whether the optimization relies on a maximum dose, mean dose, or dose to a specified volume. This information can influence how contours are edited.

In x-ray-based ART systems, another image is acquired after the adaptive process but prior to delivery to ensure that the anatomy has not deformed in the time required for adaption. As therapists will again be involved in image registration, they should be trained in how to recognize significant intra-fraction anatomical changes that would cause the adapted plan to be non-optimal. Adaptive physicians should develop a plan on how to address expected anatomical changes and what changes would require repeating the online ART workflow; this plan may be different for each disease site and should be communicated to physician-extenders to help with decision-making when the physician is not present.

The therapists should also be trained in emergency procedures to guide patient safety considerations during treatment interruptions caused by power outages, machine failures, or any other issues that can be anticipated. The emergency response plans may be different during the adaptive workflow than for IGRT treatment and may depend on exactly where in the workflow the emergency occurs. These plans should be readily available so the team has access to them quickly in case of an emergency.

20.2.2.2 Medical dosimetrists

Medical dosimetrists may be involved in developing the initial reference plan, which may also be used for adaptive plan optimization, often in an automated fashion. Some workflows may involve AI-assisted treatment planning of the initial and daily plans, and dosimetrists should be trained in the use of AI treatment planning models, their weaknesses, and on how to adjust AI plans if that is possible. Depending on the institution's adaptive workflow, a dosimetrist may also be present during the adaptive treatment to operate as a physician-extender for contouring and to assist with adaptive plan optimization or in evaluating the adaptive plan quality. Any dosimetrists participating in the adaptive workflow should have training in relevant parts of the adaptive system, with a particular emphasis on the adaptive planning system. Hands-on training on the system or in an emulator is preferred over training videos.

If they are involved in the development of the initial plan and the plan optimization goals for daily adaptive use, dosimetrists should receive instruction from adaptive physicians on expected daily anatomic variations by site and realize their potential impact on plan optimization. This will assist with developing robust plan optimization goals that remain appropriate even when the anatomy changes, which requires having clearly set priorities for whether target coverage or organ sparing take precedence. These priorities should be set by the physician but implemented in the optimization by the treatment planner. It may be beneficial for a dosimetrist to complete practice cases offline or in an emulator to confirm their understanding of the adaptive planning system.

A dosimetrist may also be present during the adaptive treatment to assist with contouring and adaptive plan optimization. In this case, dosimetrists should receive contouring training and credentialing such as that received by radiation therapists and should also be trained in using the contouring tools specific to the adaptive system. As an expert in treatment planning, dosimetrists should additionally be relied upon to recognize which contour edits will have an impact on adaptive plan optimization. To achieve the most timely and efficient adaptive workflow, edits should only be made if they impact the adaptive plan optimization, and a dosimetrist can guide other team members in that assessment.

20.2.2.3 Medical physicists

Medical physicists are often the leaders and primary implementers of AI and adaptive workflows. The responsibility of designing adaptive workflows and training programs for other role groups often falls on the physicists. The training of the physicists involved in implementing an adaptive program will primarily consist of vendor training to gain an in-depth understanding of the systems they will be using, literature review of best practices, attending specialty meetings, and site visits to learn from other users. Attendance and participation in training events should be documented. The physicists must also have knowledge of the AI used by the system and should test the properties and performance of the AI during the commissioning of the adaptive system. Depending on the system, physicists may be involved in maintaining and updating the AI and should have enough knowledge to do what is required.

Once the adaptive program is in place, physicists may be trained to assist with adaptive treatments even though they are not primarily responsible for the system and its maintenance. A training program should be devised that trains physicists on the system and provides as much information about the AI components as they need to know for safe operation. A physicist may also be called on to assist with contouring, particularly in providing peer review of physician-adjusted contours such as the target. Thus, physicists should also receive additional contouring training and credentialing such as that received by medical dosimetrists. If a dosimetrist is not present during the online adaptive treatment, a physicist may be expected to assist in adaptive plan optimization or evaluation and should be trained on how to do so in the adaptive system.

Physicists are also expected to perform pre-treatment QA for online ART. This QA may include contour review, plan review, secondary dose calculation, and possibly more depending on the systems in use. Physicists should receive training on the systems used to perform these QA checks and should be aware if any utilize AI. AI may be particularly beneficial for contour review and secondary dose calculation but must be confirmed to be operating correctly if it replaces manual checks.

Physicists may also assist the therapists in image quality assessment and image registrations, either of the daily image to the planning CT or other image sets, or of the pre-treatment image after plan adaptation. The physicist should receive training on the dosimetric impacts of anatomic changes so they can assist with determining whether a significant anatomical change has occurred which requires re-planning.

20.2.2.4 Radiation oncologists

Radiation oncologists are experts in contouring both normal organs and target structures. However, many physicians specialize by disease site, and in some adaptive coverage models, physicians may be covering adaptive treatments for disease sites outside their specialization. If this is the case, disease-site specific contour training for physicians is advised. Physicians will also need to become familiar with the contouring tools in the adaptive system and should receive hands-on training in the adaptive TPS. If the contouring or planning uses AI, physicians should also be made aware of the limitations of the AI to guide their review of its contours and treatment plans.

Radiation oncologists should also be trained in how to use the adaptive system for offline review of adaptive treatments. Particularly if the institution's workflow has a different physician than the patient's attending covering adaptive treatments, or if the attending is reviewing remotely rather than in-person, the attending physician should review each adaptive treatment. Feedback should be provided to the adaptive team for any modifications the attending wishes to see in future treatments.

20.3 End-to-end testing

End-to-end tests are an important step in any commissioning process [24, 25]. They validate that all components of the system are functioning as intended and test the connections and data transfer between components. They are also valuable for the users to practice their clinical workflows and confirm their understanding of how the system operates. For a novel system, they may be used as a training tool to introduce new staff to the workflow in a test environment. When developing new workflows such as for adaptive therapy, it is beneficial if the steps in the end-to-end test are performed by the appropriate role group (e.g. therapist, dosimetrist, physicist, and physician) rather than allowing all steps to be performed by a physicist.

For traditional radiotherapy, an end-to-end test may involve acquiring a CT scan of a phantom, developing a radiotherapy treatment plan, delivering that plan on the treatment system, and measuring the dose to a detector inside the phantom. If the measured dose agrees with the TPS's prediction, then the correct functioning of the system relating to dose delivery in a patient has been verified. For adaptive radiotherapy, however, this test is insufficient [26]. For a clinical adaptive treatment, a new plan will be developed in real time based on changes in the patient's anatomy from the original CT scan. To provide a realistic test of an ART system, the phantom should change in some way relative to the planning CT to test the generation of a new adaptive plan. Another characteristic of ART for patients is that there may be changes in density in the daily image relative to the planning CT caused by the presence or absence of gastrointestinal gas, weight gain or loss, tumor shrinkage or growth, and other possible anatomic changes. Consequently, multiple end-to-end tests may be required using different phantoms to verify the behavior of the system under different conditions [27].

End-to-end tests should be repeated after any software upgrades, focusing specifically on tests that relate to that particular software. End-to-end tests should also be considered on a monthly or annual basis for ongoing QA of system operations and for training purposes.

20.3.1 Phantom selection

Adaptive phantoms do not necessarily need to be expensive or complex, but multiple phantoms will likely be required to test different aspects of the ART workflow. Basic functionality tests may be conducted with a simple phantom, such as slabs of solid water that may be re-arranged to place the target (ion chamber or film) in a different location relative to the CT simulation scan. Tests relating to heterogeneity will require a phantom with at least two different densities. Some tests may require an anthropomorphic phantom. For some purposes, such as evaluating the accuracy of AI auto-contours, even an anthropomorphic phantom may be insufficient to provide a realistic test. Digital phantoms may be able to provide a test of systems that require realistic anatomic information. The following sections give some suggestions of physical and digital phantoms that may be useful for end-to-end tests of different features of ART AI systems.

20.3.1.1 Physical phantoms

The composition of physical phantoms used for end-to-end testing will depend on the ART system's imaging modality. MR-compatible phantoms have been developed for MR-linac commissioning [28]. Guidance also exists for commissioning clinical PET/CT systems using common phantoms [29], but phantoms allowing the injection or insertion of vials of FDG or another radionuclide would also be useful for PET-linacs. Many phantoms have been developed for x-ray guided systems and these may be used with or without modifications for adaptive testing.

Certain properties are desirable for end-to-end adaptive testing and should be considered when selecting a phantom to test a specific property. Typically, the final output of an end-to-end test is a measurement of the delivered dose, so the phantom should provide a means to acquire a measurement. This could be accomplished by having an insert that holds a detector, either an ion chamber, film, or other detector. Some progress has also been made in using gel phantoms to perform 3D dosimetry [30]. For ART specifically, it may be desirable to have a phantom that can be modified to prompt the creation of an adapted plan. Depending on the phantom, this can be achieved in several ways, such as by rearranging slabs in a slab phantom, using different density inserts, or adding bolus material over a phantom to simulate weight change [27]. There have also been advances in anthropomorphic phantoms, principally thorax, which allow internal deformation [31]. Prior to commissioning an ART system, physicists should evaluate the phantoms already available to them and decide if they can be used to perform all the necessary end-to-end testing, or if new phantoms should be acquired.

20.3.1.2 Digital phantoms

As the complexity of a delivery system increases, it becomes more challenging to find a phantom that is sufficiently advanced to provide a true clinical test of the features of the system. This is particularly true for testing AI in ART—anthropomorphic phantoms made of plastic may not be realistic enough for an AI contouring solution to work on them or to accurately test the AI's limitations. To test AI contouring and other AI solutions that require more realistic representations, digital phantoms are required [3, 26].

Digital phantoms provided by TG-132 may be useful to benchmark image registration algorithms [32]. There may also be disease-site specific digital phantoms available to evaluate rigid and deformable registration, such as the POPI 4D CT lung data sets and the Deformable Image Registration Evaluation Project head and neck data sets [33, 34]. Datasets including contour segmentations may also be suitable for evaluating AI contouring algorithms. The XCAT anthropomorphic digital phantoms (Duke University, Durham, NC, USA) provide a virtual model of male and female patient anatomy and physiology in the cardiac-torso [35].

If an appropriate digital phantom dataset is not available, institutions may need to create their own digital phantoms. Depending on the purpose of the phantom, this could be as straightforward as creating a deformed CT scan of a physical phantom [26]. The deformed CT scan could then be used as the planning CT in the adaptive TPS, so that when the phantom is scanned as part of the adaptive workflow, the daily image would not match the planning image. However, this type of simple digital phantom may not be adequate for all end-to-end tests, particularly for AI contouring tests. In cases where realistic anatomical representations are necessary, it may be preferable to use retrospective patient data as digital phantoms in an offline emulator system. If daily images using the adaptive system are available, using them in an emulator would provide a realistic end-to-end test of the system's AI capabilities on its own daily images. If daily images are not available, deformed CT images may be useful as digital phantoms, although the properties will not be identical to the daily images [36].

20.3.2 End-to-end adaptive delivery

The goal of an end-to-end test is to understand how the adaptive system operates, validate the operation performs as intended, and identify any errors or assumptions that require correction. Guidance on tolerances for adaptive end-to-end tests is not currently available but should be forthcoming from AAPM Task Group reports on specific adaptive modalities. As demonstrated in Kisling *et al* multiple end-to-end tests will be required to test the full functionality of the ART system [27]. At least one adaptive end-to-end test should be performed as part of acceptance testing so that any deficiencies can be corrected by the vendor prior to commissioning. This test will validate data transfer between different systems, such as the on-treatment imaging system, planning software, and secondary check software. A full suite of end-to-end adaptive tests, as determined by the physicists using their clinical judgment, should be performed during commissioning. It may be beneficial to use end-to-end tests as part of periodic system testing, such as on a weekly, monthly, or annual basis to confirm the stability of the system, and end-to-end tests may also be incorporated into user training programs [37].

At least one end-to-end test should test the basic functionality of the adaptive system, and this may be performed during acceptance. A simple phantom such as a stack of solid water with a Farmer chamber or film may be adequate for this test. The phantom should be set up identically to the planning CT, and the re-calculated dose on the daily image should be similar to the reference plan in terms of DVH metrics. The dose should be accurately delivered as evaluated using the detector in the phantom. This test can also be performed with a shift of the phantom relative to isocenter to verify the rigid image registration capabilities of the system. If this test fails, there may be issues with the image registration or dose calculation that must be investigated.

The behavior of the system when presented with heterogeneities must also be evaluated. Even in the pelvis, gas may be present or absent in the bowel and rectum, there may be metal implants causing artifacts, and the location of the target may change position relative to the pelvic and hip bones. A creative approach using a thorax phantom with different density inserts to simulate the presence or absence of gas and bone is demonstrated in Kisling *et al* [27]. A deformed planning CT or CT with density overrides may also be used for these tests. The system should also be tested in situations involving weight loss or tumor volume change, as these are clinical scenarios in which adaptive therapy is expected to be beneficial [27]. In all cases, the adaptive system should either be able to calculate dose correctly, or the limitations of the system should be defined and documented by the test.

As highlighted in section 20.3.1.2, digital phantoms operating in an offline emulator may be best suited to test aspects of the AI system such as image registration and contouring. Testing should be performed for all clinical disease sites and the limitations of the accuracy of these systems should be explored by the tests. For contouring end-to-end tests, the clinical environment should be simulated as much as possible with the adaptive team participating according to the planned clinical workflow.

20.4 Summary

This chapter focuses on how to successfully integrate AI-assisted adaptive radiation therapy (AI ART) into clinical practice, with an emphasis on transforming work-flows, managing risks, and preparing staff. AI ART introduces significant changes to standard workflows, making it essential to update risk management strategies, provide specialized training, and conduct thorough end-to-end testing. Collaboration among team members, regular evaluation of practices, and a strong safety culture are key to making AI ART work effectively in clinical settings.

References

[1] ASTRO 2019 Safety is no accident *Report* American Society for Radiation Oncology https://astro.org/Patient-Care-and-Research/Patient-Safety/Safety-is-no-Accident

[2] Liang J *et al* 2023 Risk analysis of the Unity 1.5 T MR-linac adapt-to-position workflow *J. Appl. Clin. Med. Phys.* **24** e13850

[3] Glide-Hurst C K *et al* 2021 Adaptive radiation therapy (ART) strategies and technical considerations: a state of the ART review from NRG Oncology *Int. J. Radiat. Oncol. Biol. Phys.* **109** 1054

[4] Huq M S *et al* 2016 The report of Task Group 100 of the AAPM: application of risk analysis methods to radiation therapy quality management *Med. Phys.* **43** 4209–62

[5] Xu A Y *et al* 2017 Failure modes and effects analysis (FMEA) for Gamma Knife radiosurgery *J. Appl. Clin. Med. Phys.* **18** 152–68

[6] Kisling K *et al* 2019 A risk assessment of automated treatment planning and recommendations for clinical deployment *Med. Phys.* **46** 2567–74

[7] Teo P T *et al* 2019 Application of TG-100 risk analysis methods to the acceptance testing and commissioning process of a Halcyon linear accelerator *Med. Phys.* **46** 1341–54

[8] Nealon K A *et al* 2022 Using failure mode and effects analysis to evaluate risk in the clinical adoption of automated contouring and treatment planning tools *Pract. Radiat. Oncol.* **12** e344–53

[9] Wegener S *et al* 2024 Prospective risk analysis of the online-adaptive artificial intelligence-driven workflow using the Ethos treatment system *Zeit. Med. Phys.* **34** 384–96

[10] Nishioka S *et al* 2022 Identifying risk characteristics using failure mode and effect analysis for risk management in online magnetic resonance-guided adaptive radiation therapy *Phys. Imaging. Radiat. Oncol.* **23** 1–7

[11] International Electrotechnical Commission 2016 Part 2: Guidance on the application of usability engineering to medical devices *Technical specification* IEC/TR 62366-2:2016 International Organization for Standardization

[12] Pawlicki T, Samost A, Brown D W, Manger R P, Kim G Y and Leveson N G 2016 Application of systems and control theory-based hazard analysis to radiation oncology *Med. Phys.* **43** 1514–30

[13] Pawlicki T, Atwood T, McConnell K and Kim G Y 2019 Clinical safety assessment of the Halcyon system *Med. Phys.* **46** 4340–5

[14] Nealon K A *et al* 2023 Hazard testing to reduce risk in the development of automated planning tools *J. Appl. Clin. Med. Phys.* **24** e13995

[15] Ford E C, Fong De Los Santos L, Pawlicki T, Sutlief S and Dunscombe P 2012 Consensus recommendations for incident learning database structures in radiation oncology *Med. Phys.* **39** 7272–90

[16] Shepherd M *et al* 2021 Pathway for radiation therapists online advanced adapter training and credentialing *Tech. Innov. Patient. Support. Radiat. Oncol.* **20** 54

[17] Picton M *et al* 2023 Introduction of radiation therapist-led adaptive treatments on a 1.5 T MR-linac *J. Med. Radiat. Sci.* **70** 94–8

[18] Li W *et al* 2023 Practice-based training strategy for therapist-driven prostate MR-linac adaptive radiotherapy *Tech. Innov. Patient. Support. Radiat. Oncol.* **27** 100212

[19] Yuen A H L, Li A K L, Mak P C Y and Leung H L 2021 Implementation of web-based open-source radiotherapy delineation software (WORDS) in organs at risk contouring training for newly qualified radiotherapists: quantitative comparison with conventional one-to-one coaching approach *BMC Med. Educ.* **21** 564

[20] Pokharel S, Pacheco A and Tanner S 2022 Assessment of efficacy in automated plan generation for Varian Ethos intelligent optimization engine *J. Appl. Clin. Med. Phys.* **23** e13539

[21] Rasing M J A *et al* 2022 Online adaptive MR-guided radiotherapy: conformity of contour adaptation for prostate cancer, rectal cancer and lymph node oligometastases among radiation therapists and radiation oncologists *Tech. Innov. Patient. Support. Radiat. Oncol.* **23** 33–40

[22] Bohoudi O *et al* 2017 Fast and robust online adaptive planning in stereotactic MR-guided adaptive radiation therapy (SMART) for pancreatic cancer *Radiother. Oncol.* **125** 439–44

[23] Price A T, Zachary C J, Laugeman E, Maraghechi B, Zhu T and Henke L E 2023 Patient specific contouring region of interest for abdominal stereotactic adaptive radiotherapy *Phys. Imaging. Radiat. Oncol.* **25** 100423

[24] Klein E E *et al* 2009 Task group 142 report: quality assurance of medical acceleratorsa) *Med. Phys.* **36** 4197–212

[25] Halvorsen P H *et al* 2017 AAPM-RSS medical physics practice guideline 9.a. for SRS-SBRT *J. Appl. Clin. Med. Phys.* **18** 10–21

[26] Chapman J W, Lam D, Cai B and Hugo G D 2022 Robustness and reproducibility of an artificial intelligence-assisted online segmentation and adaptive planning process for online adaptive radiation therapy *J. Appl. Clin. Med. Phys.* **23** e13702

[27] Kisling K, Keiper T D, Branco D, Kim G G Y, Moore K L and Ray X 2022 Clinical commissioning of an adaptive radiotherapy platform: results and recommendations *J. Appl. Clin. Med. Phys.* **23** e13801

[28] Hu Q *et al* 2020 Practical safety considerations for integration of magnetic resonance imaging in radiation therapy *Pract. Radiat. Oncol.* **10** 443–53

[29] Lopez B P, Jordan D W, Kemp B J, Kinahan P E, Schmidtlein C R and Mawlawi O R 2021 PET/CT acceptance testing and quality assurance: executive summary of AAPM Task Group 126 Report *Med. Phys.* **48** e31–5

[30] Schreiner L J 2019 End to end QA in image guided and adaptive radiation therapy *J. Phys. Conf. Ser.* **1305** 012062

[31] Tajik M, Akhlaqi M M and Gholami S 2022 Advances in anthropomorphic thorax phantoms for radiotherapy: a review *Biomed. Phys. Eng. Express* **8** 052001

[32] Brock K K, Mutic S, McNutt T R, Li H and Kessler M L 2017 Use of image registration and fusion algorithms and techniques in radiotherapy: report of the AAPM Radiation Therapy Committee Task Group No. 132 *Med. Phys.* **44** e43–76

[33] Vandemeulebroucke J, Rit S, Kybic J, Clarysse P and Sarrut D 2011 Spatiotemporal motion estimation for respiratory-correlated imaging of the lungs *Med. Phys.* **38** 166–78

[34] Pukala J *et al* 2016 Benchmarking of five commercial deformable image registration algorithms for head and neck patients *J. Appl. Clin. Med. Phys.* **17** 25–40

[35] Segars W P, Sturgeon G, Mendonca S, Grimes J and Tsui B M W 2010 4D XCAT phantom for multimodality imaging research *Med. Phys.* **37** 4902–15

[36] Meyer S *et al* 2023 Creating patient-specific digital phantoms with a longitudinal atlas for evaluating deformable CT-CBCT registration in adaptive lung radiotherapy *Med. Phys.* **51** 1405–14

[37] Lamb J *et al* 2017 Online adaptive radiation therapy: implementation of a new process of care *Cureus* **9** e1618

Chapter 21

Ethical and regulatory considerations in artificial intelligence for adaptive radiation therapy

Dandan Zheng, Megan Hyun and Andrew Fanning

This chapter explores the emerging ethical and regulatory considerations of artificial intelligence (AI) in adaptive radiotherapy (ART), a rapidly evolving field where frameworks are still in development. It begins by establishing foundational concepts in bioethics and examining the current regulatory landscape for AI in medicine. The chapter then addresses specific ethical and regulatory challenges that arise when implementing AI in ART, providing practical frameworks and approaches to ensure ethical deployment. Approaches such as explainable AI and life-cycle frameworks are discussed as methods to address these challenges throughout AI development and implementation. The chapter emphasizes the importance of mitigating bias to ensure fair treatment across diverse patient populations and underscores the need for robust regulations to protect patient data and prevent automation complacency. An ethical argument is presented for AI's role in improving resource allocation, particularly in low-resource settings, by enhancing the efficiency and accessibility of ART. Multidisciplinary collaboration and ongoing education are essential to navigate these ethical complexities, ensuring responsible AI integration that upholds patient trust and safety.

21.1 Background of ethics and regulations in AI for ART

21.1.1 A brief bioethics overview

Before discussing the specific ethical and regulatory considerations relevant to adaptive radiotherapy (ART) and the larger healthcare context, it is important to establish an understanding of a bioethics framework widely adopted in Western medicine. This framework, presented by Beauchamp and Childress [1], includes four key principles:

1. *Respect for autonomy*: fostering autonomous decision-making.
2. *Beneficence*: acting for the benefit of patients.

3. *Nonmaleficence*: refraining from acting in ways that harm patients.
4. *Justice*: seeking a just distribution of benefits.

This framework may be presented with modified organization or naming schemes [2, 3], but the core principles remain the same. Many of the codes of ethics that govern medical associations are rooted in these principles [4–6].

The application of these principles to ethical decision-making in the context of AI in radiation therapy was previously described by Hyun and Hyun, and was used to explore several ethical dilemmas, including adopting AI tools with potential biases, equitable distribution of AI benefits on a global scale, and the potential replacement of human practitioners with AI [7].

21.1.2 Regulatory state of affairs for AI in medicine

Until recent years, there has been a disturbing lack of regulatory oversight for the development and use of AI in medicine. However, as the use of the technology has grown, so has the push for effective regulation and collaboration across regulatory bodies.

In the United States, the Food and Drug Administration (FDA) published a proposed approach to pre-market review of AI-driven medical software in 2019, recognizing that their existing framework was not designed for these technologies [8]. They used the discussions surrounding this proposal to produce a five-step action plan in 2021 toward a regulatory framework for AI- and machine-learning-based software as medical devices [9].

The European Union has also proposed legislation, albeit with a more broad and comprehensive approach, through the 'AI Act' of 2021 [9]. This act expands beyond the field of medicine, aiming to develop an 'ecosystem of trust'.

Even more recently, the World Health Organization (WHO) published a document outlining six areas of regulatory considerations, including documentation and transparency, risk management and development, intended use and validation, data quality, privacy and data protection, and engagement and collaboration [10].

Another relevant document was recently released by the International Atomic Energy Agency (IAEA), endorsed by the American Association of Physicists in Medicine (AAPM), on specifically providing guidance on the roles, responsibilities, education, and training of clinically qualified medical physicists in the context of AI applications in medical physics [11]. Emphasizing the growing influence of AI in radiation oncology, diagnostic imaging, and nuclear medicine, it discusses the need for guidelines on AI use in medical physics, outlines the anticipated expansion of AI in clinical settings over the next 5–10 years, and highlights the importance of medical physicists in ensuring safe and effective clinical implementation of AI-based tools.

These efforts toward a more stable, collaborative, and effective regulatory landscape for medical AI are promising, but there is still much work to be done. Researchers, developers, and healthcare practitioners must continue to shape, monitor, and respond to regulatory changes happening around the world.

21.1.3 Ethical and regulatory concerns for AI in ART

The practical use of AI-based tools in radiation oncology faces numerous challenges, including clinical, technical, safety, ethical, privacy, and regulatory aspects. These considerations are accentuated in the context of ART, due to the heavier reliance on AI to automate and expedite the entire workflow, the need to make rapid, 'real-time' decisions, and the redefinition of roles and responsibilities among the clinical team members.

The 'black box' nature of AI tools could introduce unintended and adverse consequences when used in healthcare. In addition, AI tools are by nature data-driven, which means they can suffer from insufficient diversity, standardization, and harmonization of data elements used for AI model development. This could lead to challenges in clinical implementation, validation, and quality assurance (QA). Legal and ethical issues, coupled with a lack of specific education and training for healthcare professionals involved as described above, further contribute to the practical challenges in the clinical implementation of AI-reliant ART.

Due to the complexity, AI tools often make it difficult for users to understand how and why the AI makes certain decisions. Towards this end, recent efforts have been more focused on developing 'explainable' AIs that employ various methods to generate post hoc explanations for the decision-making process of these complex AI models [12, 13]. Regulations should be made to require vendors to be more transparent about how the AI models were trained, including what training and validation data were used. Whenever possible, vendors should also give specific instructions on their AI tools and algorithms in terms of proper implementation and testing, generalizability, the need to train on institutional data, potential pitfalls and safety features, etc

Data bias is a major ethical consideration in integrating AI into clinical practice. Inequity in healthcare and disparities in cancer survival already exist. Care needs to be taken so that data-driven AI tools will not perpetuate them [14]. For example, deep learning models have been found to discern race rather than underlying medical features from just x-ray or CT images [15]. AI has also shown under-diagnosis in under-served patient populations [16]. In developing and using AI tools for ART, we need to be mindful of potentially biased datasets underrepresenting certain patient populations in terms of age, gender, ethnicity, socioeconomic status, and geographical origin. Bias could exist in terms of technology such as device vendors or even model versions, etc, which could lead to performance bias of the developed AI products. These biases could ultimately impact treatment recommendations and patient outcomes. Having regulations to ensure data properness and transparency in model training and to monitor AI models for bias and fairness is therefore essential.

The integration of AI in radiation oncology must prioritize these ethical considerations and data privacy to maintain patient trust and safety. In data-driven AI development, robust data security measures need to be implemented to protect patient data. Although patient data privacy is an old topic in clinical research, some new considerations have become relevant in the AI era. For example, medical images, a main source of data source for these radiation oncology AIs, may not be sufficiently anonymized by conventional privacy information removals in the DICOM headers. Instead, patients may still be identifiable through 3D rendering and therefore require 'de-facing' of the images to be truly anonymous [17]. On the implementation side, patients may need to be informed or consented about the use of AI in their treatment. Transparency in AI applications and data usage is essential to maintain patient trust.

Lastly, other possible ramifications of wide adoption and over-reliance of AI include automation bias and complacency, and deskilling of the professionals [18, 19]. Automation bias refers to the tendency to favor or give greater credence to information supplied by AI, where clinicians, especially inexperienced clinicians, may be primed by the AI and predominantly seeking confirmatory information instead of engaging in a thorough and critical assessment. Automation complacency is a closely linked, overlapping concept that refers to the monitoring of AI with less frequency or vigilance because of a lower suspicion of error and a stronger belief in its accuracy (i.e. a false sense of security). In addition, increasingly wide adoptions of auto-segmentation and automatic treatment planning also introduce the risk of deskilling future generations of clinicians and planners, reducing their knowledge and expertise on performing contouring and treatment planning tasks.

Therefore, the radiation oncology community should be cautious and strategic in incorporating AI into the ART clinical practice. It requires a multidisciplinary approach, ongoing education, and a commitment to ethical principles to ensure the responsible and effective clinical use of AI. A core team of the clinical community should work closely with the researchers, vendors, and regulatory bodies to carefully evaluate these and other relevant aspects, and to together define the landscape for AI development, selection, and safe implementation into the ART clinical practice.

21.1.4 Some approaches to ethical AI in medicine

When addressing the considerations raised in section 21.1.3, several ethics approaches may be useful. The first is a strict application of the four principles laid out in section 21.1.1. When considering a question such as 'should I adopt this AI tool in my clinical practice?', a healthcare practitioner (e.g. a radiation oncologist) may consider reasons for and against from each of the principles, and see which choice has the weightiest considerations in favor of it. This approach is explored by Hyun and Hyun to address several possible ethical dilemmas in the use of AI in radiation oncology [7].

The second approach that has been proposed in the literature is the idea of a 'life-cycle' approach, which integrates ethical decision-making throughout the development and implementation of AI tools iteratively [20]. One way to take this type of approach is to ask key ethical questions at each stage of the tool's development. An available framework for this approach is the transparency, replicability, ethics, and effectiveness (TREE) framework, which lists 20 questions researchers and other stakeholders can ask at each stage [21]. For example, when a research team is at the 'inception' stage, designing a tool and planning the development of a model, researchers may ask 'what is the health question relating to patient benefit?' This question is most appropriately asked and answered early in the tool's development rather than at the end, when, say, a clinician is considering adopting the tool in patient care. At this later stage, it is important to ask questions such as 'What evidence is there that clinicians and patients find the model and its output (reasonably) interpretable?' [21] By incorporating these types of questions at the appropriate stage of development and implementation, ethical considerations are addressed throughout the process rather than as an after-thought.

Life-cycle approaches may also be combined with the four-principles approach. When asking the two questions posed above, for instance—one at the beginning of the life cycle and one at the end—the answers to the questions may be evaluated based on how well they are supported by each of the principles. It is apparent in the phrasing of the first question ('What is the health question relating to patient benefit?') that the principles of beneficence and nonmaleficence are highly relevant, and would support tools that offer potential added benefits for patients without introducing additional harms. On the other end of the cycle, the question of interpretability relies heavily on the principle of respect for autonomy, since the 'black box' nature of many AI tools may make it harder for patients to understand how the tool is being used in their care. It is possible that, at different life-cycle stages, different principles may offer weightier reasons for or against the continued development or use of an AI tool.

Another way of framing the life-cycle approach is the idea of an 'embedded ethics' framework to integrate ethics into the development of medical AI [20]. McLennan *et al* take the idea a step further than merely using a set of questions as a guide, proposing active collaboration between developers and ethicists [20]. This collaboration is recommended, not just when ethical issues are identified, but from the beginning to end of the life cycle, 'from early decision-making ... to supporting the regulatory pathway'. For this type of collaboration to thrive in radiation oncology, medical physicists and others with AI expertise must cultivate connections with ethics experts. We also see this proposed approach as a strong justification for expanding and improving ethics education in medical physics, with a focus on critical thinking and ethical analysis.

We will consider how frameworks such as these might be applied to ART in section 21.3.

21.2 Background of AI for ART

21.2.1 General workflow of ART

ART is a cutting-edge radiotherapy treatment paradigm that adapts the radiation treatment plan to the changing anatomy of the patient to maximize tumor control while minimizing normal tissue toxicity [22]. ART can be performed in varying frequencies, less frequently for cases with more gradual anatomy changes and more frequently for cases with more random anatomy changes. ART can also be performed in two different fashions—online ART and offline ART. For online

ART, the ART workflow is carried out in the same session (i.e. fraction) as the images (i.e. anatomy) used for adaptation. In contrast, for offline ART, the images are acquired, and the ART workflow is then performed between sessions generally over a longer time, and applied to future sessions.

A general workflow of ART is depicted in figure 21.1. Similar to the initial treatment planning process, it starts with acquiring images for the new anatomy. In addition to simulation images used for the original treatment planning, other in-treatment-room imaging modalities are also often utilized to generate the images for adaptive treatment planning, such as cone beam computed tomography (CBCT), in-room CT, magnetic resonance imaging (MRI), and positron emission tomography (PET). On the new images, contours need to be generated for the targets and organs at risk (OARs). With the new anatomy and contours, the dose can be reconstructed based on the original treatment plan. A decision on whether to adapt is then made after evaluating the reconstructed dose on the new anatomy. If adapting, a new treatment plan is generated on the new anatomy. Sometimes, especially for online ART, the new plan generation may take place concurrently with the old plan dose reconstruction to expedite the workflow. In either case, plan QA will need to be performed before treatment delivery.

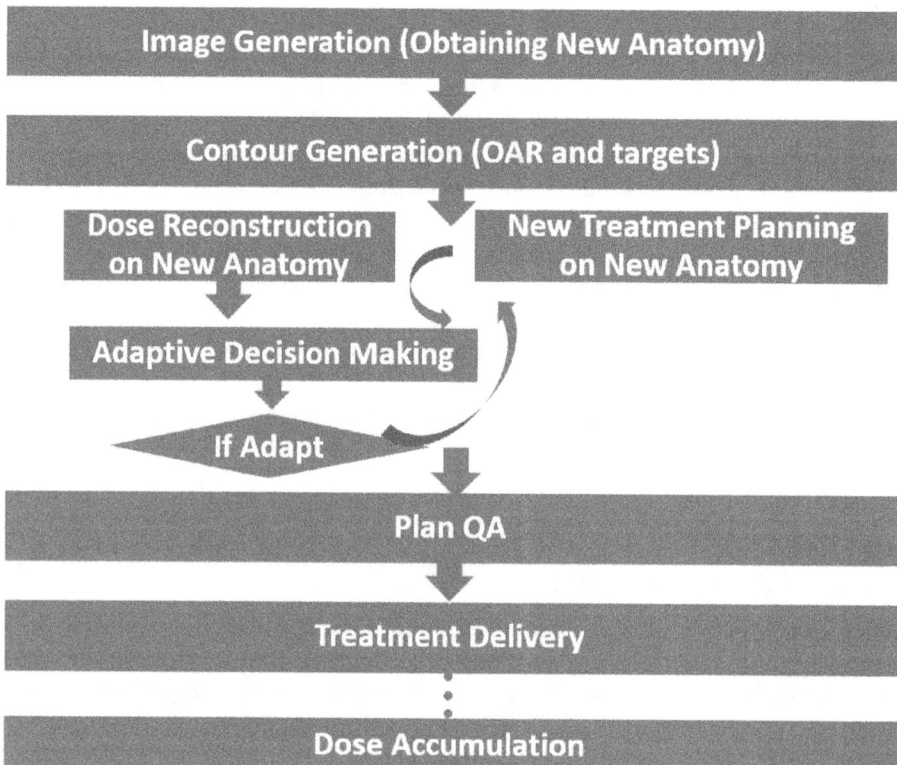

Figure 21.1. General workflow of ART. (Reproduced from [65]. CC BY 4.0.)

Because ART considers changing anatomy and creates adaptive treatment plans based on these changes, an additional ancillary step of the overall ART workflow is dose accumulation. In dose accumulation, the dose is summed considering both the anatomy and plan changes to sum up to an accurate picture of the total delivered dose.

21.2.2 AI in ART

A regular radiation therapy treatment planning process usually takes several hours to several days. A typical manual ART process would be similar in length. However, with the help of artificial intelligence (AI), some platforms have reduced this process to under 30 min, thereby allowing ART to be carried out online without the patient leaving the treatment table. This is of course a drastic time reduction of several challenging and time-consuming steps in the ART workflow, where AI has been used to automate and expedite these steps.

21.2.2.1 Image generation

Conventional simulation requires taking the patient off the treatment table and returning them to the simulation scanner (simulation CT is the most common) to acquire a new scan. In lieu of this, in-treatment-room images may be used to provide the new anatomy in ART. Current commercial systems use volumetric images such as in-room CT, CBCT, MRI, or PET. Most of these images may not be directly suited for radiation therapy treatment planning. For example, while MRI provides superior soft-tissue contrast for some anatomical regions, it does not provide electron density information required for accurate dose calculation. Similarly, although CBCT conveniently provides a patient CT on the treatment table, it generally has inferior image quality causing issues such as inaccurate Hounsfield units, lower image contrast, higher image noise, interfering image artifacts, and limited scan range or field-of-view. Despite the biological information afforded by it, PET is of poor spatial resolution and does not provide anatomical information. Therefore, to use these images for ART treatment planning, a synthetic CT is usually generated based on the new image of these modalities as well as the original planning CT. In the example of synthetic CT generation from MRI, AI-enabled methods such as deep learning (DL) are becoming the mainstay, replacing previous density-based or atlas-based methods, owing to superior speed and accuracy [23]. Similarly, AI methods are also widely adopted for synthetic CT generation from other types of images [24, 25]. Currently, many MRI-guided online ART systems use deformable registration between the session MRI and the simulation CT for density mapping, and researchers have created in-house DL-based synthetic CT generation algorithms to improve the efficiency and accuracy for this step. In a study by Hsu *et al* their DL-based synthetic CT could be generated in about 12 s as opposed to a 4 min density override and review process on ViewRay MRIdian for prostate patients [26]. Another online ART platforms, the CBCT-based Varian Ethos system, uses a synthetic CT for adaptive plan dose calculation [24]. With more advanced imaging hardware and software, direct CBCT-based adaptive dose calculation is also being introduced in Ethos with HyperSight, bypassing the need for a synthetic CT.

In addition to synthetic CT generation, AI methods can also be used in image reconstruction and image processing of the in-room image to improve its image quality and ultimately improve the accuracy and robustness of the synthetic CT. For example, AI methods have been used to reduce image noise, to improve image quality with low-dose or sparse projections, to correct for distortions, and to mitigate artifacts such as metal, beam hardening, and scatter [27–33]. Moreover, while the current clinical systems use volumetric imaging for ART image generation, research has been conducted to generate volumetric images based on limited projections, i.e. tomosynthesis from as few as a single projection and prior volumetric knowledge, using AI [34, 35]. These potential applications are perfectly suited for ART because prior volumetric knowledge does exist from the initial treatment planning.

21.2.2.2 Contour generation

Radiation treatment planning relies on accurate contour generation for the targets and OARs. Conventionally this is performed manually by the physician and the planner, and is a time- and effort-consuming process. For example, for complicated cases such as in head and neck cancers, this can be a tedious manual process of several hours. Recent advancement of AI algorithms has made major strides in automatic segmentation, considerably surpassing earlier methods of simple intensity thresholding and atlas-based contouring in terms of versatility, accuracy, robustness, and speed [36–38]. As such, these AI-powered auto-segmentation tools are rapidly being integrated into radiation therapy treatment planning clinical practice, and especially in ART to lighten the otherwise excessive workload.

These AI algorithms have shown success in organ segmentation of different anatomical sites from head to toe, and on various imaging modalities. Moreover, for target segmentation, the research has also been extended beyond solid tumors to tackle more abstract targets such as surgical beds [31, 39–41]. Although the AI-generated contours require domain experts' evaluation and sometimes modification, the availability of such tools have greatly improved the workflow efficiency and enabled the implementation of ART. In comparison with the 30–120 min spent on manual contouring of targets and OARs for usual inverse plans of different anatomical sites, the Varian Ethos ART system has been reported to shorten the volume generation, verification, and modification steps to under 10 min, sometimes under 5 min [42, 43]. Several studies reported no or minor editing needed for most AI-generated contours in the pelvic and thoracic regions on Ethos [43–47].

21.2.2.3 Plan generation

Radiation therapy treatment plan generation, especially the more sophisticated inverse treatment planning that has increasingly become the mainstream of modern radiation treatments, is a laborious process taking hours to days to complete. This is conventionally performed by a human planner who is a trained medical dosimetrist or medical physicist. The planner would choose basic planning parameters such as the number of beams, gantry angle arrangements, beam energy, and couch and collimator rotations. The planner then executes treatment planning in an often-iterative fashion to optimize the beam shaping/beam fluence to generate a not only acceptable but also optimal treatment plan for the individual case based on the anatomy. The plan generation and optimization could be a long and effort-consuming process of several hours to even days. AI has been actively researched and deployed for assisting and automating radiation therapy plan generation [48]. From the earlier implementation of simple machine learning methods on manually extracted dose overlap histogram features to the modern applications of convolution neural networks (CNNs), generative adversarial networks (GANs), and reinforcement learning methods for fully-automated treatment planning, AI has considerably sped up the plan generation process, simplified the required operator interactions, and improved the plan quality consistency, in particular for planners with less experience. For example, the Ethos ART system employs an AI-assisted intelligent optimization engine that automatically optimizes IMRT plans within minutes, and was reported to yield plans meeting desired dose objectives or with comparable plan quality with Eclipse manual plans [49–51].

21.2.2.4 Plan QA

Conventionally, a phantom-based measurement is employed to assess the dose calculation accuracy in radiation therapy plans that are developed inversely and involve complicated modulation. More recently, machine learning and AI methods have been applied to facilitate calculation-based and trajectory-log-based QA, circumventing phantom measurements [52]. Calculation-based QA enables plan QA for online ART without requiring the patient leaving the treatment table and therefore keeping the patient in the treatment position. Machine learning methods have also been applied to analyse measurement-based plan QA trends, identifying alternative markers beyond the gamma passing rate that could suggest meaningful dose deviations [53]. In addition, AI methods have also been used to predict dose calculated by advanced dose algorithms based on the dose calculated with lesser algorithms [54, 55]. These near-instantaneous and fairly accurate predictions can then be employed instead of directly performing the time-consuming, statistics-bound first-principle calculations using such advanced algorithms, making plan QA more streamlined for online ART. As such, these AI methods are applied to simplify and expedite the plan QA process as well as to improve its robustness.

21.2.2.5 Treatment delivery and decision making

AI has been explored to improve radiation therapy plan dosimetry through more sophisticated and automated treatment delivery such as incorporating couch and collimator angles as additional degrees of freedom in plan optimization [56, 57]. Moreover, AI has also permeated the research on clinical decision-making for whether and when to adapt, the escalation or reduction of radiation dose, which other therapy to combine and the timing of the combinations, and so on [58, 59]. Imaging-based delta-radiomics and other deep learning approaches have been explored to dynamically follow the patient over the radiation treatment course and have been combined with biology and lab-based markers to predict an individual patient's outcome and personalize their treatments [60, 61].

21.3 Ethical and regulatory considerations in AI for ART

21.3.1 Ethical and regulatory concerns in the uses of AI for ART

As introduced in section 21.2, the applications of AI enable ART and promise unprecedented precision in radiation targeting. However, these innovations necessitate rigorous ethical and regulatory considerations to ensure patient safety, data privacy, and equitable access, while preventing potential biases and ensuring the accountability of AI-driven decisions in clinical settings.

21.3.1.1 Anatomy and target delineation

For ART, AI utilization in anatomy and target delineation, particularly with deep learning-based auto-segmentation, presents several ethical and regulatory challenges. First, if the patient images and other data will be used for the continued improvement of the AI models, data privacy needs to be considered. Patients may also need to be consented for such usage as well as for using the AI segmentation tools in their treatments. Moreover, these systems rely heavily on pre-defined knowledge, leading to performance degradation when encountering unfamiliar anatomical variations. For instance, the top algorithm from the 2017 AAPM thoracic challenge underperformed on a UK dataset because it lacked data on patients with abdominal compression [62]. Similarly, the introduction of rectal spacers affected the efficiency of prostate auto-segmentation models [63].

Model re-training with diverse and up-to-date datasets can mitigate these issues. However, current commercial ART systems use pre-trained models, often based on limited institutional data, therefore displaying variability in the auto-generated contours. This could present challenges for ART implementation at different clinics. Based on institutional differences, AI-based auto-generation of OARs and targets could work better for some institutions than others, making standard guidelines and experience less effective. This is particularly concerning when the training data lacks diversity and is homogeneous in a certain population, which could lead to poor model performances on other populations. This could make ART reliant upon such auto-segmentation models less effective or beneficial in those populations.

Manual editing of the contours is allowed in ART systems and could improve the quality and robustness of ART. However, a few things need to be considered. First of all, the role and responsibility definition has shifted in ART. For example, therapists are often taking on more responsibilities for contour review and editing in the ART workflow, and these are not traditionally taught and practiced in their realm. While this may not necessarily compromise quality if proper training and supervision is put in place, automation bias and complacency tend to be more of an issue with less experienced users. In addition, in the traditional RT model, contours are thoroughly checked with many layers of redundancies: plan evaluation and review, physics initial and ongoing checks, IGRT review, chart rounds, etc. Much less thoroughness and crosscheck are built in for contour review in the ART process.

Lastly, even if the contours are thoroughly reviewed and edited by the attending radiation oncologist to ensure the correctness and accuracy of the contours, the extra time spent on it when AI models perform poorly could still compromise the efficacy of ART for these patients, as the dosimetric benefits are washed out by any intrafractional anatomical changes in the long duration [64].

Because of these concerns, it is important for the developers and vendors to take proactive steps in database curation and model development to minimize data bias and build effective and robust auto-segmentation models across diverse populations, devices, and protocols. Regulatory bodies should also come up with requirements for the vendors to have a rigorous process to consider and address these issues, to make information such as the demographic makeup of their training dataset transparent, and to disclose to users any potential biases or pitfalls of their AI models. The users should be aware that limitations exist in the technology. They should include such ethical considerations in the selection, evaluation, and implementation of these AI technologies, and continue to review, explore, and address them throughout the evolving clinical practice. Rigorous testing and validation, as well as ongoing monitoring, are necessary to ensure the AI models perform as intended.

Despite these challenges, AI-based anatomy and target delineation have demonstrated substantial progress, offering significant time savings and enabling online ART. This progress underscores the need for continued ethical and regulatory discussions to ensure these AI tools are used safely and effectively in ART.

21.3.1.2 Treatment planning

Similar to the discussion above, patients may need to be consented about the role of AI in their treatment planning. Furthermore, dataset size is often more limited for AI model training with treatment plans than for that with medical images and contours. Therefore, data diversity issues also exist in treatment planning similar to those discussed above for contouring. While AI methods such as RL could potentially reduce the required training dataset size compare to methods based on CNN, data diversity issues remain.

The performance of a treatment planning AI model is also more challenging to evaluate than a segmentation AI model, because of the lack of a ground truth. Dose–volume constraints similar to those used in conventional treatment planning could be used to for plan evaluation, along with standard qualitative evaluation approaches. However, it is difficult for clinicians to judge if the auto-generated adaptive plan is optimal for the new anatomy. Especially when some of the predefined dose–volume constraints fail or the spatial dose distribution is unacceptable, it is not straightforward to evaluate whether they fail because of the new anatomy, or if they fail because of an ill-performed model. In conventional RT treatment planning, the planner and the physician would have more time to optimize the plan through an iterative manner, and any automatically generated plans by AI can be manually improved. However, in a time-critical ART process, that is not an option and the clinicians can only accept or reject the automatically generated adaptive plan.

Although when an adaptive plan is not selected for a patient due to AI model performance issues, and the patient is still treated with the original plan similar to what would be in the conventional RT, this could still present ethical concerns. The patient could be subject to possible treatment inferiority due to patient set-up differences between the ART and standard RT workflows, discomfort, intrafractional anatomy and positional changes during the prolonged session, and at a minimum the loss of cost–benefit if performing the ART workflow becomes a billable service.

To improve the robustness of the treatment planning AI, vendors should improve the diversity of the training data, and make the training data and the AI's decision-making processes more transparent to users.

21.3.1.3 Plan selection

To expedite, streamline, and automate the ART workflow, AI may play an increasing role in treatment plan selection. While radiation oncologists currently still are responsible for this step in most practices, in some clinics there has been an increasing role shift to train and credential radiation therapists for more responsibilities in the ART workflow. AI would play an important role in supporting the plan selection step for less experienced users, or help even the experienced users make quicker decision. However, in addition to the ongoing improvement of the robustness and accuracy of these AIs, it is important to continue improving the transparency and explainability of these AIs. Healthcare providers and patients need to be able to understand and possibly appeal AI's recommendation. Again the informed consent of patients about the role of AI in the process needs to be considered, and it is critical that AI supports instead of replaces the decision-making autonomy of patients and healthcare providers.

21.3.1.4 Treatment QA and delivery

To maintain the patient positioning and immobilization in an ART workflow, calculation-based QA is used in place of conventional measurement-based QA. AI plays an important role in improving the speed and accuracy of this calculation-based QA, and in automating other relevant plan checks for the ART workflow that are regularly carried out for the initial treatment plan. For these applications, there needs to be continuous human oversight of the AI for accuracy and ongoing improvements. The AI-based QA results may be periodically checked and compared against those using non-AI methods.

Much of the data accumulated from treatment delivery may be potentially useful for treatment monitoring and outcome prediction, such as machine trajectory log files and patient images. AI may be used to automatically monitor these data and flag deviations. In addition, through analysing radiomics and other deep image features of treatment images, AI can also monitor the treatment toxicity and outcome. Data privacy and security, as well as AI model accuracy and robustness across diverse populations, are important ethical and regulatory considerations.

21.3.2 Applying ethics approaches to AI in ART

The previous section laid out numerous concerns that arise from both ethical and regulatory perspectives in the many ways AI can be used in ART. Much of the literature on ethics and AI, in fact, tends to focus on potential ethical pitfalls and lack of regulation. How are developers and clinicians to address this thorny ethical and regulatory landscape, then, when making decisions regarding AI and ART? In section 21.1.4, we outlined three approaches that have been suggested in the literature: an 'embedded ethics' approach, a 'life-cycle' approach, and an application of basic ethical principles (respect for autonomy, beneficence, nonmaleficence, and justice).

The most straightforward of these to apply in the ART context is the 'embedded ethics' approach, which involves ethicists in the development process of AI tools. Consider, as an example, the development of auto-segmentation tools discussed in section 21.3.1. Under the embedded ethics approach, one or more ethicists would be involved during every stage of the development process, which means they could perform ethical analyses that help developers minimize data bias and build more robust models. In the same section, we also discussed the need for model re-training with diverse and up-to-date datasets; because of this need, it seems prudent that the ethicist(s) also be involved in the continued development and maintenance of the models. Their ongoing analysis could help determine when re-training might be necessary to ensure potential benefits and risks are balanced and justly distributed among patients. This role that ethicists play under the embedded ethics approach would be relevant and beneficial for all the applications of AI in ART that we have discussed, including segmentation, treatment planning, plan selection, treatment QA, and treatment delivery.

The 'life-cycle' approach, which involves asking specific ethical questions at each stage of the AI tool development process, is similarly straightforward to apply, although it places more responsibility on the researchers, vendors, clinicians, and other stakeholders rather than taking advantage of ethicists' specific expertise. Take, for example, the use of AI for monitoring treatment toxicity and outcomes following radiation therapy, particularly on accumulated datasets over a course of ART. Similar to many other types of AI tools, we noted in section 21.3.1 that there are ethical concerns around data privacy and security. In the TREE framework of questions to ask during development, a question to ask at the 'inception' stage is 'When and how should patients be involved in data collection, analysis, deployment, and use?' [21] The authors suggest that, even when individual patient consent is not required or is impossible to acquire, patients and the public can and should still be involved in the data science cycle. For example, patient advocates can help confirm the need for a particular algorithm (e.g. one that monitors treatment outcomes following ART).

An additional question from the same framework that is relevant to data privacy and security concerns is 'How have the regulatory requirements for accreditation/ approval been addressed?' which is recommended at the 'implementation' stage [21]. As the regulatory landscape for AI (particularly AI in medicine) continues to evolve, developers will need to ensure that the latest guidelines and laws regarding data usage and security are followed. Asking this question at earlier stages of development is arguably more prudent, since addressing regulatory deficiencies after a model has been trained and validated could be much more difficult than building in compliance from the start.

The application of basic ethical principles is an approach that can be applied in a more ad hoc or decision-by-decision manner when making ethical decisions at any point in an AI tool's development or implementation, making it the most versatile of these three approaches. However, its application can also be subjective to the intuitions of the decision-maker. As described in section 21.1.4, this approach involves determining the reasons for and against a decision according to each of the four principles (respect for autonomy, beneficence, nonmaleficence, and justice), and then determining which of the reasons is weightiest. It is this second determination that can be the most controversial for any specific ethical dilemma.

Consider the data diversity issues we have discussed for AI-based segmentation and treatment planning tools used in ART. A related ethical dilemma that may be encountered by either developers or clinicians is whether a given AI tool should be kept on the market (developer perspective) or offered to patients (clinician perspective) when it is discovered to exhibit bias; i.e. the tool provides benefit only to part of the patient population [7]. The principle of beneficence generates a strong moral reason for the tool to be made available to those it may benefit. Yet, the principle of justice generates a similarly strong moral reason for the tool to be removed from the market or not offered to patients until it can be re-trained with more diverse data, thereby distributing the potential benefits of the tool more equitably in the long term.

When presenting this dilemma at conferences to members of both the American Association of Physicists in Medicine (AAPM) and the Australasian College of Physician Scientists and Engineers in Medicine (ACPSEM), chapter author Dr Hyun has conducted audience polls to gauge medical physicists' intuitions on the two facets of this dilemma. In both audiences, the majority of participants (86% for AAPM, 100% for ACPSEM) thought the clinician should continue to offer the tool to the subset of patients it may benefit (i.e. the reasons from beneficence are stronger). A slimmer majority (70% for AAPM, 63% for ACPSEM) thought the company should keep the tool on the market (i.e. the reasons from beneficence continue to prevail from the developer perspective), but the result was obviously more controversial.

It should be noted that the three approaches we discuss here can also be combined. Both the 'embedded ethics' and 'life-cycle' approaches are rooted in and rely on basic ethical principles, for example. Perhaps the best approach that will result in the most ethically robust AI tools for ART is one that relies on all three. When ethicists are embedded in the development process, teams ask key ethical questions along the entire life cycle of the tool, and basic ethical principles are relied upon for decision-making in and out of the clinic, we have a much better chance of maintaining ethical AI use in ART.

21.3.3 An ethical argument for AI in ART

Much of the existing literature on AI in medicine and AI in radiation therapy focuses on the ethical and regulatory concerns of its development and implementation. With regulation still in development and the numerous potential pitfalls including bias, transparency, and responsibility, it is obvious why this emphasis is warranted. However, the bioethics framework and approaches presented in sections 21.1.1 and 21.3.2 can also be applied to generate ethical arguments for the use of AI in the context of ART. One such argument can be made from the potential for AI to facilitate more just allocation of resources and potential benefits on a global scale.

The use of ART may improve care for patients by reducing dose to OARs and allowing margin reduction for target volumes. The use of clinical resources towards these ends is well supported by the bioethical principles of beneficence and nonmaleficence. However, the time and resource requirements associated with such use are a significant barrier to entry for many clinics. Those institutions with an existing ART program, or those considering beginning one, are often faced with difficult choices when discussing how best to use available resources. Online ART requires the use of an expensive dedicated machine, for example an MR-linac such as the Elekta Unity or a CBCT-based system such as the Varian Ethos. In addition to the monetary cost of a new machine, there are notable time investments required to successfully begin and maintain an online ART program. These purchases and time investments can easily preclude the consideration of an online ART program for low-resource clinics (e.g. those in low- and middle-income countries), preventing possible patient benefit.

In the case of offline ART, which may be more attractive to low-resource clinics, the monetary costs avoided by not purchasing a dedicated machine can be offset by the additional time-cost. This, again, leads to many difficult decisions for clinicians attempting to maximize their available resources. For instance, clinicians must decide whether they will create adaptive re-plans for all patients at a set time in their treatment course, or if they will assess the necessity of a re-plan at that time. Moreover, if they choose assessment over set re-planning, they must decide how often and when these assessments take place. This may translate to a choice between employing a low time-cost, single assessment (e.g. at the midpoint of a patient's treatment course), and a more time-costly course of assessment, such as assessing once every other week. Their choices may drastically change the time-cost associated with their offline ART program, as well as its clinical outcomes.

Given the time and resource-intensiveness of ART in all its forms, as well as the potential benefits that it promises, it is clear that the prudent and just use of resources in the ART context is ethically obligated on both an individual clinic and global level. This obligation can be more easily met when tools that support this goal are created and implemented. One study, conducted by chapter authors Hyun and Fanning, worked to create one such tool. We created a framework for the evaluation of different offline ART implementations. More specifically, the framework evaluated the performance of two different offline assessment frequencies, or assessment schemes. Our results quantify offline ART assessment schemes' performance through three metrics: their trustworthiness, their dosimetric benefit, and their time-cost-effectiveness. This framework provides information that may prove useful to clinicians when determining how best to use their resources.

In this proof-of-concept study, we applied the midpoint and biweekly assessment schemes to a small cohort of head and neck (H&N) cancer patients at the University of Nebraska Medical Center (UNMC). We used an assessment workflow based in Varian's Velocity software to perform assessments of seven physician-determined dose constraints for OARs at intervals dictated by these assessment schemes.

We found that midpoint and biweekly assessment performed very similarly when detecting whether a re-plan was needed, given by accuracies of 90% and 92%, respectively. These results show that the assessment schemes are comparable in their trustworthiness. Additionally, the false positive rate for both schemes was comparable. This means that the more frequent biweekly assessment would, on average, result in more unnecessary re-plans since more assessments take place. This is a valuable consideration when attempting to most prudently use clinical resources.

We quantified dosimetric benefit through the comparison of total dose constraint violations seen in the cohort with and without the use of adaptive re-planning. According to our best estimate, without adaptive re-planning, there were four instances in which an OAR's dose constraint would be violated. We compared this against the midpoint assessment scheme, which had two total dose constraint violations, and the biweekly assessment scheme, which had none at the end of treatment. This shows a respective 50% and 100% decrease in OARs receiving dose above the original plan objectives, which highlights the dosimetric benefit of these modes of offline ART.

The last and arguably most important result of our study describes the midpoint and biweekly assessment schemes' time-cost-effectiveness. We created estimates of the time-cost of each scheme assuming their most labor-intensive instances, meaning that we assumed that re-plans were always triggered whenever an assessment took place. We did this so that a time-cost-effectiveness floor could be established. We quantified benefit in three separate ways: the decrease in total OAR dose constraint violations, the dose decrease seen in triggered OARs when adaptive re-planning was used, and the dose decrease seen by all seven OARs when adaptive re-planning was used. We then quantified time-cost-effectiveness through dividing these benefits by the time-cost associated with the assessment scheme used. It was found that the midpoint assessment scheme was at least 48% more time-cost-effective than the biweekly assessment scheme according to these three benefits.

This set of results clearly shows that biweekly assessment provides more dosimetric benefit, while midpoint assessment provides benefit more efficiently. These results and framework act as a tool for clinics when trying to decide whether they can feasibly begin an offline ART program. This means that clinics who may have otherwise not considered an offline ART program could begin one, and those already considering a program could decide on their particular implementation in a more informed manner.

Equipping clinicians with an evaluation tool for offline ART helps them to fulfill their ethical obligation of most prudently and justly allocating the resources of their individual clinic. This is important because, in the modality's current state, ART's benefits are strongly linked to its time and resource-intensiveness. On top of providing information and clarity about this relationship, it could be argued that any tools that help detangle these two properties of ART should be invested in immediately and enthusiastically. An example of such a tool that could decrease resource and time requirements is AI. Section 21.2.2 describes many ways in which AI implementation currently speeds up and improves the ART workflow. These range from the use of auto-segmentation to calculation-based and trajectory-log-based plan QA.

Not only do these AI tools improve time/resource-cost-effectiveness for clinics with a pre-existing ART program, but it lowers the barrier to entry for low-resource clinics who may have otherwise not utilized ART. From an ethical perspective, this clearly helps to mitigate the issue of unjust distribution of the benefits of ART. When implemented alongside proper, well-developed, and well-informed regulation, AI tools can help ensure that the benefits of ART will become more accessible and more fairly distributed.

21.4 Summary

This chapter examines the ethical and regulatory considerations of AI in ART, highlighting the importance of developing frameworks to guide its responsible use. Key bioethical principles provide a foundation for addressing transparency, data bias, and privacy concerns. Based on the technical background of AI in ART, the chapter outlines key ethical concerns that arise when deploying AI in medical contexts, with a focus on ART-specific workflow steps under real-time decision-making pressure. We discuss applying ethical frameworks to ART AI development and deployment, and build a coherent ethical argument, emphasizing the necessity of balancing innovation with patient safety, privacy, and equity. Practical approaches for aligning AI practices with established ethical principles are proposed, emphasizing ongoing multidisciplinary collaboration and ethical vigilance, to ensure that the development and deployment of AI in ART remain both responsible and beneficial.

References

[1] Beauchamp T and Childress J 2019 Principles of biomedical ethics: marking its fortieth anniversary *Am. J. Bioeth.* **19** 9–12
[2] Erkal E Y, Akpınar A and Erkal H Ş 2021 Ethical evaluation of artificial intelligence applications in radiotherapy using the Four Topics Approach *Artif. Intell. Med.* **115** 102055
[3] Department of Health, Education and Welfare, National Commission for the Protection of Human Subjects of Biomedical and Behavioral Research 2014 The Belmont Report. Ethical principles and guidelines for the protection of human subjects of research *J. Am. Coll. Dent* **81** 4–13
[4] Donaldson S S 2017 Ethics in radiation oncology and the American Society for Radiation Oncology's role *Int. J. Radiat. Oncol. Biol. Phys.* **99** 247–9

[5] Riddick F A Jr 2003 The code of medical ethics of the American Medical Association *Ochsner J.* **5** 6–10

[6] Skourou C *et al* 2019 Code of ethics for the American Association of Physicists in Medicine (revised): report of Task Group 109 *Med. Phys.* **46** e79–93

[7] Hyun M and Hyun A 2023 Ethics and artificial intelligence in radiation oncology *Artificial Intelligence in Radiation Oncology* (Singapore: World Scientific) pp 337–57

[8] US Food and Drug Administration 2019 Proposed regulatory framework for modifications to artificial intelligence/machine learning (AI/ML)-based software as a medical device (SaMD) *Discussion paper* FDA-2019-N-1185 US Food and Drug Administration

[9] Vokinger K N and Gasser U 2021 Regulating AI in medicine in the United States and Europe *Nat. Mach. Intell.* **3** 738–9

[10] World Health Organization 2023 Regulatory considerations on artificial intelligence for health. Regulatory considerations on artificial intelligence for health *Report* World Health Organization, Geneva

[11] IAEA 2023 Artificial intelligence in medical physics *Training Course Series No. 83* IAEA-TCS-8 International Atomic Energy Agency, Vienna

[12] Barragan-Montero A *et al* 2022 Towards a safe and efficient clinical implementation of machine learning in radiation oncology by exploring model interpretability, explainability and data-model dependency *Phys. Med. Biol.* **67** 11TR01

[13] Huynh E *et al* 2020 Artificial intelligence in radiation oncology *Nat. Rev. Clin. Oncol.* **17** 771–81

[14] Tong M, Hill L and Artiga S 2022 *Racial Disparities in Cancer Outcomes, Screening, and Treatment* (San Francisco, CA: Kaiser Family Foundation)

[15] Gichoya J W *et al* 2022 AI recognition of patient race in medical imaging: a modelling study *Lancet Digit. Health* **4** e406–e14

[16] Seyyed-Kalantari L, Zhang H, McDermott M B A, Chen I Y and Ghassemi M 2021 Underdiagnosis bias of artificial intelligence algorithms applied to chest radiographs in under-served patient populations *Nat. Med.* **27** 2176–82

[17] Selfridge A R, Spencer B A, Abdelhafez Y G, Nakagawa K, Tupin J D and Badawi R D 2023 Facial Anonymization and privacy concerns in total-body PET/CT *J. Nucl. Med.* **64** 1304–9

[18] Grissinger M 2019 Understanding human over-reliance on technology *Pharm. Therap.* **44** 320–75

[19] Parasuraman R and Manzey D H 2010 Complacency and bias in human use of automation: an attentional integration *Hum. Factors* **52** 381–410

[20] Smith M J and Bean S 2019 AI and ethics in medical radiation sciences *J. Med. Imaging. Radiat. Sci.* **50** S24–S6

[21] Vollmer S *et al* 2018 Machine learning and AI research for patient benefit: 20 critical questions on transparency, replicability, ethics and effectiveness arXiv:1812.10404

[22] Sonke J J, Aznar M and Rasch C 2019 Adaptive radiotherapy for anatomical changes *Semin. Radiat. Oncol.* **29** 245–57

[23] Han X 2017 MR-based synthetic CT generation using a deep convolutional neural network method *Med. Phys.* **44** 1408–19

[24] Archambault Y *et al* 2020 Making on-line adaptive radiotherapy possible using artificial intelligence and machine learning for efficient daily re-planning *Med. Phys. Intl. J.* **8** 77–86

[25] Spadea M F, Maspero M, Zaffino P and Seco J 2021 Deep learning based synthetic-CT generation in radiotherapy and PET: a review *Med. Phys.* **48** 6537–66

[26] Hsu S H, Cao Y, Huang K, Feng M and Balter J M 2013 Investigation of a method for generating synthetic CT models from MRI scans of the head and neck for radiation therapy *Phys. Med. Biol.* **58** 8419–35

[27] Gottschalk T M, Maier A, Kordon F and Kreher B W 2023 DL-based inpainting for metal artifact reduction for cone beam CT using metal path length information *Med. Phys.* **50** 128–41

[28] Kulathilake K, Abdullah N A, Sabri A Q M and Lai K W 2023 A review on deep learning approaches for low-dose computed tomography restoration *Complex. Intell. Syst.* **9** 2713–45

[29] Lee H and Lee J 2019 A deep learning-based scatter correction of simulated x-ray images *Electronics* **8** 944

[30] Park H S, Lee S M, Kim H P, Seo J K and Chung Y E 2018 CT sinogram-consistency learning for metal-induced beam hardening correction *Med. Phys.* **45** 5376–84

[31] Qian H, Rui X and Ahn S (ed) 2017 Deep learning models for PET scatter estimations *IEEE Nuclear Science Symposium and Medical Imaging Conference (NSS/MIC)* **vol 2017** (Piscataway, NJ: IEEE)

[32] Shan S *et al* 2023 Distortion-corrected image reconstruction with deep learning on an MRI-linac *Magn. Reson. Med.* **90** 963–77

[33] Yeoh H *et al* 2021 Deep learning algorithm for simultaneous noise reduction and edge sharpening in low-dose CT images: a pilot study using lumbar spine CT *Korean J. Radiol.* **22** 1850–7

[34] Shen L, Zhao W and Xing L 2019 Patient-specific reconstruction of volumetric computed tomography images from a single projection view via deep learning *Nat. Biomed. Eng.* **3** 880–8

[35] Wang T, Xia W, Lu J and Zhang Y 2023 A review of deep learning CT reconstruction from incomplete projection data *IEEE Trans. Radiat. Plasma Med. Sci.* **8** 138–52

[36] Cardenas C E, Yang J, Anderson B M, Court L E and Brock K B 2019 Advances in auto-segmentation *Semin. Radiat. Oncol.* **29** 185–97

[37] Ding J, Zhang Y, Amjad A, Xu J, Thill D and Li X A 2022 Automatic contour refinement for deep learning auto-segmentation of complex organs in MRI-guided adaptive radiation therapy *Adv. Radiat. Oncol.* **7** 100968

[38] Kosmin M *et al* 2019 Rapid advances in auto-segmentation of organs at risk and target volumes in head and neck cancer *Radiother. Oncol.* **135** 130–40

[39] Balagopal A *et al* 2021 A deep learning-based framework for segmenting invisible clinical target volumes with estimated uncertainties for post-operative prostate cancer radiotherapy *Med. Image Anal.* **72** 102101

[40] Elguindi S *et al* 2019 Deep learning-based auto-segmentation of targets and organs-at-risk for magnetic resonance imaging only planning of prostate radiotherapy *Phys. Imaging. Radiat. Oncol.* **12** 80–6

[41] Ma C Y *et al* 2022 Deep learning-based auto-segmentation of clinical target volumes for radiotherapy treatment of cervical cancer *J. Appl. Clin. Med. Phys.* **23** e13470

[42] de Jong R, Visser J, van Wieringen N, Wiersma J, Geijsen D and Bel A 2021 Feasibility of conebeam CT-based online adaptive radiotherapy for neoadjuvant treatment of rectal cancer *Radiat. Oncol.* **16** 136

[43] Byrne M *et al* 2022 Varian Ethos online adaptive radiotherapy for prostate cancer: early results of contouring accuracy, treatment plan quality, and treatment time *J. Appl. Clin. Med. Phys.* **23** e13479

[44] Mao W *et al* 2022 Evaluation of auto-contouring and dose distributions for online adaptive radiation therapy of patients with locally advanced lung cancers *Pract. Radiat. Oncol.* **12** e329–e38

[45] Moazzezi M, Rose B, Kisling K, Moore K L and Ray X 2021 Prospects for daily online adaptive radiotherapy via ethos for prostate cancer patients without nodal involvement using unedited CBCT auto-segmentation *J. Appl. Clin. Med. Phys.* **22** 82–93

[46] Sibolt P *et al* 2021 Clinical implementation of artificial intelligence-driven cone-beam computed tomography-guided online adaptive radiotherapy in the pelvic region *Phys. Imaging. Radiat. Oncol.* **17** 1–7

[47] Zwart L G M *et al* 2022 Cone-beam computed tomography-guided online adaptive radiotherapy is feasible for prostate cancer patients *Phys. Imaging. Radiat. Oncol.* **22** 98–103

[48] Wang C, Zhu X, Hong J C and Zheng D 2019 Artificial intelligence in radiotherapy treatment planning: present and future *Technol. Cancer Res. Treat.* **18** 1533033819873922

[49] Pokharel S, Pacheco A and Tanner S 2022 Assessment of efficacy in automated plan generation for Varian Ethos intelligent optimization engine *J. Appl. Clin. Med. Phys.* **23** e13539

[50] Visak J *et al* 2023 Evaluating machine learning enhanced intelligent-optimization-engine (IOE) performance for Ethos head-and-neck (HN) plan generation *J. Appl. Clin. Med. Phys.* **24** e13950

[51] Byrne M, Archibald-Heeren B, Hu Y, Greer P, Luo S and Aland T 2022 Assessment of semi-automated stereotactic treatment planning for online adaptive radiotherapy in ethos *Med. Dosim.* **47** 342–7

[52] Sun B *et al* 2012 Evaluation of the efficiency and effectiveness of independent dose calculation followed by machine log file analysis against conventional measurement based IMRT QA *J. Appl. Clin. Med. Phys.* **13** 3837

[53] Valdes G, Chan M F, Lim S B, Scheuermann R, Deasy J O and Solberg T D 2017 IMRT QA using machine learning: a multi-institutional validation *J. Appl. Clin. Med. Phys.* **18** 279–84

[54] Kontaxis C, Bol G H, Lagendijk J J W and Raaymakers B W 2020 DeepDose: towards a fast dose calculation engine for radiation therapy using deep learning *Phys. Med. Biol.* **65** 075013

[55] Zhang J *et al* 2022 A feasibility study for *in vivo* treatment verification of IMRT using Monte Carlo dose calculation and deep learning-based modelling of EPID detector response *Radiat. Oncol.* **17** 31

[56] Sadeghnejad Barkousaraie A, Ogunmolu O, Jiang S and Nguyen D 2020 A fast deep learning approach for beam orientation optimization for prostate cancer treated with intensity-modulated radiation therapy *Med. Phys.* **47** 880–97

[57] Sadeghnejad-Barkousaraie A, Bohara G, Jiang S and Nguyen D 2021 A reinforcement learning application of a guided Monte Carlo tree search algorithm for beam orientation selection in radiation therapy *Mach. Learn. Sci. Technol.* **2** 035013

[58] Arimura H, Soufi M, Kamezawa H, Ninomiya K and Yamada M 2019 Radiomics with artificial intelligence for precision medicine in radiation therapy *J. Radiat. Res.* **60** 150–7

[59] Poon D J J, Tay L M, Ho D, Chua M L K, Chow E K and Yeo E L L 2021 Improving the therapeutic ratio of radiotherapy against radioresistant cancers: leveraging on novel artificial intelligence-based approaches for drug combination discovery *Cancer Lett.* **511** 56–67

[60] Nardone V *et al* 2021 Delta radiomics: a systematic review *Radiol. Med.* **126** 1571–83

[61] Zheng D *et al* 2023 radioGWAS: link radiome to genome to discover driver genes with somatic mutations for heterogeneous tumor image phenotype in pancreatic cancer *medRxiv*

[62] Feng X, Bernard M E, Hunter T and Chen Q 2020 Improving accuracy and robustness of deep convolutional neural network based thoracic OAR segmentation *Phys. Med. Biol.* **65** 07NT1

[63] Wang B *et al* 2022 Performance deterioration of deep learning models after clinical deployment: a case study with auto-segmentation for definitive prostate cancer radiotherapy arXiv:2210.05673

[64] Byrne M *et al* 2023 Intra-fraction motion and margin assessment for Ethos online adaptive radiotherapy treatments of the prostate and seminal vesicles *Adv. Radiat. Oncol.* **9** 101405

[65] Dona Lemus O M, Cao M, Cai B, Cummings M and Zheng D 2024 Adaptive radiotherapy: next-generation radiotherapy *Cancers* **16** 1206

IOP Publishing

Artificial Intelligence in Adaptive Radiation Therapy

Yi Wang and X. Sharon Qi

Chapter 22

Recent advances and future of artificial intelligence-augmented adaptive radiation therapy

Oscar Pastor-Serrano, Xianjin Dai and Lei Xing

Despite decades of effort, patient set-up errors and inter-fractional anatomy changes remain significant limiting factors for the optimal utilization of radiation therapy (RT). Current practices focus on improving patient positioning accuracy, treating patients as rigid entities, which overlooks the multi-dimensional nature of the beam targeting problem in RT. However, advances in artificial intelligence (AI) have opened new avenues for AI-augmented adaptive RT (AI-ART), where on-treatment imaging data are used as feedback for adaptive modification of treatment plans. This ensures full dose coverage of tumor targets while sparing organs at risk (OARs). AI-ART holds promise to reduce uncertainties in beam targeting, providing improved dose distributions, and enhancing tumor control probability with minimal normal tissue complication probability. In this chapter, recent advances in AI-ART are highlighted, shedding light on the roles of AI and the future of AI-ART. Research and development in this direction are expected to substantially improve patient care and enable the full utilization of modern RT's technical capabilities.

22.1 Introduction

Adaptive radiation therapy (ART) represents a significant advancement in the personalized treatment of cancer, offering the promise of highly tailored treatments that can adjust to changes in a patient's anatomy and tumor morphology over the course of therapy. The integration of artificial intelligence (AI) and deep learning (DL) technologies into ART protocols has been a game-changer, enhancing the precision, efficiency, and outcomes of radiation therapy. This chapter explores the pivotal role of AI and deep learning in transforming ART into a more dynamic, responsive, and patient-specific treatment modality.

doi:10.1088/978-0-7503-6119-4ch22
22-1

22.1.1 Clinical need for adaptive radiation therapy

With the developments of intensity modulated radiotherapy/volumetric modulated arc therapy (IMRT/VMAT) and image guided radiation therapy (IGRT), radiation therapy (RT) entered a new era [1–4]. By optimal modulation of intensity and beam sampling, highly conformal dose distribution can be planned and delivered. IMRT/ VMAT, and more generally, station parameter optimized radiation therapy (SPORT) [5], offers an enabling tool for dose escalation and/or stereotactic radio-surgery/stereotactic body radiotherapy (SRS/SBRT) with improved therapeutic ratio [6, 7]. However, the efficacy of modern RT can only be fully exploited with an effective means of eliminating the uncertainties in beam targeting caused by factors such as patient immobilization, inter- and intra-fractional organ motion/ deformation [4, 6, 7]. Clinically, because of these uncertainties, the exact locations of the tumor target(s) and adjacent sensitive structures are often not precisely known, leading to routine use of population- and disease-site-based margins to cope with the problem. However, these margins may be too large for some patients or too small for others, significantly compromising patient care.

In current RT practice, treatment plan optimization and dose delivery are two decoupled steps. A highly conformal treatment plan is generated based on a single static instance of the patient's anatomy at the time of treatment simulation. However, the patient's state during each fractional treatment often differs from the pre-treatment CT simulation, as observed in numerous publications reporting significant inter-fractional variations in the shapes, sizes, and positions of anatomic structures [8–15]. Organ motion, such as involuntary movement of structures adjacent to the digestive or urinary systems, and changes in the patient's condition, such as weight gain/loss, can further affect anatomy. Notable anatomical changes include unpredictable daily variations in the filling of the bladder or rectum, alongside progressive alterations throughout the treatment, such as tumor reduction. Administering radiation based on the initial treatment plan amidst such evolving anatomies can lead to significant discrepancies, potentially jeopardizing the efficacy of the treatment. For instance, regions intended to receive a high dose may inadvertently impact healthy tissues rather than exclusively targeting the tumor. This misalignment could critically reduce the dosage received by the tumor and elevate the risk of adverse effects on the nearby organs at risk (OARs).

For example, an analysis of routine cone beam computed tomography (CBCT) image data from rectal cancer patients revealed substantial changes in rectal volume and dosimetric coverage during a course of RT [16]. Figure 22.1 shows the planning CT (pCT) and three CBCT images of a rectum patient acquired at the beginning of every week for the first three weeks. In this case, the range of deformation changes in the lateral (LA) direction at the superior, middle, and inferior slices were 0–2.54, 0–2.6, and 0–1.98 cm, respectively. Similarly, the range in the anterior–posterior (AP) at the top, middle, and inferior slices were 0–2.44, 0–3.77, and 0.07–2.53 cm, respectively. Distances of the geometric centers of the rectal contours between the paired CTs at the superior, middle, and inferior slices were found to be 0–2.24, 0–2.07, 0–2.07 cm, respectively. For other disease sites, such as the head and neck

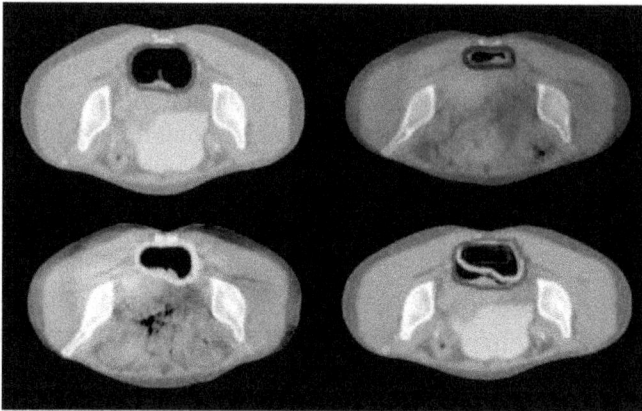

Figure 22.1. pCT and three CBCTs of a rectum patient acquired before and during the course of RT. The upper-left is pCT and the rest are CBCTs acquired one (upper-right), two (lower-left), and three weeks (lower-right) after the first fraction. The overlay of the target at different time points is shown in the bottom right image.

(H&N), prostate, lung, pancreas, and liver, similar findings have been reported [13, 17–22].

Coping with such a broad range of tumor motion by a margin-based approach is clearly difficult without significantly compromising the treatments. In general, beam targeting is a multi-dimensional problem that cannot be adequately addressed solely by translational and rotational degrees of freedom without compromising normal tissues. Consequently, the dose that the patient actually received may differ from the planned one, leading to scenarios of insufficient dose coverage of the targeted tumor volume and overdosage of normal tissues, both of which potentially compromise clinical results. The potential benefit of adaptive re-planning becomes evident when dealing with clinical cases involving significant anatomy changes, such as the one shown in figure 22.2.

22.1.2 Challenges in the clinical implementation of ART

On-board CBCT based upon flat-panel technology integrated with a medical linac has become widely available for therapy guidance. Hybrid MRI-linac units are also becoming increasingly adopted. The systems provide online 3D or even 4D [23–27] patient anatomy data that are valuable for patient set-up and, more importantly, adaptive re-planning [28–33]. In the latter case, the online volumetric imaging affords unique opportunities for us to derive the patient's on-treatment anatomic model and adaptively modify the treatment plan to cater for any anatomy changes. ART promises to achieve full dose coverage of the target through optimally adjusting the beam parameters (such as the apertures, fluences maps, and the Monitor Units (MUs)) while minimizing the doses to the OARs [28–30], and optimally compensates for any residual error after the initial patient set-up. However, there are a number of practical challenges in leveraging the concept of adaptive therapy to benefit patients.

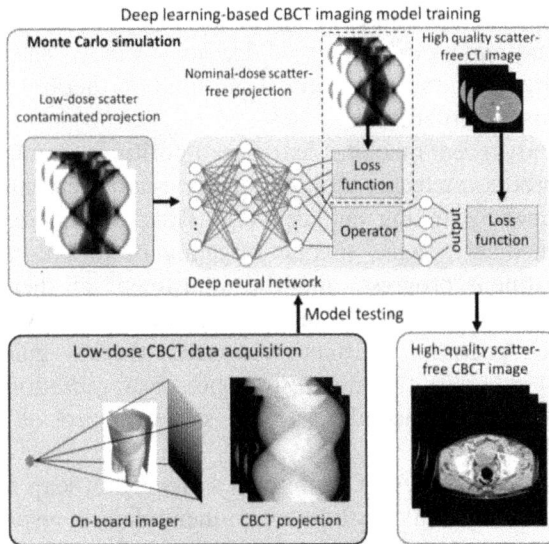

Figure 22.2. The proposed DL-based scatter-free CBCT imaging scheme. During model training, the DL model takes the low-dose scatter contaminated projection as input. The nominal-dose scatter-free projection together with the high-quality scatter-free CT images are employed as reference images to supervise the weights in the network. Once the model is well-trained, the branch of the projection-domain loss function is turned off (dashed box), and the model takes the low-dose CBCT data acquired using the OBI to yield a high-quality scatter-free CBCT image.

Technically, ART is to systematically monitor treatment variations and incorporate them to re-optimize the treatment plan during the course of treatment. ART entails adjusting dose distributions at each fraction in response to changes in the patient's anatomy or even changes in radiomics features [34] and biology [35, 36]. While the concept of ART has been around for years [28, 37, 38], its practical implementation has just begun, primarily because of the lack of technical infrastructure of adaptive planning to support a clinically meaningful ART. In reality, routine plan adaptation with the patient on the table is challenging and requires nearly real-time performance [39], which necessitates a well-integrated ART solution with fast and robust image registration, segmentation, dose optimization, and plan quality assurance (QA). These challenges are being addressed by the emerging AI technologies.

22.1.3 AI and AI in healthcare

AI has emerged as a transformative force across various industries, and its impact on healthcare is particularly profound [40]. Its application within healthcare spans a broad spectrum, significantly enhancing diagnostic precision, prognostic evaluations, treatment planning, therapeutic interventions, and even in the optimization of administrative operations, thereby elevating overall patient care standards. The power of AI lies in its ability to process and interpret vast datasets at speeds and levels of accuracy unattainable by human efforts or conventional methods alone.

This capability is instrumental in enabling healthcare professionals to derive more nuanced insights and make evidence-based decisions rapidly, ensuring tailored and effective patient care. In the specific context of radiation therapy, AI's contribution is both profound and multifaceted.

By harnessing advanced machine learning algorithms, computer vision, and natural language processing techniques, AI facilitates a more nuanced and dynamic approach to treatment planning and delivery. This encompasses the automated segmentation of medical images, precise targeting of radiation doses, real-time monitoring of treatment progress, and the adjustment of therapy protocols to accommodate changes in tumor size or location. Moreover, AI-driven predictive models can forecast potential treatment outcomes, thereby guiding clinicians in choosing the most effective treatment strategies. For radiation therapy, it can literally be leveraged to enhance almost every step or aspect of clinical workflow [40], including ART.

The integration of AI into ART represents a significant leap forward. AI-ART systems are designed to dynamically adjust treatment plans in response to changes in the patient's anatomy or tumor characteristics, ensuring that radiation therapy remains precisely targeted and maximally effective throughout the course of treatment. This adaptability is crucial for addressing inter-fraction anatomical variations, thereby minimizing radiation exposure to healthy tissues and enhancing the therapeutic ratio. Furthermore, AI's role extends beyond clinical applications to include the optimization of workflow efficiency within radiation therapy departments. By automating routine tasks and streamlining treatment planning processes, AI technologies can significantly reduce the time and resources required for each patient's treatment, thereby increasing the capacity for care delivery and improving patient outcomes. In the following, we highlight some applications of AI relevant to AI-ART.

22.2 Recent advancements in AI in ART

22.2.1 AI-augmented imaging and image analysis

One of the promising applications of AI in healthcare is in the field of medical imaging and image analysis. AI algorithms can facilitate image reconstruction [41, 42] and analyse medical images [43, 44]. Moreover, AI-powered imaging techniques can enhance the resolution and quality of medical images [47], enabling us to visualize anatomical structures and pathology with greater clarity. AI-augmented imaging has the potential to improve diagnostic accuracy, increase efficiency, and ultimately improve patient outcomes. Given the important role of CBCT in ART, here we provide some concrete examples of AI in enhancing the modality.

In CBCT, the image quality is far from satisfactory due to dramatically increased scatter contamination in cone beam geometry, making it not suitable for accurate dose calculation and ART planning. Over the years, much has been devoted in scatter correction, but a practical solution without modifying hardware remains elusive [48–56]. To solve this task a residual convolutional neural network (CNN)-based scatter correction method was proposed [57]. The CNN method is unique in two aspects: (i) it deals the sinogram data directly instead of working in the image domain and (ii) it is focused on learning the accurate behavior of scatter photon signals instead of the total projection images, thus providing an effective solution in processing the unbalanced primary and scatter signals. Training of a DL model generally requires a large number of annotated datasets, and this often presents a bottleneck in deep learning [58]. Instead of empirically measuring many paired x-ray projections and scatter distributions for supervised training, this method produced projection images and corresponding scatter-only projection images using the Monte Carlo (MC) simulation package GATE [59]. The CNN was trained to derive the scatter-only projection, so that the scatter-free (i.e. the primary) projection can be derived from the total intensity. This residual learning [60, 61] outperforms the modeling of the target image directly when the input and target images are close, which is particularly important for low-dose CBCT.

In this study [57], five digital phantoms with different inserts containing muscle, adipose, water, blood, rib bone, brain, and lung tissue were constructed to generate projections for deep learning model training. For each phantom, 360 projections were computed over a rotation with 1° angular interval, using the chemical compositions of materials in the phantoms [62, 63]. Data augmentations (90° rotations and flips) were applied during training, which increased training projection pairs to a total of 14 400. Subsequently, the proposed method was compared to a conventional method called the fast adaptive scatter kernel superposition (fASKS) method [64], and it was found to provide projections with significantly reduced scatter and CBCT images with more accurate Hounsfield units (HUs). Figure 22.3 shows a scatter-corrected image together with the ground truth image. In the CNN-corrected images, artefacts and regional errors are removed and the accuracy of HU is consistent to the ground truth value in all pixels, demonstrating that the CNN model can correct for scatter with high accuracy. The image quality of the CNN-based reconstruction was also compared with the fASKS calculation quantitatively. In the resultant images, the HU quantification, particularly in regions near the air or

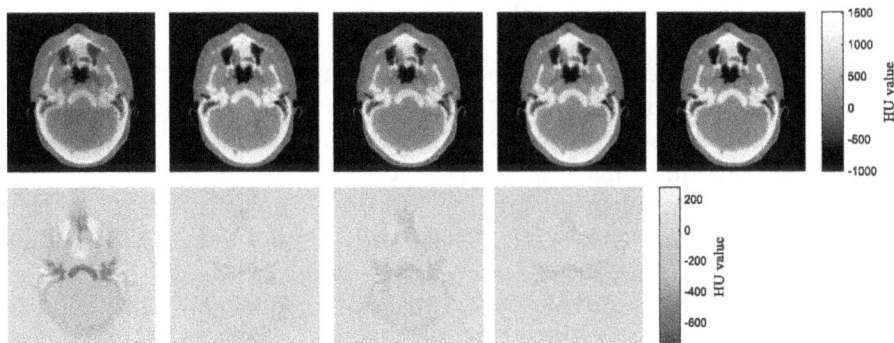

Figure 22.3. Comparison of the scatter-corrected images with the ground truth in a slice. Color maps illustrate difference maps against the ground truth. Images from left to right represent uncorrected, fASKS-corrected, CNN-corrected (MSE loss function), CNN-corrected (MAE loss function), and the ground truth image, respectively.

Table 22.1. Comparison of image quality between the fASKS- and CNN-based corrections (mean + SD). Central 40 slice images were evaluated using MAE, MSE, PSNR, and SSIM. (Adapted from [57] with permission from John Wiley & Sons. Copyright 2019 American Association of Physicists in Medicine.)

	MAE (HU)	MSE (HU^2)	PSNR (dB)	SSIM
fASKS	25.8 ± 5.4	1464 ± 651	16.9 ± 1.9	0.9992 ± 0.0003
CNN	21.8 ± 5.2	1119 ± 548	18.1 ± 2.1	0.9995 ± 0.0003
p-value	1.31×10^{-3}	1.22×10^{-2}	5.49×10^{-3}	4.04×10^{-4}

bone interfaces, and all four other quality metrics, including mean absolute error (MAE), mean squared error (MSE), peak signal-to-noise ratio (PSNR), and structural similarity (SSIM), are significantly better than that of the fASKS-corrected images (table 22.1).

Additionally, the imaging dose that results from repeated use of CBCT is also of concern [42, 65–69]. CBCT imaging can expose patients to high cumulative radiation doses and elevate individuals' lifetime risk of developing cancer or other health problems [70, 71]. In a retrospective cohort study of 178 604 pediatric patients [72], it was found that use of CT scans almost triples the risk of leukemia and brain cancers for a single CT scan (imaging dose is around 3–5 cGy). For RT patients, while imaging dose is less a concern as compared to diagnostic imaging applications, it is not negligible, because the cumulative imaging dose to the patient can be excessive when the current CBCT technique is employed. It has been reported [73] that the dose delivered to the patient is more than 3–5 cGy from a CBCT scan with current clinical protocols. When the patient is imaged daily, this amounts to more than 100 cGy dose to all tissues inside the imaging field during a treatment course of 30 fractions. Based on the ALARA (as low as reasonably achievable) principle, the unwanted CBCT dose must be minimized in order for the patient to truly benefit from the modern ART [74]. The utilization of low-dose imaging in RT effectively comes at no additional cost, as the DL strategy ensures the enhancement of low mAs scan images to high CBCT image quality without necessitating any changes to the hardware.

Further dose reduction can come from sparse sampling into the CBCT imaging scheme [42, 75–78]. Multiple groups have done extensive work in CT and MR imaging related to sparse sampling [42, 68–75, 79, 80]. Among all of these, a neural representation algorithm that quickly and accurately reconstructs CT and MR images from sparse measurement data was proposed. This approach, called neural representation with prior embedding (NeRP) [129], is a novel deep learning framework for reconstructing medical images from sparsely sampled data through implicit neural representation, embedding prior images into a neural network. NeRP significantly deviates from traditional DL methods by utilizing the prior information of a subject's image and the physics of sparse sampling to reconstruct detailed and accurate images without requiring large datasets. The methodology's main advantages include eliminating the need for extensive external training data, accurately

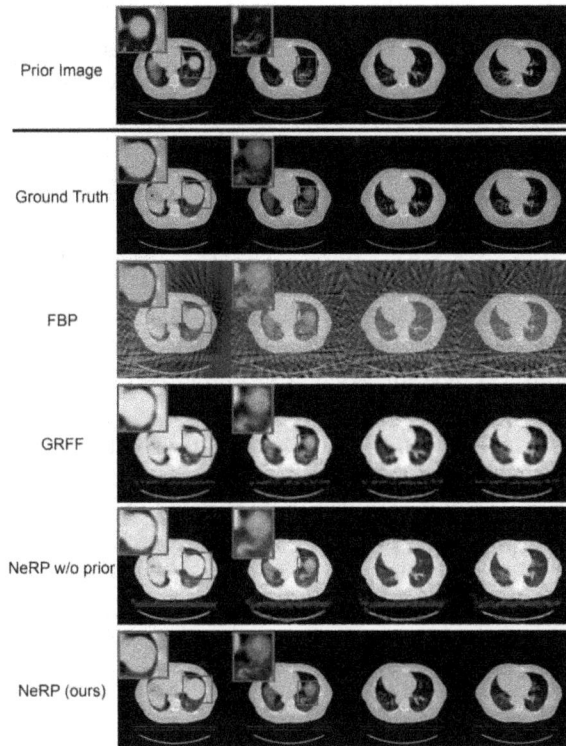

Figure 22.4. NeRP results when reconstructing lung 4D-CT scans, compared to traditional methods such as the filtered back-projection or the Fourier features (GRFF) network proposed by Tancik *et al*. (Adapted from [132]. Copyright 2023 The Author(s). Published on behalf of Institute of Physics and Engineering in Medicine by IOP Publishing Ltd. CC BY 4.0.)

reconstructing fine details, and its general applicability across various medical imaging tasks. NeRP represents a groundbreaking approach in medical image reconstruction, achieving high-fidelity images as seen in figure 22.4, being robust in capturing critical image changes such as tumor progression, and overcoming limitations of traditional reconstruction techniques. Its application demonstrates promising results across various imaging modalities, enhancing the ability to detect and monitor critical anatomical changes with minimal input data. In principle, the same approach could be applied to CBCT images, providing the speed required in ART.

Finally, for AI-based imaged processing, metal artifacts may also cause adverse effects, since they can represent out-of-distribution samples and make models fail. If needed, a DL-based artifacts removal technique can be integrated into the CBCT reconstruction system [66], resulting artifacts-free CBCT images. Moreover, if the contrast of the artifacts-free CBCT is still not sufficient for robust ART, there are two alternative solutions to further improve the image contrast. The first one is to train a DL model to map the pCT pixel values to CBCT. This so called 'synthetic'

CT technique has been well studied recently and the implementation should be straightforward. As a second option, it is possible to enhance the contrast even further by deriving dual- or multiple-energy CT images from the single-energy CBCT image.

22.2.2 AI-based image segmentation and registration

AI-augmented deformable registration and segmentation [45, 46, 81–85] holds significant potential to advance ART. In ART, the need for a robust and efficient registration algorithm to compare/fuse images acquired under different conditions or on different modalities is ever increasing. DL-based solutions have been studied for these applications [34, 86–96]. As is well known, segmentation is an important but time-consuming task [97–102]. For ART, the need for efficient and robust segmentation tools is urgent [103–107]. One solution is to propagate the contours delineated on the pCT onto CBCTs using a model. Along this line, deformable model-based contour mapping has been studied [83, 108, 109]. As such, surface mapping [86, 110–112] has been proposed, which obtains contour transformation by iteratively deforming the ROI contour-extended surface until the optimal match with the reference is found. The calculation involves only the surface and is thus efficient. However, the results depend heavily on the model, which may not be applicable for all clinical situations, as the ROI surface change is generally complex and hardly modeled by only a few parameters. Some studies introduced a regional algorithm for ROI propagation [90, 91, 113], where the deformation of an ROI contour-extended surface is not driven by an ad hoc surface model, but instead by the image features surrounding the surface. Here, the neighborhood image features of an ROI are captured by several small control volumes [113] or a narrow band [114] surrounding the ROIs. The strategy has been extended to an unsupervised learning-based contour propagation, obtaining promising results in terms of accuracy and efficiency [92].

A notable achievement in AI-enhanced image registration is the development of VoxelMorph [127], a deep learning framework initially conceived for medical image registration that has been effectively extended to segmentation tasks. VoxelMorph introduces a learning-oriented method that significantly improves the conventional medical image registration methods. Whereas traditional strategies demand optimizing a specific objective function for each image pair—a task that can be both slow and resource-intensive, particularly with sizable datasets or complex deformation models—this model conceptualizes registration as a function that associates an input image pair with a deformation field to align these images. This association is defined via a CNN, wherein the network's parameters are fine-tuned across multiple images. Upon training, VoxelMorph is equipped to instantaneously calculate a deformation field for any new set of scans, merely by applying the pre-learned function. VoxelMorph demonstrates performance comparable to top-tier registration software in terms of Dice score accuracy, but significantly reduces computation time—from hours to minutes on a CPU and to less than a second on a GPU. It offers flexibility in training with partially observed or coarsely delineated auxiliary information, enhancing Dice scores while maintaining its computational efficiency. Through amortized optimization, the model learns parameters optimal for a whole dataset, achieving state-of-the-art registration quality with as few as 100 training images. All in all, VoxelMorph can substantially accelerate the registration procedure, rendering it exponentially quicker than conventional methodologies and providing the speed needed in ART.

For online or offline ART, it is desirable to propagate contours from pCT to CBCT automatically, as well as registering doses delivered in new CBCT anatomy to the pCT for dose accumulation. While DL is powerful, there may exist special cases where a DL-based approach may not provide accurate results due to DL's sensitivity to out-of-distribution data. For example, during the course of a radiation therapy treatment, shrinkage or pathological change of the tumor may happen [115–117]. Practically, it is possible to include various special types of target and organ changes, or longitudinal data into the DL model training process, thereby increasing model robustness.

As demonstrated in the work of Pastor-Serrano *et al* [128], it is also possible to leverage longitudinal data acquired during previous treatments to train population models that generate the most likely anatomical movements in new patient anatomies. In their study, the authors presented a generative model that, based on VoxelMorph, produces deformation fields to warp the pCT and structures into different anatomies. Their proposed daily anatomy model (DAM) learns patient-specific movements between treatment sessions using population data. DAM effectively identifies deformation patterns and deformation fields from initial CT scans and delineations, and selectively applies the most plausible deformations specifically to each patient, based on end-to-end learned image features such as planning target volume (PTV) size and relative position. Based on their evaluation on multiple scans from independent test patients, DAM can accurately infer realistic CT images that mimic real anatomical variations seen in clinical patients (see figure 22.5). The resulting deformation fields are comparable to those from state-of-the-art analytical or learning-based registration methods such as VoxelMorph. Through applying DAM to real clinical data, the authors demonstrate DAM's ability to realistically simulate shifts and volume changes in the prostate, aligning well with clinical observations and previous reports. However, DAM faces challenges in simulating extreme shifts, partly due to a regularization term that restricts large deformations. Despite this, DAM shows promise in incorporating common deformations into treatment planning and evaluation, potentially enhancing ART strategies.

22.2.3 AI-augmented dose calculation

Online adaptive plan optimization necessitates a fast 3D dose calculation algorithm. Current physics-based tools for dose calculation, primarily analytical pencil beam algorithms (PBAs) and MC simulations, present a compromise between speed and accuracy. PBAs are faster but less precise in complex geometries, while MC simulations offer high accuracy at the cost of speed, making them less viable for

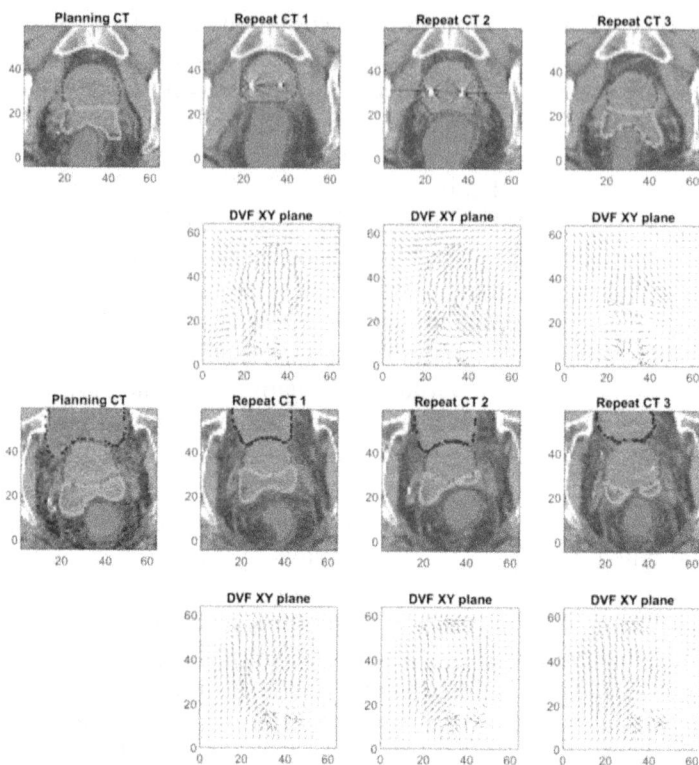

Figure 22.5. DAM predicted anatomies, starting from the planning CT, for two different patients. Each column shows a randomly generated anatomy, with its corresponding deformation field.

clinical use in adaptive proton therapy. ART requires adjustments for anatomical changes or motion, necessitating algorithms that combine MC's precision with the rapid processing of PBAs to enable near real-time adaptation.

DNNs have been applied for this purpose. Three possible approaches along the line are outlined in figure 22.6. A Deep DoseNet (DDN) model was developed for accurate and fast dose calculation and optimization [118, 119]. The DDN can be applied in three scenarios: (i) super-resolution dose calculation (similar to super-resolution imaging [120]), which maps a low resolution dose to high resolution; (ii) obtaining dose distribution by transforming the dose calculated from a fast and low-overhead analytic algorithm such as the anisotropic analytical algorithm (AAA) to that only attainable by using a more computationally expensive algorithm such as Acuros XB (AXB) algorithm or MC; and (iii) obtaining dose distribution by transforming the a raytracing grid to that only attainable by using a more computationally expensive dose calculation algorithm (such as AXB or MC).

The DDN was trained using 25 168 slices calculated using Varian Eclipse TPS on ten patient CTs whose treatment sites ranging from lung, brain, abdomen, and pelvis, using both AAA with 5 mm resolution and AXB with 1.25 mm resolution. The AAA dose slices, and the corresponding down-sampled CT slices are combined

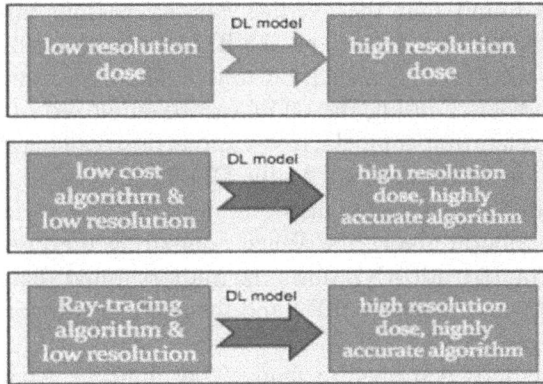

Figure 22.6. Different applications of DL to speed up dose calculation.

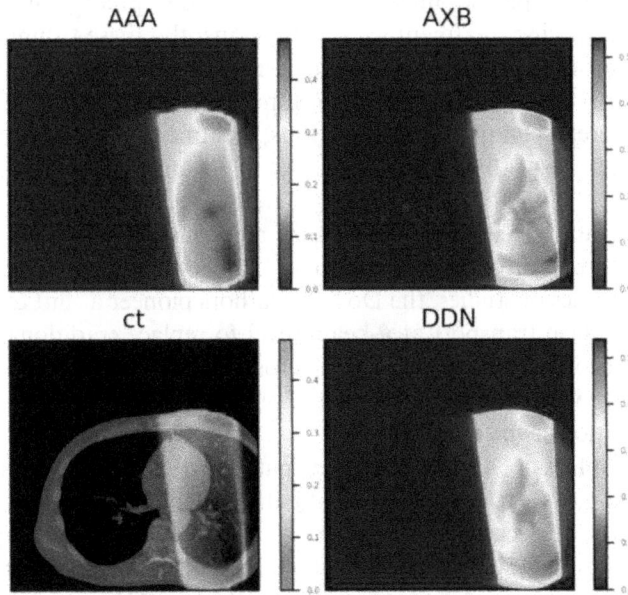

Figure 22.7. A typical dose distribution in the validation study obtained using the DDN. For visualization/comparison, the AAA, AXB, and AAA doses are overlaid on CT, and DDN doses are displayed.

to form the input to DDN with size $2 \times 64 \times 64$, which outputs the calculated Acuros dose with a higher resolution of 256×256. For evaluation, the average mean-square-error decreased from 4.7×10^{-4} between AAA and AXB to 7.0×10^{-5} between DDN and AXB, which represents a 12 times improvement.

As shown in figure 22.7, the DDN's predicted dose distribution is more consistent with the AXB calculations than AAA doses. Moreover, the DDN also reconciles the tissue density heterogeneities along the beam path and adjusts the dose accordingly. Likewise, a better agreement between the AXB and DDN calculations in the low-density lungs and in the high-density bones is clearly observed. For all the cases tested, the authors found that the average gamma passing rate at (3%, 3 mm) improved from 76% between AAA and AXB, to 91% between DDN and AXB. Most importantly, the average calculation time is less than 1 ms for a single slice using GPU hardware. As a result, the DDN can be employed as a general-purpose dose calculation acceleration engine across various dose calculation algorithms.

As demonstrated in subsequent works, the DDN can also use raytracing and CT as the input, to predict accurate dose distributions [121]. The raytracing was quickly obtained using the Siddon algorithm. When comparing the raytracing and DDN outputs with the ground truth AXB dose, the authors found that the average MSE decreased from 2.9×10^{-3} to 1.1×10^{-4} and the average gamma passing rate (3%, 3 mm) improved from 53.3% to 92.7%.

Although the methods described in figure 22.6—and, in general, practically all published deep learning models—offer significant acceleration over traditional physics-based algorithms and sometimes achieve speeds up to sub-second levels, they rely on secondary physics models or are designed to predict only complete plan or field doses for specific treatment areas. Consequently, these techniques cannot be considered universally applicable dose algorithms, lacking the flexibility to extend to various stages of the ART workflow beyond their intended use. This includes adapting to different planning configurations, treatment sites, or applications that require separate dose distributions for each beamlet, crucial for treatment adaptation.

The recently introduced dose transformer algorithm (DoTA) [131, 132], solves these problems, while offering the speed of DL methods and the accuracy of MC algorithms. In a series of studies, the DoTA's authors pioneer a shift towards learning the physics of particle transport at a beam level to replace traditional dose engines, aiming for millisecond accuracy applicable across all radiation dose calculation needs. Leveraging the forward nature of photon and proton transport, the authors conceptualize dose calculation as the modeling of a sequence of 2D geometries from the beam's eye view. DoTA integrates CNNs to extract spatial features, such as tissue and density contrasts, and employs a transformer self-attention backbone to facilitate information exchange between the sequence of geometry slices and a vector representing the beam's energy. Through extensive training on 80 000 distinct head and neck, lung, and prostate geometries, DoTA learns to predict low-noise MC simulations of proton beamlets with remarkable accuracy, achieving beamlet dose predictions in 5 ± 4.9 milliseconds, and exhibiting a remarkably high gamma pass rate of 99.37% ± 1.17% (1%, 3 mm) compared to ground truth MC calculations. Compared to PBA, the model learns to correctly predict doses in highly heterogeneous regions, as seen in figure 22.8. Notably, DoTA surpasses analytical PBAs in both precision and speed, providing MC-level accuracy 100 times faster for individual pencil beam dose prediction. Furthermore, the model can compute full treatment plan doses in only 10–15 s, depending on the number of beamlets, and maintains a 99.70% ± 0.14% (2%, 2 mm) gamma pass rate across all test patients. Outperforming all previous analytical pencil beam and deep learning-based approaches, DoTA established a new standard in data-driven dose calculation, rivaling the speed of even commercial GPU MC methodologies. Its sub-second speed fulfills the demand for ART, while its

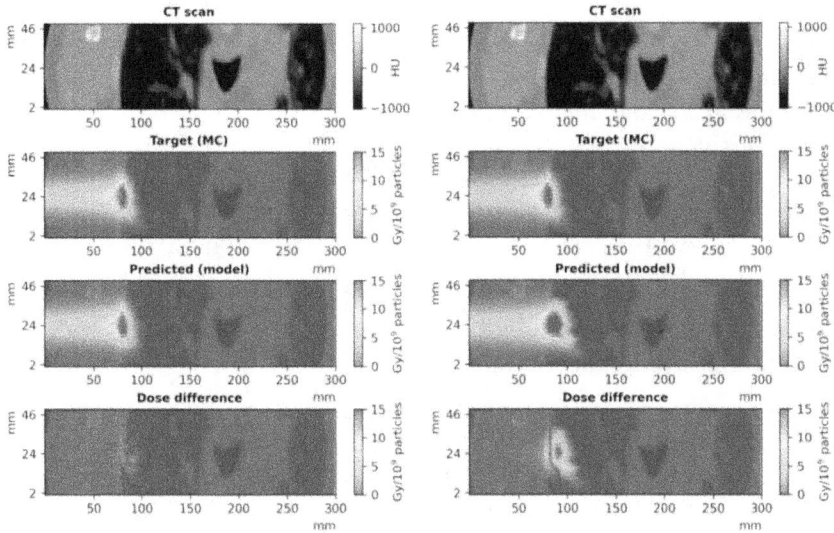

Figure 22.8. Beamlet dose distributions predicted by DoTA (left) and a PBA (right). Each column shows, in order, the CT anatomy of the lung patient, the target dose calculated with MC, the model (DoTA or PBA) prediction, and the dose difference. The example shows a beam where the Bragg peak occurs near a tissue–air heterogeneity, causing the PBA to fail. (Adapted with permission from [132]. Copyright 2022 The Author(s). Published on behalf of Institute of Physics and Engineering in Medicine by IOP Publishing Ltd. CC BY 4.0.)

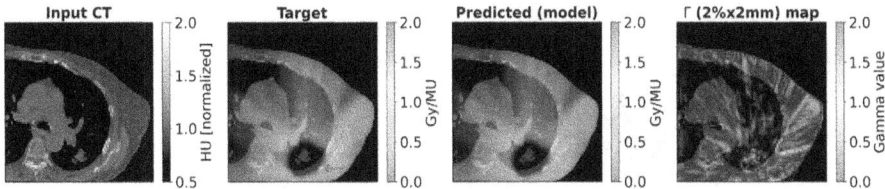

Figure 22.9. iDoTA predicted dose distribution from a lung VMAT treatment plan, including the corresponding gamma map. (Adapted from [134] with permission from John Wiley & Sons. Copyright 2023 The Authors. Medical Physics published by Wiley Periodicals LLC on behalf of American Association of Physicists in Medicine.)

straightforward implementation holds potential for enhancing other facets of the radiotherapy workflow or extending to alternative modalities such as helium or carbon treatments.

Subsequent works presented an improved version of the original algorithm, named iDoTA [133]. The model was applied to VMAT plans from prostate, lung, and H&N cancer patients with 194–354 beams per plan. iDoTA calculates full VMAT dose distributions in 6–12 s, achieving state-of-the-art performance with a $99.51\% \pm 0.66\%$ (2 mm, 2%) pass rate, as demonstrated in figure 22.9. Consequently, iDoTA is an order of magnitude faster than clinically used algorithms or MC approaches adapted to GPU hardware. While MC-GPU implementations are several orders of magnitude faster and nearly as accurate as their CPU counterparts, their total calculation times still range in the order of minutes. Furthermore, iDoTA is 20 times and 60 times faster than the Eclipse Acuros XB and AAA algorithms (Varian Medical Systems) utilized in approximately 80% of the clinics, which predict VMAT doses in 2–3 and approximately 10 min, respectively. Most importantly, the photon beams can be predicted in parallel in several batches depending on the number of GPUs and their internal memory, practically allowing for further reduction in total calculation times. The proposed model can massively speed up current photon ART workflows, reducing dose computation times from a few minutes to just a few seconds.

22.2.4 AI-augmented treatment planning

AI algorithms can speed up adaptive treatment planning by reducing the dimensionality of the dose distribution grid [122–125]. Generally, ART inverse planning involves iterative optimization of a large number of parameters, thus being time-consuming. An interesting strategy is to reduce the scale of computation and improve characterization of isodose plans. An isodose feature-preserving voxelization (IFPV) framework has been proposed to provide a concise representation of a treatment plan [123]. A dose distribution in IFPV scheme is characterized by partitioning the voxels into subgroups according to their geometric and dosimetric values while respecting the boundaries of segmented structures such as PTV, as shown in figure 22.10. The IFPV, which can be regarded as a 'smart' down-sampling instead of simply enlarging the voxel grid size in conventional down-sampling, significantly reducing the dimensionality without compromising the spatial resolution seen in traditional schemes. A k-means algorithm and support vector machine

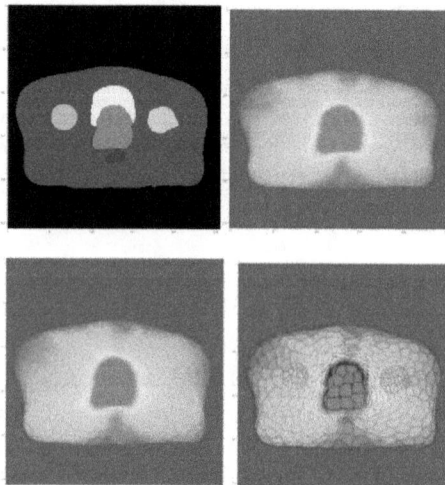

Figure 22.10. Original dose distribution and IFPV-based dose distribution of a prostate case. (a) Contours of body (blue), PTV (red), bladder (yellow), rectum (purple), and left (cyan) and right (green) femoral head. (b) Dose distributions of clinical plan. (c) IFPV distribution. (d) IFPV-based dose distribution with IFPV voxel boundaries displayed.

(SVM) runs sequentially to group the voxels into IFPV clusters. The former generates initial clusters according to the geometric and dosimetric information of the voxels and SVM is invoked to improve the connectivity of the IFPV clusters.

The authors found that the resultant plans of prostate and H&N cases compared favorably against that obtained using conventional voxelation scheme. As an example, for the case shown in figure 22.10, the number of voxels is reduced from 1.77×10^6 to 16 321 IFPV voxels, which massively reduced calculation times.

In addition to dramatically improving computational efficiency, we found that the IFPV-domain inverse planning yields equivalent treatment plans obtained using conventional approach. The IFPV provides a low parametric representation of isodose plan without compromising the plan quality, thus providing a valuable framework for various applications in RT. Moreover, the IFPV-domain transformation can be further leveraged to accelerate dose prediction with CNNs [123]. In summary, the IFPV characterization of treatment plans holds potential for various applications in ART such as plan optimization, plan data compression, and concise presentation of quality assurance data. Particularly noteworthy is the substantial reduction in dimensionality while preserving key features of the dose distribution, opening new avenues for IFPV-domain machine learning and/or other data-driven autonomous planning methodologies.

Most importantly, a prerequisite of ART is a fast and fully automated treatment planning process. To solve this task, several methods have been proposed based on a Pareto optimal projection search (POPS) algorithm [126], which combines two main search processes: (i) gradient-free search in the decision variable space and (ii) projection of decision variables to the Pareto front using the bisection method. A visualization of dose distributions at different stages of the POPS plan search is provided in figure 22.11. The PTV dose remains relatively homogeneous throughout all iterations with dose conformity being noticeably improved in the final plan when comparing to the initial plan. The POPS algorithm provides a general framework for fully automated treatment planning and addresses many key limitations of other adaptive automated planning approaches.

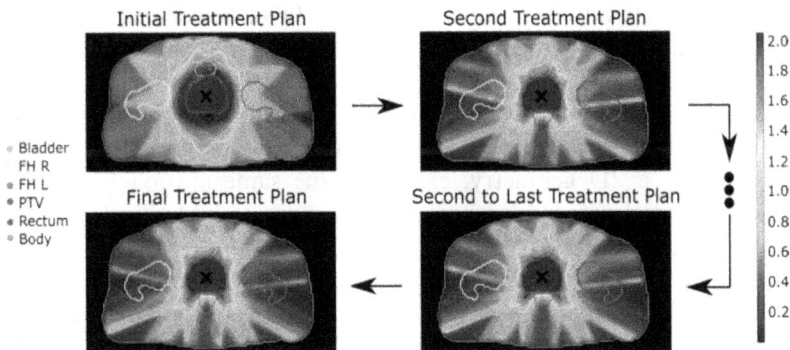

Figure 22.11. Visual comparison of initial, intermediate, and final treatment plans generated for an example patient using POPS. Dose conformity and organ sparing significantly improve from the initial plan after running POPS.

However, the most notable AI methods for automated treatment planning involve reinforcement learning (RL) algorithms. RL is a type of machine learning where an agent learns to make decisions by interacting with an environment to maximize cumulative rewards. In the context of ART, these agents can either act as clinical technicians providing the optimization parameters for the inner optimization in the TPS, or substitute the inner optimization algorithm to directly output the optimal machine parameters (e.g. multileaf collimator (MLC) leaf positions and beam intensities).

Several studies explore the use of RL agents to mimic treatment planning technicians [134–136]. A deep RL-based virtual treatment planner network (VTPN) for automating the treatment planning process in IMRT for prostate cancer was proposed for this task [134]. The VTPN mimics human planners by adjusting treatment planning parameters to generate high-quality treatment plans efficiently. The study focuses on an in-house optimization engine using a weighted quadratic objective function. VTPN learns to optimize treatment planning by adjusting weights and dose thresholds based on intermediate plan DVHs. Its effectiveness was validated on 64 additional patient cases, significantly improving the treatment plan quality score and demonstrating the network's ability to autonomously enhance treatment planning parameters for superior quality plans. The authors further proposed a knowledge-guided deep reinforcement learning (KgDRL) framework integrating human expertise with deep RL [135]. By applying this framework to prostate cancer IMRT planning, the study demonstrates how human-derived rules can effectively guide the complex decision-making process, significantly enhancing the training efficiency of the VTPN. Notably, KgDRL achieved over a 90% reduction in training time compared to conventional DRL methods, showcasing the potential for applying DRL to more complex, clinically relevant planning problems and highlighting the value of incorporating human knowledge into advanced DL approaches.

Alternatively, a deep-Q reinforcement learning (RL)-based VMAT machine parameter optimization (MPO) for prostate cancer treatment was introduced [136]. Utilizing a convolutional deep-Q network to control dose rate and multileaf collimator settings, it aimed at minimizing the Q-value measure based on dose objectives. Training on 15 patients and validating on 5, its efficacy was tested on 20 additional patients. The results showed the RL approach produced plans comparable to clinical IMRT, suggesting potential for rapid AI-based treatment plan optimization without requiring pre-optimized plans. Although the method is presented only for a 2D geometry, extending the same approach to a 3D beam model promises accelerated AI-driven optimization of VMAT plans, potentially reducing ART planning time.

Free from the domain-specific training that RL algorithms need, and the long time RL requires to gather experience, a recent study proposes using pre-trained large language models (LLMs) to automate planning. The resulting GPT-RadPlan is an innovative automated radiotherapy treatment planning tool that leverages the advanced capabilities of multi-modal LLMs [137]. By utilizing the in-context learning abilities of LLMs, GPT-RadPlan mimics experienced human planners by adjusting optimization parameters and evaluating treatment plans to meet clinical objectives without extensive domain-specific training, requiring only few reference plans and the physician's intent for the patient. It processes and understands various forms of clinical data—including text descriptions, dose–volume histogram (DVH) tables, and dose distribution images—enabling comprehensive evaluation and planning. Initial results have shown that GPT-RadPlan significantly reduces planning times and associated costs while enhancing the quality and consistency of radiotherapy plans, addressing critical limitations of existing techniques and representing a significant advancement in the integration of AI into radiation oncology practice.

22.2.5 The workflow of future AI-ART

The workflow of future AI-ART is envisioned to be highly integrated and stream-lined, with AI algorithms playing a central role in every stage of the treatment process. From image acquisition and segmentation to dose calculation and treat-ment planning, AI will automate and optimize various tasks, enabling healthcare providers to deliver personalized and precise radiation therapy to patients. Moreover, AI-driven decision support systems will help clinicians make informed treatment decisions based on real-time patient data and predictive analytics. The future workflow of AI-ART holds the promise of improving treatment efficiency, quality, and outcomes while reducing treatment-related toxicities and costs.

The journey of future AI-ART begins with the initial assessment of the patient, where AI algorithms play a crucial role in analysing diagnostic images, such as CT scans, MRI, and PET scans. These AI-driven tools are designed to enhance image acquisition, providing clearer, more detailed images that are essential for accurate tumor identification and segmentation. Advanced AI models can distinguish between tumor tissues and healthy organs with remarkable precision, automating the segmentation process that traditionally requires extensive manual effort by radiologists and oncologists. This automation not only saves significant time but also increases segmentation accuracy, laying a solid foundation for personalized treatment planning.

Following segmentation, the next critical phase in the AI-ART workflow involves dose calculation and treatment planning optimization. Here, AI algorithms excel in their ability to process complex datasets to determine the optimal radiation dose required to target the tumor effectively while minimizing exposure to surrounding healthy tissues. By leveraging machine learning models, AI-ART systems can predict the best treatment angles and radiation intensities in just a few seconds based on the patient's unique anatomy and the tumor's characteristics. This predictive capability enables healthcare providers to design highly personalized and precise treatment plans that can adapt to changes over time, ensuring the maximum therapeutic effect with the fewest possible side effects.

As the treatment commences, AI's role extends to the real-time monitoring of the therapy delivery, ensuring that the radiation dose administered aligns perfectly with the treatment plan. AI algorithms continuously analyse data from imaging done during treatment sessions to detect any changes in tumor size or position, as well as alterations in patient anatomy. This real-time analysis allows for immediate adjustments to the treatment plan, a process known as adaptive radiation therapy. By adapting the therapy to reflect current conditions, AI-ART ensures that the treatment remains as effective as possible throughout the course of therapy, even in the face of changes that would have previously required significant manual recalibration and planning.

An integral part of the AI-ART workflow involves AI-driven decision support systems that aid clinicians in making informed treatment decisions. These systems harness the power of predictive analytics, utilizing vast amounts of historical and real-time patient data to forecast treatment outcomes, potential side effects, and the likelihood of treatment success. By providing these insights, AI helps healthcare providers to tailor treatment strategies that are not only personalized but also proactive, potentially mitigating risks before they become significant problems.

22.3 Summary

In summary, RT is a major modality of cancer treatment and plays pivotal role in the management of cancer. To mitigate the uncertainties and fully utilize the technical capability of modern RT, a clinically practical ART strategy must be developed. It is critically important to establish an AI-ART framework to leverage from the state-of-the-art AI techniques and the patient's pre- and on-treatment data such as imaging and treatment plan to provide optimal adaptive plan in nearly real-time. AI holds immense potential to transform the field of radiation therapy and improve cancer care. From assisting in imaging and image analysis to optimizing dose calculation and treatment planning, AI algorithms can augment the capabilities of healthcare providers and enhance the quality and precision of radiation therapy. By integrating AI into the workflow of radiation therapy, we can expect to see significant advancements in treatment outcomes, patient experience, and overall healthcare delivery. However, challenges such as data privacy, algorithm bias, and regulatory compliance must be addressed to realize the full potential of AI-ART in radiation therapy. It is important to emphasize that, in addition to many technical and workflow issues, such as how to ensure its performance in the face of increasingly sophisticated workflow, it is critical to carry out retrospective and prospective clinical studies in the future demonstrate the benefits of emerging AI-augmented ART techniques.

References

[1] IMRT Collaborative Working Group 2001 Intensity-modulated radiotherapy: current status and issues of interest *Int. J. Radiat. Oncol. Biol. Phys.* **51** 880–914
[2] Ezzell G A, Galvin J M, Low D, Palta J R, Rosen I, Sharpe M B, Xia P, Xiao Y, Xing L and Yu C X 2003 Guidance document on delivery, treatment planning, and clinical implementation of IMRT: report of the IMRT Subcommittee of the AAPM Radiation Therapy Committee *Med. Phys.* **30** 2089–115

[3] Galvin J M *et al* 2004 Implementing IMRT in clinical practice: a joint document of the American Society for Therapeutic Radiology and Oncology and the American Association of Physicists in Medicine *Int. J. Radiat. Oncol. Biol. Phys.* **58** 1616–34

[4] Xing L, Thorndyke B, Schreibmann E, Yang Y, Li T F, Kim G Y, Luxton G and Koong A 2006 Overview of image-guided radiation therapy *Med. Dosim.* **31** 91–112

[5] Li R and Xing L 2011 Bridging the gap between IMRT and VMAT: dense angularly sampled and sparse intensity modulated radiation therapy *Med. Phys.* **38** 4912–9

[6] Timmerman R and Xing L 2009 *Image Guided and Adaptive Radiation Therapy* (Baltimore, MD: Lippincott Williams & Wilkins)

[7] Timmerman R D, Kavanagh B D, Cho L C, Papiez L and Xing L 2007 Stereotactic body radiation therapy in multiple organ sites *J. Clin. Oncol.* **25** 947–52

[8] Antolak J A and Rosen I I 1999 Planning target volumes for radiotherapy: how much margin is needed? *Int. J. Radiat. Oncol. Biol. Phys.* **44** 1165–70

[9] Hector C L, Webb S and Evans P M 2000 The dosimetric consequences of inter-fractional patient movement on conventional and intensity-modulated breast radiotherapy treatments *Radiother. Oncol.* **54** 57–64

[10] Yan D and Lockman D 2001 Organ/patient geometric variation in external beam radio-therapy and its effects *Med. Phys.* **28** 593–602

[11] Happersett L, Mageras G S, Zelefsky M J, Burman C M, Leibel S A, Chui C, Fuks Z, Bull S, Ling C C and Kutcher G J 2003 A study of the effects of internal organ motion on dose escalation in conformal prostate treatments *Radiother. Oncol.* **66** 263–70

[12] Langen K M and Jones D T 2001 Organ motion and its management *Int. J. Radiat. Oncol. Biol. Phys.* **50** 265–78

[13] Balter J M, Sandler H M, Lam K, Bree R L, Lichter A S and ten Haken R K 1995 Measurement of prostate movement over the course of routine radiotherapy using implanted markers *Int. J. Radiat. Oncol. Biol. Phys.* **31** 113–8

[14] van Herk M 2006 Errors and margins in radiotherapy *Semin. Radiat. Oncol.* **14** 52–64

[15] Vigneault E, Pouliot J, Laverdiere J, Roy J and Dorion M 1997 Electronic portal imaging device detection of radioopaque markers for the evaluation of prostate position during megavoltage irradiation: a clinical study *Int. J. Radiat. Oncol. Biol. Phys.* **37** 205–12

[16] Lee P, Xing L, Pawlicki P, Tran P, Koong A and Goodman K 2006 Image-guided radiation therapy (RT) for rectal cancer using cone beam CT (CBCT) *Int. J. Radiat. Oncol. Biol. Phys.* **66** S276

[17] Litzenberg D W, Balter J M, Lam K L, Sandler H M and Ten Haken R K 2005 Retrospective analysis of prostate cancer patients with implanted gold markers using off-line and adaptive therapy protocols *Int. J. Radiat. Oncol. Biol. Phys.* **63** 123–33

[18] Schiffner D C, Gottschalk A R, Lometti M, Aubin M, Pouliot J, Speight J, Hsu I C, Shinohara K and Roach M 3rd 2007 Daily electronic portal imaging of implanted gold seed fiducials in patients undergoing radiotherapy after radical prostatectomy *Int. J. Radiat. Oncol. Biol. Phys.* **67** 610–9

[19] Ghilezan M J *et al* 2005 Prostate gland motion assessed with cine-magnetic resonance imaging (cine-MRI) *Int. J. Radiat. Oncol. Biol. Phys.* **62** 406–17

[20] Xie Y, Djajaputra D, King C, Hossain S, Ma L and Xing L 2008 Intrafraction motion of prostate in hypofractionated radiation therapy *Int. J. Radiat. Oncol. Biol. Phys.* **51** 236–46

[21] Willoughby T R *et al* 2006 Target localization and real-time tracking using the Calypso 4D localization system in patients with localized prostate cancer *Int. J. Radiat. Oncol. Biol. Phys.* **65** 528–34

[22] Kupelian P *et al* 2007 Multi-institutional clinical experience with the Calypso system in localization and continuous, real-time monitoring of the prostate gland during external radiotherapy *Int. J. Radiat. Oncol. Biol. Phys.* **67** 1088–98

[23] Sonke J J, Zijp L, Remeijer P and van Herk M 2005 Respiratory correlated cone beam CT *Med. Phys.* **32** 1176–86

[24] Li T, Xing L, McGuinness C, Munro P, Loo B and Koong A 2006 Four-dimensional cone-beam CT using an on-board imager *Med. Phys.* **33** 3825–33

[25] Li T and Xing L 2007 Optimizing 4D cone-beam CT acquisition protocol for external beam radiotherapy *Int. J. Radiat. Oncol. Biol. Phys.* **67** 1211–9

[26] Li T, Koong A and Xing L 2007 Enhanced 4D cone-beam computed tomography using an on-board imager *Med. Phys.* **34** 3688–95

[27] Lu J, Guerrero T M, Munro P, Jeung A, Chi P C, Balter P, Zhu X R, Mohan R and Pan T 2007 Four-dimensional cone beam CT with adaptive gantry rotation and adaptive data sampling *Med. Phys.* **34** 3520–9

[28] de la Zerda A, Armbruster B and Xing L 2007 Formulating adaptive radiation therapy (ART) treatment planning into a closed-loop control framework *Phys. Med. Biol.* **52** 4137–53

[29] Wu Q, Liang J and Yan D 2006 Application of dose compensation in image-guided radiotherapy of prostate cancer *Phys. Med. Biol.* **51** 1405–19

[30] Mohan R, Zhang X, Wang H, Kang Y, Wang X, Liu H, Ang K K, Kuban D and Dong L 2005 Use of deformed intensity distributions for on-line modification of image-guided IMRT to account for interfractional anatomic changes *Int. J. Radiat. Oncol. Biol. Phys.* **61** 1258–66

[31] Hong T S, Welsh J S, Ritter M A, Harari P M, Jaradat H, Mackie T R and Mehta M P 2007 Megavoltage computed tomography: an emerging tool for image-guided radiotherapy *Am. J. Clin. Oncol.* **30** 617–23

[32] Welsh J S *et al* 2006 Clinical implementation of adaptive helical tomotherapy: a unique approach to image-guided intensity modulated radiotherapy *Technol. Cancer Res. Treat.* **5** 465–79

[33] Mackie T R, Balog J, Ruchala K, Shepard D, Aldridge S, Fitchard E, Reckwerdt P, Olivera G, McNutt T and Mehta M 1999 Tomotherapy *Semin. Radiat. Oncol.* **9** 108–17

[34] Li R, Xing L, Napel S and Rubin D 2019 *Radiomics and Radiogenomics: Technical Basis and Clinical Applications* (Abingdon: Taylor and Francis)

[35] Karava K, Ehrbar S, Riesterer O, Roesch J, Glatz S, Klock S, Guckenberger M and Tanadini-Lang S 2017 Potential dosimetric benefits of adaptive tumor tracking over the internal target volume concept for stereotactic body radiation therapy of pancreatic cancer *Radiat. Oncol.* **12** 175

[36] Yang Y and Xing L 2005 Towards biologically conformal radiation therapy (BCRT): selective IMRT dose escalation under the guidance of spatial biology distribution *Med. Phys.* **32** 1473–84

[37] Yan D, Wong J, Vicini F, Michalski J, Pan C, Frazier A, Horwitz E and Martinez A 1997 Adaptive modification of treatment planning to minimize the deleterious effects of treatment setup errors *Int. J. Radiat. Oncol. Biol. Phys.* **38** 197–206

[38] Yan D, Ziaja E, Jaffray D, Wong J, Brabbins D, Vicini F and Martinez A 1998 The use of adaptive radiation therapy to reduce setup error: a prospective clinical study *Int. J. Radiat. Oncol. Biol. Phys.* **41** 715–20

[39] Bohoudi O, Bruynzeel A M E, Senan S, Cuijpers J P, Slotman B J, Lagerwaard F J and Palacios M A 2017 Fast and robust online adaptive planning in stereotactic MR-guided adaptive radiation therapy (SMART) for pancreatic cancer *Radiother. Oncol.* **125** 439–44

[40] Xing L, Giger M L and Min J K 2020 *Artificial Intelligence in Medicine: Technical Basis and Clinical Applications* (London: Academic)

[41] Shen L, Zhao W, Capaldi D, Pauly J and Xing L 2022 A geometry-informed deep learning framework for ultra-sparse 3D tomographic image reconstruction *Comput. Biol. Med.* **148** 105710

[42] Shen L, Zhao W and Xing L 2019 Patient-specific reconstruction of volumetric computed tomography images from a single projection view via deep learning *Nat. Biomed. Eng.* **3** 880–8

[43] Seo H, Huang C, Bassenne M, Xiao R and Xing L 2019 Modified U-Net (mU-Net) with incorporation of object-dependent high level features for improved liver and liver-tumor segmentation in CT images *IEEE Trans. Med. Imaging* **39** 1316–25

[44] Chen K T *et al* 2020 Ultra-lowdose ^{18}F-florbetaben amyloid PET imaging using deep learning with multi-contrast MRI inputs *Radiology* **296** E195

[45] Chen Y *et al* 2022 Adaptive region-specific loss for improved medical image segmentation *IEEE Trans. Pattern Anal. Mach. Intell.* **45** 13408–21

[46] Seo H, Khuzani M, Vasudevan V, Huang C, Ren H, Xiao R and Xing L 2019 Machine learning techniques for biomedical image segmentation: an overview *Med. Phys.* **47** e148–e67

[47] Ye S, Shen L, Islam M T and Xing L 2023 Super-resolution biomedical imaging via reference-free statistical implicit neural representation *Phys. Med. Biol.* **68** 205020

[48] Zhu L, Xie Y, Wang J and Xing L 2009 Scatter correction for cone-beam CT in radiation therapy *Med. Phys.* **36** 2258–68

[49] Zhu L, Wang J and Xing L 2009 Noise suppression in scatter correction for cone-beam CT *Med. Phys.* **36** 741–52

[50] Lee H, Fahimian B P and Xing L 2017 Binary moving-blocker-based scatter correction in cone-beam computed tomography with width-truncated projections: proof of concept *Phys. Med. Biol.* **62** 2176–93

[51] Lee H, Xing L, Lee R and Fahimian B P 2012 Scatter correction in cone-beam CT via a half beam blocker technique allowing simultaneous acquisition of scatter and image information *Med. Phys.* **39** 2386–95

[52] Zhao W, Vernekohl D, Zhu J, Wang L and Xing L 2016 A model-based scatter artifacts correction for cone beam CT *Med. Phys.* **43** 1736

[53] Ahmad M, Bazalova M, Xiang L and Xing L 2014 Order of magnitude sensitivity increase in x-ray fluorescence computed tomography (XFCT) imaging with an optimized spectro-spatial detector configuration: theory and simulation *IEEE Trans. Med. Imaging* **33** 1119–28

[54] Boone J M and Seibert J A 1988 An analytical model of the scattered radiation distribution in diagnostic radiology *Med. Phys.* **15** 721–5

[55] Kyriakou Y and Kalender W 2007 Efficiency of antiscatter grids for flat-detector CT *Phys. Med. Biol.* **52** 6275–93

[56] Siewerdsen J H, Daly M J, Bakhtiar B, Moseley D J, Richard S, Keller H and Jaffray D A 2006 A simple, direct method for x-ray scatter estimation and correction in digital radiography and cone-beam CT *Med. Phys.* **33** 187–97

[57] Nomura Y, Xu Q, Shirato H, Shimizu S and Xing L 2019 Projection-domain scatter correction for cone beam computed tomography using a residual convolutional neural network *Med. Phys.* **46** 3142–55

[58] Wang G, Ye J C and De Man B 2020 Deep learning for tomographic image reconstruction *Nat. Mach. Intell.* **2** 737–48

[59] Jan S *et al* 2011 GATE V6: a major enhancement of the GATE simulation platform enabling modelling of CT and radiotherapy *Phys. Med. Biol.* **56** 881–901

[60] He K, Zhang X, Ren S and Sun J 2016 Deep residual learning for image recognition *Proc. IEEE Conf. Comput. Vis. Pattern Recognition* (Piscataway, NJ: IEEE) pp 770–8

[61] Hansen D C, Landry G, Kamp F, Li M, Belka C, Parodi K and Kurz C 2018 ScatterNet: a convolutional neural network for cone-beam CT intensity correction *Med. Phys.* **45** 4916–26

[62] Hudobivnik N *et al* 2016 Comparison of proton therapy treatment planning for head tumors with a pencil beam algorithm on dual and single energy CT images *Med. Phys.* **43** 495

[63] White D R, Woodard H Q and Hammond S M 1987 Average soft-tissue and bone models for use in radiation dosimetry *Br. J. Radiol.* **60** 907–13

[64] Sun M and Star-Lack J M 2010 Improved scatter correction using adaptive scatter kernel superposition *Phys. Med. Biol.* **55** 6695–720

[65] Zhang Z, Yu L, Zhao W and Xing L 2021 Modularized data-driven reconstruction framework for nonideal focal spot effect elimination in computed tomography *Med. Phys.* **48** 2245–57

[66] Yu L, Zhang Z, Li X and Xing L 2021 Deep sinogram completion with image prior for metal artifact reduction in CT images *IEEE Trans. Med. Imaging* **40** 228–38

[67] Lyu T, Zhao W, Zhu Y, Wu Z, Zhang Y, Chen Y, Luo L, Li S and Xing L 2021 Estimating dual-energy CT imaging from single-energy CT data with material decomposition convolutional neural network *Med. Image Anal.* **70** 102001

[68] Shen L, Pauly J and Xing L 2021 NeRP: implicit neural representation learning with prior embedding for sparsely sampled image reconstruction arXiv: 2108.10991

[69] Yu L, Zhang Z, Li X, Ren H, Zhao W and Xing L 2021 Metal artifact reduction in 2D CT images with self-supervised cross-domain learning *Phys. Med. Biol.* **66** 175003

[70] Bogdanich W 2009 Radiation overdoses point up dangers of CT scans *The New York Times* 15 Oct

[71] Bogdanich W 2010 After stroke scans, patients face serious health risks *The New York Times* 31 Jul

[72] Pearce M S *et al* 2012 Radiation exposure from CT scans in childhood and subsequent risk of leukaemia and brain tumours: a retrospective cohort study *Lancet* **380** 499–505

[73] Wen N, Guan H Q, Hammoud R, Pradhan D, Nurushev T, Li S D and Movsas B 2007 Dose delivered from Varian's CBCT to patients receiving IMRT for prostate cancer *Phys. Med. Biol.* **52** 2267–76

[74] Murphy M J *et al* 2007 The management of imaging dose during image-guided radiotherapy: report of the AAPM Task Group 75 *Med. Phys.* **34** 4041–63

[75] Shen L, Zhao W, Capaldi D, Pauly J and Xing L 2021 A geometry-informed deep learning framework for ultra-sparse 3D tomographic image reconstruction *Comput. Biol. Med.* **148** 105710

[76] Chen G H, Tang J and Leng S 2008 Prior image constrained compressed sensing (PICCS): a method to accurately reconstruct dynamic CT images from highly undersampled projection data sets *Med. Phys.* **35** 660–3

[77] Choi K, Wang J, Zhu L, Suh T S, Boyd S and Xing L 2010 Compressed sensing based cone-beam computed tomography reconstruction with a first-order method *Med. Phys.* **37** 5113–25

[78] Choi K, Xing L, Koong A and Li R 2013 First study of on-treatment volumetric imaging during respiratory gated VMAT *Med. Phys.* **40** 040701

[79] Wu Y, Ma Y, Capaldi D P, Liu J, Zhao W, Du J and Xing L 2020 Incorporating prior knowledge via volumetric deep residual network to optimize the reconstruction of sparsely sampled MRI *Magn. Reson. Imaging* **66** 93–103

[80] Mardani M, Gong E, Cheng J Y, Vasanawala S S, Zaharchuk G, Xing L and Pauly J M 2019 Deep generative adversarial neural networks for compressive sensing MRI *IEEE Trans. Med. Imaging* **38** 167–79

[81] Schreibmann E and Xing L 2005 Narrow band deformable registration of prostate magnetic resonance imaging, magnetic resonance spectroscopic imaging, and computed tomography studies *Int. J. Radiat. Oncol. Biol. Phys.* **62** 595–605

[82] Lian J, Xing L, Hunjan S, Spielman B and Daniel B 2004 Mapping of the prostate in endorectal coil-based MRI/MRSI and CT: a deformable registration and validation study *Med. Phys.* **31** 3087–94

[83] Schreibmann E, Chen G T and Xing L 2006 Image interpolation in 4D CT using a BSpline deformable registration model *Int. J. Radiat. Oncol. Biol. Phys.* **64** 1537–50

[84] Paquin D, Levy D and Xing L 2007 Multistage deformable image registration *Math. Biosci. Eng.* **4** 711–37

[85] Li T, Schreibmann E, Yang Y and Xing L 2006 Motion correction for improved target localization with on-board cone-beam computed tomography *Phys. Med. Biol.* **51** 253–67

[86] Liang X, Zhao W, Hristov D H, Buyyounouski M K, Hancock S L, Bagshaw H, Zhang Q, Xie Y and Xing L 2020 A deep learning framework for prostate localization in cone beam CT guided radiotherapy *Med. Phys.* **47** 4233–40

[87] Liang X *et al* 2020 Human-level comparable control volumes mapping with an unsupervised-learning model for CT-guided radiotherapy *Radiother. Oncol.* **141** 105139

[88] Chen Y, Xing L, Yu L, Bagshaw H P, Buyyounouski M K and Han B 2020 Automatic intraprostatic lesion segmentation in multiparametric magnetic resonance images with proposed multiple branch UNet *Med. Phys.* **47** 6421–9

[89] Chen Y, Xing L, Yu L, Liu W, Pooya Fahimian B, Niedermayr T, Bagshaw H P, Buyyounouski M and Han B 2021 MR to ultrasound image registration with segmentation-based learning for HDR prostate brachytherapy *Med. Phys.* **48** 3074–83

[90] Liang X *et al* 2021 Human-level comparable control volume mapping with a deep unsupervised-learning model for image-guided radiation therapy *Comput. Biol. Med.* **141** 105139

[91] Liang X, Bibault J E, Leroy T, Escande A, Zhao W, Chen Y, Buyyounouski M K, Hancock S L, Bagshaw H and Xing L 2021 Automated contour propagation of the prostate from pCT to CBCT images via deep unsupervised learning *Med. Phys.* **48** 1764–70

[92] Liang X *et al* 2020 Human-level comparable control volumes mapping with an unsupervised-learning model for CT-guided radiotherapy *Int. J. Radiat.Oncol. Biol. Phys.* **111** e95

[93] Seo H, Khuzani M, Vasudevan V, Huang C, Ren H, Xiao R and Xing L 2020 Machine learning techniques for biomedical image segmentation: an overview *Med. Phys.* **47** e148–167

[94] Seo H, Bassenne M and Xing L 2021 Closing the gap between deep neural network modeling and biomedical decision-making metrics in segmentation via adaptive loss functions *IEEE Trans. Med. Imaging* **40** 585–93

[95] Seo H, Yu L, Ren H, Li X, Shen L and Xing L 2021 Deep neural network with consistency regularization of multi-output channels for improved tumor detection and delineation *IEEE Trans. Med. Imaging* **40** 3369–78

[96] Seo H, Huang C, Bassenne M, Xiao R and Xing L 2020 Modified U-net (mU-net) with incorporation of object-dependent high level features for improved liver and liver-tumor segmentation in CT images *IEEE Trans. Med. Imaging* **39** 1316–25

[97] Pekar V, McNutt T R and Kaus M R 2005 Automated model-based organ delineation for radiotherapy planning in prostatic region *Int. J. Radiat. Oncol. Biol. Phys.* **60** 973–80

[98] Kass M R, WitKen A and Terzopoulos D 1988 Snakes: active contour models *Int. J. Comput. Vis.* **4** 321–31

[99] Coote T, Hill A, Taylor C and Haslam J 1994 The use of active shape models for locating structures in medical images *J. Image. Vis. Compution* **12** 355–66

[100] Xu C and Prince J L 1998 Snakes, shapes, and gradient vector flow *IEEE Trans. Image Process.* **7** 359–69

[101] Liu F, Zhao B, Kijewski P K, Wang L and Schwartz L H 2005 Liver segmentation for CT images using GVF snake *Med. Phys.* **32** 3699–706

[102] Weese J, Kaus M R, Lorenz C, Lobregt S, Truyen R and Pekar V 2001 Shape constrained deformable models for 3D medical image segmentation *Information Processing in Medical Imaging* Lecture Notes in Computer Science vol 2082 (Berlin: Springer) pp 380–7

[103] Li T, Schreibmann E, Thorndyke B, Tillman G, Boyer A, Koong A, Goodman K and Xing L 2005 Radiation dose reduction in four-dimensional computed tomography *Med. Phys.* **32** 3650–60

[104] Vedam S S, Keall P J, Kini V R, Mostafavi H, Shukla H P and Mohan R 2003 Acquiring a four-dimensional computed tomography dataset using an external respiratory signal *Phys. Med. Biol.* **48** 45–62

[105] Dietrich L, Jetter S, Tucking T, Nill S and Oelfke U 2006 Linac-integrated 4D cone beam CT: first experimental results *Phys. Med. Biol.* **51** 2939–52

[106] Li T, Xing L, Munro P, McGuinness C, Chao M, Yang Y, Loo B and Koong A 2006 Four-dimensional cone-beam computed tomography using an on-board imager *Med. Phys.* **33** 3825–33

[107] Rietzel E, Chen G T, Choi N C and Willet C G 2005 Four-dimensional image-based treatment planning: target volume segmentation and dose calculation in the presence of respiratory motion *Int. J. Radiat. Oncol. Biol. Phys.* **61** 1535–50

[108] Gao S, Zhang L, Wang H, de Crevoisier R, Kuban D D, Mohan R and Dong L 2006 A deformable image registration method to handle distended rectums in prostate cancer radiotherapy *Med. Phys.* **33** 3304–12

[109] Lu W, Olivera G H, Chen Q, Chen M and Ruchala K J 2006 Automatic re-contouring in 4D radiotherapy *Phys. Med. Biol.* **51** 1077–99

[110] McInerney T and Terzopoulos D 1996 Deformable models in medical image analysis *Med. Image. Anal.* **1** 91–108

[111] Chakraborty A, Staib L H and Duncan J S 1996 An integrated approach for surface finding in medical images *IEEE Workshop Mathematical Methods in Biomedical Image Analysis* (Piscataway, NJ: IEEE) pp 253–62

[112] Montagnat J, Delingette H and Ayache N 2001 A review of deformable surfaces: topology, geometry and deformation *Image Vis. Comput.* **19** 1023–40

[113] Chao M, Schreibmann E, Li T and Xing L 2007 Automated contour mapping using sparse volume sampling for 4D radiation therapy *Med. Phys.* **34** 4023–29

[114] Chao M, Li T, Schreibmann E, Koong A and Xing L 2008 Automated contour mapping with a regional deformable model *Int. J. Radiat. Oncol. Biol. Phys.* **70** 5599–608

[115] Barker J L *et al* 2004 Quantification of volumetric and geometric changes occurring during fractionated radiotherapy for head-and-neck cancer using an integrated CT/linear accelerator system *Int. J. Radiat. Oncol. Biol. Phys.* **59** 960–70

[116] Chencharick J D and Mossman K L 1983 Nutritional consequences of the radiotherapy of head and neck cancer *Cancer* **51** 811–5

[117] Donaldson S S and Lenon R A 1979 Alterations of nutritional status: impact of chemotherapy and radiation therapy *Cancer* **43** 2036–52

[118] Dong P and Xing L 2020 Deep DoseNet: a deep neural network for accurate dosimetric transformation between different spatial resolutions and/or different dose calculation algorithms for precision radiation therapy *Phys. Med. Biol.* **65** 035010

[119] Fan J, Xing L, Dong P, Wang J, Hu W and Yang Y 2020 Data-driven dose calculation algorithm based on deep U-Net *Phys. Med. Biol.* **65** 245035

[120] Liu H, Xu J, Guo Q, Ibragimov B, Wu Y and Xing L 2018 Learning deconvolutional deep neural network for high resolution (HR) medical image reconstruction *Inf. Sci.* **468** 142–54

[121] Dong P and Xing L 2020 Deep DoseNet: a deep neural network based dose calculation algorithm *Int. J. Radiat. Oncol. Biol. Phys.* **108** e344

[122] Dong P, Liu H and Xing L 2018 Monte Carlo tree search -based non-coplanar trajectory design for station parameter optimized radiation therapy (SPORT) *Phys. Med. Biol* **63** 135014

[123] Ma M, M K B, Vasudevan V, Xing L and Yang Y 2019 Dose distribution prediction in isodose feature-preserving voxelization domain using deep convolutional neural network *Med. Phys.* **46** 2978–87

[124] Ma M, Kovalchuk N, Buyyounouski M K, Xing L and Yang Y 2019 Incorporating dosimetric features into the prediction of 3D VMAT dose distributions using deep convolutional neural network *Phys. Med. Biol.* **64** 125017

[125] Deng J and Xing L 2018 *Big Data in Radiation Oncology* (Abingdon: Taylor and Francis)

[126] Huang C, Yang Y, Panjwani N, Boyd S and Xing L 2020 Pareto optimal projection search (POPS): automated treatment planning by direct search of the pareto surface *IEEE Trans. Biomed. Eng.* **68** 2907–17

[127] Balakrishnan G, Zhao A, Sabuncu M R, Guttag J and Dalca A V 2019 VoxelMorph: a learning framework for deformable medical image registration *IEEE Trans. Med. Imaging* **38** 1788–800

[128] Pastor-Serrano O, Habraken S, Hoogeman M, Lathouwers D, Schaart D, Nomura Y, Xing L and Perkó Z 2023 A probabilistic deep learning model of inter-fraction anatomical variations in radiotherapy *Phys. Med. Biol.* **68** 085018

[129] Shen L, Pauly J and Xing L 2022 NeRP: implicit neural representation learning with prior embedding for sparsely sampled image reconstruction *IEEE Trans. Neural Netw. Learn. Syst.* **35** 770–82

[130] Tancik M, Srinivasan P, Mildenhall B, Fridovich-Keil S, Raghavan N, Singhal U and Ng R 2020 Fourier features let networks learn high frequency functions in low dimensional domains *Adv. Neural Inf. Process. Syst.* **33** 7537–47

[131] Pastor-Serrano O and Perkó Z 2022 Millisecond speed deep learning based proton dose calculation with Monte Carlo accuracy *Phys. Med. Biol.* **67** 105006

[132] Pastor-Serrano O and Perkó Z 2022 Learning the physics of particle transport via transformers *Proc. of the AAAI Conf. on Artificial Intelligence* vol 36 pp 12071–9

[133] Pastor-Serrano O, Dong P, Huang C, Xing L and Perkó Z 2023 Sub-second photon dose prediction via transformer neural networks *Med. Phys.* **50** 3159–71

[134] Shen C, Nguyen D, Chen L, Gonzalez Y, McBeth R, Qin N and Jia X 2020 Operating a treatment planning system using a deep-reinforcement learning-based virtual treatment planner for prostate cancer intensity-modulated radiation therapy treatment planning *Med. Phys.* **47** 2329–36

[135] Shen C, Chen L, Gonzalez Y and Jia X 2021 Improving efficiency of training a virtual treatment planner network via knowledge-guided deep reinforcement learning for intelligent automatic treatment planning of radiotherapy *Med. Phys.* **48** 1909–20

[136] Hrinivich W T and Lee J 2020 Artificial intelligence-based radiotherapy machine parameter optimization using reinforcement learning *Med. Phys.* **47** 6140–50

[137] Liu S, Pastor-Serrano O, Chen Y, Gopaulchan M, Liang W, Buyyounouski M and Xing L 2024 Automated radiotherapy treatment planning guided by GPT-4 Vision arXiv:2406.15609